ETHICS
&ISSUES
IN CONTEMPORARY
NURSING

SECOND EDITION

ETHICS & ISSUES

IN CONTEMPORARY NURSING

NURSING ETHICS FOR THE 21ST CENTURY

Margaret A. **Burkhardt**, PhD, FNP, AHN-BC

Associate Professor, Emerita
School of Nursing
West Virginia University
Charleston, West Virginia

Alvita K. **Nathaniel**, PhD, FNP-BC, FAANP

Professor Emerita
School of Nursing
West Virginia University
Charleston, West Virginia

ELSEVIER

Elsevier
3251 Riverport Lane
St. Louis, Missouri 63043

ETHICS & ISSUES IN CONTEMPORARY NURSING, SECOND EDITION ISBN: 978-0-443-10530-2

Senior Content Strategist: Sandra Clark
Senior Content Development Specialist: Jinia Dasgupta
Publishing Services Manager: Shereen Jameel
Senior Project Manager: Beula Christopher
Senior Book Designer: Amy Buxton

Printed in India

Last digit is the print number: 9 8 7 6 5 4 3 2 1

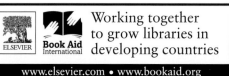

Working together
to grow libraries in
developing countries

www.elsevier.com • www.bookaid.org

To Joe and Tim.
For enduring love and support through the decades.

LIST OF REVIEWERS

Cheryl Carlin, MSN, RN, CNE
Assistant Professor
Avila University
Kansas City, Kansas

Susan C. Engle, DNP, MSN, BSN, AAS
Program Director
Eagle Gate College
Murray, Utah

Naomi Lobo, RN, BS, BSN, OCN
Chamberlain University
North Brunswick, New Jersey

Eleonor Pusey-Reid, DNP, RN, M.Ed
Associate Professor
MGH Institute of Health Professions
Boston, Massachusetts

We who lived in the concentration camps can remember the men who walked through the huts comforting others, giving away their last piece of bread. They may have been few in number, but they offer sufficient proof that everything can be taken from a man but one thing: the last of his freedoms— to choose one's attitude in any given set of circumstances, to choose one's own way.
—*V.E. Frankl,* Man's Search for Meaning

We are pleased to introduce to you this new and expanded Elsevier edition of *Ethics & Issues in Contemporary Nursing*. We believe that the ethically prepared and competent nurse is an empowered nurse. This belief has grounded the content of this text since the first edition was published in 1998 and continues to provide a framework for this current edition. It is our intention that each new edition reflects ethical considerations related to contemporary issues of importance to the delivery of health care. This edition continues to present everyday situations nurses encounter but adds content on the delivery of nursing care in crisis situations such as those we have witnessed related to natural disasters, war, and the COVID-19 pandemic. Each of these crises brings forth new moral questions and asks nurses to make decisions that might have been unthinkable in the past. If you are familiar with past editions, you will recognize the same general focus, tone, and features. If you have not used this book before, students and faculty will find some helpful advice in this preface about good ways to utilize the various features of the book.

A new feature of this edition is a more focused linking of the content of each chapter with particular sections of professional nursing codes of ethics. Specific elements of these codes that provide guidance for dealing with ethical dilemmas are regularly referenced. Nursing codes of ethics clearly state that caring in an ethical way is expected in every nursing act and encounter. Directives in these codes that address health care settings, fostering personal health and safety, advocating for healthy and collaborative work environments, promoting moral communities, and maintaining ethical competence are incorporated throughout the book.

As contemporary nurses, we face increasingly complex and challenging personal, interpersonal, professional, institutional, social, political, and global issues. Appropriate responses to these issues are seldom clear. Ethical dilemmas, in particular, involve choices with no clearly correct solutions. In this book, we aim to impose no particular perspective on the issues, rather we present compelling cases and offer the tools for readers to clarify their own values and make sound decisions. In this book, we refrain from implying "correct" answers to morally troubling questions because doing so would risk imposing our personal values on others. As nurses, we must be sensitive to this possibility and recognize that our responses to dilemmas depend on such variables as contextual factors, patient and family values, relationships, moral development, religious beliefs, spiritual perspective, cultural orientation, and legal constraints. Our intention is that you will enter each new situation prepared to make decisions with humility and moral courage.

It is our intention in this book to (1) acknowledge that each person is a moral agent, (2) raise awareness of the myriad factors that should be considered when grappling with ethical decisions, (3) present a decision-making model to help individuals process information and move toward action, (4) affirm nursing as an ethically responsible profession, and (5) highlight the critical importance of nursing codes of ethics in grounding and supporting nurses in providing ethical care. We present ethical issues from the perspective of nursing, recognizing that relationships and the authority to make decisions are affected by contextual factors such as professional status; sex; the development of the profession; personal ethical stance; social, economic, institutional, and political climate; and personal and professional empowerment.

Although acknowledging the rich and divergent history of nursing in other cultures, we have chosen to write primarily from the Western perspective. Nevertheless, we recognize that our culture is a melding of traditions and people from many other cultures. The background that we give explains the many factors that lead to social systems that either encourage or prohibit certain people from critically examining issues and making authoritative decisions. The book begins with a chapter that explores the impact of historical factors, particularly religion and sex, on the profession of nursing in Western culture. We hope that this will help you to understand more fully the context of nursing and question arbitrary and artificial barriers to ethical decision making.

Principled behavior in personal and professional situations is the organizing theme of this text. Beginning with a brief descriptive history of nursing as it relates to ethics, Part I, Guides for Principled Behavior, presents ethical theories, models, and principles that serve as guides for principled behavior. Part II, Developing Principled Behavior: Acquiring, Internalizing, and Applying Moral Values, discusses personal issues, including values clarification, moral development, and ethical decision making. Part III, Principled Behavior in the Professional Domain, presents overviews of professional and legal issues in nursing and chapters related to specific issues important to contemporary nursing. This section includes discussions about autonomy, authority, accountability, codes of practice, scholarship issues, practice issues related to health care providers, systems within which nurses work, technology, and patient self-determination. Part IV, Nursing Ethics, Global Health Care Challenges, and Social Justice, addresses 21st-century issues requiring global consciousness as a background for understanding issues that nurses encounter in the contemporary health care system. Ethical nursing practice related to global health, political, economic, social, sex, transcultural, and spirituality issues are discussed. Part V, Power to Make a Difference, focuses on attitudes, skills, and ethical grounding that empower both nurses and patients to make principled choices and act with authority and courage.

Throughout this book, we have chosen to refer to the recipient of nursing care as *patient* rather than *client*. Because nurses function as members of interdisciplinary health care teams and the term *patient* is commonly used by other health providers, using a common language fosters better communication, understanding, and collegiality. The American Nurses Association (2010) *Nursing's Social Policy Statement* notes that although the term *client* is preferred by some nurses, it implies that the recipient of care is able to choose one nurse from among many, a choice that typically does not occur. In addition, both the ICN *Code of Ethics for Nurses* and the CNA *Code of Ethics for Registered Nurses* use the term *patient*. We recognize that the term *client, person*, or *individual* may be the better choice in some circumstances and encourage the reader to make that distinction if needed.

A NOTE TO STUDENTS

This book is meant to be very personal. We encourage you to become engaged by opening your mind to new perspectives as you objectively and critically examine your values in relation to the real-life situations we present. We propose that learning is demonstrated through changed behavior. So, we hope that you will become a more sensitive, capable, courageous, mature, and responsible decision maker and citizen. We believe with Phyllis Kritek (1994) that "the measure of [one's] character and worth is not whether [one has] avoided making poor choices, but how willing [one is] to learn from these errors in an effort to not repeat them, and how [one elects] to attend to their consequences. . . . Finding meaning, discovering that which is of worth, becomes a searching process where everyone's help is welcome" (pp. 21, 33).

This book offers you the opportunity to critically examine compelling cases, to think through the related issues, contexts, and values, and to practice ethical decision making—thus doing some of the hard work before you find yourself in the midst of real-life moral challenges and problems. This book is offered as a guide to help in the process of learning to make sound choices and act in principled ways in both personal and professional realms. As you use this book, we echo the same sentiment voiced by Florence Nightingale in the preface to her *Notes on Nursing*: "I do not pretend to teach her how, I ask her to teach herself, and for this purpose I venture to give her some hints" (1859, preface).

Dealing with ethical issues requires skill in the processes of values clarification, ethical decision making, self-awareness, empowerment, transcultural sensitivity, and challenging injustice. Placing nursing within its historical context, we pose questions about contemporary issues and provide processes to help you develop sensitivity and skill and prepare you to face ethical problems. Highlighting diverse nurses and patients in a variety of settings and roles, the exercises and activities are intended to facilitate self-reflection and awareness of personal approaches to issues and decision making. Our goal is that you will become engaged in active learning through the intentional use of *Case Presentations, Think About It*, and *Ask Yourself* exercises, as well as *Discussion Questions and Activities*. We encourage you to deepen and expand your knowledge of various topics by exploring the links to online resources pertinent to chapter content. We believe that all these features are useful because they are derived from thought-provoking material or real-life case presentations.

We believe that it is essential for nurses to have a working knowledge of their professional code of ethics, thus we direct you to particular elements of these codes pertinent to the content throughout each chapter. We encourage you to have a copy of the code of ethics that is appropriate for you (available online) for reference as you use this text. Nursing codes of ethics, principles of ethics, and other concepts appear in numerous places throughout the text—each time viewed from a slightly different perspective. We ask you to return to principles, concepts, and codes of nursing ethics repeatedly to learn to apply the decision-making process in many situations. As you move through the book and explore political, professional, legal, social, and sex issues, we encourage you to examine the related ethical questions and to continually move back and forth from the concrete to the abstract, from the general to the specific, from the global to the personal, and from issue to principle—recognizing the interrelatedness of many factors.

Objectives. Each chapter begins with a list of objectives. Please read the objectives before you begin the chapter. They will help to anchor you so that you understand the focus and organization of the chapter.

Ask Yourself. You will find *Ask Yourself* questions scattered throughout the text. These questions are always related to content within the text. As you read the questions, try to balance in your mind the information presented in the text along with your own personal values and those of the profession. There are seldom clear black-and-white answers to ethics problems, so we ask you to open your mind and explore the opinions and values of other individuals and other cultures as you contemplate the questions.

Case Presentations and Think About It Questions. Nearly all case presentations in this book are derived from real-life situations. Some are seminal cases found in the literature, some are obscure cases chosen for their applicability to the content, and some reflect the experience of hands-on nurses in everyday situations. We chose these case presentations to give you a glimpse of

ethical problems that have been experienced by nurses in the past and thus to prepare you for situations that you will encounter in the future. After you have read a *Case Presentation*, thoughtfully move through the *Think About It* questions that are posed to help you explore different facets of the relevant problems. In some cases the questions help you apply ethical principles to the situation in a way that will move you toward an appropriate solution. Other questions might help you look at the problem from different perspectives or within alternative contexts. We encourage you to utilize the ethical decision-making process described in Chapter 7 to help guide you in considering your response to each case situation. Allowing yourself to explore these questions with an open mind will help you evolve into a nurse with moral integrity as you gain knowledge about nursing ethics, along with a deeper understanding of yourself and those around you.

Chapter Highlights and Summary. The *Chapter Highlights* pull out the important points made in the chapter. Even though very dramatic cases may linger in your mind as you finish a chapter, remember the cases are meant to help you understand important facets of the content. The *Summary* does not include the important points; rather, it briefly encapsulates the overarching ideas of the chapter.

Discussion Questions and Activities. The *Discussion Questions and Activities* are designed to help you further explore issues and ethics. Through further exploration, you will become more knowledgeable and adept at ethical decision making. The activities are meant to be thought provoking, but not time consuming. Questioning and exploring comprise the hard work it takes to become a mature and ethically competent nurse.

A NOTE TO FACULTY

Thank you for choosing *Ethics & Issues in Contemporary Nursing*. As we designed this book, we kept uppermost in our minds a vision of how it might be presented in the classroom. You will notice that the ethical principles and many other concepts appear in numerous places throughout the text—each time viewed from a slightly different perspective. We return to codes of nursing ethics, principles, and concepts iteratively to reinforce and strengthen previous learning. In addition to the supplementary instructor's materials, you have options as to how to use the various features of the book. If you are teaching a course online, you might ask students to post responses to the *Ask Yourself* and *Think About It* questions or the end-of-chapter *Discussion Questions and Activities* on a discussion board. In a real-time online or face-to-face classroom, you might read the case presentations and openly discuss the *Think About It* questions or the end-of-chapter *Discussion Questions and Activities*. Your role should be to encourage students to read the cases thoroughly and respond to the questions with an open mind. Case presentations may be adapted for role-play scenarios in which students get a feel for dealing with ethical situations and through which they can practice utilizing the ethical decision-making process described in Chapter 7. Exploration of online resources provided in many chapters could be incorporated into discussions or writing assignments. We acknowledge that there is a necessary, yet delicate, balance between encouraging students to understand their own values and gently moving them toward a deeper appreciation for the values of others and those promoted by the profession.

As nursing faculty you understand that nurses' professional responsibility, authority, and power to make principled choices are embedded in professional codes of nursing ethics. These codes express nursing's own understanding of its commitment to society and the ethical basis from which nurses, individually and collectively, in all roles and practice settings, can advocate for safe and ethical practice settings and safe, equitable, competent, and compassionate care for patients and communities. Through our own research and discussions with others since we published the first edition of this book in 1998, we have come to believe that nurses must become more familiar with their established professional code of nursing ethics. We have found that members of some disciplines can easily call forth specifics of their professional code of ethics, whereas this seems to occur less often with nurses. Therefore, in this edition, we refer to codes of nursing ethics throughout the book and we ask students to read pertinent sections of them when considering the case presentations and other activities. Our first reference to the codes occurs abruptly in Chapter 1, so we ask that you prepare students for this. It would benefit students to have a copy of appropriate codes (available online) for reference as they use this text. This book has international readership but is mostly marketed in the United States and Canada, so we reference the codes of nursing of the ICN, ANA, and CNA. Students in the United States should focus on the ICN and ANA codes of ethics, and students in Canada should focus on those from the ICN and CNA. Although codes of nursing ethics from around the world are very similar, we suggest that students outside North America become familiar with the nursing code of ethics in their own countries. Understanding that nurses who are firmly in touch with their own values and have internalized their professional code of ethics are better prepared to make informed decisions, we trust that this expanded edition of our text will enable you to help your students learn and internalize their code of nursing ethics as they develop or expand their moral identity and ethical nursing practice.

REFERENCES

American Nurses Association. (2010). *Nursing's social policy statement: The essence of the profession* (New edition). Author.

Kritek, P. B. (1994). *Negotiating at an uneven table: A practical approach to working with difference and diversity*. Jossey-Bass.

Nightingale, F. (1859). *Notes on nursing: What it is, and what it is not*. Harrison & Sons.

ACKNOWLEDGMENTS

Although this is the second Elsevier edition of this book, it is the sixth edition overall—four previous editions by another publisher. We began writing the first edition nearly 30 years ago. This long journey of writing and then revising the book has required solitude and the companionship and support of many people. We express gratitude to the many friends, colleagues, and mentors who have encouraged us along the way and to those who have contributed ideas and pertinent cases. Thanks go to all those who gave the time and care to review all editions of our manuscript at various stages in the writing process, providing us with helpful comments and guidance. We thank all the staff at Elsevier who have been involved with every aspect of bringing this edition to life, with special appreciation to Tamara Myers, Director of Traditional Education Content, and Sandra E. Clark, Senior Content Strategist. We continue to acknowledge in a particular way Dr. Mary Jo Butler, who encouraged and supported us many years ago as we labored to bring the first edition to life and whose resilience and positive attitude toward all that life brings continue to inspire.

Finally, we are eternally grateful to our families, Joe Golden, Tim and Josh Nathaniel, Maggie Belton, and the grandchildren who have come along since the first edition for their loving patience, humor, caretaking, and encouragement throughout this journey.

CONTENTS

Guides for Principled Behavior

Part I lays a foundation that prepares nurses to critically examine issues and systematically participate in ethical decision making. Chapter 1 gives nurses insight into the profession of nursing in Western cultures as part of an overall social system—focusing specifically on the influence of philosophy, the practice of religion, and the status of women in society. Recognizing that knowledge of ethical theories and principles can help the nurse develop a cohesive and logical system for making individual decisions, Chapters 2 and 3 describe philosophical stances, various classic ethical theories, and ethical principles.

1

Social, Philosophical, and Other Historical Forces Influencing the Evolution of Nursing Ethics

You know that the beginning is the most important part of any work, especially in the case of a young and tender thing; for that is the time at which the character is being formed and the desired impression is more readily taken.

(Plato, ca. 375/1997a)

OBJECTIVES

After completing this chapter, the reader should be able to:

1. Discuss the relationship between the social need and the origin of the profession of nursing.
2. Discuss the relationship between moral reasoning and the origin of nursing.
3. Describe the mutually beneficial relationship between the broader society and its professions.
4. Explain the effect of a culture's prevailing belief system on the practice of nursing.
5. Identify how historic spiritual beliefs and religious practices influenced evolutionary changes in nursing.
6. Discuss how the historical background of the status of women in various cultures is related to the practice of nursing.
7. Examine the effect of philosophy on beliefs and practices within society.
8. Make plausible inferences relating the evolution of the practice of nursing to the current state of the profession.
9. Begin to look at professional codes of nursing ethics as they relate to historical tradition.

INTRODUCTION

This chapter summarizes historical traditions that are critical to an examination of contemporary nursing in Western society. Customs, traditions, and beliefs flow through periods of time—some are made stronger, some are modified, and some are discarded. This chapter presents the philosophy, religion, and social structures that have shaped nursing. Knowledge of the origin and history of nursing can be an empowering experience. Through critical examination of the history of the profession, you will move beyond tradition toward thoughtful and objective reasoning and thus be better prepared to fully participate in moral discourse.

This book focuses on the traditions of the West because codes of ethics in Western countries flow from these sources. This is not to say that Eastern traditions, religions, and philosophies are of less value. We acknowledge that the East has contributed rich knowledge and wisdom. Brahmanism, Buddhism, Jainism, Confucianism, and Taoism were evolving distinctly Eastern philosophies even before many Western philosophies became popular. Eastern traditions are important, and we encourage you to learn more about them. In an increasingly multicultural environment, it is important that we fully appreciate the beliefs and traditions of others.

In general, human nature leads people to accept the beliefs and practices of those around them. Most people internalize the values, traditions, and cultural practices of their families and social groups. To secure a sense of belonging, people tend to believe what those around them believe and act in ways that are congruent with those beliefs. Social groups value actions compatible with their beliefs. Because people naturally gravitate toward membership in social groups and desire the approval of their group, traditions become self-perpetuating. The American philosopher Charles Sanders Peirce (1839–1914) discussed methods that people use to solidify or fix their beliefs.

Peirce identified four methods of fixing belief: tenacity, authority, a priori, and reasoning. He proposed that seeking truth is the goal of all human inquiry and suggested that inquiry and logic provide the way by which a person can discover truth (1877). Peirce proposed that a person only discovers truth when he or she really questions something. He believed that reasoning is the most highly evolved level of fixing belief. However, Peirce found that many people fail to question their beliefs. This allows their beliefs to be dictated by the authority method, whereby powerful persons or institutions force their version of "correct beliefs" on people by repeating rules perpetually and teaching them to the young. This method has been one of the chief means by which authorities dictate their theological and political views onto groups of people. We can broadly apply this means of fixing belief to many historical influences on the nursing profession.

Andrew Jameton called nursing the "morally central health care profession" (1984, p. xvi) because the spirit and substance of nursing spring from social and individual moral codes. There have always been people who cared for the sick and attempted to cure illness. Compassion, coupled with moral reasoning, is the historical basis for the creation, evolution, and practice of nursing. In this chapter, we will look at four historical influences on nursing as a moral discipline: social need, spirituality/religion, philosophy, and the role of women in society.

Moral beliefs of groups of people produce rules of action or ethics. These culturally accepted rules are an integral part of both the experience and the profession of nursing. Expressions of ideals, discussions of moral issues, statements of moral principles, and codes of ethics are found throughout the history of nursing. As modern technology extends the boundaries of what is possible, all of society is challenged to examine emerging ethical issues. We are faced with ethical tension in a healthcare system that requires moral decision-making yet sometimes restricts nurses from legitimate decision making roles. One of the purposes of this text is to encourage nurses to make morally defensible decisions.

We hope to present nursing ethics in a manner that will encourage empowered decision making. Manojlovich (2007) argues that there are compelling reasons to empower nurses. Powerless nurses are ineffective and are unable to influence patients, physicians, other healthcare professionals, and each other. Examining nursing empowerment, Fulton proposed that nurses' perspectives are distorted and constrained by historical forces that impart negative messages (1997). These distortions and constraints impede autonomous decision making and set the stage for authorities to coerce nurses. Congruent with Manojlovich's arguments, Hedin (1986) and Roberts (1983) suggested that as nurses struggle to cope with impossible situations, they internalize negative messages and behave in ways that are neither constructive nor empowered. Harden (1996) proposed that nurses can only understand the present healthcare culture in relation to nursing's social and professional history. These concepts flow from critical social theory as proposed by Habermas (1979) and Freire (2000). The basic principle of critical social theory is that we can only understand a social phenomenon in relation to the history and structure in which it is found. The significance of ideas can be grasped only when we objectively view them in the context of historical and social practices and webs of power and interest. Habermas (1979) proposed that, as individuals, we can assess the evidence and fully participate only when we are aware of, and free ourselves from, the hidden oppressions that affect our lives. Insights gained from the study of nursing history enable us to see conditions for what they are and to find ways of interpreting them and releasing ourselves from false narratives so we can move forward. To this end, we present some selected historical and social forces that have shaped the contours of our profession.

It is difficult to establish a clear picture of the development of the profession of nursing through history because the early emergence of the professions of medicine and nursing are so closely interwoven (Donahue, 2011).

Even so, we know that the history of nursing is one in which people—usually women—have attempted to relieve suffering. From the beginning, the motivation of nurses to care for others came from practical, moral, or spiritual influences. Our history is also the story of a profession inescapably linked to the status of women. The history of healers, and subsequently that of nurses, has gone through many phases and has been an important part of social movements.

INFLUENCE OF SOCIAL NEEDS

The helping professions find their origin, purpose, and meaning within the context of culturally accepted moral norms, individual values, and perceived social needs. Serving others and responding to their needs is an expression of moral belief. The term moral relates to what is considered right and wrong, good and bad. Moral reasoning includes an examination of behaviors and attitudes in light of their moral implications. Moral reasoning may be complex and well developed, or it may be rudimentary. Why do we care about moral issues? Some moral philosophers propose that empathy is a motive for moral reasoning and action. For example, if we visualize the suffering of another person, we begin to imagine ourselves suffering. Some describe the desire to help others as a natural outcome of social consciousness and motivation similar to the Golden Rule, the principle of treating others as one would wish to be treated. A universally popular precept, the Golden Rule is found in some form in most major moral traditions, including Christianity, Judaism, Islam, Confucianism, Hinduism, Buddhism, and Taoism. Some say that we follow the Golden Rule both to help someone in need and, to some degree, in the hope that someone will show us compassion if we are unfortunate enough to find ourselves in similar circumstances. On the other hand, if we base our moral reasoning on pure religious belief, we may be motivated by a desire to obey a commandment, fulfill what we believe to be a duty to a higher being or gain spiritual rewards. As the morally central healthcare profession, nursing has historically responded to human suffering. So, whether our original motivation for ethical action is based on a desire to help others or on a religious duty, the outcome of the action is the same: meeting the health needs of others.

ASK YOURSELF

What Is the Motivation for Helping?

Imagine a beautiful, perfect world in which all people are happy and healthy and have satisfying relationships. In this world, there is no hunger, pain, illness, or death. Each person's needs are immediately and entirely met without the help of other people. Within this society, because everyone is satisfied, healthy, and happy, there is no social disorder and no need for any helping profession: no police, doctors, nurses, lawyers, or social workers. People do not need to think about moral issues. Now imagine the social disorder that would follow the introduction of serious disease. Diseased individuals become ill and suffer pain. Their situation would seem to be hopeless. They would be unable to care for themselves, to meet their own basic needs.

- How do you imagine the "perfect" society would deal with this problem?
- Should the ill be entirely responsible to care for themselves?
- Do you think unaffected people would ignore the suffering of others and continue to live the perfect existence, or would the whole of society be responsible for helping those in need?
- Should society allow the diseased members to suffer, or should healthy people help those afflicted, thus altering their own "perfect" lives—and in turn the prevailing social order?
- What social structures would need to be created to care for those who are ill?
- Read the preface of the codes of nursing from the ANA (2015) or the CNA (2017) and the ICN (2021). How do you think the ideas in the documents were developed as the nursing needs of the people in society explicitly became the domain profession of nursing?

It is likely that at least some members of the hypothetical community described in the accompanying *Ask Yourself* exercise will recognize the importance of helping those in need. The people who respond will begin to exercise moral reasoning as they examine their beliefs. Ethics will emerge in the form of rules of action that are specifically related to solving the moral problem. Those committed to helping the ill will devise methods to utilize individuals' abilities to the best advantage and to fairly distribute the burden of providing services and resources. As this example implies, nursing is a profession that exists to meet certain needs of individuals and groups and thus is a product of the moral reasoning of people in society.

As we will see in later chapters, the needs of a society at a given time combined with its technological capabilities and available knowledge determine the existence and parameters of a profession. Societies establish dynamic professional boundaries that move and change as needs change. Nursing is a part of society. To continue to exist, our professional interest must continue to be (and must be perceived as) serving the interests of the larger society of which it is a part. The landmark document *Nursing: A Social Policy Statement* (ANA, 1980) was the profession's first description of its social responsibility. We can use both this document and subsequent revisions and guidebooks (ANA, 1980, 1995, 2003, 2010; Fowler, 2015) as a framework for understanding the profession's relationship with society and the obligation to those who receive nursing care. These documents express the mutually beneficial relationship between the broader society and its professions as follows:

> *A profession acquires recognition, relevance, and even meaning in terms of its relationship to that society, its culture and institutions, and its other members. Professions acquire recognition and relevance primarily in terms of needs, conditions, and traditions of particular societies and their members. It is societies (and often vested interests within them) that determine, in accord with their different technological and economic levels of development and their socioeconomic, political and cultural conditions, and values, what professional skills and knowledge they most need and desire. By various financial means, institutions will then emerge to train interested individuals to supply those needs. Logically, then, the professions open to individuals in any particular society are the property not of the individual but of society.*
>
> (ANA, 1980, p. 3)

ASK YOURSELF

What Makes People Service Oriented?
- Why do you think people are motivated to help those in need?
- The basis of action of those who choose to help others might be described self-interest, altruism, or a combination of other motives. How would you describe the motivation to care for others within the healing professions today?
- Nursing is a service-oriented profession. What motivated you to become a nurse?

The nursing profession was created by society to meet specific health needs. In response, the profession has made an implicit promise to ensure that members are competent to provide nursing service. That promise is assured through mechanisms such as mandatory licensure, specialty certification of nurses, continuing education, and accreditation of nursing education programs. Further, the *only* members of society that qualify to provide nursing service are nurses. That is, only nurses can legally practice nursing. The relationship between social needs and our motivation to care for others is complementary. It is fortunate that human nature is such that some of us, for whatever reason, are interested in serving others.

SPIRITUAL, RELIGIOUS, GENDER, AND PHILOSOPHICAL INFLUENCES

Spiritual/Religious Influences

The spiritual and religious foundations of past and present cultures determine many aspects of health care. Spiritual beliefs and religious practices contributed significantly to the moral foundation of nursing and other healing professions; they also influenced both the gender and, to some degree, much of the activity of healers. Spirituality and religious doctrine influenced beliefs about the value of individuals, life, death, and health. Historically, many of the dominant religious institutions made judgments about the origin and essence of healing and defined who would hold positions as legitimate healers. The path that nursing has taken since ancient times has not been smooth. There have been advances and setbacks, libraries have been destroyed, widely diverse groups have held the title of nurse, and those who were the nurses in some early cultures left few records. Nevertheless, nursing in some form has existed in every culture and has been influenced by spiritual beliefs, religious practices, and related cultural values.

Gender Influences

We celebrate nurses of all genders; however, the role of women in society is one of the most critical factors that influenced the evolution of nursing practice. Women have been healers in every culture. Though there is a rich history of men in nursing, nursing has generally been thought of as a profession of women. Even today, only 11 percent of nurses in Western countries are men (WHO,

2022). Thus, women's status in society is central to determining the extent of freedom and respect granted to nurses. Boundaries of the profession have been shaped, in large part, by social forces that determine gender roles in society. Gender stereotyping has always been a problem for nurses. Because of the perception that women are more humane and more caring by nature, they have been viewed as naturally endowed with nursing talents. Even Florence Nightingale wrote, "Every woman has, at one time or another of her life, charge of the personal health of somebody, whether child or invalid—in other words, every woman is a nurse" (Nightingale, 1860, preface).

Society either permits, limits, or prohibits women to hold roles of authority, roles that allow independent decision making or limited participation in the decision-making process. There were periods in the history of Western civilization in which women were the honored sole practitioners of the healing arts, and there were periods in which women were limited to submissive and subservient healing roles.

Philosophical Influences

From ancient times until today, philosophers have asked important questions and proposed theories that helped shape cultures. Philosophers ask questions about the nature of truth and reality. They propose theories about morality and the characteristics of the good life. They develop theories of action, interaction, cause, and effect that affect the scientific method. Since ancient times, philosophers have influenced every aspect of society. The purpose of studying the history of philosophy is to discover the most important philosophical perspectives of the great philosophers of the past and to understand how their ideas affected nursing. In this book, you will see reference to important figures in Western philosophy, including Socrates (469–399 B.C.E.), Plato (427–347 B.C.E.), Aristotle (384–322 B.C.E.), St. Jerome (ca.342–429), Thomas Aquinas (1225–1274), René Descartes (1596–1650), David Hume (1711–1776), Immanuel Kant (1724–1804), Jeremy Bentham (1748–1832), and John Stuart Mill (1806–1873).

Ancient Times
Religious Influences and the Role of Women in Ancient Times

The cosmology of a culture indirectly determines specific beliefs about the origin of disease and healing.

Cosmology is the overarching belief system of a culture. It describes how people of a particular culture view the structure, origin, laws, and processes of the universe as an ordered whole. Cosmology includes beliefs about the gods. The nature of the gods worshiped in any culture directly affects prevailing healing beliefs. Regarding ancient cultures, Achterberg wrote:

When gods lived in the Earth, the whole planet was worshiped as the manifestation of the divine. The rivers, the rocks, and especially humans were the inhabitants of a sacred place. All—what we call living and nonliving alike—was alive and related. All humans breathed the breath of the spirit and drank the waters of the spirit.

(Achterberg, 1990, p. 188)

Thus, in ancient cultures, the healer was involved with the sacred elements of the Earth and the spirit in healing practices.

Early cultures viewed the vocation of healer in terms associated with the sacred. In ancient times, the position of healer was practiced by those who were thought to have special spiritual gifts. Through the study of relics, we learn that healing arts in the ancient cultures of Sumer, Denmark, Greece, and other societies were performed in sacred ceremonies by priests, priestesses, or shamans. These ancient healers represented the embodiment of a culture's gods on Earth (Achterberg, 1990). In ancient Persia, there are indications that there were three types of healers: those who healed with the knife, those who healed with herbs, and those who healed with sacred words. Practitioners who used sacred words were considered to have the greatest prestige (Dolan et al., 1983). Archeological evidence suggests that in all early cultures the position of the healer was associated with the sacred.

Many diverse and widely placed ancient cultures left evidence that there was a time when women served in the esteemed roles of healer and priestess. Whenever the reigning deity in ancient times had a feminine, bisexual, or androgynous nature, women were leaders in the healing arts. As the world became a harsher place and the gods assumed a masculine nature, the role of women as independent, primary healers was taken away (Achterberg, 1990).

Asclepius, or Asklepios, was the ancient Greek god of medicine and healing. Asclepius was regarded as a deity, but some believe that he may have been a real person known for his humane remedies. It is said that Asclepius learned the art of surgery; the use of drugs, incantations, and love potions; and the secrets to raising the dead. According to mythology, Asclepius had several children, including Hygieia, the goddess of health (from whose name comes the word *hygiene*); Panacea, the goddess of healing (from whose name comes the word *panacea*, which means universal remedy); and Iaso, the goddess of medicine. Although the provision of nursing care in ancient Greece was considered an internal affair of families, and especially women, Asclepius's followers established temples of healing, sometimes referred to as *asclepieia*, where the sick spent the night while the proper remedies were "revealed" to the priests of the temple. In the asclepieia, health care was delivered by a servant nurse (Theofanidis & Sapountzi-Krepia, 2015). Patients who were cured made a sacrifice to Asclepius, usually a rooster (Hart, 2000).

Romans worshiped Asclepius from about 800 B.C.E. to 400 C.E., but his influence continued throughout the centuries. Some believe that Hippocrates may have studied at an asclepieion. The Hippocratic Oath begins with the words, "I swear by Apollo, the physician, Asclepius, Hygieia, and Panacea, and I take to witness all the gods, all the goddesses, to keep according to my ability and my judgment, the following Oath and agreement" (Hippocrates, ca. 450-350 B.C.E/1943). Plato, the ancient philosopher most revered by Florence Nightingale, paid homage to Asclepius in *Phaedo* when he reported that Socrates's last words were "Crito, we owe a cock to Asclepius; make this offering to him and do not forget" (Plato, ca. 353 B.C.E./1997b). Even today, the official symbol of medicine recognized by the American Medical Association and the American Osteopathic Association is the Staff of Asclepius, a depiction of one snake ascending a roughly hewn staff (Fig. 1.1). Perhaps the relationship between Asclepius and his daughters Hygieia, Panacea, and Iaso contributed to the paternalistic, male-dominated system perpetuated through much of history.

Having a great influence on Western thought, early Hebrew teaching codified health practices as an integral part of the Hebrew religion. The Mosaic health code applied to every aspect of individual, family, and Jewish community life. It included principles related to food, rest, sleep, cleanliness, hygiene, and childbearing (Dolan et al., 1983; Forst, 1994). The code required inspection

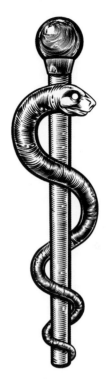

Fig. 1.1 Rod of Asclepius. (©iStock.com/ChrisGorgio.)

of food, detection and reporting of disease, methods of disposal of body excretions, feminine hygiene, and isolation of those with communicable illness. It specified particular methods of hand washing and care of food. The Hebrew high priest served in the capacity of priest/physician, and the people were admonished to honor him. Thus, for the early Hebrews, health practices were mandated by religious doctrine.

The ancient physician Hippocrates (ca.460–ca.377 B.C.E.) is universally recognized as the father of Western medicine. Hippocrates synthesized what was then known about medicine and added his own observations in a 72-book text, the *Corpus Hippocraticum*, which was the first written medical text in the Western world (Suvajdžić et al., 2016). Hippocrates was the first to develop a plan of assessment, diagnosis, treatment, and prognosis. He advocated physical examinations, emphasizing the use of the senses of sight, hearing, taste, and touch to assess the afflicted. His teachings revolutionized the healing arts in ancient Greece and established medicine as a profession, distinct from other disciplines. Differing from the prevailing superstitions that illness and healing originate from religious or magical sources,

Hippocrates believed that care of the sick should include observation of symptoms, rational conclusions, and predictable prognoses (Suvajdžić et al., 2016; Yapijakis, 2009). He approached healing passively, relying on the healing power of nature. Hippocrates was influenced by Pythagoras's theory that proposed that nature was made of four elements: water, earth, wind, and fire. Thus, he proposed that the body consisted of the corresponding four humors: black bile, yellow bile, phlegm, and blood. He proposed that it was the physician's purpose to reinstate a healthy balance of humors by promoting the healing work of benevolent nature (Yapijakis, 2009). In his writings, Hippocrates proposed strict professionalism. Most sources attribute the Hippocratic Oath to Hippocrates himself.

Philosophy in Ancient Times

Between the 6th and the 4th centuries B.C.E., in every corner of the globe, an extraordinary development was occurring. Some brilliant, creative thinkers were dissatisfied with popular beliefs and explanations. Early philosophers began to question the religious beliefs, mythologies, and folklore that had been established for centuries. Seeking wisdom, philosophers employed abstract thinking and ambitious questions. They questioned popular notions about nature and its relationship to the whims of gods and goddesses. They asked questions about the origin and the nature of all things. They pondered the essence of reality and truth. They explored ideas about the right way for humans to live (Solomon & Higgins, 1996). The ideas generated by ancient philosophers have influenced all facets of society throughout the centuries.

Socrates, Plato, and Aristotle proposed new and exciting ideas about truth, reality, relationships, ethics, and the good life. Socrates (470–399 B.C.E.) was arguably the greatest philosopher of ancient times. The first recorded full body of philosophical work was Plato's dialogs between Socrates and various other people. Socrates believed that knowledge leads to the "good life." Socrates proposed that one must seek knowledge and develop the inner self to experience a good life. He believed that a person should do what is right, even when opposed by others. Socrates and Plato believed that there was one specific type of good life that was not dependent on humans' desires, wishes, or opinions. They believed people could acquire it only through study and contemplation (Solomon & Higgins, 1996).

One of Socrates's contributions to education was the *Socratic method* of teaching. Demonstrated throughout Plato's dialogs, the Socratic method consists of a *dialectic* in which two people present opposing opinions. In contrast to an argument or debate, however, revelations occur as the two people talk and ask each other questions, and their ideas move closer to the *truth*. In this way, a teacher can lead students to think through problems in a systematic and objective manner. Teachers today commonly use the Socratic method. Class discussions and the *Ask Yourself* elements of this textbook can be used for students to learn via the Socratic method.

Aristotle, a student of Plato, proposed ideas that were different from those of his teachers. He believed that virtuous behavior consisted of attaining the "golden mean." For example, he believed that the virtue of courage is the mean between cowardice and foolhardiness. Aristotle proposed that the aim of a good life is *eudaimonia* (translated as happiness or flourishing). He proposed that eudaimonia can only occur through a life of virtue and excellence, one in which the person fulfills the aim of life. Aristotle wrote that the aim of a flautist is to play the flute, of the carpenter is to build, and so forth. Although this is a simplification of Aristotle's teachings, these examples seem to indicate that happiness or flourishing only occurs when the person focuses on excellence toward a goal. He wrote, "in life it is those who act rightly who will attain what is noble and good" (Aristotle, ca. 340 B.C.E./2000, p. 14). Elements of Aristotle's philosophies can be found in modern nursing.

The Early Christian Era
Religious Influences and the Role of Women in the Early Christian Era

Arguably the most profound religious influence on healing beliefs and practices in Western civilization occurred with the advent of the Christian era. The effect of Christian belief and organized Christian religion on the history of healing is multifaceted. It is interesting to closely examine textbooks on nursing history and recognize divergent opinions among authors. The pendulum swings from some authors' biases that present only the compassionate aspects of the Christian influence on the history of nursing to those that condemn Christianity as a misogynistic force that hindered nursing progress.

In a text on nursing history originally published in 1916, Dolan discussed caring in terms of the Christian religion when she wrote, "Man and the universe were made to exist in the profound execution of the plan of Creation" (Dolan, 1973, p. 3). Dolan used the New Testament of the Bible to describe Jesus's message about caring for others in the following way: (1) caring for others represents caring for Jesus; (2) there is spiritual reward to be gained by caring for others; (3) even in a world of selfishness and hatred one should love God and one's neighbor; (4) every person, even the "poorest and most miserable," is an important member of the Kingdom of God; and (5) every person has worth and dignity (Dolan, 1973). As this example shows, nursing texts in Western culture often reflect the prevailing influence of religious teaching on healing practices and the nursing profession.

During this era, nurses were frequently women of high social status and often became independent practitioners. Monks and women, called *deaconesses*, provided care for patients, primarily the elderly and the needy (Theofanidis & Sapountzi-Krepia, 2015). Many set aside special places in their homes for hospitality and care of the sick. These places were called *Christrooms* (Dolan et al., 1983). Others in deaconess orders can be regarded as the first visiting nurses, tending to patients in their homes, prisons, and other places. Early Christians were often compassionate, respecting the intrinsic value of each human.

As centuries passed, the path of healing practices assumed a winding course. Jeanne Achterberg describes the first 500 years after the birth of Christ as the "calm before the storm." She says, "These were fluid times, when religion was a satisfying and exotic blend of ingredients taken from pre-Christian, pagan, and folk traditions" (1990, p. 39). As time passed, war, disease, and the influence of religious dogma effectively altered the course of the healing traditions.

When religious belief moved toward a single male god, women's healing role changed from that of sacred healer to subservient caregiver. By the time Jesus lived, the place of women in the healing arts was minimal. Jesus challenged the patriarchal tradition by associating freely with women. He selected the most "compassionate, maternal images from the Jewish tradition, creating a Christian god as androgynous as any male god in history. In some of the early sects, God was even seen as a dyadic being (mother-father), rather than the trinity (father-son-holy spirit)" (Achterberg, 1990, p. 38). As a result, women enjoyed renewed acceptance as healers.

Their intellect and contribution to the religious movement were respected by the early Christians. This resurgence of power and respectability, however, only lasted for a few centuries after the birth of Christ.

Philosophy in the Early Christian Era

Many Western philosophers of the early Christian years were struggling with the challenges and practical concerns of the new religion. The most influential philosopher of these years was St. Paul. Educated in the Greek tradition, Paul agreed with earlier, non-Christian moral philosophers that there is a natural law of conscience inherent in each person (Solomon & Higgins, 1996). St. Augustine was another important philosopher. He devoted himself to integrating Christian doctrine with Plato's philosophy. He contributed to Western philosophy with an emphasis on one's personal, inner life, such as examination of the passions of the soul, including love and faith, as well as the urges, impulses, and vices such as lust, pride, and curiosity that occur in every person.

The Middle Ages
Philosophy in the Middle Ages

Sometimes labeled the Age of Faith and sometimes the Age of Superstition, the Middle Ages was a period of social disruption and cultural deterioration. The Church maintained a stronghold on society, so what little philosophy did emerge was almost entirely theological. St. Augustine's writings were highly regarded. During this period, Thomas Aquinas synthesized Greek rationalism and Christian doctrine. His work during this time became a cornerstone of religious philosophy (Russell, 2008). Later in the Middle Ages, energy was invested in retranslating Plato and Aristotle.

Religious Influences in the Middle Ages

In the early Middle Ages, many people believed that the world was falling into ruin. During this time, disease, large-scale food shortages, and war interacted to produce a predictable sequence: war drove farmers from their fields and destroyed their crops; destruction of the crops led to famine; and the starved and weakened people were easy victims of the onslaught of disease (Cartwright & Biddiss, 2020). The established social structure was deteriorating, and disorganized communities turned to feudalism, monasticism, and, in certain regions, Islam as solutions to the chaos they were experiencing. The Church was the only significant Western institution to survive the fall of the Roman Empire and the clergy held the first rank of honor in society (Pavlac, 2009).

During this time, monasticism and other religious groups offered the only opportunities for men and women to pursue careers in nursing. Much of hospital nursing was carried out by repentant women and widows called sisters and by male nurses called brothers. Deaconesses, matrons, and secular nursing orders were among the organized groups that had religious foundations and offered nursing services.

These early nurses believed they were following the command of God to imitate Jesus, who had spent his life ministering to those in need. For many, this service was viewed as a means of securing salvation. Women who entered nursing orders donated their property and wealth to the Church and devoted their lives to service. Believing that "charity" was synonymous with "love," many early Christians sold their possessions and gave everything to the Church or the poor. Although in many cases "nursing" care was delivered by slaves or servants, religious orders offered the only route through which respectable women and men could serve as nurses.

The overall belief system of a culture influences the extent to which members accept various healing methods and healthcare practices. An example of this can be seen in historical accounts of the healing arts in the Middle Ages. The term **empirical** relates to knowledge gained through the processes of observation and experience. Many people, especially those devoted to the Church, had deeply antiempirical beliefs. Consequently, people were more likely to seek healing through religious interventions such as touching religious relics, visiting sacred places, chanting, and other methods approved by the Church. Because of the religious fervor at the time, empirical treatment (particularly if provided by anyone not explicitly sanctioned by the Church), even if it was successful, was thought to be produced by the devil, because the position of the Church was that only God and the devil had the power to cause illness or promote healing.

An increasingly influential Christian doctrine led to a constant war waged against the flesh. People during the Middle Ages believed that they should "mortify the flesh" in the name of honoring the spirit. People neglected physical needs. They were dirty and covered with rashes and "foul eruptions." These problems were made worse by rough, dirty, woolen clothing and the constant presence of ticks and fleas (Achterberg, 1990). Thus, as a direct result of religious teaching, healthcare practices during the Middle Ages caused the spread of disease, intensified health problems, and limited effective empirical healing practices.

The Crusades, which began in 1096 and lasted nearly 200 years, brought many changes in the health of the population. These holy wars led to deplorable sanitary conditions, fatigue, poor nutrition, diarrhea, and the spread of communicable diseases. Health problems led to a demand for more hospitals and greater numbers of healthcare providers. Military nursing orders, formed in response to the compelling need, drew large numbers of men into the field of nursing (Dolan, 1973).

Another direct result of the Crusades was the collection of relics by the Church. Believed to offer the potential of healing miracles, the spoils of war included body parts of Crusade martyrs. The Church obtained significant wealth and power through the sale of these relics. Achterberg (1990) compares this time with the time of an earlier Roman mythology in which large numbers of deities or sainted mortals, their relics, and pilgrimages to their sacred sites were believed to hold the key to health.

For most of the Middle Ages, the Church held tremendous influence over the people and governments of all European countries. Powerful leaders within the Church determined the appropriateness of various healing practices. Official credentialing of physicians, nurses, and midwives was left in the hands of the Church. After civic legislation became common, the Church continued to enforce the law and monitor practitioners. This power was also used to enforce religious doctrine that influenced the status of women in society.

Accounts of the actual treatment of patients in early times vary. In some hospitals operated by religious orders, patients were treated as welcome guests. People sometimes pretended to be ill to be admitted. In contrast, some groups of patients were treated inhumanely, even by members of nursing orders. If nurses believed that their duty was to God and to the spiritual rather than physical needs of the patients, they may have been less attentive to physical, emotional, and comfort needs.

The treatment of the mentally ill was based for centuries on the idea that they were possessed by devils or that they were being punished for their sins (Dolan, 1973). They were often put in chains, starved, and kept in filthy conditions. There was even a time when it was thought that torture was useful in driving out madness. The mentally ill were treated inhumanely because the public perception of mental illness was based on religious beliefs about demon possession and punishment for sin.

Women in the Middle Ages

During the Middle Ages, the status of women also declined. In many ways this was directly related to Church doctrine, which institutionalized gender discrimination. Because religion was a crucial part of the lives of the people in the Middle Ages, the Church exerted power over the people's lives and ideology. St. Thomas Aquinas, ironically known within the Church as the "angelic doctor," wrote that women should be in subjugation to men. He proposed that men have higher intellectual and reasoning abilities. He wrote that women are "defective and misbegotten" and must serve men. Further, Aquinas believed that the only purpose of women was to produce children for the benefit of men, since other men could be better helpmates in all other capacities (Aquinas, ca. 1274/1920). Centuries earlier another Church leader, St. Jerome, who was paradoxically recognized for his support of matrons in their calling as nurses, remarked, "woman is the gate of the devil, the path of wickedness, the sting of the serpent, in a word a perilous object" (St. Jerome as cited by Heer, 1962, p. 322). Religious leaders in the Middle Ages were setting the stage for the persecution of women that would last for hundreds of years and leave a persistent legacy of misogyny.

Religious and Church-sanctioned secular nursing orders afforded the only legitimate avenue for women wishing to be nurses during the Middle Ages. The Church popularized the ideals of virginity, poverty, and a life of service. By the end of the 13th century, an estimated 200,000 women served as nurses within these orders (Achterberg, 1990). Caring for pilgrims in improvised infirmaries and clinics, women's nursing orders were particularly welcome during the Crusades. As was often the case, women's orders were subordinate to the men's communities (Donahue, 2011). Nevertheless, some speculate that within the structure of the Church, religious women, particularly those who were virgins (Jerome, ca. 383/1867), exercised a degree of independence and autonomy. There is no doubt that they made a great contribution to the health care of the time.

Also during the Middle Ages, the Church and the newly formed medical profession were actively engaged in the elimination of lay female healers. Women were excluded from universities. Except for those devoting their lives to serving in religious nursing orders, women were not allowed by the Church to practice the healing arts. During a revival of learning in the 13th century, the Church imposed strict controls on the new profession of medicine and officially prohibited women from its practice (Achterberg, 1990). Nevertheless, some women continued to secretly practice the healing arts, both within and outside the home. They used knowledge handed down for generations, empirical knowledge, and intuition.

People in the Middle Ages held the pervading religious view that women were essentially evil by nature. The pain of childbirth was believed to be punishment for Eve's transgression and served the purpose of reminding women of their original sinful nature (Jerome, ca. 383 B.C.E./1867). Those who dared provide pain relief to others during childbirth were severely punished (Achterberg, 1990). Later, the original sin of Eve would be used to justify torturing and murdering thousands of women during the witch hunts.

The medical profession was officially sanctioned by the Church, and male physicians began to be trained in the university setting. Even so, there was very little scientific knowledge. The physician relied solely on superstition (Ehrenreich & English, 2010). University-trained physicians used bloodletting, astrology, alchemy, and incantations. Their patients were almost exclusively wealthy. Physicians' treatments were usually ineffective, often dangerous, and inaccessible to the poor. Lay healers were often more successful than physicians.

Women Healers and Social Turmoil

Peasant women were often the only healers for people who suffered from poverty and disease. Folk healers had extensive knowledge about cures that had been handed down for generations via the oral tradition. They constantly improved their practice through empirical methods of observation, trial, and evaluation. Whereas physicians continued to rely on superstition, peasant women developed an extensive understanding of bones and muscles, herbs, drugs, and midwifery (Barstow, 1995; Ehrenreich & English, 2010). Some authorities at the time believed that folk healers were actually practicing some form of magic or witchcraft (Barstow, 1995). Others speculated that these women were honoring the old pagan religions and worshiping the old gods who (according to Church authorities) had assumed the persona of the devil (Achterberg, 1990). It is likely that lay women healers were simply caring for others in a manner that was consistent with prevailing folk belief. After all, almost everyone in medieval Europe believed in the reality of magic (Barstow, 1995). The Church itself acknowledged that magic was part of the natural world, yet instructed people in the community to avoid it. They acknowledged both acceptable miracles and evil magic (Pavlac, 2009). This atmosphere set the stage for Church-sanctioned crimes against women in the form of witch hunts.

The witch hunts swept across Europe from the 14th to the 17th centuries. The atmosphere that led to the witch hunts was a critical mixture of war, disease, and poverty combined with religious fervor, superstition, and political unrest. The witch trials were carried out through an organized partnership among the Church, state, and emerging medical profession. Women, particularly women healers, represented a political, religious, and sexual threat to both Church and state. An atmosphere of misogyny, superstition, and the widespread belief in magic set the stage that would allow terrible crimes to be perpetrated against women (Achterberg, 1990; Barstow, 1995; Ehrenreich & English, 2010).

Armed with authorization to purge Germany of witches, inquisitors Kramer and Sprenger (1486/1971) wrote *Malleus Maleficarum*, also known as the *Hammer of Witches* (Fig. 1.2). Kramer and Sprenger defined witchcraft as treason against God and described it as female rebellion. Used as a witch hunters' manual, the *Malleus Maleficarum* expressed virulent antifeminine and antisexual opinions. Kramer and Sprenger claimed that women were "more bitter than death." They described women as naturally more impressionable and superstitious than men, liars, evil, impulsive, having slippery tongues, in need of male supervision, and "given to witchcraft." Like other religious leaders before them, they believed that women were "intellectually like children." They wrote that women came under the spell of witchcraft because they were "feebler both in mind and body." Kramer and Sprenger wrote that any woman who dared to cure disease was a witch and further, that men should choose to die rather than be cured by a witch. They believed that midwives were the most wicked. *Malleus Maleficarum* was printed in four languages and at least 29 editions between the years 1486 and 1669.

What were the crimes of which the women were accused? Any woman who treated an illness, even if she

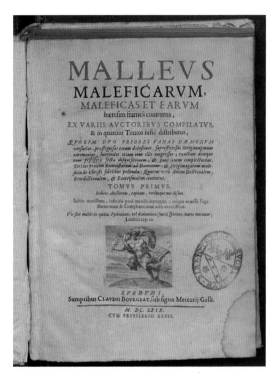

Fig. 1.2 Malleus Maleficarum 1487. Google Images at https://commons.wikimedia.org/wiki/File:Malleus_maleficarum,_Lyon_1669,_Titelseite.jpg#filehistory

applied a soothing salve to the diseased skin of her child, was likely to be accused of witchcraft. If the treatment failed, she was thought to have cursed the patient. If the treatment succeeded, she was believed to be in consort with the devil. Although women were permitted to practice midwifery (no one else wanted to do it), midwives were accused of witchcraft if anything went wrong with either the mother or the baby.

ASK YOURSELF

Healing or Witchcraft?

Imagine yourself the parent of a small child in the 16th century. You believe the Church doctrine about the origin of the knowledge of healing. Your family and neighbors are aware of the growing problem of witchcraft in the region. Your child becomes ill, and you recall a remedy that your mother used successfully with the same ailment.

- Would you openly attempt to alleviate your child's suffering and risk being accused of witchcraft?
- How would you feel about having to make this decision?

It is difficult to comprehend the effect of the witch hunts on European society. The most authoritative estimate of the number of executions is between 50,000 and 100,000 (Chollet, 2022), with some estimates as high as 10 million. Women comprised 85–95 percent of those killed (Barstow, 1995). Women silently watched the public humiliation, torture, disfigurement, and death of other women. Barstow believes that this public acknowledgment of the evil nature of the female sex left all women humiliated and frightened. Because both the accused and those viewing the proceedings were powerless to prevent the torture and executions, the witch craze served to undermine women's belief in the ability and power of women. Indeed, this was likely the inference made by all of society. Achterberg writes, "women were never again given full citizenship in any country, nor was their role in the healing professions reinstated" (1990, p. 98). Even after the end of the witch hunts, women were prohibited from the independent healing professions by law in every country in Europe. This created a climate by which males became the authoritative medical professionals (Ehrenreich & English, 2010). Although accounts of the witch hunts are absent in most popular nursing history texts, these events probably influenced the future of the profession more than any other single factor.

The Renaissance and the Reformation

The 14th through the early 16th centuries were known for two great movements: the Renaissance and the Reformation. The Reformation was a religious movement precipitated by the widespread abuses that had become part of Church life and doctrinal disagreement among religious leaders. This period left little of the old Church intact (Collinson, 2004). The Renaissance, sometimes called *the Enlightenment*, produced an intellectual rebirth that ushered in the scientific era.

The 16th-century Reformation was one of the greatest religious revolutions of all time. At the start of the 16th century, Western Europe had only one religion—Roman Catholicism. During the Middle Ages, the Church had amassed remarkable wealth and perpetrated many kinds of abuses. Martin Luther sparked a movement in the 16th century that resulted in the establishment of Protestantism. Gradually releasing people from the oppressive control of the Church, the Reformation allowed new types of thinking and opened the door for the Renaissance. Philosophy and science no longer needed to justify themselves to religion.

The Reformation produced unrest. Widespread abuses and differences in belief among church leaders led to a struggle between Catholic and Protestant groups across Europe. One outcome was that the laws and customs in Protestant countries discouraged the humane care of the poor and vulnerable (Donahue, 2011). Religious nursing orders were driven out of hospitals, and many orders were ultimately closed. During this era, hospitals became places of horror. No qualified group took the place of the religious nursing orders. Unqualified and undesirable women were assigned nursing duties. Conditions were at their very worst between 1550 and 1850—the "Dark Period of Nursing"—when convalescent patients, prostitutes, prisoners, and drunkards provided hospital nursing care (Donahue, 2011).

The Renaissance fostered the scientific revolution and a new era in the healing arts. Beginning its gradual escape from the control of the Church, the scientific community made advances in mathematics and the sciences. Philosophical humanism emerged during the Renaissance. Humanism established humans, rather than God, as a focus of interest. This new perspective enabled a scientific outlook that viewed the universe as governed by general laws. Copernicus theorized that the Earth was not the center of the universe. The philosopher and scientist Galileo used direct observation to gain new knowledge about astronomy. Advances in science during the Renaissance inspired the philosophers of the time. They came to believe that genuine knowledge was accessible to individuals through careful observation of empiric phenomena and subjective reasoning (Solomon & Higgins, 1996).

Some have argued that the Renaissance benefited men but not women. Although released from the grip of fear produced by the witch hunts, women of the Renaissance continued to live in subordination to men. Their day-to-day lives changed little. Most women were denied educations and, for the most part, none were allowed to become legitimate members of any profession.

ASK YOURSELF

Who Has the Right to Make Ethical Decisions?
Ethical decision making is not the sole domain of the physician. Nurses may be better prepared and have more opportunities to discuss moral problems with patients and families.
- Can you describe an instance in which a physician assumed the authority to make an ethical decision,

denying nurses (and perhaps the patient and family) participation in the decision-making process?

- If you feel you had an important contribution to make in a particular circumstance and your opinion was not considered, how would you react?
- How do you think nurses can overcome the strong heritage of subjugation?
- How does the language about advocacy in the codes of nursing ethics from the ANA (Provision 1.4), ICN (Element 2.7), and CNA (p. 5) support nurses' involvement in ethical decision making?

Modern Era

The **modern era** immediately followed the Renaissance and is generally thought to include the late 16th through the late 18th centuries. This era ushered in tremendous advances in science, politics, and philosophy. Many modern philosophers' ideas directly influenced the profession of nursing as we know it today. Among these philosophers were Immanuel Kant (1724–1804), who proposed an ethical system based on duty and moral imperatives, and John Stuart Mill (1806–1873), who described a new way of thinking about ethics and justice. Kant and Mill are discussed in depth in Chapters 2 and 3. Another philosopher, René Descartes (1596–1650), proposed new theories that changed the course of science for all time.

Descartes is credited with proposing a theory that quickly altered philosophical beliefs about the separation of mind and body. Descartes claimed that all life phenomena can be explained solely in terms of mathematics and physical/chemical laws of matter and motion. He proposed that the universe is a physical thing and that everything in the universe is like a machine, which can be analyzed and understood. Descartes further theorized that the mind and body are separate entities and that people are set against a world of objects that they must seek to master (Descartes, 1614/2013). Based on Descartes's work, **Cartesian philosophy** began to replace religious beliefs related to physical and spiritual realms.

Cartesian philosophy resulted in a perceived separation between the acts of caring and curing in the healing arts. Descartes's philosophy elevated the sciences and made scientific inquiry possible, yet it failed to improve the status of nursing. Achterberg identifies this time as an important turning point. She says in regard to Cartesian philosophy, "When spirit no longer is seen to abide in matter, the reverence for what is physical departs. Hence medicine no longer regarded itself

as working in the sacred spaces where fellow humans find themselves in pain and peril, and where transcendence is most highly desired" (1990, p. 103). Nursing as we know it today began to emerge in the modern era. Cartesian philosophy effectively created a clear distinction between nurses and physicians and formalized their hierarchical relationship. Nurses' place in the modern-era healthcare system was limited to the "caring" realm. Caring was given lower status than curing within the hierarchy of the healing arts. Some would argue that this legacy remains today.

Although the antebellum era in nursing is often referred to as "lost decades" in American history, there is evidence that nurses practiced within faith communities. Although there were no structured nursing education programs in America prior to the Civil War, both Protestants and Catholics had organized nurses. Examples of faith communities that had nurses recognized for their skill and devotion include Shaker villages, the settlements of Church of Jesus Christ of Latter Day Saints (LDS), and the Catholic orders of the Sisters of Charity and the Sisters of St. Joseph.

Examples of American Protestant groups of women dedicated to nursing include the Shakers and the Church of Jesus Christ of Latter Day Saints. Nurses in Shaker villages in the antebellum period were appointed by spiritual leaders to be the main providers of health services in their communities. Shaker nurses cared for patients in infirmaries called "Nurses' Shops" or "Sick Rooms" and administered emetics, cathartics, injections, enemas, steams, and sweats (Libster, 2018). Nurses were also an important group within the LDS church. The Women's Relief Society educated LDS nurses who, in turn, established extensive healing networks to comfort and care for people in the community. These women were honored and "set aside" in their communities because they were nurses. In caring for the ill, LDS nurses dispensed herbs and prepared mild foods, in keeping with their religious beliefs (Libster, 2018).

The number of Catholic women's orders in America increased quickly during the last years of the antebellum period from 82 orders in 1845 to 381 in 1860 (Howe & Berennan, 2013). Sisters of Charity was founded in France in 1633 by Vincent de Paul and Louise de Marillac. Opening their first infirmary in America in 1815, the community of women was not cloistered but allowed to go into the homes of the sick poor. They performed hands-on care of the sick, spiritual instruction, bleeding, administering remedies, and preparing the sick for death (Libster, 2018). Along with many other Catholic nursing orders, the Sisters of Charity established infirmaries and hospitals. Founder Louise de Marillac wrote, "The girls … who are asking to enter the Company of the Daughters of Charity…must have no other intention when entering the Company, than the pure desire to serve God and their neighbor. They must be willing to live in the Company in a constant state of interior and exterior mortification and be determined to observe their Rules (sic) faithfully, especially those requiring absolute obedience" (de Marrilac, 1658, p. 583/1991). The Sisters of St. Joseph were also caring for the poor and infirm during this period. In 1853 six Sisters of St. Joseph arrived in Wheeling, Virginia (now West Virginia) and immediately began to caring for the congregation and the ill and poor in the community, mostly immigrants (Joseph, 2022). In 1859 the General Assembly of Virginia granted a charter to Wheeling Hospital and invited the Sisters of St. Joseph to operate the institution (Howe & Berennan, 2013). Although they had no formal nursing training, the sisters cared for and provided comfort to patients. During the Civil War, the sisters cared compassionately for both Union and Confederate soldiers in the Wheeling Hospital (Howe & Berennan, 2013, p. 22).

In England, the founder of modern nursing, Florence Nightingale (1820–1910), reflected the influence of the Renaissance and Reformation. As a person, Nightingale (Fig. 1.3) remains an enigma. She viewed nursing as a profession separate from the Church, yet she began her career as the result of a mystic experience. According to Nightingale, God spoke to her four times, calling her into his service when she was 16 years old (Selanders, 2010). Her experience in the Crimean War was the direct result of her second revelation, which she termed a call from God (Dossey, 2010; Showalter, 1981). Although she was opposed to using Church affiliation as a criterion for admission to nursing programs, her religious beliefs were evident in her dealings with students, whom she admonished to work diligently because "if there is no cross, there is no crown" (Achterberg, 1990; Selanders, 2010). In addition, Nightingale's description of nursing as caring for the mind and the body implies a rejection of Descartes's philosophy on the separation of these two human spheres.

Florence Nightingale became a model for all nurses. She was a nurse, statistician, sanitarian, social reformer, and scholar. She opened the first secular training school

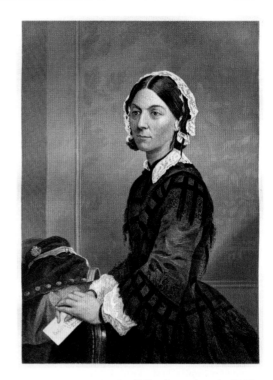

Fig. 1.3 Florence Nightingale. (©iStock.com/traveler1116.)

for nurses; initiated the first study of the occupational health of nurses; worked with a multidisciplinary team of doctors, statisticians, engineers, and architects to effect healthcare reform; and formulated the basic principles of a public healthcare system (McDonald, 2013). Nightingale was a scholar who studied Plato and helped translate some of his writings into English. She saw corollaries between nursing and Plato's conception of public service. Plato believed that the aim of education is to mold talented people into leading citizens, who will in turn care for the good of the community. Nightingale viewed this orientation to service as the basis for nursing's goal to improve the welfare of people.

Nightingale was politically astute, intelligent, and single-minded. Contrary to the accepted Victorian social order, Nightingale addressed moral issues with courage and conviction. Having strong opinions on women's rights, she was quick to challenge the established male hierarchy. Nightingale argued for the removal of restrictions that prevented women from having careers (Simpkin, 2014). Her writings instructed nurses to "do the thing that is good, whether it is 'suitable for a woman' or not" (Nightingale, 1860, p. 76). Although some argue that Nightingale was not a feminist, her writings indicate that she felt women should have a more important place in the social structure. She wrote, "Passion, intellect, moral activity—these three have never been satisfied in woman. In this cold and oppressive conventional atmosphere, they cannot be satisfied" (Nightingale, ca. 1852/1979, p. 25). Based on her life and accomplishments, it is certain that Florence Nightingale did not ascribe to the popular Cartesian notion that women do not have minds and souls and are put on the Earth solely for man's purpose and pleasure.

Lavinia Lloyd Dock (1858–1956) is another of nursing's great modern leaders. Considered a radical feminist, Dock actively engaged in social protest, picketing, and parading for women's rights (Feldman & Lewenson, 2000). She was concerned with the problems plaguing both the education and employment of nurses, warning that male dominance in the health field was the major problem confronting the nursing profession. Although she enjoyed the support of a community of like-minded nurses, Lavinia Dock's contemporaries largely ignored her concerns, and 21st-century nurses have found themselves fighting the same battles.

Contemporary Era

For the most part, philosophers in the contemporary era have analyzed, parsed, explained, and further developed views of philosophers of the past. They have explored to a greater extent some of the concepts familiar to nursing such as morality, ethics, duty, and compassion. As you will see in Chapter 2, contemporary philosophers have applied philosophical schools of thought to the healthcare field and created systems to describe and evaluate ethical behavior. As the healthcare professions have matured, so have the philosophical basis for many of their actions.

The mid-1900s brought great advances for nurses. There was a long-awaited increase in the number of men in nursing, particularly in mental health settings. Nurses entered professional, social, and political spheres. Although recurrent themes of paternalism and subjugation continued to affect the nursing profession, 20th-century women became more politically active. The women's movement encouraged political, social, and economic action to correct the wrongs suffered by women. Nursing gained acceptance as a legitimate healthcare force. In 1958 the first liaison committee was established between the American Nurses Association (ANA) and the American Medical Association (AMA). A historic joint conference was held between the two groups in 1964. Participating in federal policy making, the nursing profession was represented as Medicare was signed into law in 1965 and later enjoyed federal legislation in 1997 that authorized Medicare reimbursement for nurse practitioners and clinical specialists (AANP, 2013).

Perceiving a healthcare crisis of growing proportions and recognizing the need for comprehensive, accessible, and affordable health care, society challenged established institutions to foster greater use of nurses in expanded roles. Encouraged by a society in which health care had become a scarce resource, nurse practitioners, nurse midwives, and other advanced practice nurses began to assert themselves as independent professionals. Many nurses began to provide independent healthcare services and assume institutional and political leadership positions.

Managed care and other healthcare reform programs that emerged in the late 20th and the early 21st centuries offered nurses both opportunities and challenges. Mechanisms of payment for healthcare services reshaped the healthcare environment. Hospitals strived to streamline services through improved efficiency and reduced waste. Many healthcare services previously provided in the high-tech hospital setting were provided by nurses in the home when patients were quickly released from hospital care due to pressure from third-party payers.

By the mid-1900s, nursing had overcome many social and institutional barriers. Recognizing the legitimate need for both the caring and curing aspects of healing, nurses worked together in teams with other health professionals to improve the status of the nursing profession and to ensure that healthcare system problems are addressed. Social awareness of problems in healthcare systems led to changes that affected nursing. As you will read in subsequent chapters, organizations and policy makers based recommendations for change on well-established philosophical foundations, social ideas, beliefs, and the climate of the time. For example, four Institute of Medicine (IOM) reports, *To Err Is Human, Crossing the Quality Chasm, the Future of Nursing,* and *The Future of Nursing 2020-2030,* which directly affect nursing education and practice (IOM, 2000, 2001, 2010; National Academy of Medicine 2021), flow from ethical principles that will be discussed further in Chapter 3. Nurses, as members of the IOM, fully participated in recommendations that continue to shape nursing practice.

In 2000 the IOM (renamed the National Academy of Medicine) issued a report entitled *To Err Is Human: Building a Safer Health System.* This report pointed out the high incidence of error that leads to deaths and other serious consequences in US healthcare systems. The report included recommendations that affect nursing. Recommendations include the following: (1) increasing user-centered design to improve safety, efficiency, and effectiveness; (2) avoiding reliance on memory through such devices as standardized processes, checklists, and standardization of equipment and processes; (3) attending to work safety in such areas as work hours, workloads, staffing ratios, and sources of distraction; (4) avoiding reliance on vigilance because it is difficult to maintain vigilance for long periods; (5) developing healthcare teams to improve outcomes; (6) involving patients in their own care, such as giving greater access to personal health information and hospital discharge medication reconciliation; (7) anticipating the unexpected; (8) designing processes for recovery, such as keeping antidotes on hand; and (9) improving access to accurate, timely information (IOM, 2000). As a result of the 2000 IOM report, many institutional processes, including those involving nurses, have changed.

In 2001 the IOM released the second part of a quality initiative entitled *Crossing the Quality Chasm: A New Health System for the 21st Century*. Aims in the 2001 report likewise affect nurses. The aims included improving safety, effectiveness, timeliness, and efficiency of patient-centered care. For the first time, recommendations also called for equitable care that does not vary in quality because of personal characteristics of patients such as gender, ethnicity, geographic location, or socioeconomic status.

In collaboration with the Robert Wood Johnson Foundation in 2010, the IOM turned its focus to the profession of nursing in a report entitled *The Future of Nursing: Leading Change, Advancing Health*. Nursing represents the largest sector of the health professions, with more than three million nurses. Therefore, committee members believed support of the nursing profession would positively affect health care for the nation. Four key messages were included in the report:

1. Nurses should practice to the full extent of their education and training.
2. Nurses should achieve higher levels of education and training through an improved education system that promotes seamless academic progression.
3. Nurses should be full partners with physicians and other healthcare professionals in redesigning health care in the United States.

4. Effective workforce planning and policy making require better data collection and an improved information infrastructure (IOM, 2010, p. 29).

In the midst of the COVID-19 pandemic in 2020, the IOM again focused on the nursing workforce with a new report entitled, *The Future of Nursing 2020-2030: Charting a Path to Achieve Health Equity*. In this report, the IOM recognized the critical importance of health in all aspects of life and pointed out the necessity for nurses, who are at the forefront of health care, to address social determinants of health, health equity, and health outcomes. Reeling from the unimaginable circumstances of the COVID-19 pandemic during the International Year of the Nurse and the Midwife, the 2020 IOM report calls for social and governmental structures to support a stronger, more diverse nursing workforce so that nurses can "promote health and well-being among nurses, individuals, and communities; and address the systemic inequities that have fueled wide and persistent health disparities" (IOM, 2021). The report, which is freely accessible online, concludes with nine incremental recommendations for government, regulatory, policy, healthcare delivery, nursing education, and fiduciary bodies to devise systems to support nurses as they practice to the full extent of their education and address social determinants of health, health equity, and health outcomes.

The late 20th and the early 21st centuries have ushered in increasingly elaborate medical technology, new knowledge that elevates the level of health care, an aging population with more complex health needs, and shrinking funding sources. Pandemics, natural disasters, ideological controversies, and global conflicts have brought nurses face to face with previously unthinkable circumstances. It is encouraging, therefore, that positive contemporary social forces, such those brought about by the IOM, have made a lasting impact on the profession of nursing. Managed care and other mechanisms of payment for healthcare services have also reshaped the healthcare environment. Hospitals strive to streamline services through improved efficiency and reduced waste; fewer healthcare services are provided in the high-tech hospital setting as patients are released for healthcare support at home; nurses have established new roles; and nursing education has evolved. The position of the professional nurse within these systems is far from assured. Recalling lessons from the past, nurses remain acutely aware of newly won professional recognition.

ASK YOURSELF

When Nurses Risk Their Lives to Care for Patients
In 2020, nurses worked in COVID-19 units even though the disease was highly communicable; the death rate was high; and there was no cure, no vaccine, and insufficient personal protective equipment. Some had small children at home, some had immunocompromised family members, and some were vulnerable, themselves. Yet, they continued to show up at work—sometimes living in isolation from their families.

- What motivated these nurses?
- Why did they continue to work in these dangerous situations even at the risk of contracting the disease or taking it home to family members?
- What would have happened if nurses, *en masse*, had refused to submit themselves to the lethal dangers of COVID-19 infection?
- Codes of nursing ethics (available online) provide ethical guidelines for nursing practice. How do the codes of ethics of the ANA (2015, Provisions 5.1 and 8.4) or the CNA (2017, Parts I.A.9 and I.G.5) and the ICN (2021, Elements 2.4 and 3.7) apply to nurses' ethical responsibilities during pandemics or other emergency events?

SUMMARY

Nursing was created by society to meet the specific real and perceived health needs. The profession belongs to society and therefore is bound by the duty to competently meet the needs for which it was created. Individual nurses therefore have a duty to fulfill the promise the profession has made to society.

In all cultures, the nursing profession has been profoundly influenced by various aspects of spirituality and religious practice. The natures of both the healer and the healing act have been influenced by the prevailing cosmology. Until the past two centuries, healing was strongly associated with the sacred. Religious institutions have influenced the parameters and membership of the profession by either including or excluding particular groups.

From ancient times until today, philosophers have asked important questions and proposed theories that helped shape cultures. Even when people do not recognize it, culture is influenced by philosophers' ideas. These ideas permeate society, relationships, and professions.

Since the first philosophers emerged, no element of society has been free from the influence of philosophy.

Women have been healers in every culture. Because nursing is primarily a profession of women, the status of women in society has been an important factor in determining the role of nurses in the healthcare system. Women's status in society directly determines the freedom they are given to become educated, to think and act independently, and to participate fully in the healing arts. There were periods in history in which women were allowed freedom and responsibility, and there were dark periods in which women lived in subjugation. Nursing today is at a crossroad, free of many of the restrictions of the past yet not fully franchised as a profession with power and authority. In the 21st century, particularly in response to the exigencies of the COVID-19 pandemic, natural disasters, and global conflict, nursing has been rapidly changing and adapting. Through social initiatives such as IOM reports, major changes are occurring in healthcare systems and both the practice of nursing and nursing education.

CHAPTER HIGHLIGHTS

- Throughout history, spiritual beliefs, religious practice, cultural norms, and political factors have influenced evolutionary changes in nursing. These factors continue to influence the practice of nursing today.
- Prevailing philosophical ideas influence every aspect of culture.
- Social need is the criterion for the existence of all professions.
- Moral thinking occurs when individuals or groups desire to meet the needs of others.
- The practice of nursing is focused on meeting the healthcare needs of others; therefore, the practice of nursing originates in moral thinking.
- Professions exist to meet the needs of society.
- Society grants professionals the exclusive right to practice within defined parameters.
- Professionals have a reciprocal duty to society to practice competently.
- Because nursing is primarily a profession of women, the social status of women affects the status of the profession.

- The status of the nursing profession determines members' ability to practice with freedom and responsibility.
- Pivotal changes in the nursing profession are occurring in the contemporary era.

DISCUSSION QUESTIONS AND ACTIVITIES

1. Talk with nurses, physicians, and ministers. Ask their opinions about why some people choose to help others in need. In class, analyze and compare the responses.
2. Discuss the historical developments that caused the separation of the professions of medicine and nursing. How were the distinctions drawn as to the boundaries of the professions? How would you change the boundaries today?
3. Search the Internet for information on Florence Nightingale. Pictures and a short history can be found at the Florence Nightingale Museum web page at https://www.florence-nightingale.co.uk/.
4. What is the relationship between the role of women in history and the status of nurses?
5. What is the relationship between the role of women in the 21st century and the status of nurses?
6. Search out a few retired nurses. Ask them to describe the relationship between nurses and physicians in the mid-1900s. How was this related to the roles of women in society during the same period?
7. Search out a few nurses who were working through the COVID-19 pandemic. Ask them how their nursing role was affected by the pandemic.
8. Discuss the relationship between the role of nurses in the healthcare system today and their role in ethical decision making in the clinical setting.
9. Discuss how codes of nursing ethics support the profession of nursing related to attaining or maintaining an authoritative role in the healthcare system of the future.

REFERENCES

AANP. (2013). *Fact sheet: Medicare reimbursement*. https://www.aanp.org/legislation-regulation/federal-legislation/medicare/68-articles/325-medicare-reimbursement

Achterberg, J. (1990). *Woman as healer*. Shambhala.

ANA, (1980). *Nursing: A social policy statement*. Author.

ANA, (1995). *Nursing's social policy statement*. Author.

ANA, (2003). *Nursing's social policy statement* (2nd ed.). Nursebooks.org.

ANA, (2010). *Nursing's social policy statement: The essence of the profession*. Nursebooks.org.

ANA, (2015). *Code of ethics for nurses with interpretive statements*. Nursebooks.org.

Aquinas, T. (1920). Treatise on man. (Fathers of the English Dominican Province, Trans.). In *Summa Theologiae*. (Original work published ca. 1274)

Aristotle, (2000). Nicomache an ethics In R. Crisp (Ed.),Ed. & Trans. *Aristotle: Nicomachean ethics*. Cambridge University Press (Original work published ca.340 BCE).

Barstow, A. L. (1995). *Witchcraze: A new history of the European witch hunts* (Reprint ed.). Pandora.

CNA. (2017). *Code of ethics for registered nurses*. Available from https://cdn1.nscn.ca/sites/default/files/documents/resources/code-of-ethics-for-registered-nurses.pdf#:~:text=The%20Canadian%20Nurses%20Association%20%28CNA%29%20Code%20of%20Ethics,receiving%20care.%20The%20Codeis%20both%20aspirational%20and%20regulatory

Cartwright, F. F., & Biddiss, M. (2020). *Disease and history: From ancient tmes to Covid-19* (4th ed.). Lume.

Chollet, M. (2022). In S. R. Lewis (Ed.),Trans *In defense of witches: The legacy of the witch hunts and why women are still on trial* (English ed.). St. Martin's Press Chollet, M. (2022). In defense of witches: The legacy of the witch hunts and why women are still on trial (S. R. Lewis, Trans.; English ed.). St. Martin's Press.

Collinson, P. (2004). *The Reformation: A history*. Modern Library.

Descartes, R. (2013). *Rene Descartes meditations on the first philosophy* (J. Cottingham, Ed. & Trans. Latin-English ed.). Cambridge University Press. (Original work published 1614)

Dolan, J. A. (1973). *Nursing in society: A historical perspective* (13th ed.). Saunders.

Dolan, J. A., Fitzpatrick, M. L., & Herrmann, E. K. (1983). *Nursing in society: A historical perspective* (15th ed.). Saunders.

Donahue, M. P. (2011). *Nursing, the finest art: An illustrated history* (3rd ed.). Mosby.

Dossey, B.M. (2010). *Florence Nightingale: Mystic, visionary, healer* (Commemorative ed.). F.A. Davis.

Ehrenreich, B., & English, D. (2010). *Witches, midwives, and nurses: A history of women healers* (2nd ed.). Feminist Press.

Feldman, H. R., & Lewenson, S. B. (2000). *Nurses in the political arena: The public face of nursing*. Springer.

Fowler, M. D. M. (2015). *Guide to nursing's social policy statement: Understanding the profession from social contract to social covenant*. Nursebooks.org.

Forst, B. (1994). *The laws of kashrus: A comprehensive exposition of their underlying concepts and applications* (2nd ed.). Mesorah Publications.

Freire, P. (2000). *Pedagogy of the oppressed* (30th anniversary ed.). Continuum.

Fulton, Y. (1997). Nurses' views on empowerment: A critical social theory perspective. *Journal of Advanced Nursing, 26*(3), 529–536. https://www.ncbi.nlm.nih.gov/pubmed/9378874.

Habermas, J. (1979). *Communication and the evolution of society*. Beacon Press.

Harden, J. (1996). Enlightenment, empowerment and emancipation: The case for critical pedagogy in nurse education. *Nurse Education Today, 16*(1), 32–37. https://www.ncbi.nlm.nih.gov/pubmed/8700068.

Hart, G. D. (2000). *Asclepius: The god of medicine*. Royal Society of Medicine Press.

Hedin, B. A. (1986). A case study of oppressed group behavior in nurses. *Image: Journal of Nursing Scholarship, 18*(2), 53–57. https://www.ncbi.nlm.nih.gov/pubmed/3634752.

Heer, F. (1962). *The medieval world: Europe* (pp. 1100–1350). Weidenfeld and Nicolson.

Hippocrates. (1943). Hippocratic corpus (L. Edelstein, Trans.). In: *The Hippocratic oath, text, translation, and interpretation*. Baltimore, MD: Johns Hopkins Press (Original work published ca. 450-350 B.C.E.).

Howe, B. J., & Berennan, M. A. (2013). The sisters of St. Joseph in Wheeling, West Virginia during the Civil War. *U.S. Catholic Historian, 31*(1), 21–49. https://www.jstor.org/stable/24584777.

ICN, (2021). *The ICN code of ethics for nurses*. International Council of Nurses. https://www.icn.ch/system/files/2021-10/ICN_Code-of-Ethics_EN_Web_0.pdf.

IOM, (2000). *To err is human: Building a safer health system*. National Academies Press.

IOM, (2001). *Crossing the quality chasm: A new health system for the 21st century*. National Academies Press.

IOM, (2010). *The future of nursing: Leading change, advancing health*. National Academies Press.

Jameton, A. (1984). *Nursing practice: The ethical issues*. Prentice-Hall.

Jerome, S. (1867). The perpetual virginity of blessed Mary: Against Helvidius (Hon. W. H. Fremantle, Trans.). In: *Eternal World Television Network*. https://www.ewtn.com/catholicism/library/perpetual-virginity-of-blessed-mary-against-helvidius-11630.(Original work published ca. 383).

Kramer, H., & Springer, J. (1971). The Malleus Maleficarum (R. M. Summers, Trans.). In: *The Malleus Maleficarum of Heinrich Kramer and James Sprenger*. New York, NY: Dover (Original work published 1486).

Libster, M. M. (2018). Spiritual formation, secularization, and reform of professional nursing and education in antebellum America. *Journal of Professional Nursing: Official Journal of the American Association of Colleges of Nursing, 34*(1), 47–53.

Manojlovich, M. (2007). Power and empowerment in nursing: looking backward to inform the future. *Online Journal of Issues in Nursing, 12*(1), 2.

de Marrilac, L. (1991). Letter 561 to Brother Ducourneau. In: *Spiritual Writings of Louise de Marrilac: Correspondence and thoughts* (D. C. Sr. Louise Sullivan, Trans.). New City Press (Original work published in 1658).

McDonald, L. (2013). The timeless wisdom of Florence Nightingale. *Canadian Nurse, 109*(2), 36.

National Academies of Medicine, (2021). *The future of nursing 2020-2030: Charting a path to achieve health equity*. National Academies Press.

Nightingale, F. (1860). *Notes on nursing what it is, and what it is not*. Harrison.

Nightingale, F. (1979). *Cassandra: An essay*. Feminist Press. (Original work written ca. 1852).

Pavlac, B. A. (2009). *Witch hunts in the Western world: Persecution and punishment from the Inquisition through the Salem trials*. Greenwood.

Peirce, C. S. (1877). The fixation of belief. *Popular Science Monthly, 12*, 1–15.

Plato. (1997a). The republic (G. M. A. Grube, ref. C.D.C. Reeve, Trans.). In J. M. Cooper & D. S. Hutchinson (Eds.), *Plato: Complete works*. Hackett (Original work written ca 375).

Plato. (1997b). Phaedo (G. M. A. Grube, Trans.). In J. M. Cooper (Ed.), *Plato Complete Works*. Hackett (Original work written ca. 353).

Roberts, S. J. (1983). Oppressed group behavior: Implications for nursing. *Advances in Nursing Science, 5*(4), 21–30. https://www.ncbi.nlm.nih.gov/pubmed/6410980.

Russell, B. (2008). *History of Western philosophy: And its connection with political and social circumstances from the earliest times to the present day*. Touchstone.

Selanders, L. C. (2010). Florence Nightingale: The evolution and social impact of feminist values in nursing. *Journal of Holistic Nursing, 28*(1), 70–78. https://doi.org/10.1177/0898010109360256.

Showalter, E. (1981). Florence Nightingale: The evolution and social impact of feminist values in nursing. *Journal of Women in Culture and Society, 6*, 395–412.

Simpkin, J. (2014). *Florence Nightingale*. https://spartacus-educational.com/REnightingale.htm

Sisters of St. Joseph. (2022). *About Us*. Sisters Health Foundation. https://sistershealthfdn.org/about-us/history/

Solomon, R. C., & Higgins, K. M. (1996). *A short history of philosophy*. Oxford University Press.

Suvajdžić, L., Djendić, A., Sakač, V., Čanak, G., & Dankuc, D. (2016). Hippocrates: The father of modern medicine.

Vojnosanitetski Pregled: Military Medical & Pharmaceutical Journal of Serbia, 73(12), 1181–1186. https://doi.org/10.2298/VSP150212131S.

Theofanidis, D., & Sapountzi-Krepia, D. (2015). Nursing and caring: An historical overview from ancient Greek tradition to modern times. *International Journal of Caring Sciences, 8*(3), 791–800.

WHO. (2022). *The Global Health Observatory*. https://www.who.int/data/gho/data/indicators/indicator-details/GHO/nurses-by-sex-(-)

Yapijakis, C. (2009). Hippocrates of Kos, the father of clinical medicine, and Asclepiades of Bithynia, the father of molecular medicine. Review. *In Vivo, 23*(4), 507–514. https://www.ncbi.nlm.nih.gov/pubmed/19567383.

2

Theories of Ethics

Within Siddhartha there slowly grew and ripened the knowledge of what wisdom really was and the goal of his long seeking. It was nothing but a preparation of the soul, a capacity, a secret art of thinking, feeling and breathing thoughts of unity at every moment of life. This thought matured in him slowly, and it was reflected in Vasudeva's old childlike face: harmony, knowledgeof the eternal perfection of the world, and unity.

(Hesse, 1971, p. 131)

OBJECTIVES

After completing this chapter, the reader should be able to:

1. Discuss the purpose of philosophy.
2. Define the terms moral philosophy and ethics.
3. Discuss the importance of a systematic study of ethics to nursing.
4. Discuss the importance of ethical theory.
5. Describe utilitarianism.
6. Describe deontological ethics, defining the terms categorical imperative and practical imperative.
7. Define the terms virtue and virtue ethics.
8. Discuss moral particularism.
9. Relate principles of ethics to nursing codes of ethics.

INTRODUCTION

At its core, nursing deals with issues and situations that have elements of ethical or moral uncertainty. A spiraling dependence on complex technology and the resulting longer life spans and higher healthcare costs, coupled with increasing professional autonomy, global disease, and supply chain insufficiency create an atmosphere in which nurses are faced with problems of ever-increasing complexity. Nurses need to be able to recognize situations with troubling ethical and moral implications and make thoughtful decisions based on recognized ethical principles and theory. This text will prepare you to examine issues and come to logical, consistent, and thoughtful ethical decisions. The study of ethics will make you more rational, self-assured, self-reliant, and effective.

As nurses, we need to be able to recognize ethical components of practice and engage in a structured ethical decision-making process. We must have the willingness and courage to participate in work that is emotionally painful. Ethical problems deal with issues of great significance to those involved and, by their very nature, have no easy or obvious solutions. We must have a solid knowledge base that prepares us to identify circumstances that involve ethical components. Knowledge of and insight into personal values, cultural norms, moral development, professional ethics, and ethical theory are necessary for the practicing nurse. We must be sensitive, patient, and insightful. Recognition of subtle clues that may indicate when a situation is laden with ethical components demands that we are attentive to all facets of the case. This requires time, focused attention, and sensitivity. We need to be knowledgeable and adept in making logical, fair, and consistent decisions. Ethical decision-making models offer a variety of methods for coming to rational conclusions. Willingness, courage, knowledge, and moral sensitivity must all be present for us to participate effectively in ethical decision making.

CASE PRESENTATION

Nursing Students Face an Ethical Dilemma

A dilemma is defined as a problem that requires a choice between two options that are equally unfavorable and mutually exclusive. Ethical dilemmas occur when there is a strong moral component to the situation. Tonya and Lydia are two senior nursing students assigned to work in the intensive care unit (ICU) with a critically ill patient. The patient, Mr. Dunn, is an 87-year-old retired ironworker. He lives alone in an old two-story frame house. Mr. Dunn is diabetic. He is nearly blind and has moderately advanced prostate cancer and Alzheimer disease. Mr. Dunn was admitted to the ICU after he was discovered unconscious in his home by a neighbor. At that time, he was ketoacidotic and had a very severe necrotic wound on his left leg. The surgeon plans to amputate Mr. Dunn's left leg but has been unable to get consent from either Mr. Dunn or his next of kin, a niece who lives out of town.

Tonya is proud of her efficiency as a nursing student. She makes rapid decisions. As they discuss the case, Tonya insists that Mr. Dunn must have the amputation. She boldly suggests to the physician that he should appoint a surrogate decision maker for Mr. Dunn so that the surgery can proceed. The course is clear to her. Lydia, on the other hand, is not certain of the correct course of action. She talks to Mr. Dunn and his niece about his condition. She wonders if the amputation is the best solution to his problem. She thinks about what his quality of life will be after the surgery. She worries about his ability to care for himself and about his state of mind should he be forced to live in a nursing home. She thinks about what she would want for her own father if he were in the same situation—or what she would want for herself. Lydia falls asleep at night pondering these thoughts. She does not know how to go about solving the problem. Tonya is impatient with Lydia. She thinks that Lydia wastes her time and energy worrying about this problem when the solution is apparent to her.

Think About It
Facing Ethical Dilemmas
- What alerts you to the presence of an ethical dilemma?
- How do you feel when confronted with difficult ethical decisions?
- To what degree do you think nurses should become involved in making decisions such as the one described in this situation?
- Tonya and Lydia have different qualities. With which qualities of each nurse do you identify?
- If you were Tonya and Lydia's nursing professor, what parts of the profession's code of ethics could you use to help Tonya and Lydia think about this situation?

In this case presentation, we see nurses at both extremes. Tonya makes quick decisions. Although efficient, she probably fails to recognize the ethical nature of the problem, the affect the outcome may have on the people involved, or possible solutions that differ from her own. She has great pride in her ability to make decisions and has confidence that she is correct. Lydia, being more insightful and sensitive, recognizes intuitively that the problem presents no clear solution. She is troubled by the situation but has no tools with which to deal with the problem. Each of these nurses will benefit from a study of nursing ethics—Tonya may become more thoughtful, and Lydia may become more confident and efficient in her decision making. The two may be able to come to a mutual understanding.

Ethics and Nursing

Nursing is a profession that deals with the most personal and private aspects of people's lives. From the beginning of time, nurses—whether called healers, sisters, caretakers, nurturers, or nurses—have cared for those in need in a very personal and intimate way. Nurses are attentive to patients' needs over long periods. They may have made home visits and may know patients' families. They may care for patients at their bedside for hours and days on end. It is through the intimacy and trust inherent in the nurse-patient relationship that nurses become critical participants in the process of ethical decision making.

As members of a dynamic profession, nurses are faced with ethical choices that affect the profession itself. For example, as the needs and demands of society change, the boundaries of the domain of nursing contract and expand. This forces us to make decisions about such issues as the delegation of traditional nursing functions to nonnurse caregivers and the expanding boundaries of nursing. Because nursing is self-regulated, we review and discipline peers. This holds many ethical implications as we attempt to balance this responsibility with our desire to advance the profession, protect the public, and maintain professional cohesiveness.

Nurses may also take part in decision making on a broader scale. More than ever before, nurses are participating as members of policy-making bodies. Legislatures and government; community, state, and national task forces; committees; and boards of advisors are among those healthcare decision making groups in which nurses have become integral and respected members. Nurses participating in decision making at this level must be aware of the ethical implications of their decisions, particularly those dealing with the distribution of goods and services. These decisions are at the very heart of our society's beliefs about the value of the individual and, as such, compel those involved to cautiously deliberate every decision.

This chapter includes a discussion of some prevailing ethical theories. You may ask how you will use these theories in your practice. To be sure, you will not choose one theory to use exclusively in your career. Instead, you will have a clear awareness of the many nuances and rules that govern moral and ethical decisions. You will better understand decision-making models at the many levels of the healthcare system, and you will be ready to make clear and consistent ethical choices of your own. You will understand the language of ethics and be empowered as you engage in intraprofessional and interprofessional dialogs.

PHILOSOPHY

Philosophy is literally translated as the love of wisdom. Even though it involves abstract concepts, philosophy is intended for everyone. It is both natural and necessary to humanity. Philosophy includes an intense and critical examination of beliefs and assumptions. It gives coherence to the whole realm of thought and experience and offers principles for deciding what actions and qualities are most worthwhile. Philosophy will also show inconsistency in meaning and context. As you read in Chapter 1, throughout history, there have been many philosophical schools of thought. Because of the nature of philosophy, it is impossible to verify philosophical beliefs or theories; nevertheless, the study of philosophy helps give order and coherence to beliefs and assumptions. It gives shape to what would otherwise be a random chaos of thoughts, beliefs, assumptions, values, and superstitions.

ASK YOURSELF

Socratic Questioning

As you learned in Chapter 1, the ancient philosopher Socrates used questioning to help his students. His questions challenged the accuracy and completeness of their thoughts. Socrates used common language and called on his students to confront and examine their own beliefs through the use of common sense. Professors today may use the Socratic method to demonstrate new perspectives and to help students organize their thoughts. Professors may use any one of the following types of questions: conceptual clarification questions, questions that explore assumptions, questions that explore reasons and evidence, questions about viewpoints and perspectives, questions about contradictions, and questions about implications and consequences. Consider the following scenario.

James is a registered nurse who works evenings in the emergency department while completing his bachelor's degree. During a class discussion about professional responsibility, he says, "I would like to see the legislature pass a law to make it illegal to prescribe narcotics to drug addicts." The professor wants to make sure James fully

understands the nature of the problem and the implications of such a law. To shed light on the factors that might not have been considered, the professor might pose the following questions to James and then open discussion to the entire class:

- "Are you saying that no controlled substance should ever be prescribed to a person who has an addiction?"
- "What evidence do you use to classify a person as a drug addict?"
- "Can you imagine a situation in which your judgment about whether a person is a drug addict could be wrong?"
- "Do you agree that it is possible for a person who has a drug addiction to also have severe pain?"
- "Which classes of people deserve pain relief?"
- "Can you think of a situation in which it might be okay to prescribe controlled substances to a drug addict?"
- "What would be the long-term social consequences if people who are drug addicts could never receive controlled substances through legitimate sources?"
- "Who would benefit from such a law? Who would be harmed?"

Philosophers such as Socrates examine questions that deal with the most important aspects of life (Fig. 2.1). Typical questions include the following: What is the meaning of life? Is there a God? What is reality?

What is truth? What is the essence of knowledge? How can something be known? How can one describe the relationships among persons, or between humans and the Divine? What is happiness? What is the ideal or

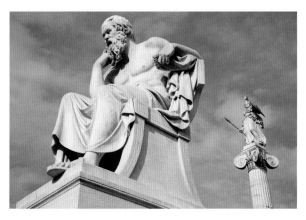

Fig. 2.1 Marble Statue of Ancient Greek Philosopher Socrates. (©iStock.com/chatsimo.)

virtuous human character? How can one understand human beliefs, values, and morals? Questions such as these have been asked by the most widely studied philosophers. Buddha asked, "How can one find the path that leads to the end of suffering?" Confucius asked, "What is the remedy for social disorder?" Socrates asked, "How should one live?" Aristotle asked, "What is a virtuous life?" Through the centuries, philosophy has concerned itself with topics that define the essence of human life. Martin Buber said, "With soaring power [man] reaches out beyond what is given him, flies beyond the horizon and the familiar stars, and grasps a totality" (1965, p. 61). Ayn Rand, author and social philosopher, eloquently expressed her thoughts when she wrote the following:

> *A philosophic system is an integrated view of existence. As a human being, you have no choice about the fact that you need a philosophy. Your only choice is whether you define your philosophy by a conscious, rational, disciplined process of thought and scrupulously logical deliberation—or let your subconscious accumulate a junk heap of unwarranted conclusions, false generalizations, . . . undefined wishes, doubts and fears, thrown together by chance, but integrated by your subconscious into a kind of mongrel philosophy and fused into a single weight: self-doubt, like a ball and chain in the place where your mind's wings should have grown. (1982, p. 5)*

Philosophy is divided into subcategories that include abstract ideas about knowledge and how people should live their lives. Authorities organize the branches of philosophy in a variety of ways. For the purposes of this book, we organize philosophy into three areas that include ideas about the general nature of the world (metaphysics), justification of belief (epistemology), and the conduct of life (ethics). Metaphysics is the branch of philosophy concerned with questions about the nature of existence, being, becoming, and reality. Metaphysical questions include, for example, "What is the nature of reality?" "Is there a God?" Cosmology, mentioned in Chapter 1, falls under the broad category of metaphysics. Epistemology is the study of the nature of knowledge and how we acquire it. Epistemology seeks to answer questions such as, "What can be known?" What is the difference between knowing and believing?" "How does one learn?" "Why do we believe some things and not others?" Ethics (also called moral philosophy) deals with concepts of right or wrong conduct. Ethics seeks to answer questions about what makes actions or laws right or wrong, good or bad, just or unjust, good or evil, fair or unfair. This branch of philosophy seeks answers to questions such as "Are actions right in themselves, regardless of consequences or do consequences matter more than the actions?" and "What is justice?" Although metaphysics and epistemology provide an important foundation for nursing research, in this text we focus on ethics because it provides the groundwork for a discussion of many of the troubling moral issues facing nurses.

Theories consist of unified and logical systematic statements that explain something. Theories are based on general principles. Moral theories provide a framework for cohesive and consistent ethical reasoning and decision making. There are many moral theories. Some theories are more fully developed than others, and some consist of combinations of other theories. The most mature moral theories are part of more comprehensive and integrated philosophies. Most of them clearly reflect earlier ideas proposed by historical figures such as Socrates, Plato, or Aristotle. This chapter is devoted to an examination of the two moral theories that have had the greatest influence on contemporary bioethics and nursing: utilitarianism and deontology. We also include a description of virtue or character ethics. Theories related specifically to resource allocation, such as libertarianism, are described in Chapter 15. Nurses who are interested in a more detailed examination of specific theories should read works by the original theorists as well as analyses by contemporary writers.

MORALS AND ETHICS

Moral philosophy is the philosophical discussion of what is considered good or bad, right or wrong, in terms of moral issues. Moral issues are those that are essential, basic, or important. They deal with important social values or norms, such as respect for life, freedom, and love; issues that provoke the conscience or such feelings as guilt, shame, self-esteem, courage, or hope; issues to which we respond with words such as *ought, should, right, wrong, good*, and *bad;* and issues that are uncommonly complicated, frustrating, nonresolvable, or difficult in some indefinable way (Jameton, 1984). Morality is less structured than moral philosophy. It refers to traditions or beliefs about right and wrong conduct. Morality includes social and cultural conventions with a history and code of learnable rules. It exists before we are taught its rules—we learn about morality in our culture as we grow up (Beauchamp, 2001).

Ethicists generally distinguish four levels of moral discourse, based upon a 1952 paper by Henry David Aiken (Fig. 2.2). The levels of **moral discourse** include **casuistry**, rules and rights (codes of ethics), **normative ethics**, and **metaethics**, moving up the ladder of abstraction from the former to the latter. Casuistry occurs at the level of the case or story. For example, sources of authority for new judgment may proceed from someone's experience of a similar case in the past or from a paradigm case, such as the Karen Ann Quinlan case (Dengrove Collection, n.d.) or the Tuskegee syphilis study (Jinbin, 2017). The next level of moral discourse, rules, and rights includes codes of ethics and relies upon rule-like maxims or claims of rights. Nursing codes of ethics and declarations of patients' rights are examples of this level of discourse which can help to guide nurses when making ethical decisions. When the discussion of rules and rights as demonstrated in codes of ethics, for example, does not solve a moral problem, people may move to normative ethics in which norms of behavior, character, and moral relations are discussed. Normative ethics is a form of moral discourse that seeks to set norms or standards for conduct. Normative ethics focuses on intrinsic values such as truth, moral goodness, and happiness; guides for right action such as principles of bioethics and duty-based ethics; and virtues, including professional, secular, and religious virtues (Veatch & Guidry-Grimes, 2020). Deontology, utilitarian, and virtue ethics that follow are competing theories of normative ethics. The highest and most abstract level of moral discourse is that of metaethics, which includes discussions about the source of ethics (secular or religious) and how one knows what is ethical. Discussions about naturalism and rationalism that follow are examples of metaethics. Throughout this book, you will be asked to look at

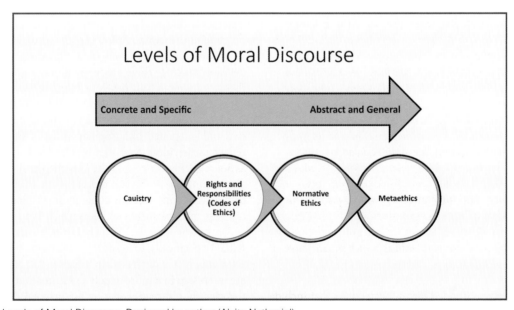

Fig. 2.2 Levels of Moral Discourse. Designed by author (Alvita Nathaniel).

situations and discuss cases at any one of these four levels of moral discourse.

Ethics is concerned with the study of social morality and philosophical reflection about society's norms and practices. Ethics furnishes us with the practical application of moral philosophy, asking the question, "What should I do in this situation?" Professional codes of ethics are tools that offer a formal process for applying moral philosophy. The study of ethics gives us a groundwork for making logical and consistent decisions. These decisions may be based on morality or formal moral theory. Ethics offers structured guidelines, but it seldom tells us what we ought to do in specific situations. We must become familiar with our professional codes of ethics, so we are prepared to make well-informed ethical decisions in each case.

Philosophical Basis for Ethical Theory

Similar to the way in which each person's experiences and values contribute to the development of personal ethics, professions committed to a common ideal strive to develop discipline-specific rules of behavior. **Professional codes of ethics** generally appear when occupations organize themselves into professions. Codes of professional ethics govern professional behavior. They embody core values shared by members of the profession. Codes of ethics formalize professional values, promote accountability, give the profession legitimacy, and provide the profession and the public with frameworks to evaluate situations and aid decisions. Professions have a vested interest in the conduct of their members for several reasons including protecting people the profession serves, ensuring the competence of members, and safeguarding the integrity and trustworthiness of the discipline. Most ethics codes dictate that members conduct themselves honestly, fairly, competently, and benignly, and they provide guidance for ethical conduct in morally ambiguous situations (Bullock & Panicker, 2003; Goldman, 2019; Pipes et al., 2005). As illustrated throughout the following chapters, nursing codes of ethics provide guidance to nurses in their relationships with patients, colleagues, the profession, and society. Specific codes of ethics for nurses, such as those developed by the American Nurses Association (ANA), the Canadian Nurses Association (CNA), and the International Council of Nurses (ICN), serve as guides for nurses in practice. Nursing codes of ethics derive from coherent philosophical foundations and established ethical theories.

ASK YOURSELF

What Are Your Beliefs?
- Do you believe that some actions are always wrong in all circumstances? Give examples.
- Do you believe that you have an innate knowledge of right and wrong?
- How did you learn right and wrong? What was the influence of your parents? Society? Other forces?
- What are your thoughts about how beliefs concerning right and wrong originate?
- To what degree do you believe that rules about right and wrong originate from a universal source? From within yourself?

Unlike mathematics or other empirical sciences, there are no absolute rules governing ethics. Mathematicians can say for certain that two plus two equals four, regardless of the time of day, circumstances, feelings, or beliefs of those involved in the calculations. Ethical rules are less clear and difficult or impossible to prove. For example, whereas some people believe that killing for any reason is always wrong, others argue that euthanasia can be beneficial either for the individual or the society, that abortion to save the life of the mother is permissible, or that killing during war is justified. There are reasonable arguments based on opposing viewpoints that support any of these beliefs. How can rational people reach such different conclusions? The answer to this question may lie in the background and perspectives of the individuals involved.

Ethical theories are derived from either of two basic schools of thought: naturalism or rationalism. An examination of these perspectives will help clarify the various theories.

Naturalism

Naturalism is a view of moral judgment that regards ethics as dependent on human nature and psychology. The naturalism approach to morality requires that humans have the ability to be moral and think intelligently about morality in a way that is compatible with science, nature, and other humans. Naturalists do not hold supernatural beliefs, rather that people can judge what is moral through sensory experience, without reliance on a higher authority (Shook, 2010). Naturalism attributes differences in moral codes to social conditions and proposes that nearly all people have similar underlying psychological tendencies (Raphael, 1994). These similarities suggest that there is universality (or near-universality) in moral judgment. This viewpoint allows each group or person to make judgments based on feelings about particular actions in particular situations. It further suggests that in similar circumstances most people will make similar judgments. Naturalism does not explain aberrant, selfish, or cruel choices that are made by people who seem to be otherwise rational.

Naturalism holds that, collectively, all people tend to make similar ethical decisions. Though there are many value differences among cultures, the variations are not as great as they may seem. Most people desire to be happy, to experience pleasure, and to avoid pain. There seems to be a natural tendency to sympathize with the wishes and feelings of others and, therefore, to approve of helping people in need. Raphael outlines similarities among cultures:

All societies think that it is wrong to hurt members of their own group at least (or to kill them unless there are morally compelling reasons); that it is right to keep faith; that the needy should be helped; that people who deliberately flout the accepted rules should be punished (1994, p. 16).

Empathy is a motivating factor in moral decision making. Empathy is the sharing in imagination of others' feelings. Derived from the Greek, the word literally means to *suffer with*. This entails imagining oneself in the shoes of another and consequently sharing their feelings. The Dalai Lama (1999) proposed that empathy enables us to enter into, and to some degree participate in others' pain and is, therefore, one of humans' most significant characteristics. "It is what causes us to start at the sound of a cry for help, to recoil at the sight of harm done to another, to suffer when confronted with others' suffering" (p. 64). It can be as simple as the "tingly feeling" you get when you hear about someone's pain and the accompanying capacity to access associated emotions (Boddice, 2016). Empathy, according to some, is a natural tendency and is the basis for moral reasoning. Others believe that empathy has somewhat of a social origin and can be learned. The Dalai Lama (1999) proposes that humans' capacity for empathy is the source of the most precious human quality—compassion. Compassion, as he describes it, encompasses a wealth of meaning including affection, kindness, gentleness,

gentleness of spirit, and warm-heartedness. The Scottish philosopher David Hume (1738) suggested further that sympathy (closely related to empathy) is the main source of moral distinctions, particularly because of the resulting tendency to improve the public good.

ASK YOURSELF

What Would You Do?

If theories about naturalism are true, most people would have similar reactions in certain situations. Think about what you would do in the following situations, and ask yourself if most people would act in the same way as you:

- A toddler wanders into a busy intersection with no parent in sight.
- A woman trips and falls into a fountain and lies face down without moving.
- A coworker inadvertently reaches for an adult strength of heparin (10,000 u/mL) to administer to a premature infant rather than a pediatric strength of heparin (1.0 u/mL).

Rationalism

The opposing school of thought is **rationalism**. Rationalism is a view appealing to intellectual and deductive reason, rather than sensory experience, as the source of knowledge or justification. Rationalists argue that feelings or perceptions may not actually be similar in all people. Rationalists believe, as did Socrates, that there are absolute truths that are not dependent on human nature. They argue that ethical values have an independent origin in the universe or, perhaps, from God and that they can be known to humans through the process of reasoning. Rationalists believe there are truths about the world that are necessary and universal and that these truths are superior to the information that we receive from our senses.

To rationalists, moral rules are necessarily true. Rationalists see the knowledge gained through the senses as only contingently true (Raphael, 1994). For example, the grass is perceived as green, but the actual color may be different—or may be seen as different by some. Likewise, one who feels bad when hearing of the misfortune of a friend may not feel the same way when misfortune occurs to an enemy. On the other hand, rationalists propose that moral or ethical rules are always true. For example, rationalists argue that it is always good to help those in need, regardless of the circumstances.

Differences between naturalism and rationalism revolve around the question of the origin of ethics. Is ethics a matter of feeling and sensory experience or of deductive reasoning? Are individuals free to make ethical choices based on a predictable human nature, or is the foundation of ethics based on universal truth? The comparison between naturalism and rationalism is seen clearly in the study of ethical theories. We challenge you to consider these two viewpoints when reading ethical theory.

THEORIES OF ETHICS

Moral philosophy is the branch of philosophy that examines beliefs and assumptions about human values. Ethics is the practical application of moral philosophy. Given the moral context of good or bad, right or wrong, ethics will answer the question, "What should I do in this situation?" The philosopher reveals an integrated system of principles in which elements, like pieces of a puzzle, have a logical fit. By developing a theory of morality, the philosopher hopes to explain values and behavior related to cultural and moral norms. Each theory is based on the viewpoint of the individual philosopher and maintains philosophical consistency within itself. The discussion related to naturalism and rationalism explains one basic difference among moral philosophers. The ethical theories of utilitarianism and deontology are included in this chapter because they are practical and complete; internally and morally coherent; and are the major theories central to medical ethics, nursing ethics, and bioethics.

The following case implies the differences among various ethical theories. Remember, there are no clear answers to ethical dilemmas. The reader's basic viewpoint is reflected in responses to the questions. If your answers are inconsistent, you may need to identify and strengthen a cohesive ethical basis for practice.

Utilitarianism

As you will see throughout this book, **utilitarianism** is a useful form of moral philosophy that is often employed in healthcare policy. Sometimes called **consequentialism**, utilitarianism is a type of teleological theory. *Telos* comes from the ancient Greek language and literally means *end*: Utilitarianism is the moral theory that holds that an action can be considered good or bad in relation

---

CASE PRESENTATION

Conflicting Duties

Anthony is a nurse and director of a local hospice service. Unrelated to his work with hospice, he serves on a statewide advisory board that makes recommendations about the allocation of Medicaid services. In response to a dramatic decrease in federal funding, the board must discontinue some programs. Anthony and other board members are asked to choose between eliminating funding for some immunization programs that serve tens of thousands of youths or eliminating a single costly program that provides catastrophic assistance to only a few individuals. Because of his experience with hospice patients, Anthony recognizes the importance of programs to help with catastrophic illness. He knows that catastrophic illness can lead to death when families cannot pay for care or can totally bankrupt families. However, he is hesitant to advise eliminating immunization programs because immunizations are proven to save more lives than any other healthcare intervention.

Think About It
Resolving Conflicting Duties
- What facet of this situation leads to the ethical bind Anthony is experiencing?
- To what degree does Anthony have a primary duty to see that catastrophic programs benefiting his hospice patients continue to be funded?
- As an advisory board member, what is Anthony's responsibility to the large number of children who would be denied the benefit of lifesaving immunizations?
- What ethical basis should Anthony use for making his decision?
- How would you decide what to do in this situation?

---

to its end result. Utilitarianism is an important ethical philosophy that has its basis in naturalism. According to the utilitarian school of thought, the right action is that which has the greatest **utility**, or usefulness. Utility holds that an action is morally right if it increases the net amount of good, taking into account the harm that may occur as well (Veatch & Guidry-Grimes, 2020), so that no action is, in itself, either good or bad. Utilitarians hold that the only factors that make actions good or bad are the outcomes, or end results, that are derived from them. Bykvist (2010) proposes that a basic tenet of utilitarianism is that we should make the world as good as we can by making the lives of people as good as we can.

Jeremy Bentham (1748–1832), a leading political philosopher, is considered the father of modern utilitarianism. His theories laid the foundations of modern government and social science. According to Bentham's theory, actions are right when they increase happiness and diminish misery and wrong when they have the opposite effect. Following is Bentham's definition of the "principle of utility:"

> *By utility is meant that property in any object, whereby it tends to produce benefit, advantage, pleasure, good, or happiness ... or ... to prevent the happening of mischief, pain, evil, or unhappiness to the party whose interest is considered: if that party be the community in general, then the happiness of the community: if a particular individual, then the happiness of that individual (1948, p. 2).*

Bentham attempted to create a science derived from the principle of utility. He proposed that we should measure the product of an act in terms of the value of a proposed pleasure. Six criteria used to measure pleasure include intensity, duration, certainty, propinquity (nearness in place or time), fecundity (the chance of it being followed by sensations of the same kind), and purity (the chance of it not being followed by sensations of the opposite kind). Bentham proposed that each criterion be given a value and that the sum of the values related to pleasure be weighed against a similar sum of values related to the pain that might result from any given act. In essence, the person should act in accordance with a mathematical formula, resolving ethical decisions based on the sum of the value of a given act. Because Bentham's formula to measure utility is complex and cumbersome, it is not used today. Nevertheless, when choosing a course of action, a person will tacitly consider some of Bentham's criteria such as the likely intensity, duration, and certainty of the anticipated outcome.

Though many critics describe Bentham as having a hedonistic tendency (his theory is often referred to as hedonistic utilitarianism), it is clear from his writings that his interest extended far beyond physical pleasure. He wrote that *pleasure* is synonymous with many other terms, such as *good, profit, advantage*, and *benefit*. In fact, his interest in the common good of the community refutes those who charge that his theory is hedonistic. He describes a type of justice in which action should tend to augment the happiness of the community as a whole, rather than diminish it.

John Stuart Mill (1806–1873) was a leading 19th-century British moral philosopher. Like Bentham, Mill was a utilitarian. He described utilitarianism in terms of judging acts according to their end results. He wrote, "All action is for the sake of some end; and rules of action, it seems natural to suppose, must take their whole character and color from the end to which they are subservient" (1910/2011, p. 2). The phrase *the end justifies the means* relates to Mill's theory. According to Mill, the only right actions are those that produce the greatest happiness. His "greatest happiness principle" holds that the right action in conduct is not the agent's own happiness, but the happiness of all concerned. He further believed that sacrifice is good only when it increases the total sum of happiness. For Mill, the object of virtue is the multiplication of happiness. He cautioned, however, that we must carefully attempt to avoid violating the rights of some people in the process of maximizing the happiness of others.

Mill defined his concepts in ways that make the meaning of this theory clearer. He described happiness as a state of pleasure that is not restricted to physical pleasure alone. Consistent with Aristotle's ancient philosophy, Mill made a strong argument in favor of prioritizing pleasure, with intellectual pleasure having greater priority than physical pleasure. Further, Mill condemned those who chose sensual indulgences to the injury of health. He described the greatest sources of physical and mental suffering as "indigence, disease, and the unkindness, worthlessness, or premature loss, of objects of affection" (1910, p. 14).

Although Mill disagreed with the notion that rules of ethics are edicts from God, he related utilitarianism to Judeo-Christian doctrine. He believed utilitarianism to be in the spirit of the Golden Rule: "Do unto others as you would have them do unto you." Thus, the Golden Rule depicts the ideal perfection of utilitarian morality. Mill further believed that the happiness of humankind is within the interest of a benevolent God and that people are given the opportunity to make ethical choices according to these precepts.

Although the works of Bentham and Mill are the most frequently quoted, there are many other utilitarian theories. There are two basic types of utilitarianism. **Act-utilitarianism** suggests that people choose actions that will, in any given circumstance, increase the overall good. **Rule-utilitarianism**, on the other hand, suggests that people choose rules that, when followed consistently, will maximize the overall good.

CASE PRESENTATION

Making Decisions Based on the Situation

Many years ago, as a junior nursing student, Mary was assigned to observe the labor and delivery department of a small rural hospital. As frequently occurs in small towns, the nurses and physicians were acquainted with many of the women—they knew their backgrounds, home situations, and so forth. During her second day on the unit, Mary attended the delivery of a set of premature twins. After delivering the tiny babies, the physician walked to a nearby room and placed them on a metal utility table. He turned and said to those in attendance, "Nobody is to touch them. This woman has nine children at home. She doesn't need any more babies."

Because these babies were very premature, it is possible that they would not have survived in the best of situations. The physician may have correctly believed that the babies were delivered too early to survive. Nevertheless, the nurses struggled with the moral implications. This example raises many ethical questions and illustrates a case of paternalism and utilitarianism taken to the extreme.

Think About It
Does the End Justify the Means?
- Utilitarianism holds that an action is judged good or bad in relation to the consequences or outcomes that are derived from it. If the physician were thinking in terms of utilitarianism, what could have been the arguments to support his actions?
- Assume that the twins were rescued. Name as many possible outcomes as you can imagine.
- Name four arguments for and four arguments against the physician's decision.
- Considering her position as a student in the hospital, what were Mary's options?
- What thoughts would have gone through your mind if you were in this situation?
- Return to this situation after you have read the following section on deontology and ask yourself the same questions.
- How should Mary, as a student, look to a code of nursing ethics to help her understand the appropriate role she should play in this situation?

Act-Utilitarianism

Act-utilitarianism allows for different, sometimes opposing, actions in different situations. For example, although act-utilitarians probably believe that it is best to tell the truth (or keep promises, or avoid killing, and so on), they recognize that there are times when the overall consequences will be better for everyone concerned if this guideline is not followed, even if the rights of some individuals are violated (Beauchamp & Childress, 2019; Smart, 1997). Act-utilitarians recognize that tenets should be used as rough guidelines rather than as strict rules.

Rule-Utilitarianism

Rule-utilitarianism, on the other hand, suggests that people should act according to rules that tend to maximize happiness and diminish unhappiness. Rule-utilitarianism requires that people in all circumstances tell the truth, keep promises, avoid killing, and so on because the overall good is maximized by consistently following such rules. The rules are consistent and easy to learn. For example, there may be times when you wonder if deceiving a patient is acceptable. If an elderly patient involved in an automobile accident is critically injured and unstable, should you temporarily deceive him about his wife's death? A rule-utilitarian would argue that you should not deceive the patient. Even though you are afraid that this patient's health might be threatened if you tell the truth, a widespread use of deception will eventually cause more harm than good. Thus, though rule-utilitarians recognize that in some instances good might result from a particular act that violates the rules, in the end, the overall good is maximized by following strict rules in all situations.

Utilitarianism is widely used in the healthcare system. It is the basis for many policy-level decisions about the distribution of a large portion of healthcare resources and services. Utilitarianism can be especially integral to medical emergency triage decisions, such as those found in a variety of triage protocols (Aacharya et al., 2011). Governmental and institutional policymakers attempt to wisely distribute funds. Debates about funding are often in the news and include topics on a variety of public programs, such as the Affordable Care Act, Medicare, Medicaid, managed care, family planning, pediatric services, mental health, drug treatment, and others. Although these programs focus on delivering cost-effective healthcare to large numbers of people through the application of utilitarian principles, they serve specific populations and thus might use resources that could have been used by others.

One dramatic example of the need for utilitarian ethics is a mass casualty incident. A Mass Casualty Incident is defined as an event that overwhelms healthcare systems by generating a large number of casualties at one time, vastly exceeding resources and capabilities (DeNolf & Khawaji, 2021; Lomaglio et al., 2020). Types of mass casualty incidents include building collapses, train and bus collisions, earthquakes, floods, plane crashes, fires, shootings, and terrorist attacks. Indeed, COVID-19 in 2020 can be thought of as a slowly developing mass casualty event because of its overwhelming impact on healthcare systems worldwide. Hospital emergency departments and ICUs were inundated, personal protective equipment and medication were scarce, and healthcare providers were overwhelmed.

Mass casualties have occurred to diverse groups of people in every part of the world. In emergency situations such as war or natural disasters, utilitarianism may become the default method of making decisions. Consider this e-mail message from a Dallas physician who served on a disaster assistance team set up at the New Orleans airport in the days immediately following Hurricane Katrina. He writes,

Our team was the first to arrive at the airport and set up our field hospital. We watched our population grow from 30 … personnel taking care of six patients … to around 10,000 people in the first 15 hours. These people had had no food or water or security for several days and were tired, frustrated, sick, wet, and heartbroken. People were brought in by trucks, buses, ambulances, school buses, cars, and helicopters. We received patients from hospitals, schools, homes…the entire remaining population of New Orleans, funneled through our doors…. Our busiest day, we off-loaded just under 15,000 patients by air and ground. At that time, we had about 30 medical providers and 100 ancillary staff. All we could do was provide the barest amount of comfort care. We watched many, many people die. We practiced medical triage at its most basic—"black-tagging" the sickest people and culling them from the masses so that they could die in a separate area. (Vankawala, 2006, p. 65)

Hurricane Katrina is only one of many recent mass incidents that have required swift judgments about how and to whom to deliver emergency care. Mass casualties have been seen in a number of natural disasters in the recent past. Examples include the Indian Ocean earthquake and tsunami (2004), Hurricane Katrina (2005), the Haiti earthquake (2010), and the Indonesia earthquake (2018). Examples of highly publicized terrorist attacks with mass casualties in the recent past include the terrorist attacks in New York and Pennsylvania (September 11, 2001), and the Boston Marathon bombing (2013). Examples of shootings with mass casualties were those in Virginia Tech classrooms (2007); a movie theater in Aurora, Colorado (2012); Sandy Hook Elementary School in Connecticut (2012); Pulse nightclub in Orlando, Florida (2016); the Harvest music festival in Las Vegas (2017); the Highland Park, Illinois Fourth of July parade (2022); Tops supermarket in Buffalo, New York (2022); and Robb Elementary School in Uvalde, Texas (2022). After each of these mass casualty incidents, healthcare facilities were overwhelmed, and people were forced to make rapid decisions about how and to whom to distribute scarce resources.

Devastating mass casualty events lead to a need for swift action by healthcare providers in official positions, as well as those who struggle to give care at ground zero (Fig. 2.3). In each event listed above, swift life-altering decisions were made about medical care for large numbers of people. What rules can be used to guide how on-the-spot decisions are made? The Federal Emergency Response Agency of the US Department of Homeland Security publishes a guidebook to be used by agencies at

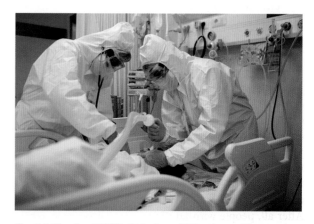

Fig. 2.3 Treating COVID-19 Patient. (©iStock.com/Tempura.)

all levels of the public and private sector (FEMA, 2017). State and local governments and the armed services have protocols in place for mass casualty incidents. So healthcare professionals should be prepared for mass casualties. The purpose of the protocols is to ensure the best outcome for the largest number of people. The first responders will ask themselves questions such as the following: Which victims can survive without immediate care? Which victims need urgent care to survive? Which victims will not survive even with immediate care? As demonstrated during Hurricane Katrina, extensive emergency care given to people with no chance of survival was predicted to expend valuable time and overwhelm scarce medical resources at the expense of those with potentially survivable injuries. According to the most widely used protocol, those who have severe injuries that are likely to be fatal without rapid intervention should be the first priority for treatment, while those with injuries so extreme that survival is impossible should be separated from other victims, intermittently reassessed, and given comfort care.

Mass casualties are the most dramatic illustrations of utilitarianism in practice. However, utilitarianism serves as the basis for the distribution of services in everyday situations. For example, whenever there is a shortfall of critical care beds, someone (likely a nurse) will use utilitarian principles to assign bed space or schedule emergency surgeries. These choices became everyday events during the height of the COVID-19 pandemic when ICU beds, ventilators, and medications were so very scarce.

Though utilitarianism is widely accepted, there are a few problems inherent in its use. Utilitarianism does not give sufficient thought to respect of persons. In fact, it is possible that harm can be done to minority groups or individuals in the name of the overall good. For example, most countries have rather strict criteria to determine who is eligible to receive a heart transplant. The number of patients with failing hearts far exceeds the number of donor organs, so someone must decide which candidates have the best chance of a good outcome. Utilitarianism gives little recognition to the principle of autonomy, particularly when we consider utilitarian decision making relative to distributive justice, the ethical principle that relates to fair, equitable, and appropriate distribution of goods and services. After all, people with failing hearts cannot have donor hearts simply because they want them. They must meet the standardized criteria. Critics of utilitarianism argue that these types of decisions sacrifice the rights of individuals in favor of the overall good.

ASK YOURSELF

Is Utilitarianism Useful?
- What useful guidelines does utilitarianism provide in terms of distributing resources?
- To what degree is it permissible to sacrifice the rights of one to provide for the welfare of many?
- Is it ever permissible to sacrifice the rights of many to provide resources for one person?
- What examples of utilitarianism in healthcare have you noticed in the recent past?

Even though there are problems inherent in utilitarianism, this ethical theory captures the imagination as an attractive moral philosophy. Its appeal lies in the simple precept of promoting benefits to as many people as possible. It is particularly useful as a method of deciding issues of distributive justice.

Deontology

Deontological theories of ethics are based on the rationalist view that the rightness or wrongness of an act depends on the nature of the act, rather than its consequences. The term **deontology** is taken from the Greek word for duty. Occasionally, deontology is called **formalism**; some writers refer to this type of ethical theory as **Kantianism**. Deontology is based on the writings of the German philosopher Immanuel Kant, who shaped many deontological formulations. The terms **deontology** and *Kantian ethics, and formalism* are often used interchangeably.

Kant was born in Königsberg, Prussia, in 1724. After an uninspiring academic career, he surprised the world with his groundbreaking ethical theory. Late in his life, Kant published volumes of philosophical writings that shook the religious and political systems of his day and continue to have a strong influence on contemporary ethical philosophy. Kant proposed that ethical rules are universal and that humans can derive certain consistent principles to guide action. As Socrates suggested centuries earlier, Kant believed that awareness of moral rules is the product of pure reason, rather than experience, as the naturalists would maintain. Kant asserted that moral rules are absolute and apply to all people, at all times, in all situations. He believed that ethical rules could be known by rational humans. Knowledge of the right course of action in any given situation could be gained by following a maxim that he called the **categorical imperative**. *Categorical* refers to moral rules that have no exceptions; *imperative* denotes a command that is derived from principle. Kant said there is only one categorical imperative:

> *Act only according to that maxim by which you can at the same time will that it should become a universal law.* (Kant, 1785/1959, p. 39)

In other words, if an action is morally right, it can reasonably be imagined to be a strict universal law. As an example, Kant related a moral problem in which a man needs to borrow money to feed his family. He knows that he will not be able to repay it but knows that he will not receive the loan if he does not promise to repay it at a certain time. To satisfy himself that the act of making a false promise to repay the money is morally correct, the man asks himself the question, "Should every person always make promises that they know will not be fulfilled?" Reasoning it through, the man can see that this could not become a universal law, because no one would ever believe what has been promised. Consequently, promise making would hold no meaning. On the other hand, truth telling could be a universal law. Kant gave similar examples of situations related to suicide, squandering of talent, and helping others. Rather than compile a list of specific ethical rules, Kant proposed that each rational person should use the test of the categorical imperative to guide his or her actions.

Following the categorical imperative, Kant also described the **practical imperative**:

> *Act so that you treat humanity, whether in your own person or that of another, always as an end and never as a means only (1785/1959, p. 47).*

To treat another person as an "end," according to Kant, is to make his or her ends your own and to act toward his or her goals as you naturally do toward your own. For example, if a patient's goal is to get well, that should also be the nurse's goal. The nurse should not use this patient simply as a means to a paycheck (a means to an end). Raphael (1994) makes the point that Kant's practical imperative automatically shows that domination of one person over another is morally wrong.

Domination makes no allowance for the dominated person's power of decision-making. He also notes that acting toward another as you would toward yourself mandates that, whenever possible, you must help people who need help. The practical imperative requires that we must fulfill certain duties owed to others.

When the categorical imperative and the practical imperative are merged, there is a strong implication that each person is a member of a *realm of ends*—a politically organized society. Kant calls this "a systematic union of rational beings through common objective laws" (1785/1959, p. 51). This requires that we should act as members of a community of equal and autonomous individuals and that each member should treat all others as moral beings. Each person should have regard for the desires of others and allow them the freedom to make decisions about themselves. In Kantian theory, there is an inherent recognition that all people are equal and equally competent to make universally legislative decisions. Kantian ethics is an ethics of democracy because it requires "liberty, equality, and fraternity" within a politically organized society (Raphael, 1994, p. 57).

Deontology also implies that ethics are derived from fulfilling duties. One must act for the sake of duty or obligation. Kant believed that all *imperatives of duty* can be deduced from his categorical imperative (one should act as if one's actions could become universal law for all people) and must also comply with his practical imperative (treat all people as ends, none as means to an end). He also believed that an action done from duty has its moral worth based on reverence for the law and for doing one's duty, rather than the results or outcomes of the act (Kant, 1785/1959).

Most professional codes of ethics are based on Kant's principles. Nurses' codes of ethics stress both the importance of fulfilling duties that are inherently owed to patients and the importance of preserving the dignity and autonomy of each individual patient. For example, the 2015 ANA Code of Ethics for Nurses notes that "Nurses establish relationships of trust and provide nursing services according to need, setting aside any bias or prejudice. Factors such as culture, value systems, religious or spiritual beliefs, lifestyle, social support system, sexual orientation or gender expression, and primary language are to be considered when planning individual, family, and population-centered care" (ANA, 2015, p. 1). This statement presumes that the nurse has a duty to respect and care for the patient in terms of the patient's unique qualities, needs, and values. It illustrates the principles of respect for person, beneficence, and autonomy, which are covered in detail in Chapter 3. These principles are so pervasive in the profession that they often go unnoticed. When you maintain confidentiality, when you advocate for a patient, when you keep promises, when you tell the truth, and when you practice with skill, you are utilizing deontic principles.

The practical application of deontological ethics carries with it some acknowledged problems. Deontology allows for no exceptions—it is rigid. It does not assist us in choosing among conflicting alternatives or principles and, in fact, may present a conflict between two equally compelling duties. In addition, disregarding the consequences of any given action can occasionally lead to disastrous results when the needs of an individual are given higher consideration than the needs of a larger group.

Like utilitarianism, deontology is an attractive ethical theory. It is, in fact, a most popular foundation for many contemporary beliefs. It provides clear guidelines for judging the rightness or wrongness of action. It recognizes the dignity and autonomy of individuals and allows all people equal consideration. It serves as a basis for much of the contemporary ethical thinking that guides healthcare delivery and influences nursing codes of ethics.

CASE PRESENTATION

Weighing Rights and Duties in Questions of Justice
Rina is the home health nurse for Mrs. B., an 89-year-old widow who lives in the home that she and her husband shared until his death five years earlier. Mrs. B. suffers from severe rheumatoid arthritis and has a new colostomy. The colostomy was performed as a last resort for severe ulcerative colitis. Mrs. B. is unable to care for herself because of the advanced state of her arthritis. Mrs. B. does not have dementia. Her daughter, son-in-law, and two teenage grandchildren moved into her home to take care of her daily needs. After many months, the family expresses to Rina that caring for Mrs. B. has become an untenable burden. They ask her to help them arrange long-term care in a local nursing home. Overhearing the conversation, Mrs. B. expresses to Rina that she wants to continue to live in her home at any price.

Think About It
Whose Rights Are More Important?
- Does Mrs. B. have the right to stay in her home, even if the entire family is made unhappy by her presence?

- According to Kantian ethics, what factors must the family consider in deciding?
- Kantian ethics is duty oriented. Assuming that a Kantian basis for ethical decision making is used, to whom does Rina owe a duty?
- To what degree should the rights of the other family members bear on the decision that Rina makes?
- How do nursing codes of ethics offer Rina guidance as she responds to this situation?
- Apply the categorical imperative to Rina's decision.
- Whose decision is this to make? Why?
- What would you do if you were Rina? On what basis would you make your decision?
- How might cultural factors influence decisions in this situation?
- How will nursing codes of ethics from the ANA (Provisions 1 and 2), ICN (Elements 1.1 and 2.7), and CNA (Parts I.B.1 and I.B.3) help Rina to clarify her responsibility?

Virtue Ethics

Virtue ethics, sometimes called **character ethics**, represents the idea that individuals' actions are based on a certain degree of innate moral virtue. First noted in the writings of Plato, Aristotle, and early Christian philosophers, there has been a contemporary resurgence of interest in virtue ethics. Relying on Aristotle's *Nicomachean Ethics* (ca. 350 B.C.E./2000) and more recent philosophy, Löfquist (2017) identified four notions associated with virtue ethics: (1) one should act in a way that a virtuous person would act, (2) virtues are part of a good life, (3) virtues must be developed over time, and (4) virtues do not provide simple answers to morally difficult situations. Beauchamp and Childress (2019) add that the person must also desire and be motivated and to act in a virtuous manner. Western moralism emerged with the idea of the cardinal virtues of wisdom, courage, temperance, justice, generosity, faith, hope, and charity (Kitwood, 1990). Modern and contemporary writers also include such virtues as honesty, compassion, caring, responsibility, integrity, discernment, trustworthiness, and prudence. Though nearly absent in nursing ethics texts at the end of the 20th century, virtue ethics is reemerging in the 21st century as an important framework for examining moral behavior.

The concept of virtue ethics presents a challenge to deontological and utilitarian theories. Deontology and utilitarianism conceive of the demands of morality similarly; ethics provides guidelines that seek the morally correct solution. In contrast, virtue ethics posits that morality rests on the character of persons. Beauchamp and Childress (2019) define virtue as a character trait that is valuable to society and reliably present in the individual. There are no principles or rules to follow in virtue ethics. Rather it is thought that the virtuous person will naturally choose the morally correct action. For example, the reason you should not lie is not because it is against the moral law, nor because it will not maximize well-being, but rather because you know that it is *dishonest* (Crisp & Slote, 1997). Beauchamp (2001) suggests that virtue should not be thought of as a moral requirement, because this confuses it with a principle or rule. Rather we could say that a *moral* virtue is a character trait, such as truthfulness, kindness, or honesty, that is morally valued. A person with moral virtue has both morally appropriate desire and consistent moral action.

Plato and Aristotle were the first Western philosophers to write about virtue ethics. Both believed that human well-being is the highest aim of morality and that virtues are necessary character traits for the good person. In fact, the term *ethics* was derived from Aristotle's word *ethika*, which refers to matters having to do with character. Aristotle (384–332 B.C.E.) considered goodness of character to be produced by the practice of virtuous behavior, rather than virtuous acts being the end result of a good character. According to Aristotle, virtues are tendencies to act, feel, and judge that are developed from a natural capacity by proper training and exercise. He believed that practice creates a habit of acting in a virtuous way and that virtue can be learned and improved. Virtue, according to Aristotle, is equal to excellence of character and depends on motivation, deliberation, clear judgment, self-control, and practice (ca. 350 B.C.E./2000). He considered virtue to be the fruit of intelligent pursuit—the achievement of wise and mature experience in the fully developed person. Aristotle believed that virtue could

only be achieved by training and habituation—thus, a virtuous character is created by repeatedly acting in a virtuous manner. Aristotle's traits of a virtuous character provided three criteria:

1. Virtuous acts must be chosen for their own sake.
2. Choice must proceed from a firm and unchangeable character.
3. Virtue is a disposition to choose the mean.

The *golden mean* of virtuous behavior, for Aristotle, meant practicing moderation: avoiding both excess and deficiency. For example, Aristotle conceived of courage as the golden mean between cowardice and foolhardiness and generosity as the golden mean between stinginess and extravagance. Aristotle did not list a number of moral principles. For him, the basic moral question is not "what should one do," but rather "what should one be" (Aristotle, ca. 350 B.C.E./2000). Interestingly, the Dalai Lama (1999) agrees with Aristotle's philosophy on virtue and further states that wisdom is the only virtue that is always good—never requiring moderation.

Phillipa Foot, one of the founders of contemporary virtue ethics, added another perspective to Aristotle's concept of a virtuous person. Foot proposed that virtue lies not only in engaging in virtuous acts but also in will. She defined will as "that which is wished for as well as what is sought." According to Foot, a positive or moral will is sometimes the necessary ingredient for success. She wrote,

> Sometimes one man succeeds where another fails not because there is some specific difference in their previous conduct but rather because his heart lies in a different place; and the disposition of the heart is part of virtue. ... What this suggests is that a man's virtue may be judged by his innermost desires as well as by his intentions and this fits with our idea that a virtue such as generosity lies as much in someone's attitudes as in his actions. (Foot, 2002, p. 4)

According to Foot, virtue is not like a skill or an art. It cannot merely be a practiced and perfected act. It must actually engage the will. In other words, an act, for example, although apparently kind or generous, cannot be considered virtuous if the intention is not good. Although Aristotle's idea of virtue is one of hope (everyone has the capacity to learn virtuous action), Foot makes the road to virtuous character less easily traveled.

Focal Virtues

Discussing virtue, Beauchamp and Childress (2019) define character as being made up of a set of stable traits that affect a person's judgment and action. Like Aristotle, Beauchamp and Childress suggest that although people have different character traits, all have the capacity to learn or cultivate those that are important to morality. They propose that five focal virtues are more pivotal than others in characterizing a virtuous person: compassion, discernment, trustworthiness, integrity, and conscientiousness.

Compassion. **Compassion** is the ability to imagine oneself in the situation of another. Beauchamp and Childress (2019) define the term *compassion* as a trait combining an attitude of active regard for another's welfare with an awareness and emotional response of deep sympathy and discomfort at the other person's suffering. This virtue embodies the Golden Rule. Compassion is so important that many times the patient's need for a compassionate and caring presence outweighs the need for technical care. We must be careful, however, that compassion does not impede our ability to make objective decisions.

Discernment. The virtue of **discernment** is related to the classical concept of wisdom. Discernment rests on sensitive insight involving acute judgment and understanding, and it results in decisive action (Beauchamp & Childress, 2019). Discernment gives us insight into appropriate actions in given situations. It requires sensitivity and attention attuned to the demands of a particular context. For example, a discerning nurse will recognize when a patient needs comfort and reassurance rather than privacy. Discernment requires that one continually strives to recognize and understand important nuances in human behavior.

Trustworthiness. **Trustworthiness** is another focal virtue for nurses. Trust is a confident belief in the moral character of another person. Trust entails confidence that another will act with the right motives consistent with moral norms (Beauchamp & Childress, 2019). Trustworthiness is measured by others' recognition of the nurse's consistency and predictability in following moral norms. In practical terms, trustworthiness is accounted for in the reputation we have among coworkers. This virtue is important for us in our relationships with patients, physicians, and other nurses.

Integrity. **Integrity** is perhaps the cardinal virtue. **Moral integrity**, according to Beauchamp and Childress (2019), means soundness, reliability, wholeness, and an integration of moral character. It also refers to our continuing to follow moral norms over time. Beauchamp and Childress describe integrity as the character trait of a rational and stable integration of moral values coupled with judgments and actions that are consistently faithful to those values. A person with integrity has a consistency of convictions, actions, and emotions and is trustworthy. Integrity is compromised when the nurse acts inconsistently or in a way that is not supported by professed moral beliefs. Deficiencies in moral integrity may include such vices as hypocrisy, insincerity, and bad faith.

Conscientiousness. Many people think of **conscientiousness** simply as a person's tendency to do a job well, but the virtue of conscientiousness is closely related to questions of morality. The term *conscientious* is derived from *conscience*. Conscience involves an awareness of morality or of what is considered right, fair, and just. It includes self-reflection and judgment about whether an act is required or prohibited, right or wrong, good or bad. Conscientiousness, then, is an internal acknowledgment or of one's motives and actions and a sense of right and wrong, particularly as related to things for which one is responsible. It includes an ability to judge the moral quality of one's motives and actions. Beauchamp and Childress (2019) propose that a person is conscientious if he or she is motivated to do what is right, has thought rationally and diligently about the action, intends to do what is right, and exerts effort to do so. As you will learn in Chapter 17, nurses are sometimes presented with situations in which their conscience conflicts with some role obligation or official order from an authority. In such cases the nurse may be able to refuse the activity through professionally accepted means but should not obstruct others from performing the act.

Virtue Ethics in Nursing

How does the concept of virtue or character ethics fit with nursing as a principled profession? It is likely that principled behavior, although not the sole domain of a good moral character, is more likely to occur in the presence of one. Certainly, Florence Nightingale thought virtue was an important trait of the good nurse. Nightingale learned Greek as a child. She was inspired by

Plato and translated parts of *Phaedo, Crito*, and *Apology*. Nightingale was intrigued by Plato's description of elite people with rare gifts who command many kinds of knowledge. The characteristics, or virtues, of these people, resonated with Nightingale and were reflected in her writings throughout her life (Dossey, 2010). She believed that one of the aims of philosophy was to cultivate in gifted people their potential intellectual and moral qualities.

The Nightingale Pledge, composed by Lystra Gretter In 1893 and traditionally recited by graduating nurses, implies virtue of character as nurses promise purity, faith, loyalty, devotion, trustworthiness, and temperance. It is reasonable to say that good character is the cornerstone of good nursing and that the nurse with virtue will act according to principle. If Aristotle was correct in his belief that virtue can be practiced and learned, then we can learn, through practice, those acts that, by their doing, create a virtuous person.

Moral Particularism

Moral particularism utilizes the principles and rules of different moral theories. It is a form of moral theory that embraces the uniqueness of cases, the culturally significant ethical features, and ethical judgment in each particular case (O'Neill, 2001). The moral particularist enters a situation fully aware of the ethical principles and maxims of the profession and appreciates them as illuminators of moral problems (Fletcher, 1966). Particularism would recognize the principles of utilitarianism and deontology, for example, but would view them as generalizations, rather than rules.

Most moral theories are not sensitive to the particulars of each case such as the context, situations, relationships, and individuals. Moral particularists claim that this failure represents a fundamental flaw in these theories. Even in the face of generally accepted moral theory, health professionals' moral decisions are shaped by the practical circumstances of their work (Anspach, 1987). This may be especially true for nurses.

Little (2001) suggests that theory is essential to the moral life. Generalizations are useful for teaching and justifying, for understanding the "why." Moral particularism recognizes the need for rules that allow for exceptions in terms of what Aristotle might have meant when he called for "for the most part" generalizations. Little calls these *defeasible* generalizations—ones that are useful, yet capable of being annulled or invalidated

in certain situations. Exceptions to these generalizations occur only in situations that deviate from the norm. Following Aristotle's lead, the moral particularist can make explicit what types of actions have a moral nature, as well as what sort of conceptual priority, centrality, or evaluative privilege is relevant in particular situations. Because every situation contains unique elements, most of the moral generalizations we make in everyday life turn out to be irreducibly porous, "shot through" with inevitable exceptions. Nevertheless, these generalizations are explanatory and insightful in that they situate particular cases within a framework (Little, 2001).

O'Neill (2001) suggests that there are bona fide practical ethical principles that do not require uniform action; rather, they are indeterminate—constraining but not regimenting action. They are more likely to recommend *types* of action rather than offer detailed instructions for living. The extent of uniformity or differentiation to be stipulated in particular aspects of life is a matter of practical reasoning and judgment—what Aristotle would call *deliberation*. Sensitivity to particulars may originate in perception, intuition, or practical judgment. Because of its sensitivity to the uniqueness of each situation, moral particularism cannot be prescriptive. It must rely on certain relevant principles, such as those of utilitarianism and deontology, for the starting point of judgment. Always difficult and often not wholly successful, practical judgment is a matter of finding some act that adequately meets many requirements (O'Neill, 2001).

ASK YOURSELF

Are You a Moral Particularist?

Moral particularism is seldom discussed but often used. You will see it practiced every day. In the next chapter, you will learn more about ethical principles. One of the principles is autonomy, the principle that demands that we respect people's right to freely make decisions about themselves. Another principle is beneficence, which requires us to "do good." In some situations, autonomy and beneficence conflict. A moral particularist will suggest that the "particulars" should determine to what degree we follow these principles. Think about the principles of autonomy and beneficence in the following situations. If you cannot uphold both principles, you might be a moral particularist.

- An 84-year-old patient with Alzheimer disease was admitted to the hospital yesterday with left lower lobe pneumonia. He is on oxygen and intravenous

(IV) antibiotics. He telephones the taxi company for a ride home.

- A 68-year-old hospitalized patient with atrial fibrillation has become dramatically symptomatic with fluid retention, fatigue, and dyspnea. When asked about her medication history, she says, "I have been taking hydroxychloroquine that my husband got at the barber shop. I have a right to get it there and I have a right to take it!" Hydroxychloroquine is known to cause atrial fibrillation, elongated QT interval, and fatal atrial tachycardia.
- A 20-year-old woman who is 20 weeks pregnant is admitted to the emergency room after an auto accident. Her liver and spleen are ruptured, and she is hemorrhaging. Her blood pressure is 70/30 mm Hg. The fetus is alive but will be nonviable outside the uterus. Fetal demise is certain if the mother continues to hemorrhage. The woman whispers, "I am a Jehovah's Witness. Do not give me any blood products."

Nurses cannot function properly if they do not know something about their patients. Nurses' relationships with patients include closeness, touch, and proximity (Fig. 2.4). Criticisms of formal or "formula" ethics include distinctions of "distant" versus "close-up" ethics. Abstract ethical principles and rules are emphasized in distant ethics, whereas close-up ethics attends to the primacy of human relationships and recognizes the importance of feelings, values, and individual and family conscience (Penticuff, 1991).

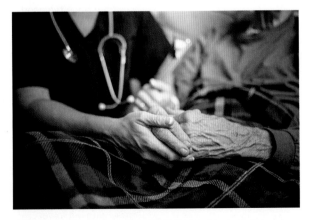

Fig. 2.4 Nurses' Relationships With Patients Include Closeness, Touch, and Proximity. (©iStock.com/LPETTET.)

Nursing's views of what it means to do good for patients accumulate through recognition of the particulars in nurses' stories about caring for patients up close as they experience illness, recovery, and death. Nurses attend to the concrete details of everyday experience. Nurses' perspectives on doing what is good for the patient originate from the unique viewpoints of the nurse and patient within arm's length of each other (Penticuff, 1997). This arm's-length type of relationship is necessary because human touch and close scrutiny of patients' responses are integral to nursing care. According to Donchin (2001), within this relationship, the nurse and patient share a common goal unique to the circumstances and choices of the patient, recognizing that the individual cannot be abstracted from an "entwinement in particulars." The close-up nature of nursing sets the stage for a special type of relationship based on intimacy. Intimacy begins when the patient reveals feelings and information to the nurse. If the nurse listens supportively, the patient feels understood, validated, and cared for (Kirk, 2007). Thus, the nurse's simple act of listening while near creates an opportunity for doing good within a moral particularist framework.

SUMMARY

Ethical theory helps us understand the origin and process of ethical and moral thinking and behavior. Two important theories are particularly important to nursing ethics. The ethical theory of utilitarianism was developed in part by Jeremy Bentham and later refined by John Stuart Mill. Utilitarianism suggests that ethical decisions should be based on the anticipated outcome or end result. Accordingly, no action is inherently right or wrong. This theory also provides for the greatest good for the greatest number. Utilitarianism is particularly useful in situations of distributive justice but tends to ignore the rights of the minority or the individual.

Deontology, or Kantian ethics, was initially developed by Immanuel Kant. This theory, revolving around the categorical imperative, assists one in making ethical decisions. The categorical imperative demands that the person ask the question, "Can this action be a law for all people in all circumstances?" Additionally, the theory presents the practical imperative, which requires that we treat all individuals as if they were ends only, rather than means. Kantian ethics provides clear guidelines for making ethical decisions but does not provide for making decisions when duties or obligations conflict.

Virtue, or character, ethics, as described by Aristotle, depicts each person as capable of practicing and learning virtue through the repetition of virtuous acts. Thus, the virtuous person is one in whom virtue becomes a habit. Virtue ethics complements other ethical theories and can be used to nurture or predict character in individuals. Ethical theories can help us understand ethical decision-making models and assist in developing a cohesive and logical system for making individual decisions.

Particularism utilizes the principles and rules of other moral theories. It is a form of moral theory that embraces the uniqueness of cases, their culturally significant ethical features, and ethical judgment in each particular case. Because of its sensitivity to the uniqueness of each situation, moral particularism cannot be prescriptive. It must rely on certain relevant principles, such as those of utilitarianism and deontology, for the starting point of judgment.

CHAPTER HIGHLIGHTS

- Philosophy is the intense and critical examination of beliefs and assumptions.
- Moral philosophy is the philosophical discussion of what is considered good or bad, right or wrong, just or unjust.
- Ethics is the product of a formal process for making logical and consistent decisions based on moral philosophy.
- Ethical theories explain values and behavior related to the cultural and moral norms.
- As the morally central healthcare profession, nursing requires astuteness in moral and ethical issues.
- Utilitarianism holds that the right action is that which has the greatest utility or usefulness and that no action is in itself either good or bad.
- Deontology is based on the rationalist view that the rightness or wrongness of an act depends on the nature of the act, rather than its consequences.
- Kantianism is a particular deontological theory developed by Immanuel Kant.
- The categorical imperative is the Kantian maxim requiring that no action can be judged as a right that cannot reasonably become a law by which every person should always abide.

- The practical imperative is the Kantian maxim requiring that one always treat others as ends and never as a means.
- Virtue ethics, usually attributed to Aristotle, represents the idea that individuals' actions are based on innate moral virtue.
- Moral particularism takes into account the unique aspects of each case and utilizes appropriate generalizable moral principles from different moral theories.
- Nursing codes of ethics offer guidelines for action with many complex moral issues.

DISCUSSION QUESTIONS AND ACTIVITIES

1. Read either the ANA *Code of Ethics for Nurses with Interpretive Statements*, the ICN *Code of Ethics for Nurses*, or the *Canadian Code of Ethics for Registered Nurses* (whichever is most appropriate for your situation) and discuss how the various statements in the codes relate to each of the principles discussed in this chapter.
2. Go to the Kennedy Institute of Ethics Bioethics Library website. Do a literature search for recent articles on ethical theory. Report your findings to the class.
3. Describe the differences in naturalist and rationalist beliefs about the origin of ethical rules.
4. Describe a hypothetical situation in which an ethical dilemma exists and discuss solutions to the dilemma in terms of act-utilitarianism and rule-utilitarianism.
5. Identify specific healthcare funding policies and discuss them in terms of utilitarian theory.
6. Discuss how Kantian or deontological ethics apply to codes of nursing ethics (ANA, ICN, or CNA, whichever is more appropriate for your situation).
7. Describe a real or hypothetical situation in which there is an ethical dilemma. Use the rule of the categorical imperative to solve the dilemma.
8. List and describe the virtues that you feel are important for nurses.
9. Consider the following situation: Two nursing students are discovered to have collaboratively cheated on several assignments. After being questioned by the instructor, both students deny having cheated, even though the evidence is irrefutable. Discuss these students in terms of virtue ethics and Kantian ethics. Do these students have integrity? Do these students have the character to become good nurses? How would you apply the categorical imperative?

REFERENCES

Aacharya, R. P., Gastmans, C., & Denier, Y. (2011). Emergency department triage: An ethical analysis. *BMC Emergency Medicine, 11*(1), 16. https://doi.org/10.1186/1471-227x-11-16.

Aiken, H. D. (1952). The levels of moral discourse. *Ethics, 62,* 235–248.

ANA. (2015). *Code of ethics for nurses with interpretive statements*. http://nursingworld.org/DocumentVault/Ethics-1/Code-of-Ethics-for-Nurses.html

Anspach, R. R. (1987). Prognostic conflict in life-and-death decisions: The organization as an ecology of knowledge. *Journal of Health and Human Behavior, 28,* 215–231.

Aristotle. (2000). *Nicomachean ethics* (R. Crisp, Trans.). Cambridge University Press (Original work published ca. 350 B.C.E.).

Beauchamp, T. L. (2001). *Philosophical ethics: An introduction to moral philosophy* (3rd ed.). McGraw Hill.

Beauchamp, T. L., & Childress, J. (2019). *Principles of biomedical ethics* (8th ed.). Oxford University Press.

Bentham, J. (1948). *An introduction to the principles of moral legislation*. Hafner Press.

Boddice, R. (2016). *The science of sympathy: Morality, evolution, and Victorian civilization*. University of Illinois Press.

Buber, M. (1965). *The knowledge of man: A philosophy of the interhuman*. Harper & Row.

Bullock, M., & Panicker, S. (2003). Ethics for all: Differences across scientific society codes. *Science and Engineering Ethics, 9*(2), 159–170. https://www.ncbi.nlm.nih.gov/pubmed/12774648.

Bykvist, K. (2010). *Utilitarianism: A guide for the perplexed*. Continuum International.

Crisp, R., & Slote, M. (Eds.). (1997). *Oxford readings in philosophy*. Oxford University Press.

Dalai Lama. (1999). *Ethics for the new millennium*. Riverhead.

Dengrove Collection. (n.d.). Karen Ann Quinlan and the right to die. UVA Law Special Collections. https://archives.law.virginia.edu/dengrove/writeup/karen-ann-quinlan-and-right-die

DeNolf, R. L., & Khawaji, C. I. (2021) EMS mass casualty management. In: StatPearls. https://www.ncbi.nlm.nih.gov/books/NBK482373/

Donchin, A. (2001). Understanding autonomy relationally: Toward a reconfiguration of bioethical principles. *Journal of Medicine and Philosophy, 26*(4), 365–386.

Dossey, B. M. (2010). *Florence Nightingale: Mystic, visionary, healer* (Commemorative ed.). F.A. Davis.

FEMA. (2017). *National incident reporting system*. Washington, DC. Retrieved from https://www.fema.gov/emergency-managers/nims

Fletcher, J. (1966). *Situation ethics: The new morality*. Westminster Press.

Foot, P. (2002). *Virtues and vices and other essays in moral philosophy*. Oxford Scholarship Online. https://doi.org/10.1093/0199252866.001.0001.

Goldman, A. (2019). Moral epistemology and professional codes of ethics In A. Zimmerman, K. Jones, & M. Timmons (Eds.), *The Routledge handbook of moral epistemology*. Routledge.

Hesse, H. (1971). *Siddhartha*. Bantham.

Hume, D. (1738). *A treatise of human nature*. Clarendon Press.

Jameton, A. (1984). *Nursing practice: The ethical issues*. Prentice-Hall.

Jinbin, P. (2017). Historical origins of the Tuskegee experiment: The dilemma of public health in the United States. *Uisahak, 26,* 545–578. https://doi.org/10.13081/kjmh.2017.26.545.

Kant, I. (1959). *The moral law: Foundations of the metaphysics of morals* (L. W. Beck, Trans.). Bobbs-Merrill (Original work published 1785).

Kirk, T. W. (2007). Beyond empathy: Clinical intimacy in nursing practice. *Nursing Philosophy, 8*(4), 233.

Kitwood, T. (1990). *Concern for others: A new psychology of conscience and morality*. Routledge.

Little, M. O. (2001). On knowing the "why": Particularism and moral theory. *The Hastings Center Report, 31*(4), 32–40.

Löfquist, L. (2017). Virtues and humanitarian ethics. *Disasters, 41*(1), 41–54. https://doi.org/10.1111/disa.12191.

Lomaglio, L., Ansaloni, L., Catena, F., Sartelli, M., & Coccolini, F. (2020). *Mass casualty inident: Definitions and current reality*. Springer.

Mill, J. S. (2011). *Utilitarianism*. Andrews UK Limited. (Original work published 1910).

O'Neill, O. (2001). Practical principles and practical judgment. *The Hastings Center Report, 31*(4), 15–24.

Penticuff, J. H. (1991). Conceptual issues in nursing ethics research. *Journal of Medicine and Philosophy, 16*(3), 235–258. http://www.ncbi.nlm.nih.gov/entrez/query.fcgi?cmd=Retrieve&db=PubMed&dopt=Citation&list_uids=1880464.

Penticuff, J. H. (1997). Nursing perspectives in bioethics In K. Hoshino (Ed.), *Japanese and Western Bioethics* (pp. 49–60). Khower Academic Publishers.

Pipes, R. B., Holstein, J. E., & Aguirre, M. G. (2005). Examining the personal-professional distinction: Ethics codes and the difficulty of drawing a boundary. *American Psychologist Journal, 60*(4), 325–334. https://doi.org/10.1037/0003-066X.60.4.325.

Rand, A. (1982). *Philosophy: Who needs it*. Bobbs-Merrill.

Raphael, D. D. (1994). *Moral philosophy* (2nd ed.). Oxford University Press.

Shook, J. (2010). *The naturalistic approach to mortality.* Center for Inquiry. https://centerforinquiry.org/blog/the_naturalistic_approach_to_morality/

Smart, J. J. C. (1997). Utilitarianism In C. Sommers & F. Sommers (Eds.), *Vice and virtue in everyday life: Introductory readings in ethics* (pp. 110–123). Cambridge University Press.

Vankawala, H. (2006). A doctor's message from Katrina's front lines. *Baylor University Medical Center Proceedings, 19*(1), 65–66. https://doi.org/10.1080/08998280.2006.11928130.

Veatch, R. M., & Guidry-Grimes, L. K. (2020). *The basics of bioethics* (4th ed.). Routledge.

3

Ethical Principles

The quality of mercy is not strain'd
It droppeth as the gentle rain from heaven
Upon the place beneath. It is twice blest:
It blesseth him that gives, and him that takes.
(William Shakespeare, The Merchant of Venice)

OBJECTIVES

After completing this chapter, the reader should be able to:

1. Discuss the principle of respect for autonomy in terms of patients' rights, informed consent, advocacy, and noncompliance.
2. Discuss the principle of beneficence as it relates to nursing practice.
3. Define the principle of nonmaleficence, and weigh actions in terms of harm and benefit.
4. Relate the principle of veracity to nursing practice.
5. Examine the principle of confidentiality in nursing practice, recognizing legal implications and reasonable limits to confidentiality.
6. Discuss the principle of justice as it relates to the distribution of healthcare goods and services.
7. Relate the principle of fidelity to nursing's promise to society.
8. Discuss situations in which there is a conflict between two or more ethical principles.
9. Discuss the relationship between ethical principles and codes of nursing ethics.

INTRODUCTION

The most common means of approaching ethical problems is through careful examination in light of established ethical principles. Ethical principles are basic and obvious moral truths that guide deliberation and action (Box 3.1). Major ethical theories utilize many of the same principles, though the emphasis or meaning may be somewhat different in each. For example, respect for autonomy is a dominant principle in deontological theory but is less important in utilitarian theory. To make consistently appropriate decisions, nurses must understand ethical principles and be adept at applying them in a meaningful and consistent manner. Attention to principles is an essential foundation of ethical practice in nursing, even though principles sometimes conflict, and none are absolute. This chapter examines the following fundamental ethical principles: respect for autonomy, beneficence, nonmaleficence, veracity, confidentiality, justice, and fidelity.

Respect for Persons

All principles discussed in this chapter presuppose that nurses have respect for the value and uniqueness of persons. Occasionally viewed as an ethical principle in its own right, respect for persons implies that one considers others to be worthy of high regard. Genuine regard and respect for others is the moving force behind all caring professions. All Western codes of nursing ethics explicitly state that respect for persons is a cornerstone of

---

BOX 3.1   Ethical Principles at a Glance

Respect for Autonomy: Respect for autonomy denotes honoring people's freedom to make choices about issues that affect their lives, free from lies, restraint, or coercion.

Beneficence: The principle of beneficence means to do good. It requires nurses to act in ways that benefit patients. Beneficence includes doing good, preventing harm, and removing evil or harm.

Nonmaleficence: Nonmaleficence directs one to avoid causing harm, including deliberate harm, risk of harm, and harm that occurs during the performance of beneficial acts.

Veracity: The ethical principle of veracity means telling the truth.

Confidentiality: The ethical principle of confidentiality demands that one not disclose private, sensitive, or secret information.

Justice: Justice is the ethical principle that relates to fair, equitable, and appropriate treatment in light of what is due or owed to persons, recognizing that giving resources to some people will mean that others will not receive them.

Fidelity: The ethical principle of fidelity relates to the concept of faithfulness and the practice of keeping promises.

---

professional ethics. Discussion of the ethical principles in this chapter is based on the belief that nurses value the principle of respect for persons.

RESPECT FOR AUTONOMY

As you would expect, the ethical principle of **respect for autonomy** denotes an obligation to honor the autonomy of other persons. The word "autonomy" literally means self-governing and is sometimes called *the right to self-determination*. Autonomy denotes having the freedom to make choices about issues that affect one's life, free from lies, restraint, or coercion. Respect for autonomy is closely linked to the notion of respect for persons and is an important principle in cultures where all individuals are considered unique and valuable members of society.

Three basic elements are implied in the concept of autonomy. First, the autonomous person must be able to determine personal goals. These goals may be explicit and of a global nature or may be less well defined. For example, the patient with an ankle injury may have a goal to return to athletic play within two weeks of the

injury or may simply wish to be pain free. In either case, the patient develops personally chosen goals consistent with a particular lifestyle. Second, the autonomous person has the capacity to decide on a plan of action. The person must be able to understand the meaning of the choices and deliberate on the various options, while understanding the implications of possible outcomes. Imagine, for example, ordering from a restaurant menu written in a language you do not understand. You have the freedom and responsibility to make a choice but cannot make a meaningful choice without understanding the language. When we believe that a patient is not able to comprehend the meaning of choices, goals, or outcomes, we say that the person is incompetent to make decisions or lacks decision-making capacity. Certain groups of patients are generally thought of as unable to make informed choices. Children, fetuses, and those with mental impairments are among these groups. Third, the autonomous person has the freedom to act on the ultimate choice. In situations where persons are capable of formulating goals, understanding various options, and making decisions, yet are not free to implement their plans, autonomy is either limited or absent. Autonomy may also be limited in situations where the means to accomplish autonomously devised plans do not exist. An example is seen in the case of the indigent person who has no healthcare insurance. This person may choose to have, for example, a pancreas transplant in lieu of insulin injections but has no financial means to meet this goal. To ensure autonomy, each of the four elements must be present to a reasonable degree.

The American Nurses Association (ANA) *Code of Ethics for Nurses* strongly supports patients' right to self-determination. The ANA declares that autonomy is a fundamental right that must be respected by nurses as follows:

Patients have the moral and legal right to determine what will be done with and to their own person: to be given accurate, complete, and understandable information in a manner that facilitates an informed decision; and to be assisted with weighing the benefits, burdens, and available options in their treatment, including the choice of no treatment. They also have the right to accept, refuse, or terminate treatment without deceit, undue influence, duress, coercion, or prejudice, and to be given necessary support throughout the decision-making and treatment process.

(ANA, 2015, p. 2)

A number of factors may threaten patient autonomy. The patient is in an inherently dependent role. The patient seeks healthcare assistance because of a real or perceived need and, as a result, can be perceived as dependent on the healthcare provider. The role of the healthcare professional, on the other hand, is one of power, which is based on knowledge and authority. This complementary relationship, although a necessary one, can lead to violations of patient autonomy when the patient does not or cannot exert autonomy.

Healthcare professionals are often insensitive to the ways in which the healthcare industry systematically dehumanizes and erodes the autonomy of patients. Patients are forced to comply with rules that require

---

ASK YOURSELF

Is the Patient Role a Dependent One?

- Describe a time when you or a family member was hospitalized.
- How did you or your family member feel when interacting with members of the healthcare team who were standing in a hospital room, dressed in professional clothing, while you or your family member was lying in a bed in pajamas or a hospital gown or, worse yet, naked?
- As a patient, have you or a family member ever felt unheard or not respected in a healthcare setting?
- Describe the degree to which you or your family member was able to maintain dignity and autonomy.
- How does the ANA *Code of Ethics for Nurses with Interpretive Statements* (Provision 1.1), the International Council of Nurses (ICN) *Code of Ethics for Nurses* (Element 1.2), or the *Canadian Code of Ethics for Registered Nurses* (Part C.4) apply to nurses' actions when delivering care?

---

them to be and act dependent. Immediately on admission to a hospital, patients are disrobed, asked questions about personal and private matters, forced to relinquish money and belongings, and expected to remain in a bed, emphasizing the dependency of the patient role. We place patients in rooms with doors that are seldom closed and ask them to wear bed clothing. Workers, who are strangers to patients, freely enter and leave patients' rooms and talk among themselves, making privacy impossible. Regardless of their personal habits or knowledge of their own healthcare, patients are forced to bathe at certain times, eat at certain times, take medications at certain

times, and are often prohibited from practicing self-care measures that may have been their habits for many years. Patients are expected to follow each plan that is made. Otherwise, they will be labeled difficult or non-compliant. For all the lip service given the importance of autonomy, healthcare professionals are often guilty of creating a climate of dependency for patients—of coercing otherwise autonomous, intelligent, and independent adults into an essentially dependent role.

There is one caveat—North Americans generally value personal agency and independence and Western researchers have assumed that most people want to make decisions based upon their own preferences, but many cultures do not place the same value on individualism. Nurses should respect those from other cultures where collectivism is valued, and autonomous decision making may include seeking advice from family or healthcare providers. For instance, in a review of cross-cultural research on decision making, Yates and de Oliveria (2016) found that people from East Asia, Russia, and India are more likely to call on others for help in making decisions, rather than confronting challenges alone. Indeed, working-class Americans were found to be more likely than middle-class Americans to seek the advice of others when making decisions. Similarly, Thompson et al. (2022) found that Mexicans were more likely than White Americans to seek advice when making decisions. Thus, nurses should be aware that a patient's culture can determine the way that autonomous decisions are made.

Autonomy is seen as less important in cultures that do not regard all people as being of equal worth and in cultures that respect social structure above individual rights. Where slavery exists, where women are expected to be subservient to men, where minority races are not respected, or where children are exploited, the notion of autonomy is meaningless. Autonomy cannot thrive in a climate that does not allow for either the independent planning of personal goals or the privilege of examining and choosing options to meet goals.

Subtle Violations of Patient Autonomy

Often nurses and other healthcare workers fail to recognize subtle violations of patient autonomy. This especially occurs when nurses perceive choices to be self-evident. At least four factors are related to this failure. First, nurses may falsely assume that patients have the same values and goals as themselves. This state of mind compels some nurses to believe that the only reasonable course of action is the one that is consistent with their own values. This leads to faulty conclusions. For example, if an elderly person chooses to stay in her own home, even though to others she seems incapable of caring for herself, her choice might be viewed as unreasonable and might become grounds to believe the patient is incompetent to make decisions. In other words, "If you don't make the choices that seem correct to me, you must be incompetent to make decisions." In truth the elderly person may recognize that life is drawing to a close and may want to remain in familiar surroundings, maintain dignity, remain independent, and prevent needless depletion of her life savings. The decision is based on her thoughtful consideration of the consequences of staying home versus the consequences of living in a long-term care facility. There are some who would insist that she should be allowed to stay at home, even if she places herself in considerable danger, as long as she does not jeopardize the autonomy of others.

The second potential violation of patient autonomy lies in a failure to recognize that individuals' thought processes are different. Discounting a particular decision as incorrect may not take into consideration the fact that people process information in different ways. There are those whose thought processes are very linear, logical, and methodical, and there are others who think in ways that are creative and free flowing. For example, Yates and de Oliveria (2016) found that Koreans favor intuitive decision making while Canadians tend to use a mix of logic and intuition, and Japanese prefer a slower decision-making process. It is particularly important to recognize these types of differences when several people are working together to come to a common decision. What is obvious to one will not be obvious to all—not necessarily because of a difference in values, knowledge base, or intellect, but because of different ways of processing information. This is an important consideration when collaborating with patients, families, and other professionals.

The third potential violation of patient autonomy occurs when nurses make false assumptions about patients' knowledge levels. It is easy for nurses to forget that we have gained a specialized body of knowledge through years of nursing education and work experience. Nursing language and knowledge about basic anatomy and physiology, disease processes, the mechanism of action of drugs, and so forth are so ingrained

in our minds that it is easy to presume everyone has at least some of the same type of knowledge. We often assume patients have more knowledge than is reasonable for them to have. Consequently, we may unreasonably discount or criticize patients' decisions. Recall that an understanding of the options, outcomes, and implications of health problems is inherently necessary for patients to make autonomous decisions. Therefore, the nurse should assess the patient's level of understanding and offer necessary teaching to foster autonomy.

Most people subscribe to the concept of autonomy, but few are prepared to accept total autonomy for every person in every situation. The ethical principle of respect for autonomy does not require you to respect all autonomous actions no matter how irrational the decision seems or how costly or damaging the results might be. Although you value patients' autonomy, you must simultaneously uphold responsibilities to yourself and to other people who could be harmed by the patient's choices. This can be a difficult distinction to make. For example, when assessing the decision-making capacity of an alcohol- or drug-impaired patient, healthcare providers ask themselves questions such as how impaired must this person be to lose the capacity to make rational decisions. To the extent that it is unreasonable to accept the autonomous decisions and actions of all people in all circumstances, we are called to uphold the principle of autonomy, rather than to respect each autonomous choice patients may make.

Fourth, nurses sometimes violate patient autonomy in subtle ways when caught up in the "work" of nursing. This produces a climate of industrious habit. As we go about our work—doing procedures, giving medications, writing care plans, and trying to keep up a frantic pace—attentiveness to patient autonomy is sometimes neglected. When nurses are working around them, patients may feel objectified, unseen, unheard, and not cared for. In today's climate of advanced technology, fiscal uncertainty, staffing reductions, and bottom-line management, nurses should constantly remind themselves to center their attention on the patient as the focus of nursing care.

Patient autonomy is more frequently discussed in terms of related issues such as informed consent, paternalism, advocacy, compliance, and self-determination. Let us review this principle as it relates to these and other recurrent themes.

Informed Consent

Informed consent is a term used to describe the process by which competent patients give voluntary consent for medical or surgical treatments or biomedical research after receiving information about potential risks and benefits. Informed consent is a practical application of the principle of respect for autonomy. It demonstrates legal protection of a patient's right to personal autonomy related to specific treatments and procedures. The concept of informed consent has come to mean that patients are given the opportunity to autonomously choose a course of action for medical care. This is usually discussed in relation to surgery, complex medical procedures, and research (Fig. 3.1).

Our contemporary practice of informed consent is a direct outcome of past research atrocities. Although research focusing on the human body, illness, and injury has its roots in the ancient world, it was not until after World War II that organizations and governments began to create policies to protect human subjects of medical research. World War II created a perfect storm in which ethical research violations seemed to occur on a large scale in many countries. Voluntary and nonvoluntary medical experiments to ostensibly improve medical practice during the war included infecting participants with pathogens, inflicting mortal wounds, and exposing subjects to high altitude, freezing conditions, radiation, and biological and chemical agents (Harris, 1999; United States Holocaust Memorial Museum, n.d.; Weindling, 1996). Highly publicized accounts of atrocious human rights violations spurred the development of policies that now affect every aspect of healthcare delivery.

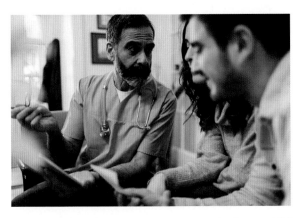

Fig. 3.1 Nurse Discusses Informed Consent for Surgery With Patient and Family. (©iStock.com/vgajic.)

When Nazi physicians were charged with war crimes, there were no established guidelines for ethical conduct in research. Therefore, while the trial was ongoing and with the assistance of physicians, the judges developed a set of 10 ethics guidelines by which to compare the conduct of the Nazi physicians (Alliance for Human Research Protection, 2022; Nuremberg Military Tribunal, October 1946–April 1949; Shuster, 1997; Weyers, 2007). The first and most prominent guideline established that research must be voluntary, as follows:

> *The voluntary consent of the human subject is absolutely essential. This means that the person involved should have legal capacity to give consent; should be so situated as to be able to exercise free power of choice, without the intervention of any element of force, fraud, deceit, duress, over-reaching, or other ulterior form of constraint or coercion; and should have sufficient knowledge and comprehension of the elements of the subject matter involved as to enable him to make an understanding and enlightened decision. This latter element requires that before the acceptance of an affirmative decision by the experimental subject there should be made known to him the nature, duration, and purpose of the experiment; the method and means by which it is to be conducted; all inconveniences and hazards reasonably to be expected; and the effects upon his health or person which may possibly come from his participation in the experiment.*
>
> (Nuremberg Military Tribunal, October 1946–April 1949, pp. 181–182)

After the Nuremberg trials, international governments and professional bodies began to institute policies and guidelines for informed consent that spilled over from research into medical and surgical care. These policies include many ethical and legal requirements. Nurses, who are often highly involved in obtaining informed consent, must understand the process and the legal requirements for each step. More specific details about informed consent are found in Chapters 11 and 12.

Paternalism

Paternalism is a gender-biased term that literally means acting in a fatherly manner. The traditional view of paternal actions includes such role behaviors as leadership, benevolent decision making, protection, and discipline. **Paternalism** means acting in a way that one believes will benefit, protect, or advance the interest of a person, even when this action goes against the person's expressed desires or limits his or her freedom of choice (Munson & Lauge, 2016). As commonly used in nursing, the term *paternalism* generally carries negative connotations, particularly related to implied dominant male versus submissive female roles. For example, before the age of informed consent, physicians advocated a "fatherly" role that allowed them to make decisions regarding the best form of treatment. An early leader in medical ethics, Dr. Thomas Percival, advocated this authoritative role when he wrote, "Physicians should study, also, in their deportment, so to unite tenderness with steadiness, and condescension with authority, as to inspire the minds of their patients with gratitude, respect, and confidence" (1803, p. 27). Apparently not an advocate of informed consent, he also advocated withholding information from the patient when he wrote, "As misapprehension may magnify real evils or create imaginary ones, no discussion concerning the nature of the case should be entered into before patients" (p. 29).

As viewed today, this gender-biased concept of paternalism has negative connotations, particularly as viewed by nurses. This is due in part to recognition that in the past the autonomy of patients was frequently violated in the name of beneficence. Recent research demonstrates that whether a person exhibits paternalistic behavior depends partly on the perception of the other person's mental capacities. Assertive people see paternalism as effective when they view other people are less mentally capable (Schroeder et al., 2017). Some professionals assume that they are uniquely qualified to make healthcare decisions by virtue of their professional knowledge and, further, that professional knowledge is the only knowledge needed to make healthcare decisions. Shiffrin, in fact, proposes that for an action to be paternalistic, the healthcare provider must believe that his or her judgment is better than the patient's (Shiffrin, 2000). This kind of paternalistic thinking ignores multiple factors that might be unrelated to physical outcomes yet affect the whole person. These factors include, among others, economic considerations, lifestyle, values, role, culture, and spiritual beliefs. In making decisions, all possible factors must be taken into consideration. This dictates that the patient must be autonomously engaged in the decision-making process.

In some cases, patients may communicate a wish to place decision making in the hands of family or healthcare providers. The patient may make an autonomous choice to rely on the provider's discretion. After all, the patient seeks healthcare and needs the knowledge and skills of providers. In their dependence on healthcare professionals, patients willingly surrender some measure of autonomy. Culture plays an important part in the measure of autonomy patients willingly yield. One research study, for example, clearly demonstrated that Mexican patients prefer paternalism as compared to White Americans, who prefer autonomy. Mexican patients described their physicians' paternalism in overwhelmingly positive terms while White Americans described their physicians' paternalism as overwhelmingly negative. Thus, the nurse should be aware that there is diversity among cultural groups when it comes to the exercise of autonomous decision making and the perception of paternalism in healthcare.

Advocacy

Advocacy is the act of supporting, speaking for, defending, or interceding on another's behalf, while honoring the other's autonomy. As a function of moral authority, patient advocacy is central to nursing and is implicitly or explicitly included in nursing codes of ethics. The act of advocacy in nursing is generally an informal, implicit function of the nurse-patient relationship. The goal of nursing advocacy is to ensure the welfare of the patient. Differing from paternalism, advocacy works toward the patient's own goals or goals the nurse believes the patient would have chosen. Virginia Henderson was one of the first nursing scholars to describe the advocacy role of nurses. She described advocacy as nurses helping patients do what they would ordinarily do for themselves when they lack the strength, will, or knowledge to care for themselves (Henderson, 1966).

Nursing advocacy occurs in many different types of situations. The nurse who communicates the patient's wishes in a staff meeting and the one who supports the patient in decision making are both advocates. Nurses can be advocates in the presence of patients, when patients are not present to express their own wishes, or when patients have diminished decision-making capacity.

Advocacy is especially appropriate when a patient has diminished decision-making capacity or is unable to communicate. The bedside nurse is often in the best position to know the patient's wishes. Nurses advocate for what we believe the patient would have chosen for themselves if that were possible. For example, we assume that a person would choose to be protected from injury. Within that context, when we believe an elderly, agitated patient is incompetent, we might employ means to eliminate falls or wandering. This type of advocacy should not be evoked simply because the nurse senses a risk of harm, but rather when patients cannot advocate for themselves. Ironically, Virginia Henderson, the well-known nursing leader who first defined nursing advocacy, recounts her experience as a hospitalized patient:

> *I was in the room with another patient, and I couldn't stand being in bed any longer, and I would sit in a chair. This nurse came in and saw me sitting in the chair, and she said, "Ms. Henderson if you keep doing that, we are going to have to tie you down." I thought, you just try it.*
>
> (Goldsmith, 1992, p. 4)

Even though Virginia Henderson was 94 years old at the time of her hospitalization, she was certainly competent to make decisions for herself. Patients who are competent must be allowed to act autonomously—even if the choices can be predicted to cause them harm or render them incompetent. One exception is that even competent persons cannot be allowed to act in ways that cause harm to others. Advocacy combines genuine concern for the patient with careful consideration of the patient's ability to make autonomous decision.

ASK YOURSELF

Who Should Make Decisions?

- How do you feel when someone else makes a decision about you without your input?
- Because nurses and doctors know more about the science of healthcare, when, if ever, is it appropriate for them to make decisions about the healthcare plan without input from the patient or family?
- How should you respond if a patient says, "Tell me what to do?"
- What guidance does the ANA *Code of Ethics for Nurses with Interpretive Statements* (Provisions 1.4 and 2.1), the ICN *Code of Ethics for Nurses* (Elements 1.1, 1.2, and 1.7), or the *Canadian Code of Ethics for Registered Nurses* (Part C.5) give the nurse in regard to advocacy?

Especially when patients are unable to communicate or have diminished decision-making capacity, there can be a thin line between advocacy and paternalism (Zomorodi & Foley, 2009). We suggest that the difference lies in the locus of power. Paternalism places power in the hands of the person who is making the decision for the patient. It implies that the decision maker knows what is best. With true advocacy, the patient retains the power. Advocacy expresses respect for the patient's autonomy because it aims to act according to the patient's own values. Zomorodi and Foley (2009) warn that nurses may not know patients' wishes and may not have access to family members who can act as surrogates. In these situations, it is possible for nurses to act in what they believe would be the best interests of patients, but they can unwittingly move toward medical paternalism. Therefore, nurses must constantly evaluate their actions to enhance the advocacy role and avoid unwanted paternalism.

Noncompliance

The term *noncompliance* is generally thought of as denoting a stubborn unwillingness of the patient to participate in healthcare activities. This commonly entails a lack of participation in a regimen that has been planned by the healthcare professional but must be carried out by the patient. Examples of such activities include taking medication as scheduled, maintaining a therapeutic or weight-loss diet, exercising regularly, and quitting smoking. The use of the term *noncompliance* is just as likely to represent failure of the nurse as it represents failure of the patient. Discussions about noncompliance and care of noncompliant patients center around two basic factors. First, the autonomous participation of the patient in the healthcare plan is essential to success. When patients are fully aware of the choices in healthcare therapies and the consequences of nontreatment and are encouraged to make healthcare decisions, they are more likely to participate in their own care. Often nurses formulate plans of care that are consistent with a scientific base of knowledge but seem bewildering or unreasonable to patients. Nurses are remiss if patients are not autonomous participants in the formulation of the plan. Second, nurses and other healthcare professionals must assess patients' abilities to follow plans of care. Patients may be unable to comply with plans for a variety of reasons, including lack of resources, lack of knowledge, lack of support from family members, psychological factors, and cultural beliefs that are not consistent with proposed plans of care. An example of patients' inability to comply with a plan of care is seen every day in physicians' offices and emergency departments. Often patients are given prescriptions for medications that are prohibitively expensive. When they return with the same symptoms, not having taken the prescribed medication, they are invariably labeled as noncompliant. The problem is not one of compliance, but rather the healthcare professionals' negligence in assessing their patients' ability to follow a plan of care.

What are we to do when patients are well informed and apparently able to follow plans of care yet do not? One hears stories of physicians who dismiss patients who do not comply with instructions—smoking cessation, for example. In a climate of limited resources, this is a question worthy of contemplation. Codes of ethics

for nurses universally support respect for individuals and individual choice and are not restricted by considerations of social or economic status (ANA, 2015; CNA, 2017; Gillon, 1985; ICN, 2021). Further, nurses must not be affected by patients' individual differences in values, backgrounds, customs, attitudes, gender, and beliefs. Because healthcare practices are an integral part of patients' backgrounds, customs, and beliefs, refusal to participate in a plan of care, regardless of the outcome, is the prerogative of the patient and must not affect the care given by the nurse. Ultimately, choices about healthcare practices belong to patients. If allowed to choose, patients should not be labeled in a negative way when nurses do not agree with their choices. It is not appropriate for professionals who express the belief that all competent patients have the right to autonomous choices to make value judgments about the choices made and subsequently label patients as noncompliant.

CASE PRESENTATION

Noncompliance Versus Autonomy

Cora is a 45-year-old woman who looks years older than her stated age. She has a very limited monthly income and no health insurance. Cora smokes 2½ packs of cigarettes per day. She has severe chronic obstructive pulmonary disease with constant dyspnea and frequent exacerbations. The nurse who sees her at a local free clinic speaks to Cora often about the importance of quitting smoking because he is interested in slowing the progression of Cora's disease. Cora continues to smoke and returns repeatedly for increasingly severe problems. The staff label Cora as noncompliant. During a particularly severe exacerbation, the frustrated nurse says to Cora, "You know you are committing suicide by continuing to smoke." Cora replies, "You don't understand. I live alone. I have no money, no friends, no family, and will never be able to work. I know the damage I'm doing, but smoking is the only pleasure I have in life."

Think About It

Do Nurses Coerce Patients?

- In attempting to persuade Cora to stop smoking, to what degree is the nurse violating Cora's right to autonomy?
- Does Cora have the right to choose to continue smoking?
- If rights and responsibilities are correlative, how should the clinic respond to Cora continuing to smoke? Would you suggest that the clinic continue to serve Cora, even though she is not following the plan of care?
- To what degree is coercion employed in situations such as Cora's? Is coercion an appropriate strategy?
- What would you do if you were the nurse?
- Which provisions, elements, or parts of nursing codes of ethics apply to the nurse caring for Cora?

BENEFICENCE

The principle of **beneficence** means to do good. It requires nurses to act in ways that benefit patients. Beneficent acts are morally and legally demanded by the professional role (Beauchamp et al., 2013). The objective

of beneficence provides nursing's context and justification. It lays the groundwork for the trust that society places in the nursing profession, and the trust that individuals place in particular nurses or healthcare agencies. Perhaps this principle seems straightforward, but it is actually very complex. As we think about beneficence,

BOX 3.2 Elements of Beneficence

- Do or promote good
- Prevent harm
- Remove evil or harm

certain questions arise: How do we define beneficence—what is good? Should we determine what is good by subjective or objective means? When people disagree about what is good, whose opinion counts? Is beneficence an absolute obligation and, if so, how far does our obligation extend? Does the trend toward unbridled patient autonomy outweigh the obligations of beneficence? Veatch (2012) asks whether the goal is really to promote the total well-being of the patient or to promote only the medical well-being of the patient. We must keep these questions in mind as we practice.

The ethical principle of beneficence has three major components: to do or promote good, to prevent harm, and to remove evil or harm (Box 3.2). Beneficence requires that we do or promote good as a positive act (Beauchamp & Childress, 2019). The underlying purpose of the profession is, in fact, to do good. Every expert performance of nursing functions and every act of kindness demonstrate beneficence. Listening to patients, administering medication, and providing comfort—all are beneficent acts. Even with the recognition that *good* might be defined in several ways, it seems safe to assume that the intention of nurses in general is to do good. Questions arise when those involved in a situation cannot decide what is *good*. For example, consider the case of a patient who is in the process of a lingering, painful, terminal illness. There are those who believe that life is sacred and should be preserved at all costs. Others believe that a natural and peaceful death is preferable to an extended life of pain and dependence. The definition of *good* in each case will determine, at least in part, what action should be taken.

The principle of beneficence, which is a major focus of nursing codes of ethics, also requires nurses to prevent or remove harm (Beauchamp & Childress, 2019). For example, the ICN *Code of Ethics for Nurses* says, "Nurses take appropriate actions to safeguard individuals, families and communities, and populations when their health is endangered by a co-worker, any other person, policy, practice or misuse of technology" (ICN, 2021, p. 12). Similarly, the Canadian Nurses Association (CNA) *Code of Ethics for Registered Nurses* says, "Nurses question and intervene, report and address unsafe, non-compassionate, unethical or incompetent practice or conditions that interfere with their ability to provide safe, compassionate, competent and ethical care; and they support those who do the same" (2017, p. 8). As you can see, the codes of ethics require nurses to courageously guard patients against harm, even harm that can occur as the result of problems in the organization or the acts of people who have authority.

Likewise, the ANA *Code of Ethics for Nurses with Interpretive Statements* requires that nurses must prevent or remove harm. "Nurses must be alert to and must take appropriate action in all instances of incompetent, unethical, illegal, or impaired practice or actions that place the rights or best interests of the patient in jeopardy" (ANA, 2015, p. 12). In regard to removing harm, the ANA *Code of Ethics for Nurses* is quite specific, requiring the nurse to focus on the patient's best interests "as well as on the integrity of nursing practice" (p. 12). Steps include the following: expressing concern to the person carrying out the questionable practice; reporting the practice to the appropriate authority within the institution; and, if not corrected, reporting the problem to other appropriate authorities, such as practice committees of the pertinent professional organizations or licensing boards. The ANA *Code of Ethics for Nurses* also calls for all nurses to actively assist whistleblowers whose reports are supported by facts.

Nurses perform positive acts of beneficence related to doing good with every nursing action. It is easy to imagine sensational acts of beneficence related to preventing or removing harm. For example, a nurse might dramatically stop a drug-impaired coworker from administering the wrong medication. Recall the Utah nurse who appropriately refused to give a police officer permission to draw blood from an unconscious patient who was not under arrest and was not a suspect (Ortiz & Siemaszko, 2017). Video of the nurse's forcible arrest was the topic of national news stories for days. However, preventing or removing harm is not always dramatic. It occurs every day and can be subtle, as seen in the following Case Presentation.

CASE PRESENTATION

Preventing or Removing Harm

Quinn was a young charge nurse in a cardiac telemetry unit. One patient on the unit was Reese, an 18-year-old popular high school athlete who had attempted suicide using a drug that affected cardiac function. Because of the sensitive nature of Reese's condition and the fact that he was a popular local figure, his parents and family physician decided to restrict visitors to immediate family and treating providers. While on evening rounds, Quinn saw an unfamiliar man dressed in an army uniform walk away from the nurses' desk and quickly move toward Reese's

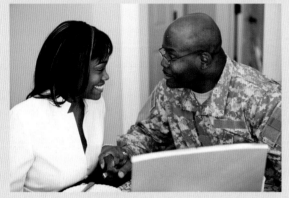

Fig. 3.2 Army Psychiatrist and Nurse. (©iStock.com/video1.)

room. Quinn entered the room and quietly asked the man to step into an adjacent office. Quinn said, "I'm sorry, but visitors are restricted. Are you a family member?" The man answered that he was Reese's psychiatrist and that he had come from an army function. Undeterred, Quinn asked for identification. Seeing his hospital credentials, Quinn realized that the man was, indeed, a psychiatrist affiliated with the hospital. The psychiatrist smiled, grasped her hand, and said, "I understand why you would be concerned and I'm very impressed" (Fig. 3.2).

Think About It
Preventing Harm
1. Why was Quinn's act considered beneficent?
2. Does it matter that Quinn's suspicions were unfounded?
3. Would you have the courage to call a person out of a room and ask for credentials if you experienced a similar incident?
4. The psychiatrist's reaction was positive—in fact, it was beneficent. What other reaction might Quinn have anticipated?
5. Imagine at least four other potential risks of harm for which Quinn should have been vigilant.
6. Did Quinn correctly apply codes of ethics from ANA (2015, Provisions 1.5 and 6.2) or CNA (2017, Parts I.A.1 and I.A.4) and ICN (2021, Elements 1.4 and 1.9) to this situation?

NONMALEFICENCE

The principle of **nonmaleficence** is so related to beneficence that some nurses become confused. Whereas beneficence requires us to prevent or remove harm, nonmaleficence requires us to avoid actually causing harm. This principle includes avoiding deliberate harm, risk of harm, and harm that occurs during the performance of beneficial acts. Most ethicists today tend toward placing this principle above others, as suggested by the Hippocratic tradition to "first do no harm." Nonmaleficence prohibits, for example, experimental research when it is fairly certain that participants will be harmed, and the performance of unnecessary procedures for economic gain or solely as a learning experience.

At first glance, it seems obvious that nurses must not cause harm. Isn't it unthinkable that a nurse would

harm patients? However, nonmaleficence also means avoiding harm as a consequence of doing good. When harm can occur as a result of a beneficial act, the harm or risk of harm must be carefully weighed against the expected benefit. For example, sticking a child with a needle for the purpose of causing pain is always bad—there is no benefit. Giving an immunization, on the other hand, although causing pain, results in the benefit of protecting the child from serious disease. The harm caused by the pain of the injection is easily outweighed by the benefit of the vaccine. In day-to-day practice, we encounter many situations in which the distinction is less clear, either because the harm caused may appear to be equal to the benefit gained because the outcome of treatment cannot be assured or as a result of conflicting beliefs and values. For example, consider analgesia for patients with painful terminal illness. Opioids may be the only type of medication that will relieve very severe pain. Opioids, however, may result in dependence and can hasten death when given in amounts required to relieve pain. Cammon and Hackshaw (2000) offer another common example. Orders for patients to have nothing by mouth (NPO) before diagnostic tests and surgical procedures are common practice and are unquestioned by most nurses. The authors cite real examples in which elderly patients were denied food for up to six days as tests and

procedures were completed. The tests and procedures were likely ordered or performed by several consulting physicians who were not aware of the total duration of NPO orders. The consequences of starvation in the elderly can be devastating, yet the practice of following NPO orders for long periods is seldom questioned. As nurses, we must be alert to situations such as these in which harm may outweigh the benefit, considering our own values and those of patients.

CASE PRESENTATION

Beneficence Versus Nonmaleficence

A retired nurse recounts an incident that she believes relates to the principle of nonmaleficence. As a senior nursing student, she was responsible for the care of a man who had a shotgun wound to his abdomen. Surgery had been performed, and the surgeon was unable to adequately repair the damage. The man was not expected to survive the day. He was, however, awake and strong, though somewhat confused. He had a fever of 107°F. He was receiving intravenous fluids and had continuous nasogastric suction. The man begged for cold water to drink. Following the accepted protocol after surgery, the physician ordered nothing by mouth in the belief that electrolytes would be lost through the nasogastric suction if water were introduced into the stomach. The student had been taught to follow the physician's orders. She repeatedly denied the man water to drink. She worked diligently—giving iced alcohol baths, taking vital signs, monitoring the intravenous fluids, and being industrious. The patient felt as if he were being tortured.

He begged for water. The student nurse followed orders perfectly. After six terrible hours, she turned to find the man quickly drinking the water from one of his ice bags. She left the room, stood in the hallway, and cried. She felt she had failed to do her job. As a result of the gunshot wound, the man died the next morning. Today her view of the situation is different.

Think About It
Weighing Harm Against Benefit
- Was this patient harmed? Discuss your answer.
- What was the benefit of the NPO order?
- Discuss whether the harm of thirst or the benefit of maintaining nothing by mouth should take precedence.
- What other ethical principles are relevant?
- Why did the student experience such extreme distress?
- What do you think an experienced nurse would do in a similar circumstance?
- Identify a provision, element, or part of any code of nursing ethics that applies to this situation.

The Case Presentation of the man mortally wounded by a gunshot wound illustrates the difficulty encountered when attempting to honor the principles of beneficence and nonmaleficence when they conflict.

VERACITY

The term **veracity** means telling the truth. Truthfulness is widely accepted as a universal virtue. Most of us were taught as children to always tell the truth. Philosophers, in general, favor openness and honesty. The philosophers most frequently cited in nursing literature,

Immanuel Kant and John Stuart Mill, agree in favor of truth-telling. Nursing literature promotes honesty as a virtue and truth-telling as an important function of nurses. However, there are some differences in perspective among healthcare professionals. Bioethicists disagree on the absolute necessity of truth-telling in all instances.

We can support nurses' practice of telling the truth in many ways. Although it is not always the easy option, truth-telling engenders respect, open communication, trust, and shared responsibility. It is promoted in all professional codes of nursing ethics.

Truth-telling and Virtue

1. If nursing literature promotes honesty as a virtue and truth-telling as an important function of nurses, how should one view a student nurse who cheats on assignments?

2. Nurse practitioners and physicians have been known to "fudge" on physical examination data, diagnoses, or time spent with patients to receive payment (or higher payment rates) from Medicare, Medicaid, or other third-party payers. Do you consider this a violation of the ethical principle of veracity?

3. What are the nursing implications in regard to veracity in the ANA *Code of Ethics for Nurses with Interpretive Statements* (Provisions 2.1 and 4.2), the ICN *Code of Ethics for Nurses* (Elements 1.3 and 1.8) or the *Canadian Code of Ethics for Registered Nurses* (Part A.5) apply to nurses' responsibility to address these disparities?

A very general interpretation of the ideas of the philosopher Martin Buber (1965) suggests that true communication between people can take place only when there are no barriers between them. Lying or deception creates a barrier between people and prohibits both meaningful communication and the building of relationships. Recognizing that communication is the cornerstone of the nurse-patient relationship, an argument can be made that nurse must be truthful to communicate effectively with patients.

Violating the principle of veracity shows a lack of respect. As suggested by Carter (2016), lying and deceit are instruments of power. Telling lies or avoiding disclosure implies that the nurse or other person involved assumes power over the patient or, at the very least, disrespects the patient's autonomy. Jameton (1984) suggests that manipulating information for the purpose of controlling others is like using coercion to control them. In essence, this keeps them from participating in decisions on an equal basis.

Jameton (1984) also suggests that deceiving others may constitute an unnecessary assumption of responsibility. When unfortunate consequences occur, the person responsible for the deception can also be assumed to be responsible for the consequences. On the other hand, when bad consequences occur after the patient has been told the truth, the outcome can be attributed to unfortunate circumstances.

Truth-telling engenders trust. We can make the argument that truth-telling is imperative to ensure that patients continue to trust nurses. By virtue of the trust inherent in the nurse-patient relationship, patients are willing to suspend some measure of autonomy and seek help in meeting healthcare needs. Without this trust, the nurse-patient relationship would be destroyed.

Veracity is now included in the formal relationship between hospitals and patients. Veracity is explicit in US federal law ("Conditions of Participation for Hospitals: Patient's Rights C.F.R. 42 § 482.13", 2006, Amended 2019; "Patients' Rights, 38 C.F.R. § 17.33," 1982, Amended 2005), and the AHA brochure, *The Patient Care Partnership* (2003), which replaced the original American Hospital Association's *Statement on a Patient's Bill of Rights*. According to these documents, providers are expected to care for patients with skill, compassion, and respect. Each of these directives indicates that patients have the right to obtain complete, current information concerning diagnosis, treatment, and prognosis in terms they can be reasonably expected to understand and specifies that physicians, nurses, and other healthcare professionals are responsible for ensuring that patients' rights are honored.

As with other principles, there is a dramatic discrepancy between nursing and medical literature with regard to veracity. Recognizing that nearly all healthcare is an interdisciplinary effort and that disclosure of information to patients involves both nurses and physicians, it is important for us to understand the medical perspective.

Physicians often make the claim that patients do not want bad news and that some truthful information has the potential to harm them. In the name of beneficence, some physicians occasionally proceed with either nondisclosure or outright lies. Lipkin (1991) argues that physicians should sometimes deceive their patients or withhold information from them. It is his view that patients do not have sufficient information about how their bodies function to interpret medical information accurately, and sometimes they do not want to know the truth about their illness. Joseph Ellin (1991) discusses special considerations that have been posed by the medical profession in relation to truth-telling. He suggests that it does not seem beneficent to adopt an ethic of absolute veracity in which it is an obligation to cause avoidable anguish to someone who is already ill, especially when hope and positive outlook may promote healing and help prolong life.

He writes, "One could hope to avoid this dilemma by holding that the duty of veracity, though not absolute, is to be given very great weight, and may be overridden only in the gravest cases" (p. 82). Ellin draws a distinction between lying and deception: lying is the purposeful telling of untruths, whereas deception is usually accomplished through nondisclosure. He argues that there is an absolute duty to avoid lying to patients; however, there is no duty not to deceive. Examples he

gives include withholding information about a poor prognosis or giving placebo medication. Consider the following situation: A mother of four is admitted to the emergency department after an automobile accident in which two of her children are killed. Recognizing that she is in very serious condition, it would be appropriate, according to Ellin, to avoid telling her of the death of her children. If, however, she asks about their condition, she must be told the truth.

ASK YOURSELF

Is Truth Telling Always Required?

Codes of nursing ethics require truth-telling. However, bioethicists disagree on the absolute requirement to tell the truth in every situation. As a nurse, you must anticipate that you will be faced with difficult on-the-spot decisions. Consider the following scenarios and think about how you would respond if you were the nurse:

- A 91-year-old woman with dementia repeatedly and urgently asks the nurse to call her father to pick her up and take her home. Whenever anyone tells the woman that her father is no longer alive, she becomes agitated, angry, and more confused.
- A patient with schizophrenia comes to a clinic with complaints of a terrific rash all over his body. He asks for a salve to heal his rash, even though there is no evidence of any type of skin condition. To satisfy the man, the nurse practitioner prescribes a petroleum-based ointment often used for diaper rash. The nurse practitioner believes there is little evidence to substantiate the use of the ointment, but also believes there is almost no risk of harm. The nurse dispenses a handful of sample packets of the ointment.

- A two-year-old is admitted to the hospital for an overdose of acetaminophen, which the father mistakenly administered. The nurse knows that acetaminophen overdoses sometimes result in liver failure. Crying, the father says, "Please tell me everything will be okay."
- A hospitalist orders a placebo for a hospitalized patient. The patient says to the nurse, "This medicine is helping me so much. Please tell me the name of it so I can ask my family doctor to prescribe it when I go home."
- A 22-year-old college student is diagnosed with an aggressive inoperable brain tumor. The student's parents ask the staff to tell the patient that she will be fine if she follows the doctor's orders.
- A pregnant woman tells the nurse that her friend's cousin recommends a certain pediatrician, Dr. T., for her expected baby. The nurse knows that Dr. T. bases her care on her 1970s medical school education and has several lawsuits against her. The woman asks, "Do you think she would be the best doctor for my baby?"

All situations in the "Ask Yourself: Is Truth Telling Always Required?" scenarios present difficult decisions that call for thoughtful responses. Can you devise a response to each situation in a way that is therapeutic, does not deceive the patient, and does not consist of "Ask your doctor"? For instance, the woman with dementia cannot understand that her father is no longer alive. If she could, she would already know it. So, telling her that he died many years ago serves no therapeutic purpose. The solution might be to divert her attention to another topic.

Bok (1991) examines the practice of physicians deceiving patients in the name of beneficence. Although

many would classify deceiving patients as paternalism, Bok writes that lying to patients has historically been seen as an excusable act. "Some would argue that doctors, and only doctors, should be granted the right to manipulate the truth in ways so undesirable for politicians, lawyers, and others" (p. 75). In fact, truth-telling has never been a principle that was given consideration in physicians' literature. Veracity is absent from virtually all medical oaths, codes, and prayers. Even the Hippocratic Oath makes no mention of truthfulness. The 1847 version of the American Medical Association Code of Ethics poetically endorses deception by physicians when the results might discourage the patient. The Code also instructs the physician to delegate the responsibility to give bad news to others, if possible.

> *For, the physician should be the minister of hope and comfort to the sick; that, by such cordials to the drooping spirit, he may smooth the bed of death, revive expiring life, and counteract the depressing influence of those maladies which often disturb the tranquility of the most resigned, in their last moments. The life of a sick person can be shortened not only by the acts, but also by the words or the manner of a physician. It is, therefore, a sacred duty to guard himself carefully in this respect, and to avoid all things which have a tendency to discourage the patient and to depress his spirits.*
> (American Medical Association, 1847, p. 106)

Nursing and medicine view veracity from two different perspectives. It is clear that physicians have traditionally seen disclosure or nondisclosure to be a facet of medical care that has implications for patient welfare. Physicians may consider withholding bad news to be a beneficent act if they think disclosing the information will harm the patient. Nursing, on the other hand, generally upholds veracity as supporting individual rights, respect for persons, and the principle of respect for autonomy. To collaborate successfully, however, one must recognize the viewpoints of others. Chapter 6 discusses methods of making decisions about ethical problems when there are differences of perspective among those involved.

CONFIDENTIALITY

The ethical principle of **confidentiality** relates closely **privacy**. There are at least two basic ethical arguments in favor of maintaining confidentiality. The first of these is the individual's right to control personal information and protect privacy. The second argument is one of *utility*—the weighing of good versus harm.

Privacy refers to the right of an individual to control the personal information or secrets, images, motivations, and relationships that are disclosed to others. Privacy includes the capacity to choose what others know about us, particularly intimate personal details. In Western cultures, privacy is thought to be a fundamental right of individuals and the precursor to the ethical principle of confidentiality. The ability to maintain privacy is an

expression of autonomy. A person has a right to decide what information to disclose and to whom. Privacy is important because it enables us to maintain dignity and preserve a measure of control over our own lives. There are five forms of privacy that involve limited access to the person: **informational privacy**, which includes information both in writing, such as medical records, and given orally, even in casual conversation; **physical privacy**, which focuses on individuals' bodies and their personal space; **decisional privacy**, which includes how people make personal choices, including cultural and religious preferences; **proprietary privacy**, which involves property interests including a person's image or biological materials; and **relational privacy**, which includes the family and similarly intimate relations (Allen, 1977; Beauchamp & Childress, 2019). Patients should be able to expect that personal, private, or embarrassing information will not be shared unnecessarily among healthcare providers, the privacy of their bodies and personal space will be respected, their method of making decisions will be honored, their image or biological specimens will not be shared unnecessarily, and their personal relationships will be respected.

Whereas privacy refers to the right of an individual to control personal intimate details and information, the ethical principle of confidentiality relates to a responsibility to avoid violating another person's privacy. In the healthcare setting, confidentiality is invoked whenever a patient discloses information to another, and the person to whom the information is disclosed promises, either implicitly or explicitly, not to communicate that information to others without the patient's permission. The ethical principle of confidentiality is made explicit in the nurse-patient relationship by virtue of its inclusion in nursing codes of ethics, federal law, and institutional policy. Confidentiality demands that the nurse respect personal confidence and refrain from prying or disclosing private information. Because nurses' work brings them into close contact with patients, they are often aware of sensitive and intimate personal information. Nurses should not casually discuss private patient matters, nor should they inadvertently share patients' personal information. Patient information is never an appropriate topic for elevator or dinner conversation. Maintaining confidentiality is an expression of respect for persons and is essential to the nurse-patient relationship. Consider the following Case Presentation about making the best choice.

CASE PRESENTATION

Making the Best Choice

Lora is a 17-year-old cheerleader. She comes to the local family-planning clinic requesting birth control pills. Lora is a very attractive, neat, and pleasant patient. In the process of completing the initial physical examination, the nurse practitioner finds evidence of physical abuse, including a recent traumatic perforated eardrum. Lora hesitantly and tearfully admits that her biological father slapped her across her left ear before she came to the clinic. She reports that she recently moved into his home after living most of her life with her mother and stepfather. She tearfully reports that her stepfather was sexually abusive to her and that she wishes to remain with her biological father. She says that she can tolerate being slapped around occasionally, and she does not want to get her biological father in trouble or be forced to move back to her stepfather's home. The nurse feels in a bind because the nursing code of ethics and federal law require that the nurse maintain confidentiality, yet state law requires that the nurse report any suspicion of child abuse.

Think About It
To Tell or Not to Tell
- What ethical principles are involved?
- Does Lora's obligation to report the incident of child abuse supersede the obligation to maintain confidentiality—particularly considering that the patient requested confidentiality? What if Lora were 14 years old?
- What are the options for the nurse?
- What are the possible outcomes of the different options?
- Does Lora's autonomy outweigh the nurse's responsibility to report the abusive situation?
- What provisions, elements, or parts of the ANA *Code of Ethics for Nurses with Interpretive Statements*, ICN *Code of Ethics for Nurses*, or the *Canadian Code of Ethics for Registered Nurses* address this complex issue?

Codes and oaths of nursing and medicine dating back many centuries support the principle of confidentiality. The ICN, ANA, and CNA codes of nursing ethics require that nurses maintain confidentiality of patient information, stating that the nurse must keep that information confidential, sharing only the information necessary to provide patient care. Confidentiality is the only facet of patient care mentioned in the Nightingale Pledge. This

oath has been recited for decades by graduating nurses: "I will do all in my power to elevate the standard of my profession and will hold in confidence all personal matters committed to my keeping and all family affairs coming to my knowledge in the practice of my profession" (Gretter, 1893). Like nurses, physicians are required to maintain confidentiality. Although they list instances in which confidentiality may be breached by physicians, both the American Medical Association (AMA) (2017) and the World Medical Association (2022) include confidentiality as a cornerstone of medical ethics. The centuries-old first code of medical ethics, the Hippocratic Oath, is very clear: "Whatever, in connection with my professional practice, or not in connection with it, I see or hear, in the life of men, which ought not to be spoken of abroad, I will not divulge, as reckoning that all such should be kept secret" (Hippocrates, ca. 400 BCE/1849).

Medical records can be a source of confidentiality breach. When adding information to patient records, nurses must keep in mind the type of information needed and the number of people who have legitimate access to the records. In a hospital situation, patient charts are accessible to many personnel. Nurses, physicians, dietitians, respiratory therapists, utilization review staff, financial officers, students, secretaries, physical therapists, and others have legitimate reasons to view patient records. Inappropriately recorded information of a sensitive and private nature that the patient intends for the nurse alone can become widely known in a large healthcare facility if it is included in the medical record. Thus, care must be taken in choosing information to be recorded in patients' charts.

Confidentiality is particularly important when revelations of intimate and sensitive information have the potential to harm the patient. Harm can take various forms, such as embarrassment, ridicule, discrimination, deprivation of rights, physical or emotional harm, and loss of roles or relationships. Consider the plight of early AIDS victims whose diagnoses became public knowledge.

The second argument in favor of upholding confidentiality is one of utility, which holds that an action is morally right if it increases the net amount of good, taking into account the harm that may occur as well (Veatch & Guidry-Grimes, 2020). If patients suspect that healthcare providers reveal sensitive and personal information indiscriminately, they may be reluctant to seek care, thus increasing potential harm. For example, it is well documented that veterans often hesitate to seek healthcare. When they do initiate healthcare, they are often reluctant to report physical and mental health concerns because of shame or fear of stigmatization if others learn about their problems (Malmin, 2013; Simmons & Yoder, 2013). Government policymakers recognize that patients may be reluctant to seek necessary healthcare if they believe private information will be disclosed. For example, because of the intimate and private nature of reproductive health issues, policies regulate stringent confidentiality procedures for certain health issues such as family planning and sexually transmitted infections. Nurses must be aware that revealing some health conditions can harm the patient. Inappropriately disclosing diagnoses such as mental illness, alcoholism, drug addiction, sexual orientation, and sexually transmitted diseases can lead to stigmatization and subsequently discourage others from seeking care.

Contemporary Issues of Confidentiality

The expansion of information technology poses new risks to confidentiality. Patient information and images can be stored on tablets, laptops, CDs, DVDs, thumb drives, and cell phones; transmitted to cloud storage or industry platforms; or shared via e-mail or text. Handheld electronic devices, although convenient, are easily misplaced or stolen. Confidential patient information on these devices can be compromised. Likewise, social media poses a risk to patient confidentiality. See Chapter 8 for more about the confidentiality of electronic records and the National Council of State Boards of Nursing social media guidelines.

The US government made the delicate balance between ethical principles more complex when confidentiality of patient information became a legal mandate. In 1996 Congress enacted the Health Insurance Portability and Accountability Act (HIPAA). The HIPAA Privacy Rule made confidentiality of medical records a legal requirement. See Chapter 8 for more complete information about HIPAA privacy requirements.

Limits of Confidentiality

Should the principle of confidentiality be honored in all instances? There are arguments related to harm and vulnerability that favor questioning the absolute obligation of confidentiality in certain situations. The nurse who recognizes that maintaining confidentiality will result in preventable wrongful harm to innocent others should weigh the harm to the patient if confidentiality is waived versus the harm that might occur to the innocent other if the nurse maintains confidentiality. Although it has been repealed in most states, premarital testing for syphilis was once mandatory. States intended to prevent the spread of a serious communicable disease to innocent babies and spouses. In this instance, society chose to override the privacy of the individual to protect the health of the innocent. Though directing nurses to maintain confidentiality, the ANA Code of Ethics for Nurses (2015) recognizes that duties of confidentiality are not absolute and may need to be modified to protect the patient, other innocent people, and, in cases of mandatory disclosure, for public safety.

In rare instances, case law supports the harm principle. In a crucial case from July 1976, the California Supreme Court ruled that a psychologist, his supervisor, and their facility were liable for the wrongful death of Tatiana Tarasoff. Prosenjit Poddar killed Tatiana Tarasoff in October 1969. Two months earlier, Poddar had confided his intention to kill Tatiana to his psychologist. Though the psychologist initially tried to have his patient involuntarily committed, his supervisor intervened and allowed Poddar to return home. Neither Tatiana nor her parents were informed of the patient's threats. The court found that the therapist and his supervisor were responsible for the wrongful death of Tatiana because they knew in advance of Poddar's intentions. The court decided that the therapist's obligation to protect the innocent third party, now termed a "duty to warn," superseded the obligation to maintain confidentiality (Siddharth et al., 2016).

Foreseeability is an important consideration when confidentiality conflicts with the duty to warn. The nurse should be able to reasonably foresee harm or injury to another person to violate the principle of confidentiality in favor of a duty to warn. The Tarasoff case exemplifies the reasonable application of the harm principle. Subsequent court cases support the decision in the Tarasoff case. Courts have found that privacy is not absolute and is subordinate to the state's fundamental right to enact laws that promote public health.

The duty to protect others from harm is stronger when the third party is dependent on others or is in some way especially vulnerable. Vulnerability implies risk or susceptibility to harm when vulnerable individuals are relatively unable to protect themselves. For example, nurses have an absolute duty to report child abuse—nurses are *mandatory reporters*. Mandatory reporting varies across jurisdictions but usually includes reporting harm to children, disabled adults, and senior citizens. Because these groups are dependent and vulnerable, they are at greater risk of harm. Coupling the potential of harm with vulnerability produces a strong argument for violating the principle of confidentiality in certain instances. However, it is clear that there is a dynamic tension between the patient's right to confidentiality and the duty to warn innocent others. Nurses need to recognize that careful consideration of the ethical implications of actions will not always be supported in bureaucratic and legal systems.

Nurses must ensure all forms of privacy and maintain confidentiality, except when patients give permission to disclose information, when state or federal law requires disclosure, or when the patient is unable to give consent and disclosure of private information is in the best interest of the patient. Even then, the information disclosed must be the minimum necessary and must be shared only with those who need it to benefit the patient or for legal purposes.

ASK YOURSELF

Can Nurses Violate Confidentiality?
- How do you think confidentiality and the harm and vulnerability principles can be reconciled?
- How would you feel if a relative contracted HIV from a source who public health officials knew was infected and had reason to believe would infect your relative but neglected to warn?
- How would you feel if you were diagnosed with drug-resistant tuberculosis and the director of the clinic talked about your diagnosis with his golf partners?
- Is confidentiality specifically addressed in nursing codes of ethics?

JUSTICE

Justice is the ethical principle that relates to fair, equitable, and appropriate treatment in light of what is due or owed to persons, recognizing that giving resources to some people will mean that others will not receive them. Within the context of healthcare ethics, the most relevant application of the principle focuses on distribution of goods and services. This application is called **distributive justice**, which relates to fair, equitable, and appropriate distribution in society, determined by justified norms that structure the terms of social cooperation. Its scope includes policies that allot diverse benefits and burdens such as property, resources, taxation, privileges, and opportunities. Unfortunately, there is a finite supply of goods and services, and it is impossible for all people to have everything they might want or need. So, one of the primary purposes of governing systems is to formulate and enforce policies that deal with fair and equitable distribution of scarce resources.

Decisions about distributive justice are made on different levels. The government is responsible for creating policies about broad public health access issues, such as influenza vaccine supplies, children's immunization programs, and Medicare for the elderly. Professional organizations such as the ANA or AMA articulate some distributive justice guidelines such as those for triage. Hospitals and other organizations formulate policies on an institutional level and deal with issues such as how decisions will be made concerning who will occupy intensive care beds and which types of patients will be accepted in emergency rooms. Nurses and other healthcare providers frequently make decisions of distributive justice on an individual basis. For example, having assessed the needs of patients, nurses decide how best to allocate their time (a scarce resource). In emergency situations, nurses may be responsible for life-and-death triage decisions.

There are three basic areas of healthcare relevant to questions of distributive justice. First, what percentage of overall resources is reasonable to spend on healthcare? Second, recognizing that healthcare resources are limited, which aspects of healthcare should receive the most resources? Third, which patients should have access to the limited healthcare staff, equipment, and so forth (Jameton, 1984)?

In making decisions of distributive justice, one must ask the question, "Who is entitled to these goods or services?" Philosophers have suggested a number of different ways to choose among people. Box 3.3 lists some of the ways that people have historically made distributive justice decisions. Some believe that all people should receive equally, regardless of need. On the surface, nationalized healthcare systems would seem to meet this criterion because all citizens would be eligible for the same services. However, because some citizens would necessarily require more healthcare services than others, nationalized systems also meet the criterion of need.

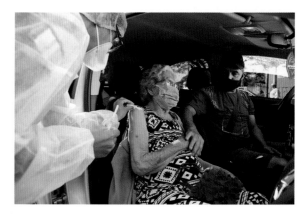

Fig. 3.3 Elderly Woman Receives COVID-19 Vaccine at a Drive-Through Immunization Clinic. (©iStock.com/Jair Ferreira Belafacce.)

The German philosopher Friedrich Nietzsche had a different perspective. He believed that society's goal should be to support and enhance superior individuals. For Nietzsche, the choice of distribution was a clear one—to each according to his present contribution or potential for future contributions essential to society (Ward, 2011; Wells, 2013). The idea that each should receive according to effort is a common belief in our culture and indicates the traditional "work ethic." To each according to that person's rights indicates a libertarian viewpoint, and to each as he or she would wish to be treated reflects the Golden Rule. Entitlement programs in the United States generally award benefits based on a combination of need and the greatest good that can be accomplished for the greatest number of people, such as with immunization programs. Chapter 15 discusses the application of the principle of distributive justice in greater detail.

The COVID-19 pandemic forced institutions and governments to rapidly write guidelines on how distributive justice decisions should be made. Meier (2022) gathered information on decisions made by governments of many countries and found that the countries' guidelines flowed from varied perspectives. Some suggested giving priority healthcare services (such as ICU beds and ventilators) to those with the greatest need, such as the elderly, while others called for distributing services in a way that created the greatest benefit for the greatest number of people by giving priority to those with the best chance of survival. Some countries gave preference to healthcare workers who contracted COVID-19 through their work, while others preferred a more egalitarian approach—giving each person an equal chance at receiving healthcare services. There were discussions in some countries about giving lower priority to patients who had not followed mask, social distancing, and immunization precautions and there were discussions about distributing resources and services on a "first come first serve" basis, though neither of these methods ended up in major guidelines. For the most part, guidelines in the United States were piecemeal and varied from location to location, with state, local, and even institutional decisions affecting the distribution of healthcare goods and services. Fig. 3.3 shows an elderly woman receiving a COVID-19 vaccine at a drive-through vaccination clinic.

CASE PRESENTATION

The Case of COVID-19

The COVID-19 pandemic provides a dramatic example of distributive justice in healthcare. In late December 2019 a novel strain of an old virus emerged and by March 2020 the World Health Organization had declared a worldwide pandemic. Because of a rapid spread and extreme morbidity and mortality of the disease, governments and healthcare organizations around the world scurried to develop, mobilize, and distribute scarce resources and to make morally pertinent decisions about how to ration them. When discussing the ethics of distributive justice, it is important to examine all factors and look to the past for lessons learned.

In 1918 an estimated 500 million people worldwide were infected with an influenza virus, often called the "swine flu." The strain of the disease was exceptionally severe, with total deaths estimated to be 50 million (Taubenberger et al., 2019). The virulent, highly contagious virus produced three pandemic waves in rapid succession. Before the pandemic receded, one-third of the world's population had been infected.

In 1976 US Public Health officials identified a handful of cases, similar to the 1918 influenza. Recalling the severity of the 1918 pandemic, CDC officials called for rapid mass immunizations. The first vaccines were administered in October 1976, and 40 million Americans received the vaccine within three months. Unfortunately, vaccinated individuals had an 11 times greater chance of developing Guillain-Barré syndrome than those who were not vaccinated. The predicted pandemic never materialized, and those who were infected experienced low morbidity and almost no mortality. The vaccine appeared to have been more dangerous than the disease (Neustadt & Fieneberg, 2005).

When similar cases emerged in April 2009, the CDC again recalled the high death toll of the 1918 pandemic. Officials recognized the potential for rapid spread of the disease, high morbidity and mortality, unusual morbidity age distribution, and multiple pandemic waves. They also remembered the disastrous results of the poorly tested 1976 swine flu vaccine. The CDC quickly began pursuing multiple high-yield methods to develop a vaccine. Within six months, millions of doses of antiviral medications were distributed, with the first available vaccines administered to high-risk groups and healthcare workers. As it turned out, the 2009 virus was not as virulent as anticipated, and the dollar cost of the vaccine campaign was tremendous. It is impossible to know how many lives were saved by the mass campaign. Balancing potential harm against potential benefit seemed like a juggling act done in the dark.

Then in 2020 the worldwide medical community became alarmed at the rapid spread and virulence of the COVID-19 virus with press coverage comparing COVID-19 to the 1918 influenza pandemic. After a sputtering governmental response in the United States, scientists began rapid research and development of a new vaccine aimed at preventing the disease. Vaccines were developed in record time and rolled out incrementally as production allowed, beginning in early 2021. By the time vaccine distribution began, hospitals were overwhelmed with critically ill and dying patients, the nursing shortage had reached crisis level, and some critical supply chains were failing. With the guidance of the CDC, state governments made decisions about incremental distribution of the scarce COVID-19 vaccines, initially through various public health efforts. Recipient groups were prioritized in the United States with nursing home residents and first-line healthcare workers given the first priority for vaccination. As more vaccines became available, priority groups were expanded to include older adults, immunocompromised, and "essential workers" (which were defined differently in different locations). Because of children's vulnerability, research, development, and distribution to children occurred after other population groups. By November 2021 the death rate had been lowered as much as 40.6 percent as a result of vaccination efforts (Rhyne, 2022). As the United States and other Western countries rolled out millions of COVID-19 vaccine doses in the early days, third-world countries had little or no available vaccine.

Think About It
Judge the COVID-19 Vaccine Response
- What potential large-scale harms and benefits were inherent in this situation?
- If you were a government official, what factors would you have taken into consideration to make decisions about the rollout of the COVID-19 vaccine?
- Front-line healthcare workers and people at known high risk were given first access to the vaccine. How would you describe this distributive justice decision? Was it fair?
- Considering the 1918 pandemic, would you have done anything differently in 2020 to protect large numbers of people?
- Thinking back to the discussions of deontology and utilitarianism in Chapter 2, which theory more closely applies to this case study?
- Since lack of immunity allows the virus to mutate and spread further, what are your thoughts about the scarcity of vaccines in third-world countries?
- Research has shown that there are racial, ethnic, and rural vs urban disparities in delivery of COVID-19 vaccines (Ndugga et al., 2022; Saelee et al., 2022). How does the ANA *Code of Ethics for Nurses with Interpretive Statements* (Provision 8.3), the ICN *Code of Ethics for Nurses* (Element 4), or the *Canadian Code of Ethics for Registered Nurses* (Parts B.2 and F.6) apply to nurses' responsibility to address these disparities?

FIDELITY

The ethical principle of **fidelity** relates to the concept of faithfulness and the practice of keeping promises. Beauchamp and Childress (2019) call fidelity a central and often underappreciated moral norm (p. 353). Fidelity establishes that a professional is morally obligated to act faithfully for the benefit of another, particularly when implicit or explicit promises are made. Society has granted nurses the right to practice nursing through the processes of licensure and certification, which is "based on a social contract that acknowledges professional rights and responsibilities as well as mechanisms for public accountability" (ANA, 1995, p. 3). The process of licensure is one that ensures no other group can practice within the domain of nursing as defined by society and the profession. Thus, when nurses accept licensure and become legitimate members of the profession, they must uphold the responsibilities inherent in the contract with society. Members are called to be faithful to the society that grants the right to practice—to keep the promise of upholding the profession's code of ethics, to practice within the established scope of practice and definition of nursing, to remain competent in practice, to abide by the policies of employing institutions, and to keep promises to individual patients. To be a nurse is to make these promises. In fulfilling this contract with society, nurses are responsible for faithfully and consistently adhering to these basic principles (Fig. 3.4).

On another level, the principle of fidelity relates to loyalty within the nurse-patient relationship. It gives rise to an independent duty to keep promises or contracts (Veatch, 2012) and is a basic premise of the nurse-patient relationship. Problems sometimes arise when there is a

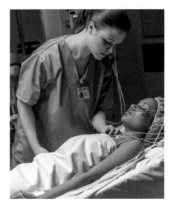

Fig. 3.4 Fidelity Implies That Nurses Must Remain Competent to Practice. (©iStock.com/simonkr.)

conflict between promises that have been made and the potential consequences of those promises in cases when carrying them out will cause harm in other ways. Though fidelity is the cornerstone of a trusting nurse-patient relationship, most ethicists think there are no absolute, exceptionless duties to keep promises—that in every case the harmful consequences of the promised action should be weighed against the benefits of keeping the promise.

CASE PRESENTATION

Consider the case of 15-year-old Lewis Blackman. Lewis was an exceptional student and athlete. In November 2000 Lewis and his parents decided that he would undergo an elective surgery for a congenital condition called *pectus excavatum* in which the chest wall is concave rather than convex. He entered a large university teaching hospital anticipating a relatively minor surgery and rapid recovery. When Lewis woke from anesthesia on Thursday, November 2, he reported his pain was a 3 on a 1–10 pain scale. Around the same time, nurses recorded that Lewis wasn't producing any urine. Nevertheless, nurses administered an intravenous dose of a nonsteroidal antiinflammatory drug (NSAID) that requires good kidney function and carries many risks, including the potential for perforated ulcers and internal bleeding. On Friday evening, Lewis's surgeon left for the weekend. Saturday morning, Lewis was visited by another surgeon whose documentation indicated no unusual or alarming signs. After Saturday morning, interns and residents took charge of Lewis's care. On Saturday night Lewis began to run a slight fever, and his feet were cold to the touch. He was still on the intravenous NSAID.

On Sunday morning Lewis began experiencing horrific pain in his upper abdomen. A nurse alerted to severe abdominal pain would ordinarily contact an attending physician. However, the nurse told Lewis and his mother that the abdominal pain was gas. Lewis's mother recalls the nurse saying, "There is nothing I can do for gas pain" (Monk, 2002). Even though Lewis was pale and getting weaker, one nurse suggested a bath, and another asked Lewis's mother to help him walk in the hallway. On Sunday afternoon, Lewis's abdomen became hard and distended—a well-known indication of a potentially lethal condition such as a perforated ulcer and internal bleeding. As Lewis's temperature dropped, he became paler, had a cold sweat, was exhausted, and was in severe pain. Lewis's mother called the nurse many times and repeatedly asked for an experienced physician, rather than a resident. The nurse argued with her and became offended, as did the intern caring for Lewis. By Sunday afternoon, Lewis's pulse was 126 and his temperature was dropping. Sunday night his pulse increased to 142 and his temperature dropped to 95°F. For two hours, while Lewis was bleeding to death from a perforated ulcer, no one was able to find a detectable blood pressure. Nevertheless, nurses were not alarmed. Trying one blood pressure device after another, they believed the problem was with the equipment. Shortly after noon, the chief resident entered the room and called a code. After 60 minutes of cardiopulmonary resuscitation, Lewis was declared dead—five hours after his blood pressure was undetectable and 31 hours after he first complained of severe abdominal pain.

In a series of videos, which are posted on the QSEN website, Lewis's mother, Helen Haskell, describes the nurses as young, inexperienced, and task oriented, rather than goal or patient oriented (QSEN Institute, 2018). Nurses decorated the hallway and laughed in the nurses' lounge as her young son was dying. She was aware that the nurses documented Lewis's vital signs and symptoms that would alarm most experienced nurses, yet they failed to act, even after her repeated entreaties. Although Lewis's mother gives credit to one nurse who tried to advocate for Lewis, she lays much of the blame on the nurses who should have had the knowledge, critical thinking, and moral authority to have acted in a way that could have prevented Lewis's death.

Think About It
Task Oriented Versus Patient Oriented
A litany of practice issues surrounds Lewis Blackman's care. However, we turn our attention here to the applicable ethical and moral issues.

1. How does the ethical principle of fidelity relate to the nursing care delivered to Lewis Blackman?
2. How does the ethical principle of respect for persons relate to the nursing care delivered in this case?
3. Because Lewis was a minor, his parents held decision-making authority. How was the principle of respect for autonomy violated in this case?
4. Identify problematic issues of beneficence and nonmaleficence in the case of Lewis Blackman. How might the nurses have better demonstrated these principles as they cared for Lewis?
5. Aside from a lack of knowledge, why do you imagine the nurses failed to act on Lewis's behalf?
6. How might a nurse have effectively advocated for Lewis and his mother?
7. Justice is the ethical principle that relates to fair, equitable, and appropriate treatment in light of what is due or owed to persons. How does the nurse's refusal to contact an attending physician constitute a distributive justice issue?
8. The identifiers of Lewis Blackman's name, age, city, hospital, and private health information pertaining to his condition and care were made public. Considering the ethical principle of confidentiality and the HIPAA Privacy Rule, how do you think this information was legally shared with the public?
9. Lewis Blackman's complex case touches on several important ethical issues. Identify at least two provisions, elements, or parts of a nursing code of ethics that apply to this case.

SUMMARY

As we participate in meeting the healthcare needs of society, we must be constantly aware of the ethical implications inherent in many situations. Each nurse must develop a philosophically consistent framework from which to base contemplation, decision, and action. It is this framework that gives shape to our concept of various ethical principles. The principles discussed in this chapter presuppose nurses' innate respect for persons. Ethical principles include respect for autonomy, beneficence, nonmaleficence, veracity, confidentiality, justice, and fidelity. Ethical principles are generally complementary; however, at times they may conflict. Nurses must be prepared to thoughtfully examine situations in the light of established ethical principles.

CHAPTER HIGHLIGHTS

- Ethical principles are basic and obvious moral truths that guide deliberation and action.
- All ethical principles presuppose a basic respect for persons.
- Respect for autonomy denotes respecting another person's freedom to make choices about issues that affect his or her life.
- Various intrinsic and extrinsic factors threaten patient autonomy.
- The principle of beneficence maintains that one ought to do or promote good, prevent evil or harm, and remove evil or harm.
- The principle of nonmaleficence requires one to avoid causing harm, including deliberate harm, risk

of harm, and harm that occurs during the performance of beneficial acts.

- The principle of veracity relates to the universal virtue of truth telling.
- Privacy is the capacity to choose what others know about us, particularly intimate personal details.
- Confidentiality is the ethical principle that requires nondisclosure of private or secret information with which one is entrusted.
- Justice is the ethical principle that relates to fair, equitable, and appropriate treatment in light of what is due or owed to persons, recognizing that giving to some will deny receipt to others who might otherwise have received these things.
- Fidelity is the ethical principle that relates to faithfulness and promise keeping. Fidelity requires trustworthiness and expertise.
- Nursing codes of ethics offer guidelines for action with many complex moral issues.

DISCUSSION QUESTIONS AND ACTIVITIES

1. Read either the ANA *Code of Ethics for Nurses with Interpretive Statements*, the ICN *Code of Ethics for Nurses*, or the *Canadian Code of Ethics for Registered Nurses* (whichever is most appropriate for your situation) and discuss how the various statements in the codes relate to each of the principles discussed in this chapter.
2. Read the following hypothetical situation and answer the questions that follow:
3. An elderly man presents himself to the emergency department of a small community hospital. The patient has contractures and paralysis of his left hand; he apparently has complete expressive and at least partial receptive aphasia. Upon questioning, the man takes off his right shoe and points to his right great toe and grimaces, apparently indicating a problem in that area. The nurse is unable to gather any further information from him because of his difficulty in communicating. In attempting to help him, she asks if he has a neighbor or friend accompanying him. He shakes his head, indicating that he is alone. Curious, the nurse asks him how he came to the hospital. The patient smiles and proudly produces a driver's license from his shirt pocket. Subsequently, the nurse leaves the room and

returns a few minutes later to find that the patient left the hospital, having received no care. The nurse suspects that because of his current physical condition the man is unsafe to drive a motor vehicle.
   - What are the ethical implications of this situation?
   - What ethical principles are involved?
   - Should the nurse pursue avenues to locate the patient and ensure that he is not endangering himself or others by driving? Would this be a breach of confidentiality? Autonomy?
   - How does the nurse express fidelity in this situation?
   - What is the beneficent action?
4. Describe situations you have witnessed in which decisions were made for patients in a paternalistic manner. Discuss your perception of the difference between paternalism and advocacy. Give examples.
5. Read the following hypothetical case and answer the questions that follow:
6. Martha is a 75-year-old woman who has terminal cancer of the bladder. During the course of her therapy in a small rural hospital, she sustains third-degree radiation burns to her lower abdomen and pelvic area. Her wounds are extensive and deep, involving her abdominal wall, bladder, and vagina. The physician orders frequent medicinal douches and wound irrigations. These treatments are quite painful, and the patient wants the treatments discontinued but is too timid to actually refuse them. The physician will not change the order.
   - Discuss the situation in terms of beneficence and nonmaleficence.
   - How does this patient express her autonomy?
   - What is the nurse's responsibility in assisting the patient to maintain autonomy?
   - How does the nurse deal with conflicting loyalties and principles?
7. Do you think healthcare professionals should disclose information to patients related to a poor prognosis, for example, even though the information may cause distress? Discuss your views in depth.
8. Jameton (Jameton, 1984) says that for nurses to be less than competent is unethical. Discuss this statement in terms of fidelity.
9. Read the following hypothetical case and answer the questions that follow:
10. Nels Gruder is a 40-year-old disabled truck driver. He was injured several years ago in a

trucking accident. He subsequently has had back surgery but continues to have severe pain. He has been seen by every local neurosurgeon and, for one reason or another, is not pleased with the care he has gotten. Because of the seriousness of his initial injuries, there is little doubt that Mr. Gruder has chronic back pain. Even though the local emergency room policy of not prescribing opioid analgesics for chronic pain is clearly stated on signs in the waiting area, Mr. Gruder comes there frequently complaining of severe back pain. He reports a history of gastric ulcers and allergy to NSAIDs. The nurse practitioner who sees Mr. Gruder is faced with a man who is in obvious pain. She wishes to help him relieve the pain he is experiencing. At the same time, she realizes that opioid analgesia is not appropriate for this type of problem and is unable to prescribe NSAIDs because of his reports of gastric ulcers and allergy. He says he has tried exercises and a local pain clinic, neither of which was effective. He is aware of the emergency room policy regarding opioid analgesics for chronic pain, but he comes there in desperation. He insists that his pain is relieved only by opioid analgesia.

- What ethical principles are involved?
- Does the benefit of pain relief outweigh the harm potentially caused by long-term opioid analgesic use for this patient?
- Should Mr. Gruder's perceived need for opioid pain medications be honored even though the nurse practitioner is concerned that he might have a problem with drug dependence?
- How does the nurse do what she thinks is right and yet respect Mr. Gruder's autonomy?
- Is it important that the nurse's actions please the patient?

11. Perform an Internet search for the HIPAA Privacy Rule. What are the 18 patient identifiers that must be removed from research, teaching, and quality improvement documents to maintain patient confidentiality and privacy?

12. View Helen Haskell's six-minute video, *Part Two: A Mother's View of Lessons Learned* on the QSEN Institute Lewis Blackman Story (http://qsen.org/publications/videos/the-lewis-blackman-story/) webpage. Answer the website questions that accompany the video.

REFERENCES

Allen, A. L. (1977). Genetic privacy: Emerging concepts and values In M. A. Rothstein (Ed.), *Genetic secrets: Protecting privacy and confidentiality in the genetic era* (pp. 31–59). Yale University Press.

Alliance for Human Research Protection. (2022). *The significance of the Nuremberg Code.* https://ahrp.org/the-significance-of-the-nuremberg-code/.

AMA. (2017). *Code of medical ethics.* https://www.ama-assn.org/delivering-care/ethics/code-medical-ethics-overview

American Hospital Association. (2003). *The patient care partnership.* https://www.aha.org/other-resources/patient-care-partnership

American Medical Association. (1847). *Code of medical ethics.* https://www.bioethicscourse.info/codesite/1847code.pdf

ANA. (1995). *Nursing's social policy statement.* Author.

ANA. (2015). *Code of ethics for nurses with interpretive statements.* Nursebooks.org. http://nursingworld.org/DocumentVault/Ethics-1/Code-of-Ethics-for-Nurses.html.

Beauchamp, T. L., & Childress, J. (2019). *Principles of biomedical ethics* (8th ed.). Oxford University Press.

Beauchamp, T. L., Walters, L., Kahn, J. P., & Mastroianni, A. C. (2013). *Contemporary issues in bioethics* (8th ed.). Cengage.

Bok, S. (1991). Lies to the sick and dying In T. A. Mappes & J. S. Zembaty (Eds.), *Biomedical ethics* (pp. 74–81). McGraw Hill.

Buber, M. (1965). *The knowledge of man: A philosophy of the interhuman.* Harper & Row.

Cammon, S. A., & Hackshaw, H. S. (2000). Are we starving our patients? *American Journal of Nursing, 100*(5), 43–46.

Carter, M. (2016). Deceit and dishonesty as practice: The comfort of lying. *Nursing Philosophy, 17*(3), 202–210.

CNA. (2017). *Code of ethics for registered nurses.* https://cdn1.nscn.ca/sites/default/files/documents/resources/code-of-ethics-for-registered-nurses.pdf#:~:text=The%20Canadian%20Nurses%20Association%20%28CNA%29%20Code%20of%20Ethics,receiving%20care.%20The%20Code is%20both%20aspirational%20and%20regulatory.

Conditions of Participation for Hospitals: Patient's Rights C.F.R. 42 § 482.13 (2006, Amended 2019). https://www.ecfr.gov/current/title-42/chapter-IV/subchapter-G/part-482/subpart-B/section-482.13

Ellin, J. S. (1991). Lying and deception: The solution to a dilemma in medical ethics In T. A. Mappes & J. S. Zembaty (Eds.), *Biomedical ethics* (pp. 81–87). McGraw-Hill.

Gillon, R. (1985). Autonomy and the principle of respect for autonomy. *British Medical Journal, 290,* 1806–1808.

Goldsmith, J. (1992). Virginia Henderson, RN: Humanitarian and scholar. *Reflections, 18*(1), 45.

Gretter, L. (1893). *Nightingale pledge.*

Harris, S.H. (December 10–12, 1999). *Japanese medical atrocities in World War II: Unit 731 was not an isolated aberration. International citizens' forum on war crimes and redress: Seeking reconciliation and peace for the 21st century, Tokyo, Japan*. http://www.vcn.bc.ca/alpha/speech/Harris.htm

Henderson, V. (1966). *The nature of nursing: A definition and its implications for practice, research, and education.* MacMillan.

Hippocrates. (1849). *Hippocratic oath* (F. Adams, Trans.). (Original work published ca. 400 BCE).

ICN. (2021). *The ICN code of ethics for nurses.* https://www.icn.ch/system/files/2021-10/ICN_Code-of-Ethics_EN_Web_0.pdf

Jameton, A. (1984). *Nursing practice: The ethical issues.* Prentice-Hall.

Lipkin, M. (1991). On lying to patients In T. A. Mappes & J. S. Zembaty (Eds.), *Biomedical ethics* (pp. 72–73). McGraw-Hill.

Malmin, M. (2013). Warrior culture, spirituality, and prayer. *Journal of Religion and Health, 52*(3), 740–758. https://doi.org/10.1007/s10943-013-9690-5.

Meier, L. J. (2022). Systemising triage: COVID-19 guidelines and their underlying theories of distributive justice. *Medicine, Healthcare and Philosophy: A European Journal*, 1–12. https://doi.org/10.1007/s11019-022-10101-3.

Monk, J. (June 16, 2002). Special Report: How a hospital failed a boy who didn't have to die. *The State, 8*, 9. http://www.lewisblackman.net/.

Munson, R., & Lauge, I. (2016). *Intervention and reflection: Basic issues in bioethics* (10th ed.). Cengage.

Ndugga, N., Hill, L., Artiga, S., & Haldar, S. (July 14, 2022). *Latest data on COVID-19 vaccinations by race/ethnicity.* https://www.kff.org/coronavirus-covid-19/issue-brief/latest-data-on-covid-19-vaccinations-by-race-ethnicity/#:~:text=Across%20the%2036%20states%20for,for%20Black%20people%20(59%25).

Neustadt, R. E., & Fieneberg, H. V. (2005). *The swine flu affair: Decision-making on a slippery disease.* University Press of the Pacific.

Nuremberg Military Tribunal. (October 1946–April 1949). *Trials of war criminals before the Nuremberg Military Tribunals.* Washington, DC: U.S. Government Printing Office. https://www.loc.gov/item/2011525338/.

Ortiz, E., & Siemaszko, C. (2017). Utah nurse arrested for refusing to give patient's blood to police. *NBC News.* https://www.nbcnews.com/news/us-news/utah-nurse-arrested-refusing-give-patient-s-blood-police-n798021

Patients' Rights, 38 C.F.R. § 17.33, (1982, Amended 2005). https://www.ecfr.gov/current/title-38/chapter-I/part-17/subject-group-ECFR8cadb005766bd82/section-17.33

Percival, T. (1803). *Medical ethics: A code of institutes and precepts adapted to the professional conduct of physicians and surgeons* (3rd ed.). Shrimpton.

QSEN Institute. (2018). *The Lewis Blackman Story [Video].* http://qsen.org/publications/videos/the-lewis-blackman-story/

Rhyne, B. M. (2022). Estimating lives saved by COVID vaccines. *The Digest, 5.* https://www.nber.org/digest/202205/estimating-lives-saved-covid-vaccines.

Saelee, R., Zell, E., Murthy, B. P., Castro-Roman, P., Fast, H., Ment, L., Shaw, L., Gibbs-Scharf, L., Chorba, T., Harris, L. Q., & Murthy, N. (2022). Disparities in COVID-19 vaccination coverage between urban and rural counties – United States. *Morbidity and Mortality Weekly Report, 71*(9), 335–340. https://doi.org/10.15585/mmwr.mm7109a2.

Schroeder, J., Waytz, A., & Epley, N. (2017). Endorsing help for others that you oppose for yourself: Mind perception alters the perceived effectiveness of paternalism. *Journal of Experimental Psychology. General, 146*(8), 1106–1125. https://doi.org/10.1037/xge0000320.

Shiffrin, S. V. (2000). Paternalism, unconscionability doctrine, and accomodation. *Philosophy & Public Affairs, 29*(3), 205–250.

Shuster, E. (1997). Fifty years later: The significance of the Nuremberg Code. *New England Journal of Medicine, 337*, 1436–1440. http://www.nejm.org/doi/full/10.1056/NEJM199711133372006.

Siddharth, S., Rajesh, S., & Tamonud, M. (2016). The story of Prosenjit Poddar. *Journal of Mental Health and Human Behaviour, 21*, 138–140.

Simmons, A., & Yoder, L. (2013). Military resilience: A concept analysis. *Nursing Forum, 48*(1), 17–25. https://doi.org/10.1111/nuf.12007.

Taubenberger, J. K., Kash, J. C., & Morens, D. M. (2019). The 1918 influenza pandemic: 100 years of questions answered and unanswered. *Science Translational Medicine, 11*, eaau5485. https://www.science.org/doi/10.1126/scitranslmed.aau5485?url_ver=Z39.88-2003&rfr_id=ori:rid:crossref.org&rfr_dat=cr_pub%20%200pubmed.

Thompson, G. A., Segura, J., Cruz, D., CArnita, C., & Whiffen, L. H. (2022). Cultural differences in patients' preferences for paternalism: Comparing Mexican and American patients' preferences for and experiences with physician paternalism and patient autonomy. *International Journal of Environmental Research and Public Health, 19*, 10663. https://doi.org/10.3390/ijerph191710663.

United States Holocaust Memorial Museum. (n.d.). *The doctors trial: The medical case of the subsequent Nuremberg proceedings.* https://encyclopedia.ushmm.org/content/

en/article/the-doctors-trial-the-medical-case-of-the-sub-sequent-nuremberg-proceedings

Veatch, R. M. (2012). *The basics of bioethics* (3rd ed.). Pearson Education.

Veatch, R. M., & Guidry-Grimes, L. K. (2020). *The basics of bioethics* (4th ed.). Routledge.

Ward, J. (2011). Nietzxche's value conflict: Culture, indivudual, synthesis. *Journal of Neietzxche Studies, 41*, 2–23.

Weindling, P. (1996). Human guinea pigs and the ethics of experimentation: The BMJ's correspondent at the Nuremberg medical trial. *British Medical Journal, 313*(7070), 1467–1470. https://www.ncbi.nlm.nih.gov/pubmed/8973237.

Wells, K. (2013). Nietzsche's society. *Stance, 6*, 53–61.

Weyers, W. (2007). *The abuse of man: An illustrated history of medical experimentation*. Ardor Scribendi.

World Medical Association. (2022). *WMA international code of medical ethics*.

Yates, J. F., & de Oliveria, S. (2016). Culture and decision making. *Organizational Behavior and Human Decision Processes, 136*, 106–118.

Zomorodi, M., & Foley, B. J. (2009). The nature of advocacy vs. paternalism in nursing: Clarifying the 'thin line'. *Journal of Advanced Nursing, 65*(8), 1746–1752. https://doi.org/10.1111/j.1365-2648.2009.05023.x.

Developing Principled Behavior: Acquiring, Internalizing, and Applying Moral Values

Acquiring and internalizing moral values is a developmental process that occurs in the context of relationships within family, society, culture, and other groups such as religious, educational, and professional organizations. Understanding and applying these values in various life situations requires conscious reflection and practice. Part II discusses processes of values clarification, moral development, and ethical decision making with its application to clinical situations. Because personal values and moral development influence perceptions and decisions, readers are encouraged to become aware of their own values and to examine perspectives of moral development in light of the ethical theories and principles presented in Part I. This knowledge enables readers to be more conscious of personal values and begin to be more sensitive to the perspectives, decision-making abilities, cultural context, and tendencies of self and others. Understanding personal values enables nurses to more clearly identify how their values and beliefs align with the moral norms of the nursing profession.

4

Values Clarification for Ethical Nursing Practice

*As your actions are informed by your awareness of values, your thinking and your ideas
are shaped and changed by your experiences with those actions.*

(Chinn, 2013)

OBJECTIVES

After completing this chapter, the reader should be able to:

1. Define and differentiate personal values, societal values, professional values, organizational values, and moral values.
2. Discuss how values are acquired.
3. Discuss self-awareness as a tool for living an ethical life.
4. Explain the place of values clarification in nursing.
5. Describe values conflict and its implications for nursing care.

6. Describe the interaction among personal, professional, and institutional values.
7. Discuss the importance of attending to both personal values and patient values.
8. Discuss elements of codes of nursing ethics that speak to the importance of awareness of and adherence to personal and professional values.

INTRODUCTION

Principled behavior flows from personal values that guide and inform our responses, behaviors, and decisions in all areas of our lives. Professional values are embedded in professional codes of ethics and standards of practice for nurses and form the foundation of ethical nursing practice. Ethical decision making requires a keen awareness of self that includes knowing what we value, believe, or consider important, as well as knowledge of ethical theories, principles, and the moral values of the profession. Nurses need to be grounded in strong personal values that are aligned with the standards of the profession to competently address ethical challenges that arise from societal changes, globalization, health disparities, and issues of equity, equality, diversity, and social justice (ANA, 2015, Provisions 1.2, 5.6, 9.9; CNA, 2017, Part I.G.1; ICN, 2021, Elements 1.8, 2.5). The branch of philosophy that studies the nature and types

of values is called **axiology**, a word that comes from the Greek meaning *worth* or *worthy*. Axiology includes the study of values in art, known as *esthetics;* in human relations and conduct, known as *ethics;* and in relation to beliefs regarding the relationship with the divine, known as *religion*. This chapter asks readers to conscientiously examine personal values and beliefs, how they influence the way we relate to self and others within personal and professional arenas, and how congruent they are with the values of the nursing profession.

WHAT ARE VALUES?

Values are ideals, beliefs, customs, modes of conduct, qualities, or goals that are highly prized or preferred by individuals, groups, or society. They are abstract concepts that reflect what is meaningful and important to us. Values are learned in both conscious and unconscious ways and become part of a person's makeup.

They manifest as subjective preferences or dispositions that motivate and guide behavior and decisions. Values become "real," or actualized, when they are expressed through the ways we behave and the choices we make in the context of daily life. Our preferences and the hierarchical nature of values become evident when we are faced with choices. For example, if both comfort and appearance are valued in how we dress, the hierarchy becomes evident when a person chooses to wear a more restrictive suit rather than a more relaxed casual outfit for a professional interview. Our values influence choices and behavior, whether or not we are conscious that the values are guiding the choices. Values provide direction and meaning to life and a frame of reference for integrating, explaining, and evaluating new experiences, thoughts, and relationships. Values may be expressed overtly, as espoused behaviors or verbalized standards, or they may manifest in an indirect way through verbal and nonverbal behavior.

Moral Values

As previously noted, moral thought implies thoughtful reflection about what is right and wrong, good and bad. **Moral values** are the standards or principles that guide individuals in evaluating what is considered right and good or wrong and bad. They are acquired within family and cultural groups, through religious or philosophical orientation, and through aligning with professional norms and values. Moral values reflect our character and govern the choices we make when faced with ethical issues or dilemmas.

ACQUIRING VALUES

Personal ethical behavior flows from values held by an individual that develop over time. Cultural, ethnic, familial, environmental, educational, and other experiences of living help shape our values. We begin to learn and incorporate values into our beings at an early age and continue the process throughout our lives. As noted earlier, values are acquired in both conscious and unconscious ways. Values may be learned in a conscious way through instruction by parents, teachers, religious leaders, educators, and professional and social group leaders. Many values are formally adopted by groups and are written in professional codes of ethics, religious doctrines, societal laws, and statements of an organization's philosophy. Socialization and role modeling,

which are other ways in which values are acquired, lead to more subconscious learning. Some values stay with us throughout much of our life, and others may change or be altered in response to personal development and experiences. Freely choosing those values that we most cherish and relinquishing those that have little meaning is an important step in values formation (Howard, 2016; Lewis, 2007).

Because values become part of who we are, they often enter into our decision making in less-than-conscious ways. We constantly make judgments that reflect our values, though not always realizing that we have a given set of values or that these values are affecting our decisions (Engebretson & Ahn, 2022; Sastrawan et al., 2021; Schoof & Clark, 2018). Becoming aware of our values is an important step in being able to make clear and thoughtful decisions and is an essential component of developing the moral integrity needed for professional nursing practice. In the area of ethical decision making, knowing our own values in a conscious way and being able to help others name their values clearly are particularly important.

ASK YOURSELF

How Have Your Values Developed?

Think of three ideals or beliefs that you hold dear in your personal life. Try to trace each belief or ideal back to the earliest time in your life when you were aware of its importance or presence.

- When and how did you learn to view each belief or ideal as important?
- How have they changed or evolved?
- Where do you find your support for them?
- How prevalent do you think these beliefs or ideals are among other people?
- What do you think of people who hold different beliefs or ideals?
- Think of a time in your life when one of these beliefs or ideals was challenged. How did you feel? How did you react? Were your beliefs modified due to this challenge?

SELF-AWARENESS

Ethical relationships with others begin with self-knowledge and the willingness to honestly and appropriately express that awareness to others. Self-knowledge is an ongoing, evolving process that requires us to make a commitment to know the truth about ourselves and to be aware of how our perceptions affect our sense of what we consider true in a given situation. This is not an easy commitment to make. Although the truth can be painful at times, paradoxically, it can also set us free. As our perceptions change, our idea of what is true may also change. Keep in mind that most situations are not black and white. All sides are present in each experience. Like the aperture of a camera, what we see in any situation depends on the lens we are using, how close or far we are standing, and the angle from which we are looking. From this perspective, there can be many views of a situation, depending on how many people are picturing it. Awareness of the particular lens through which we view the world enables us to identify and better understand our own responses in a situation. Understanding that there can be different views and openly sharing individual perspectives help us appreciate the truth inherent in each perspective.

The term *values clarification* refers to the process of becoming more conscious of and naming what we value or consider worthy. It is an ongoing process that is grounded in our capacity for reflective, intelligent, self-directed behavior (Burkhardt, 2022; Lewis, 2007; Wocial, 2018). By focusing time, energy, and attention to reflecting on our values, we shed light on our personal perspective and discover our own answers to many concerns and questions. Reflecting on what we hold dear or consider worthy requires us to pay attention to what we think (the cognitive self), what we feel (the affective self), and, ultimately, how we act (the behavioral self). Values clarification can be approached in a variety of ways that engage both our thinking and feeling sense. For example, we can ponder what is meaningful in our lives, consider what we believe about what is right or wrong, or identify characteristics of people whom we admire. This reflection helps us become aware of what we hold dear. A more structured way of identifying values is to review a list of value words such as *integrity, peace, love, kindness, health, family, justice, caring, autonomy, truth*, and *friendship* and then list them in order of importance or select the two or three values from the list that are most important to us. Developing a personal value portrait (Gibson, 2008) offers another approach to identifying values. This process, which focuses on delineating personal and professional values, begins with writing down characteristics we admire in

ourselves and others, characteristics we respect in others, and characteristics we consider undesirable in others. The next part of the process is to rank the values on each list in order of importance and, after reflecting on these lists, to develop a brief statement or description of personal values. The process continues with identifying and rank-ordering personal and professional responsibilities, obligations, and loyalties in relation to the identified personal values. After reflection, these are combined into a statement that provides a personal value portrait.

Engaging in deep reflection regarding our values requires us to consider both what we think or believe is right and valuable, and also to pay attention to how we feel about these beliefs. As we become more aware of our core values, we also realize that we make choices about what we consider most worthy and that these choices may shift to some degree in level of importance over time. Although identifying and naming what we value is essential to values clarification, the process also requires that we observe and reflect on how we live these values and whether our beliefs and actions are internally consistent with these beliefs. Is there congruence between what we say we hold dear and how we behave? Awareness of circumstances in which our actions are not fully aligned with our values enables us to take corrective action. This may mean adjusting our behavior in the situation or choosing to remove ourselves from the situation, if possible.

ASK YOURSELF

Internal Consistency Among Beliefs, Choices, and Actions

A report in WebMD on September 18, 2021, noted that a hospital system in Arkansas that required COVID-19 vaccine as part of employment received a large number of vaccine exemption requests for the vaccine that was significantly disproportionate to what they had seen with the flu vaccine. The majority of these requests cited religious exemption due to the use of fetal cell lines in the development of the vaccine. Noting that many commonly used drugs used fetal cell lines during research and development the hospital provided a religious attestation form for individuals requesting a religious exemption that included a list of 30 of these drugs (including medications such as Tums, aspirin, ibuprofen, acetaminophen, albuterol, and Claritin). They ask these employees to attest that their religious belief is "consistent and true" and that they will not use any of the medications listed (https://www.webmd.com/vaccines/covid-19-vaccine/news/20210918/some-medications-also-tied-to-religious-vaccine-exemption).

- In your understanding what does being internally consistent between beliefs/values and choices/actions mean?
- What choices and actions would demonstrate internal consistency with the stated beliefs underlying the request for religious exemption noted in the example above?
- Consider a challenging situation in your life in which you demonstrated internal consistency between your strongly held beliefs and your actions or choices. What factors contributed to your choosing actions consistent with your values?
- Identify areas in your life in which some of your choices and behaviors are inconsistent with strongly held values and beliefs. What factors contribute to this inconsistency?
- What would help you become more aware of where there is congruence or incongruence among your values, motivations, and behaviors?

No one set of values is appropriate for everyone; we must appreciate that values clarification may lead to different insights for different people (Engebretson & Ahn, 2022; Gibson, 2008). The extent to which we appreciate our own values is the foundation from which we can begin to understand the values of another. Engaging in values clarification promotes a closer fit between our words and actions, enabling us to more clearly "walk our talk," thus enhancing personal integrity. As noted in Chapter 2, integrity refers to adherence to moral norms that is sustained over time. Trustworthiness and consistency of convictions, actions, and emotions that are implicit in integrity are addressed in numerous ways in nursing codes of ethics (examples include ANA, 2015, Provisions 1.2, 5.4; CNA, 2017, Part I A.3, G.2; ICN, 2021, Element 1.8, 2.8).

As previously noted, the process of gaining clarity about what we treasure addresses both the cognitive and the affective domains. By becoming more conscious of our own behavior and feelings, we learn to discern whether our choices flow from chosen values or are the result of preconditioning and following the values of others. Assessment of personal values requires a readiness and willingness to take an honest look at our ideals and behaviors; at our words, actions, and motivation; and at the congruence and incongruence among them. One goal of the process is to be aware of and choose our own values rather than to merely act out prior conditioning.

Enhancing Self-Awareness

Self-awareness is the ultimate tool for living a personally ethical life (Fig. 4.1). Values clarification and self-awareness go hand in hand. The first and most important step in awareness of the self is the conscious intention to be aware. Being conscious of our thoughts, feelings, physical and emotional responses, and insights in various situations can promote appreciation of our values. Conversely, by identifying and analyzing personal values, we become more self-aware (Burkhardt & Nagai-Jacobson, 2022; Schoof & Clark, 2018). We can enhance insight by developing the ability to step back and observe what is going on in a particular situation—being aware of self and aware of our reactions in the present moment. Self-awareness can begin with as simple an act as tuning in to our breathing—noting its

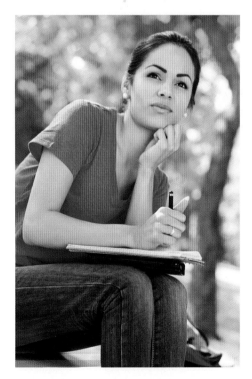

Fig. 4.1 Self-Reflection Regarding Personal Values. From (©iStock.com/Steve Debenport.)

rate, rhythm, depth, and other characteristics without any effort to change it. It is a way of becoming conscious of an act that usually occurs quite unconsciously. Another way to become more aware is to pay attention to how we are feeling physically and emotionally in a given circumstance—to name the feelings without judging them. We might ask, "What do I think I am reacting to here, and can I identify where that reaction comes from?" For example, when you see a beautiful sunset, you might note a feeling of peace, exhilaration, or relaxation and realize you are responding to beauty, with an ensuing memory that your mother was always one to be observant of beauty in her world. You thus recognize that you learned this value, at least in part, from your mother. Introspection, observation, reflection, meditation, journaling, art, writing, therapy, reading, discussion groups, and feedback from others assist us in expanding self-awareness.

Individual reflection and discussion with another person or in small groups help us to become more aware of and to analyze our values. Group discussion enables us to react and to hear the reactions of others. Such processes may lead us to see more clearly those values we have accepted because of conditioning and to articulate better those values we have chosen for ourselves. These processes may also lead us to modify our perspective based on the insights of others. Other tools that open our perspective include taking the other side of a debate, interviewing people with differing opinions, walking in another's shoes and defending their position, and asking for feedback on our own positions. Another way to look at values is to ask general questions such as:

- If I knew I would die in six weeks, what would I be doing today?
- If I had to leave my house and could only take three things with me, what would they be?
- Where would I like to be 5, 10, or 20 years from now?

Journaling

Journals are personal records or notes that may include thoughts, feelings, experiences, ideas, reactions, dreams, drawings, and other expressions related to what is going on in one's life. They may be kept on a regular or periodic basis, may be structured or unstructured, and may include art as well as words. For many people, keeping a diary or journal of experiences and personal reactions to situations is a useful tool for developing awareness. Many books are available to guide someone new to

journaling, and readers are encouraged to explore these resources. Box 4.1 offers guidelines that may help students utilize the journaling process to gain insight into personal values. When writing in a journal, let your thoughts flow as freely as possible without censoring or judging what you are writing. Allow yourself time and privacy when you are journaling, and keep the journal in a place where you feel comfortable that you can control who has access to it. Commit to journaling on a regular basis. Recognize that journaling is a personal process and go with your own style. If a format such as that suggested in Box 4.1 helps you, go for it! If not, write as the thoughts flow from you.

BOX 4.1   Journaling for Values Awareness

- Describe a situation in your personal or professional experience in which you felt uncomfortable or felt that your beliefs or values were being challenged, or in which you felt your values were different from those of others involved.
- As you record the situation, include how you felt physically and emotionally at the time you experienced the situation.
- Write down your feelings as you remember the situation. Are your reactions now any different from when you were actually in this situation?
- What personal values do you identify in the situation? Try to remember where and from whom you learned these values. Do you totally agree with the values, or is there anything about them that you question or wonder about their validity?
- What values do you think were being expressed by others involved? Were they similar to or different from your values?
- What do you think you reacted to in the situation?
- Can you remember having similar reactions in other situations? If yes, how were the situations similar or different?
- How do you feel about your response to the situation? Is there anything you would change if you could repeat the scene? Rewrite the scene with the changes. What might be the consequences of these changes?
- How do you feel with the new scenario?
- What do you need to do to reinforce behaviors, ideals, beliefs, or qualities that you have identified as personal values in this situation? When and how can you do this?

VALUES IN PROFESSIONAL SITUATIONS

Ethical codes delineate the moral values of a profession. Although these codes may vary somewhat in different counties, the moral fabric of nursing remains congruent worldwide (Ilaslan et al., 2021; Sastrawan et al., 2021; Weis & Schank, 2017).

Ethical codes for nursing worldwide delineate core values that underlie the ethical practice of nursing with individuals, groups, and society both locally and globally. These values include caring, honesty, integrity, autonomy, accountability, human dignity, responsibility, advocacy, maintaining competence, reducing health disparities, and social justice. Nurses are expected to be familiar with and "adhere to the values, moral norms, and ideals of the profession, to embrace them as part of what it means to be a nurse" (ANA, 2015, p. vii).

The ethical nature of nursing decisions, behaviors, and overall quality of care are measured in so far as they are congruent with nursing codes of ethics. Professional identity as a nurse is grounded in internalizing the moral norms and values of the profession (ANA, 2015, p. vii; CNA, 2017, Part A. G. 1; ICN, 2021, Element 1.8). An instrument such as *The Nurses Professional Values Scale-3* (Weis & Schank, 2017) can be used to identify the level of importance nurses ascribe to various components of the ethical standards of the nursing profession. The scale consists of 28 items, each of which is a short statement reflecting a provision in the *Code of Ethics for Nurses with Interpretive Statements* (ANA, 2015). The score received upon completing the scale is an indication of a nurse's professional values. Although this scale is based on the *American Nurses Association Code of Ethics* (ANA, 2015), the values identified in the scale are pertinent to nursing practice globally (Asiandi et al., 2021; Ilaslan et al., 2021; Sastrawan et al., 2021). As noted above, personal and professional values both influence our behaviors and decisions as we engage in the ethical practice of nursing. Articulating personal beliefs and values along with our level of commitment to professional values enables us to more consciously integrate the two.

Developing insight into our values improves our ability to make value decisions and enhances our **moral agency**. Moral agency refers to a nurse's ability to act morally and promote positive outcomes for patients, basing actions and decisions on internalized principles and knowledge of right and wrong, good and bad. Because these values are internalized, they become part of our identity. Shedding light on our values enables us to be more conscious in exercising our moral agency and in being accountable for our actions.

A fundamental aspect of ethical behavior is being conscious of our motives. Knowing and appreciating our own value system provide a basis for understanding how we respond within decision-making situations. It also enables us to acknowledge similarities and differences in values when interacting with others. This ultimately promotes more effective communication and care. Commitment to developing greater awareness of personal values enables us to be more effective in facilitating the process with others. In the professional realm, these others may be staff, patients, families, or institutions.

Values Conflict

When personal values are at odds with those of patients, colleagues, or the institution, internal or interpersonal conflict may result. This can subsequently affect patient care. Dealing in an effective way with values conflict requires conscious awareness of our own values, as well as awareness of the perceived values of the others involved. Such awareness enables us to be more alert to situations in which we are judging the behaviors of others according to our own values, or in which our personal values are being imposed upon another. When differences in values are identified, we can choose to respond to another's viewpoint in a way that seeks understanding and common ground, rather than reacting in a "knee-jerk" fashion. In this way, the integrity of the caring relationship can be maintained. In situations of values conflict, codes of ethics direct nurses to examine the source of the conflict and work toward resolution where possible while preserving professional integrity. When there is a serious conflict with the nurse's moral beliefs, the nurse provides compassionate and competent care while facilitating alternative care arrangements (ANA, 2015, Provision 2.2; CNA, 2017, Part I.G.7; ICN, 2021, Element 2.8).

The following Case Presentation provides an example of values conflict. As you read the case, think about the values that are evident in the situation. Put yourself in the position of each of the participants and ask yourself what you might do if you were in their shoes.

CASE PRESENTATION

Impact of Beliefs and Values on Care

Nine-year-old Benton is a patient in the pediatric unit with a diagnosis of terminal-stage Ewing sarcoma. He has three sisters, ages seven, six, and three, who are presently being cared for by a grandmother. His father is self-employed and works long hours. His mother has never worked outside the home. Both parents have high school educations, and their primary activities outside of family are church related. They belong to a small nondenominational rural church and state that they hold fast to what is taught in the Bible and put their faith in the word of God.

Before his illness, Benton, a healthy child, had been brought to the clinic only for acute health concerns. Shortly after entering second grade two years ago, he began limping. The family attributed the limp to a playground injury. When he continued to complain of pain and the limp persisted after three months, his mother took him to a local health clinic. Above-the-knee amputation followed diagnosis, but metastasis was evident in nine months. Chemotherapy has only been palliative.

The physician has discussed Benton's poor prognosis with the parents, recommending comfort care. The parents say they want everything possible to be done for him, and the father conducts nightly prayer sessions at Benton's bedside, affirming that God is healing Benton. His father refuses to allow staff to speak with Benton regarding fears or concerns about his condition. This directive has presented concerns for nurses, especially when Benton asked the nurse whether he is going to die. When asked what Benton has been told, the father responds,

"He knows God is trying us and we must have faith." The mother, who appears less confident of healing, is there 24 hours a day. She supervises Benton's care relentlessly, at times irritating staff with questions and demands. She keeps a notebook record of her son's care, including medication, times of care, intake and output, and personal assessments. Although Benton used to talk to staff, he now appears frightened and remains quiet, sleeping off and on.

Think About It
Dealing with Values Conflict
Respond to these questions from the vantage point of the nurse in the preceding Case Presentation:

- What is your first personal reaction to this situation? Identify your values relative to the situation.
- What do you perceive to be the values of each person involved? Which values might you support or affirm and why?
- Identify value differences that might lead to conflict. Give specific examples of how such a conflict can potentially affect relationships and patient care.
- Describe specific nursing interventions aimed at managing the conflict in a professional manner, and give examples of how codes of nursing ethics would guide such actions.
- Describe your own strengths and limitations as you consider dealing with this situation.

Impact of Institutional Values

Nurses need to be conscious of both the spoken and unspoken values in their work settings. **Overt values** of individual institutions and organized healthcare systems are explicitly communicated through philosophy and policy statements. Values may also be implicit in expectations that are not in writing; these are called **covert values**. Covert values may be unspoken and sometimes unconscious expectations that are often discovered only as one encounters attitudes or controversies within a particular work setting. For example, a new nurse may learn of an expectation on the unit to regularly skip lunch and breaks to avoid overtime (even though nurse self-care is part of the written

philosophy of the institution) only after working in the setting for several days.

The obligation to attend to patient care and well-being is embedded in both personal and professional nursing ethics. However, nurses may find that the ability to act on their values is restricted within healthcare institutions where they work. For example, a nurse who values personalized care that focuses on patient needs may be at odds with the attitudes and expectations of an institution that places institutional goals, such as doing more with less, above providing excellent nursing care. The complex organization and multiple goals of these institutions, particularly large healthcare corporations, may create expectations that subordinate patient care goals to institutional goals and limit a nurse's ability to provide care the nurse believes to be for the moral good of patients (Kelly & Porr, 2018; Liaschenko & Peter, 2016). Readers are encouraged to review how ethical codes address a nurse's responsibility for the safety and integrity of both self and patient when faced with such situations (ANA, 2015, Provision 5.4; CNA, 2017, Part I.A.7, A.8. B.5; ICN. 2021, Element 2.10).

Accepting employment implies a willingness to work within the value system of the organization—both overt and covert. Thus, when seeking employment, nurses should identify how their personal values align with or are different from those of the institution. Consider, for example, Anton, a nurse who accepts a position at a health center because the center publicizes a commitment to providing quality care to all patients. Within two months he notices that patients with Medicaid cards are kept waiting longer than those with private insurance and are treated rudely by many of the staff. When he initiates teaching with Medicaid patients, he is told not to waste his time because "those people won't change their ways." Overtly, the health center is committed to quality care for all patients; however, the covert values reflect different attitudes toward and levels of care for those receiving Medicaid. Anton's values of providing quality care for all may prompt a variety of responses in this situation. He may compromise his values if he wants to get along with other staff and do well in the job, he may expend much energy challenging the institutional value system, or he may decide that he cannot continue to work in this system.

What we believe and how we think about a job are important and have a direct impact on job performance (Demarest & Schoof, 2011). Such internal belief systems tend to shape people's thinking and direct them to do what they think is right, regardless of the employer's philosophy. These authors suggest that it is better to identify what is valued by employers, that is, where they stand and what they pay attention to and reward, and then to decide whether one can work in that environment. In healthcare settings, for example, there are three primary ways to approach patient care: focus on meeting patient needs (intrinsic care), focus on doing all the tasks (extrinsic care), and focus on following the rules (systemic care). If there is a conflict between our values regarding patient care and the values of the institution, physician, and family, we may experience moral distress. **Moral distress** is the reaction to a situation in which there are moral problems that seem to have clear solutions, yet we are unable to follow our moral beliefs because of external restraints. This distress is often evidenced in anger, dissatisfaction, frustration, and poor performance in the work setting and may lead to burnout. Moral distress is discussed further in Chapter 7.

ASK YOURSELF

How Should Values Influence Job Selection?

Maria, a recently divorced mother of three, desperately needs to return to work, but nursing jobs in her area are scarce. There is one opening at a nursing home that allows physician-assisted death. The job, which has excellent salary and benefits, including onsite child care, looks great to Maria, except that ending one's own life is against her religious and personal beliefs. A friend who works at the nursing home said that, unless they are short staffed, Maria would not have to attend to these patients if she had objections.

- What dilemmas are evident in this situation?
- What are the value differences? What guidance can Maria find in nursing codes of ethics?
- What are your values related to this situation?
- What factors should Maria consider in deciding whether to take the job?

CASE PRESENTATION

Differences in Personal and Organizational Values

Joan has been the nurse manager of her unit for the past 10 years and is highly regarded by the hospital's administration. For the past several months, however, she has been feeling more frustrated and less satisfied with her work because of staffing cuts and other institutional decisions related to patient care priorities. Attending to patient needs has always been the most rewarding part of her job. However, recently she feels that she has been forced to overlook these needs and attend more to the needs of the organization. She considers leaving, but she has seniority, good benefits, and two children to support. She is also aware that her distress at work is affecting her family because she carries a lot of the frustration home with her.

Think About It
How Values Affect Choices
- Identify values evident in this situation. Which of these reflect your personal values?
- What conflicts might arise from these values?

- What do you think Joan should do? Support your decision with ethical reasoning.
- If you were in Joan's position, what beliefs, ideals, or goals would guide you in deciding to stay or leave? Identify the potential consequences of each choice.
- What guidance might Joan receive from ethical codes such as ANA (2015, Provision 5), CNA (2017, Part I.B.5), and ICN (2021, Element 2.4)?

Clarifying Values with Patients

Values of both nurses and patients influence patient care situations. Because patients are the recipients and consumers of healthcare, it is good to know what they expect or value. Patient and healthcare provider perceptions of what constitutes quality of care can be quite different. Great discrepancies in these perceptions may lead to patient dissatisfaction. This can have a variety of consequences, including affecting a patient's attitude and decisions regarding following recommendations for care and treatment (which may affect recovery), marring the reputation of the agency, and increasing the potential for malpractice litigation. Consider the possible conflict of values and resulting dissatisfaction when patients expect nurses to spend time with them and the institution puts more emphasis on getting the tasks done, or when patients need to share their stories and nurses are focused on entering standard history data into the computer.

ASK YOURSELF

What Would You Do?

- You are busy, and two call lights go on at the same time. What factors enter into deciding which one you respond to first?
- Consider that in this situation one patient is in serious condition and has been verbally abusive to staff, whereas the other is not quite as serious and is someone you really enjoy being with. Which patient would you respond to first and why?
- Your patients let you know how much they appreciate the extra care and time you give them compared with the other nurses. At the same time, your evaluation is coming up, and your supervisor has indicated that you need to be more efficient with your time. What would you do in this situation and why?
- How would nursing codes of ethics inform your decision in these situations? Be specific.

When working with patients regarding healthcare decisions, nurses need to be aware of their personal values and patients' values pertaining to health. When the health values of the nurse and those of the patient are different, the patient may become labeled as uncooperative, self-destructive, noncompliant, ignorant, or unwilling to take responsibility for her or his own health. Attentiveness to cultural and religious values is especially important in this regard. Refer to Chapter 18 for a discussion of transcultural and spiritual issues.

Nurse theorist Dr. Nola Pender and colleagues (Murdaugh et al., 2018) discuss the role of values in health promotion. They note that it is important for nurses to know their personal values and to avoid imposing their values on patients. Consider, for example, an obese patient with terminal lung cancer and a prognosis of three to six months to live, who continues to smoke and is a confirmed agnostic. If priorities on the care plan include weight loss, smoking cessation, and facilitating the patient's making peace with God, the nurse must consider whether personal values are being imposed on the patient.

Self-awareness enables the nurse to be more effective in helping patients identify what is important to them without passing judgments about differences between patient and nurse values. Gaining greater clarity about values lessens the chance of inconsistency, confusion, misunderstanding, and inadequate decision making on the part of patients and families, and enables them to establish and work toward health goals that are aligned with what is important to them. The ability to make informed choices, including the process of informed consent, is enhanced by being clear about what we value.

Assisting patients to identify and to act from what they believe and value related to health, health promotion, and healthcare options is a key aspect of nursing care. Patient values become evident as nurses listen carefully to what patients say; observe their behaviors and reactions; and thoughtfully support their exploration of questions, issues, and concerns. Pender's *Health Promotion Model* (Murdaugh et al., 2018) provides a focused process of identifying patient values related to health beliefs and behaviors and incorporating these values in care planning. The goals of this process include helping patients achieve greater consistency among values, attitudes, and behaviors and to understand the personal and social consequences of acting on current values. Grounded in the understanding that persons have the capacity for reflective self-awareness and that they value growth in directions they view as positive, the model guides nurses in planning health-related activities with patients that are congruent with their current values and allow for the possibility for self-initiated changes in value hierarchies that may lead to healthier lifestyles.

SUMMARY

This chapter has discussed the importance of self-awareness regarding values and the valuing process. Values are learned and change in response to life situations as a person develops. The process of values clarification enables persons to begin to identify and choose their own values rather than merely act according to prior conditioning. The interaction between personal values and those of patients, organizations, and the nursing profession can affect job satisfaction and patient care. The reader is encouraged to explore various processes that facilitate values clarification, both those presented in this chapter and those found in other resources.

CHAPTER HIGHLIGHTS

- Values are highly prized ideals, behaviors, beliefs, or qualities that are shaped by culture, ethnicity, family, environment, and education and are acquired in both conscious and unconscious ways.
- The process of incorporating values into one's life begins at an early age and continues throughout life. Some values remain consistent, whereas others change in response to growth and life experiences.
- Awareness of personal values undergirds the ability to make clear and thoughtful decisions and enables us to acknowledge similarities and differences in values when interacting with others, thus promoting more effective communication, care, and facilitation of values clarification with others.
- Values clarification is not intended to instill values; rather, the aim is to facilitate awareness of personal values to move toward the point of choosing our own values rather than merely reacting from prior conditioning.
- Nurses need to be grounded in strong personal values that are aligned with the ethical standards of the profession to competently address ethical challenges that arise from societal changes, globalization, health

disparities, and issues of equity, equality, diversity, and social justice.
- Dealing effectively with values conflict requires attention to personal values, the perceived values of others, and the ability to recognize both overt and covert expressions of values in a situation.
- Congruence between personal values and those of an institution is an important consideration for a nurse seeking employment.
- Assisting patients to articulate their values and beliefs is an important part of nursing care and may help prevent confusion and misunderstanding when there are differences in values between patients and healthcare providers.
- Nursing codes of ethics address the importance of awareness of and adherence to personal and professional values.

DISCUSSION QUESTIONS AND ACTIVITIES

1. A nonnursing classmate asks you why nursing students have to study values. How would you respond? Incorporate your understanding of the nature of values and how they become part of us into your response.
2. What values guide your personal life? How did you learn these values? Select something that you consider important in professional nursing practice and trace how you learned this value.
3. Discuss why values clarification is important both personally and professionally.
4. Identify the overt values of your healthcare agency and identify the overt and covert values of nurses and others within the agency. Explain the importance of knowing about both.
5. Describe a situation in which you experienced someone (it could be you) reacting from values that were not conscious at the time. How did this affect the interaction?
6. Determine the health values of three patients or people you do not know well and discuss why nurses need to be attentive to what others, particularly patients, value.
7. Describe a situation in which you experienced values conflict and how you dealt with the conflict.
8. Find current examples of public or professional figures whose personal values seem at odds with their

professional or public trust. Discuss your reaction to the discrepancy in values that you identify and the interplay between personal values and professional integrity.

9. Review the code of ethics from the ANA (2015), the CNA (2017), or the ICN (2021), whichever is most appropriate for your situation, and discuss how pertinent statements in the codes guide nurses in dealing with situations of values conflict.

10. Use values clarification exercises to help you reflect on your own values. Examples of these exercises can be found in many self-help books and online at websites such as:

http://www.ethicalleadership.org/uploads/2/6/2/6/26265761/1.4_core_values_exercise.pdf

https://carleton.ca/mentoring/wp-content/uploads/Values-Assessment-Community-College-of-Vermont.pdf

http://kathycaprino.com/wp-content/uploads/2014/04/WBDC-Values-Exercise.pdf

REFERENCES

ANA. (2015). *Code of ethics for nurses with interpretive statements.* http://nursingworld.org/DocumentVault/Ethics-1/Code-of-Ethics-for-Nurses.html

Asiandi, A., Erlina, M., Lin, Y. -H., & Huang, M. -C. (2021). Psychometric evaluation of the Nurses Professional Values Scale-3: Indonesian version. *International Journal of Environmental Research and Public Health, 18,* 8810. https://doi.org/18168810.

Burkhardt, M. A. (2022). Holistic ethics In M. A. B. Helming, D. Shields, K. A. Avino, & W. E. Rosa (Eds.), *Dossey & Keegan's Holistic nursing: A handbook for practice* (8th ed., pp. 107–120). Jones & Bartlett Learning.

Burkhardt, M. A., & Nagai-Jacobson, M. G. (2022). Spirituality and health In M. A. B. Helming, D. Shields, K. A. Avino, & W. E. Rosa (Eds.), *Dossey & Keegan's holistic nursing: A handbook for practice* (8th ed., pp. 121–144). Jones & Bartlett Learning.

Chinn, P. L. (2013). *Peace and power: Building communities for the future* (8th ed.). Jones & Bartlett Learning.

CNA. (2017). *Code of ethics for registered nurses.* https://cdn1.nscn.ca/sites/default/files/documents/resources/code-of-ethics-for-registered-nurses.pdf#:~:text=The%20Canadian%20Nurses%20Association%20%28CNA%29%20Code%20of%20Ethics,receiving%20care.%20The%20Code-deis%20both%20aspirational%20and%20regulatory

Demarest, P. D., & Schoof, H. J. (2011). *Answering the central question: How science reveals the keys to success in life, love, and leadership.* Heart Lead Publications.

Engebretson, J. C., & Ahn, H. (2022). Cultural engagement In M. A. B. Helming, D. Shields, K. A. Avino, & W. E. Rosa (Eds.), *Dossey & Keegan's holistic nursing: A handbook for practice* (8th ed., pp. 417–426). Jones & Bartlett Learning.

Gibson, P. A. (2008). Teaching ethical decision making: Designing a personal value portrait to ignite creativity and promote engagement in case method analysis. *Ethics & Behavior, 18,* 340–352.

Howard, J. P. (2016). *Values at work: Clarifying and focusing on what is most important.* CentASC Press.

ICN. (2021). *The ICN code of ethics for nurses.* https://www.icn.ch/system/files/2021-10/ICN_Code-of-Ethics_EN_Web_0.pdf

Ilaslan, E., Geçkil, E., Kol, E., & Erkul, M. (2021). Examination of the professional values of the nurse and the associated factors. *Perspectives in Psychiatric Care, 57,* 56–65. https://doi.org/10.1111/ppc.12524.

Kelly, P., & Porr, C. (2018). Ethical nursing care versus cost containment considerations to enhance RN practice. *Online Journal of Issues in Nursing, 23*(1) 10913734. https://doi.org/10.3912/OJIN.Vol23No01Man06.

Lewis, H. (2007). *A question of values: Six ways we make the personal choices that shape our lives.* (Rev. ed.). Axios Press.

Liaschenko, J., & Peter, E. (2016). Fostering nurses' moral agency and moral identity: The importance of moral community. Nurses at the table: Nursing, Ethics, and Health Policy, special report. *Hastings Center Report, 46*(5), S18–S21.

Murdaugh, C. L., Parsons, M. A., & Pender, N. J. (2018). *Health promotion in nursing practice* (8th ed.). Pearson.

Sastrawan, S., Weller-Newton, J., Brand, G., & Malik, G. (2021). The development of nurses' foundational values. *Nursing Ethics, 28*(7–8), 1244–1257. https://doi.org/10.1177/09697330211003222.

Schoof, H., & Clark, K. (2018). Living a richer life: It's all in your head. CreateSpace Independent Publishing Platform. Retrieved from www.LivingaRicherLifebook.com.

Weis, D., Schank, M.J. (2017). Development and psychometric evaluation of the nurses professional values scale-3. *Journal of Nursing Measurement.* 25(3), 400–410 https://doi.org/10.1891/1061-3749.25.3.400.

Wocial, L. D. (2018). In search of a moral community. *Online Journal of Issues in Nursing, 23*(1), 2,. 10913734.

5

Moral Development: Acquiring Moral Reasoning, Values, and Behaviors

What is firmly established cannot be uprooted.
What is firmly grasped cannot slip away.
It will be honored from generation to generation.
(Lao Tsu, Tao Te Ching, trans. 1972)

OBJECTIVES

After completing this chapter, the reader should be able to:

1. Discuss the influences of culture on values development.
2. Contrast theoretical approaches to moral development.
3. Describe and differentiate the ethic of care and the ethic of justice.
4. Evaluate the influence of moral development on ethical decision-making capacity.
5. Discuss nursing considerations related to moral development.

INTRODUCTION

Nurses frequently encounter situations that present ethical dilemmas. In some situations the "right" choice seems quite evident, whereas in other circumstances a considerable lack of clarity about what is "right" may exist. How do we come to know what is right or how to respond in a principled way in a given situation? This chapter addresses the question of how a person develops as a moral being and how values may change over time. The chapter reviews factors that influence values formation, theoretical perspectives related to moral development, and nursing considerations regarding moral development.

TRANSCULTURAL CONSIDERATIONS IN VALUES DEVELOPMENT

The worldview, or cosmology, that is characteristic of a particular culture is rooted in the culture's shared story. Cosmology is an organizing way of looking at the nature of the universe as a whole and the role of humans in it that incorporates both the physical plane and the interconnected, multidimensional universe. It is a set of assumptions about perceived reality that guide, support, and empower members of the culture. Beginning with the culture's origin story, the shared story provides a context for ascribing meaning to and determining relationships with all aspects of human experience. It is the big picture that explains how and why things are as they are and helps people understand how they can live in the world and deal with the various experiences and events of life. The worldview reflected in a culture's cosmic story influences roles and relationships among its members, between its members and other humans, and between its members and the natural and supernatural worlds. Cosmology is the way people of all cultures address the big questions of life:

- Where did we come from?
- Where are we going?
- Why am I here?
- What is the meaning of life?
- What is right and wrong?
- What is good and bad?

Moral development is a product of the sociocultural environment in which we live and develop. The sociocultural environment includes cultural, historical, familial, social, interpersonal, institutional, racial, socioeconomic, and religious influences through which we process deep experiences and acquire insights and tools that help us develop an ethical stance (Andrews, Boyle & Collins, 2020; Jensen, 2015; McFarland & Wehbe-Alamah, 2015; Srivastava, 2023). All societies have ethical systems that are developed within and shaped by the mores and worldview of the culture. Rules and principles that guide behavior and determine right and wrong vary across, and even within, different cultures (Jensen, 2015; Johnstone, 2012). In his now classic work, *The Silent Language*, Hall (1973) notes that we learn what is considered right and wrong within the culture in *formal* ways such as by precept and admonition, through *informal* processes such as role modeling, and by *technical* learning in a teacher-to-student process. Norms for etiquette and ethical behavior that are "known" within the culture may be acquired by an outsider through technical learning; however, they are often appreciated by a neophyte only when a transgression has occurred and corrections to, or sanctions for, the behavior have been imposed. An innate human capacity for developing an ethical stance to life congruent with the sociocultural world in which one lives emerges through this process.

Moral values need to be viewed from a cultural perspective (Fig. 5.1). *Culture* refers to the totality of the lifeways of a group of interacting individuals consisting of learned patterns of values, beliefs,

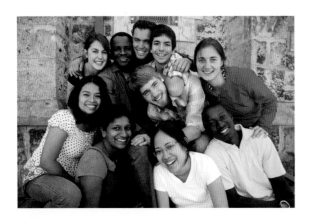

Fig. 5.1 What Is Your Cultural Identity? (From ©iStock.com/adl21.)

behaviors, and customs that are shared by that group (Engebretson & Ahn, 2022; McFarland & Wehbe-Alamah, 2015; Ray, 2016; Spector, 2017; Srivastava, 2023). Cultural communities include any groups whose members share important beliefs, values, and practices, for example, religious groups, ethnic groups, civic and professional organizations, social clubs, gangs, and healthcare institutions. Many aspects of cultural identity, reactions, and responses are unconscious; thus, self-awareness is fundamental to approaching values development from a sociocultural perspective. We begin by identifying our own cultural perspective and how it affects our nursing care. This process involves understanding that we are shaped by the shared worldview of the sociocultural groups to which we belong, as well as reflecting on our values, biases, assumptions, beliefs, attitudes, prejudices, and sense of status in relation to someone from a different culture (Doutrich et al., 2014; Srivastava, 2023). In this way, we come to better appreciate that moral constructs and approaches to moral reasoning and decision making in one culture cannot necessarily be applied universally to another culture. A value such as individual autonomy may be regarded highly in a culture that prizes independence and individualism. However, the same value may be considered contrary to the norm in a society in which persons are defined by their relation to others and high value is placed on the well-being of the group. For example, Doutrich and colleagues (2014) note that in the general Japanese population, a sense of self and self-identity derives from interconnectedness and being in relationship with others. For a person from this culture, approaching decisions from the perspective of the autonomy principle may seem uncomfortable and be perceived to be against moral norms. Similarly, understandings of principles such as justice and care may vary in different cultures. As you explore the following theories regarding the process of values development, be aware that the norms described in the early work of Kohlberg and Gilligan were derived primarily from Anglo-American and Anglo-European populations. Jensen's (2015) work offers insight into key elements of moral development in different cultures around the world. Continued exploration of moral development and what it means to be a moral person within a transcultural context such as that presented in Jensen's (2015) book is needed.

What Is Your Cultural Identity?

Our culture is part of the fabric of who we are and helps fashion our identity. Culture often influences our lives and behavior in subtle and unconscious ways. Self-reflection helps us become aware of ways that culture influences our attitudes and behaviors personally and professionally.

- How would you describe your cultural background?
- How did you develop your cultural identity? How has this identity changed over time?
- Do you consider yourself part of a dominant culture or a nondominant culture?
- Name two or three important values or beliefs that most people in your culture hold dear. How did you learn these values?
- Is there anything about your culture's history that you are proud of or ashamed of?
- Can you think of a time when your cultural norms or beliefs made it difficult for you to relate to someone from another culture?

BELIEFS AND VALUES

How does a person come to have certain values? In Chapter 4, we defined values as ideals, customs, modes of conduct, qualities, or goals that are highly prized or preferred by individuals, groups, or society. A person's values are the internalized ideas about the worthiness or desirability of something. Our view of life shapes what we value. Values derive from beliefs—ideas that one holds to be fact. Beliefs may flow from empirical observation, logic, tradition, feelings, faith, or other sources. Beliefs form our conception of the world, and they provide a framework within which perceptions occur. Together with other mental and emotional states, beliefs function as reasons for action.

How does one develop beliefs, and why does one hold onto beliefs that may seem to be illogical to other people? Plato's famous cave metaphor gives us the opportunity to think about how people begin to imagine meaning and derive beliefs, even when based on false-hoods. In *The Republic*, Socrates makes the point that people tend to hold onto beliefs even when they have no facts to back them up. People tend to attach meaning when none exists and tend to continue to believe, regardless of contradictory evidence. In Plato's "cave" analogy, Socrates envisions a dreadful scene in which

some humans have lived their entire lives underground in a cave. The entrance is high up in the cave and open to the daylight. The prisoners have been chained there since childhood, restrained in one place with their arms and legs tied. They cannot turn their heads and can only see the cave wall in front of them. There is a fire burning far up and behind them, and there are other people walking upward toward the cave opening carrying large items. The prisoners who are tied cannot see the other people or the fire, but they can see the flickering shadows of the people and the items they are carrying on the wall in front of them. Socrates asks us to imagine, if the prisoners could talk to one another, wouldn't they start to create names for the things they see on the wall and wouldn't they start to imagine what the shadows and noises might mean? They would become convinced that their beliefs were "truth." Socrates also asks what would happen if the prisoners were released and able to see the actual items being carried upward. Wouldn't they resist changing their beliefs (Plato, ca. 375 B.C.E./1997)?

What does this metaphor mean? For Socrates, the light at the opening of the cave represents truth. The people chained at the bottom of the cave are located far from the truth. Endlessly sitting there, they begin to interpret random clues and attach meaning and value to them. Given enough time, they would develop beliefs based on these fabricated meanings. The other people in the cave are climbing to the opening, moving toward knowledge of the truth. Coming out of the cave, or even moving toward the opening, the people who have been moving forward can see what is true—not a flickering shadow obscured by smoke, but objects as they really exist. Plato thus suggests that anyone who seeks knowledge must strive and move forward. He also implies that one must be careful about establishing and holding onto beliefs based primarily on imagination or tradition.

Values are derived from belief, and belief drives action. With this in mind, it is helpful to examine ideas about the origin and development of beliefs. Charles Sanders Peirce, a prolific American philosopher who was introduced in Chapter 1, proposed that doubt and belief are two states of mind that feel entirely different: belief is satisfactory and doubt is unsatisfactory. Peirce (1877) suggested that self-assurance and absolute belief (even in the presence of total ignorance) may be a satisfying mode of living to which one clings tenaciously. On the other hand, the state of doubt is intolerable. It forces a person to act until belief is attained. Peirce identified "truth" as the goal of all human inquiry. Yet the only condition that produces inquiry is one that begins when a person really questions something. Real inquiry begins with genuine doubt and ends when belief is established. Peirce proposed four basic methods of fixing belief: tenacity, authority, a priori, and reasoning.

The tenacity method of fixing belief is one in which the person obstinately adheres to beliefs already held. "The instinctive dislike of an undecided state of mind, exaggerated into a vague dread of doubt, makes [people] cling spasmodically to the views they already take" and further that "the pleasure he [or she] derives from his calm faith overbalances any inconveniences resulting from its deceptive character" (Houser & Kloesel, 1992, p. 116). The person believes what was previously believed, does not question it, and does not recognize the validity of others' beliefs.

Peirce's second method of fixing belief is the authority method. This method occurs when some institution forces its doctrines on people by repeating them perpetually and teaching them to the young. This method has been one of the chief means of upholding doctrines. Theological or political institutions sometimes have the power to prevent contrary doctrines from being taught, advocated, or expressed. This method is often accompanied by atrocities and forces people "to adopt one belief, to massacre all who dissent from it and burn their books" (Kloesel, 1986, p. 16).

Peirce calls the third method of fixing belief the a priori method. This method occurs when one sees that other people, communities, or countries have totally different beliefs. One may then begin to think about his or her own view in terms of a higher value (Houser & Kloesel, 1992). A wider sort of social feeling and understanding is generated in which previous beliefs are questioned. The willful adherence to beliefs forced by authority is given up. People talk with each other and gradually develop beliefs consistent with what Peirce calls "natural causes" (Houser & Kloesel, 1992). When the a priori method of fixing belief does not work, Peirce believes there is a tendency for people to begin inquiry based on true induction and thus begin to practice reasoning.

Reasoning is based on discovering what is real: it seeks truth. Peirce (1877) proposes that reasoning is the only method that presents a distinction between a right and a wrong way, and it fixes belief more surely than the other three methods. According to Peirce, truth is the conclusion that would be reached by every person who would pursue the same method of reasoning if taken far enough. This reasoning process is one way that moral development occurs.

ASK YOURSELF

How Do Life Experiences and Culture Influence Decision Making?

Think about a professional or personal situation in which you were faced with an ethical dilemma.

- What made it a dilemma for you?
- What life lessons or experiences helped you decide on the best course of action?
- What sociocultural factors can you identify that may have affected your decision?
- What personal cultural values or principles guided you in this process?
- When and how did you learn these values or principles?
- Are these values and principles congruent with the sociocultural world in which you grew up? In which you now live?

THEORETICAL PERSPECTIVES OF MORAL DEVELOPMENT

Discussions of moral development found in nursing literature flow primarily from frameworks developed by Kohlberg (1981) and Gilligan (1982). An overview of the work of each of these scholars is presented in this section, followed by a discussion of how they contribute to understanding moral reasoning within nursing. Fowler's (1995) work on faith development is briefly discussed regarding insights relative to values development. Kohlberg's theory, which suggests that cognitive development is necessary, though not sufficient, for moral development, draws on Piaget's (1963) work on cognitive development in children. Thus, a brief review of Piaget's theory is also included here. Jensen's (2015) cultural-developmental approach that addresses the relationship between moral development and culture is briefly described. As you review the models highlighted in this section, remember that a theory is a proposed explanation for a class of phenomena. A given theory is not necessarily truth or reality, but it does shed light on truth. Engage in critical thinking and intuitive knowing as you read, being attentive to what rings true in your

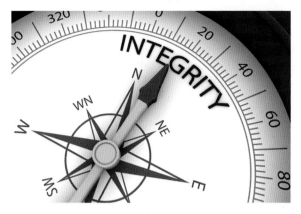

Fig. 5.2 Moral Compass. (From ©iStock.com/akinbostanci.)

own experience. Consider what each of these theories contributes to an understanding of how we develop our own moral compass to guide our ethical decisions, thus expanding our *moral intelligence*, which is the ability to process ethical information, to know right from wrong, to align personal moral values, behaviors, and goals with universal ethical principles, and to apply them in a consistent way to ethical problem solving and conflict resolution (Hadian Shirazi & Sabetsarvestani, 2021; Shabib et al., 2022; Fig. 5.2).

Piaget's Stages of Cognitive Development

Piaget's (1963) description of stages of cognitive development addresses how the mind works, that is, the development of intellectual capacities through the time of childhood, from birth to about 15 years of age. He notes that cognitive development progresses through four stages, provided there is an intact neurologic system and appropriate environmental interaction and stimuli. Although Piaget suggests specific ages for each stage, there may be variation due to environmental factors or innate intellectual capacities. Piaget's stages are:

- Sensorimotor (birth to 24 months), including six substages
- Preoperational (age two to seven years), including the preconceptual and intuitive stages
- Concrete operations (age 7–11 years)
- Formal operations (age 11–15 years)

Piaget believes that there are no further quantifiable changes in cognitive abilities after age 15. According to his theory, cognitive development progresses from thought dominated by motor activity and reflex, through

the development and use of symbolic representations such as language, to logical thought applied to concrete and then to abstract situations.

Kohlberg's Theory of Moral Development

Kohlberg's (1981) theory of moral development was derived initially from interviews conducted with boys ranging in age from early childhood to late adolescence. In these interviews, he asked participants to respond to hypothetical ethical dilemmas, such as a man considering stealing a drug to save his dying wife because he cannot afford the drug and has exhausted other possibilities of paying for it. The pattern of the responses that he observed, coupled with inferences about the reasoning behind the responses, suggested a progression in moral reasoning spanning three levels, each of which includes two stages. These levels and stages are summarized as follows.

Level I

The Preconventional Level has an egocentric focus and includes two stages. In Stage 1, The Stage of Punishment and Obedience, rules are obeyed to avoid punishment. In Stage 2, The Stage of Individual Instrumental Purpose and Exchange, conformity to rules is viewed to be in our own interest because it provides rewards. Fear of punishment is a major motivator at this level.

Level II

The Conventional Level is focused more on social conformity and includes two stages. In Stage 3, The Stage of Mutual Interpersonal Expectations, Relationships, and Conformity, concern about the reactions of others is a basis for decisions and behavior, and being good to maintain relations is important. In Stage 4, The Stage of Social System and Conscience Maintenance, we conform to laws and to those in authority because of duty, both out of respect for them and to avoid censure. For persons in this level, fulfilling our role in society and living up to the expectations of others are important, and guilt is more of a motivator than the fear of punishment noted in Level I.

There is a transitional phase between Stages 4 and 5 in which emotions begin to be recognized as a component of moral reasoning. This transition includes an awareness of personal subjectivity in moral decision making and recognition that social rules can be arbitrary and relative.

Level III

The Postconventional and Principled Level has universal moral principles as its focus. It includes two stages. In Stage 5, The Stage of A Priori Rights and Social Contract or Utility, the relativity of some societal values is recognized, and moral decisions derive from principles that support individual rights and transcend particular societal rules such as equality, liberty, and justice. In Stage 6, The Stage of Universal Ethical Principles, internalized rules and conscience reflecting abstract principles of human dignity, mutual respect, and trust guide decisions and behaviors. Persons at this level make judgments based on impartial universal moral principles, even when these conflict with societal standards.

This model proposes a linear movement through hierarchical stages, whereby each stage presupposes having completed the prior stage and is the basis for the subsequent stage. It is the pattern of a person's utilization of a particular level of reasoning that determines the stage, noting that each successive stage requires more advanced levels of moral reasoning. Research utilizing this framework indicates that not everyone moves through all the stages and that few people actually progress to the postconventional level. It is also evident within this framework that women seem to plateau in Stage 3, and most men never move beyond Stage 4 (Colby & Kohlberg, 1987; Held, 2006). Kohlberg's model is generally considered an **ethic of justice** because it is an approach to ethical decision making based on objective rules and principles in which choices are made from a stance of separateness.

Gilligan's Theory of Moral Development

Gilligan (1982, 1987) and Gilligan et al. (1994) studied the psychological development of women, arguing that women approach moral decision making from a different perspective than men do. In contrast to the justice ethic described by Kohlberg, in which personal liberty and rights are prime, Gilligan noted that women tend to utilize an ethic of caring, in which the moral imperative is grounded in relationship with and responsibility for one another. "Women's construction of the moral problem as a problem of care and responsibility in relationship rather than of rights and rules ties the development of their moral thinking to changes in their understanding of responsibility and relationship, just as the conception of morality as justice ties development to the logic of equality and

reciprocity" (Gilligan, 1982, p. 73). Gilligan's research indicated that the care perspective is the default perspective that women use and feel most comfortable with and would turn to first. Her research did not say that most women think in the care perspective, whereas most men think in the justice perspective. Rather, she suggested that many women think from the justice perspective, about one-third of the adult population are mixed between them, and, when pressed, all people can shift to the other perspective. However, the primary group who start off from the care perspective are women, so if you leave women out of a study, you leave out the care perspective.

Gilligan's research suggests a progression of moral thinking through three phases, each of which reflects greater depth in understanding the relationship between self and others, and two transitions that involve critical reevaluation of the conflict between responsibility and selfishness. The sequence described proceeds from an initial concern with survival, to focusing on goodness, to reflectively understanding care as the most adequate guide for resolving moral dilemmas.

Phase 1

In this phase, the concern for survival, the focus is on what is best for the self and includes selfishness and dependence on others. The transition to Phase 2 involves an appreciation of connectedness and that responsible choices consider the effect they have on others.

Phase 2

The phase of focusing on goodness includes a sense of goodness as self-sacrifice, in which the needs of others are often put ahead of self, and there is a sense of being responsible for others so that one is regarded positively. This focus on goodness reflects an awareness of relationship with others and may be used to manipulate others through a "see how good I have been to you" attitude. In the transition to Phase 3, there is a shifting from concern about the reactions of others to greater honesty about personal motivation and the consequences of choices and actions. Responsibility to self is considered, along with responding to the needs of others.

Phase 3

The phase of the imperative of care reflects a deep appreciation of connectedness, including responsibility to self and others as moral equals, and a clear imperative to harm no one. We take responsibility for choices, in which projected consequences and personal intention are the motivation for actions, rather than concern for the reactions of others.

Although Gilligan does not clearly associate particular ages with each phase of development, she suggests a linear process moving from one phase to the next through the transitions. This process may be associated with cognitive and emotional development as they interface with experiences of connectedness. Gilligan's model is generally considered an **ethic of care**.

Fowler's Stages of Faith Development

Fowler's (1995) discussion of faith development incorporates reflections on the development of values. His insights offer another perspective on the process of moral development. Fowler refers to faith as "a generic feature of the human struggle to find and maintain meaning, a dynamic existential stance, a way of leaning into and finding or giving meaning to the conditions of our lives" (p. 92). He notes that faith is not synonymous with religion and that it may or may not find religious expression. He suggests that faith development flows from an integration of ways of knowing and valuing. This perspective is different from the work of Piaget and Kohlberg, who conceptually separate cognition or knowing from emotion or affection, suggesting that logical knowing is separate from other important modalities of knowing. Fowler writes, "in moral judgments the valuations of actions and their consequences as well as evaluations of self in relation to the expectations of the self and others are difficult to conceive, even in formal and structural terms, apart from inherent affective or emotive elements of knowing" (1995, p. 102).

Fowler proposes six stages of faith, beginning with an intuitive faith in early childhood and progressing to universalizing faith. He notes that movement through the stages may not be limited to a linear pattern, recognizing that spiraling back to earlier stages may occur in response to various life experiences.

Stage 1

Occurring after the undifferentiated faith of infancy, Intuitive-Projective faith is image and fantasy filled. The child's understanding and feelings toward the ultimate conditions of life are intuitive and shaped by the stories, actions, moods, and examples of those around them.

Stage 2

Mythic-Literal faith reflects beliefs and moral rules and attitudes that symbolize belonging within a community or family and that are taken on with literal interpretations. Story provides a major source of meaning, and a worldview based on reciprocity and fairness is developed.

Stage 3

Synthetic-Conventional faith reflects a movement into a world beyond the family in which values and beliefs derive from experiences in interpersonal relationships. Expectations and judgments of significant others are very influential in determining the values one holds. Although a personal clustering of values and beliefs is emerging in this stage, reliance on those in traditional authority roles or on the consensus of a valued group for validation of beliefs and actions is common. Fowler notes that although this stage arises in adolescence, many adults remain here.

Stage 4

In the stage of Individuative-Reflective faith, persons must begin to take responsibility for their own beliefs, values, and commitments, differentiating personal identity and worldview from that of others. In this way, one's own values become recognized as factors in judgments on and reactions to the actions and decisions of self and others.

Stage 5

Conjunctive faith requires an opening to our inner depths in which we are able to recognize values, beliefs, and myths developed within our particular cultural, social, or religious tradition that separate one from others. This stage requires an attitude of openness to that which formerly might have been perceived as threatening, different, and other, appreciating that although our own values provide a framework for ascribing meaning, they are only relative and partial apprehensions of transcendent reality.

Stage 6

With Universalizing faith, the imperatives of absolute love and justice become primary, and we focus energy on transforming the present reality toward a transcendent actuality inclusive of all beings. Fowler notes that persons in Stage 6 are quite rare, frequently being honored more after death than in life.

Cultural-Developmental Theory

Jensen (2015) discusses the cultural-developmental approach to moral reasoning. This theory derives from a growing focus in moral psychology regarding the development of diverse kinds of reasoning across the life span and how this developmental process varies across cultures. The aim of the theory is to shed light on how culture and moral development influence and inform each other. This approach suggests a template that charts trajectories for moral development across the life span for three kinds of moral reasoning: the *Ethics of Autonomy, Community, and Divinity*. This template can accommodate different cultures, allowing for variations in the development and expression of the three ethics across the life span (Guerra & Giner-Sorolla, 2015).

The *Ethic of Autonomy* focuses on self as an individual, emphasizing concepts such as justice, fairness, and the well-being, interests, and rights of individuals and between individuals.

The *Ethic of Community* focuses on persons as members of groups, emphasizing the moral authority of the family and social or other groups, roles within families, the importance of conforming to norms and social rules, duty to others, concern with the welfare and interests of the group, and how identity is defined by social groups.

The *Ethic of Divinity* focuses on persons as spiritual or religious beings, emphasizing moral norms and values based on divine and natural law, religious rules, sacred lessons, spiritual purity, and how actions might affect one's soul or spiritual self.

Jensen (2015) notes that this approach looks at moral development with regard to both consistencies and changes in the degree to which each of the three ethics is used over the life span. In addition, the approach addresses the types of moral concepts related to each ethic used by persons of various ages. The template of the cultural-developmental approach suggests that, whereas *autonomy* reasoning remains generally stable from childhood through adulthood, the type of autonomy reasoning may change over the life span—for example, the focus on self-interest in childhood expands to include a sense of fairness and justice in relation to others as the person matures. In cultures with a strong emphasis on the interests of the group, however, elements of autonomy reasoning may decline with age as individuals align more with group identity and values. The template suggests that moral reasoning related to *community* (which includes family and other groups) rises from childhood through adulthood in degree, usage, and types of reasons. As involvement in groups beyond family increases, moral reasons expand beyond focus on roles and relationships within the family to include concern for friends, relationships with authority figures, and influences of various social groups. According to the template, moral reasoning related to *divinity* is generally lower in childhood and rises in adolescence. This occurs as adolescents develop a sense of spirituality or religiosity, which may include increased knowledge of spiritual or religious teachings and a sense of moral responsibility related to these teachings. In cultures in which divinity concepts are associated with everyday objects and activities, however, children may incorporate moral reasoning related to divinity at earlier ages. Research utilizing this theory indicates that in some groups there may be equal emphasis on two or even all three ethics. Also, an individual may link one or more of these ethics together in certain cultural contexts (Hickman & Fasoli, 2015).

Kohlberg and Gilligan suggest that values development moves from a focus on self and survival, through responding to external forces such as perceived authority or opinions of others, toward being motivated and guided by universal considerations. They also note that it is more common to find adults functioning in the middle phases of relying on external authority as guideposts for moral decisions than to find adults who base their actions and decisions on internalized universal guides that transcend codified rules. Fowler's model acknowledges that both reason and emotional response are factors in moral decision making and includes the suggestion that development may follow a pattern more spiral than linear. Within this pattern it is conceivable that, in response to life-changing experiences, persons may spiral back to an earlier stage and move through the stages again from a renewed perspective. Jensen's approach offers a broader view of moral development that takes into consideration the impact of the ethics of autonomy, community, and divinity in the development of moral reasoning within and across cultures. Cultures vary in the emphasis placed on each ethic in determining what is right or wrong. This model recognizes that the process of development of each of these ethics across the life span may differ from one culture to another. Table 5.1 provides an overview of each of these theories.

TABLE 5.1 Moral Development Theories			
Kohlberg Ethic of Justice	**Gilligan Ethic of Care**	**Fowler Faith Development**	**Jensen Cultural-Developmental**
Level I *Preconventional Level* Stage 1—Stage of punishment and obedience Stage 2—Stage of individual instrumental purpose and exchange	Phase 1 *Concern for Survival*—Focus on what is best for self Transition to Phase 2 Appreciation of connectedness and how choices affect others	Stage 1 *Intuitive-Projective Faith* Image and fantasy filled Stage 2 *Mythic-Literal Faith* Literal beliefs and rules learned from family	Ethic of Autonomy Focuses on self as an individual—justice, fairness, rights as individuals
Level II *Conventional Level* Stage 3—Stage of Mutual Interpersonal Expectations, Relationships, Conformity Stage 4—Stage of Social System and Conscious Maintenance	Phase 2 *Focusing on Goodness* Sense of self-sacrifice and being responsible for others so one is regarded positively Transition to Phase 3 Increased awareness of personal motivations and less concern about the reactions of others	Stage 3 *Synthetic-Conventional Faith* Values and beliefs derived through interpersonal relationships Stage 4 *Individuative-Reflective Faith* Begin to take responsibility for one's own faith	Ethic of Community Focuses on persons as members of groups—moral authority of family and social groups
Level III *Postconventional and Principled Level* Stage 5—Stage of A Priori Rights and Social Contract or Utility Stage 6—Stage of Universal Ethical Principles	Phase 3 *The Imperative of Care* Deep appreciation of connectedness and responsibility to both self and others	Stage 5 *Conjunctive Faith* Recognize values and beliefs of own tradition that separate one from others Stage 6 *Universalizing Faith* Imperative of absolute love and justice—focus on inclusiveness of all beings	Ethic of Divinity Focuses on persons as spiritual or religious beings—moral norms and values based on divine and natural law and religious/spiritual guidance

Because we develop values within a sociocultural context, incorporating cultural sensitivity and cultural humility into the assessment, study and evaluation of values development are imperative. As you will read in Chapter 18, **cultural sensitivity** considering sociocultural factors that support and encourage the process of moral development within the context of each person's culture, including our own culture. **Cultural humility** involves approaching people from other cultures with dignity and respect, a willingness to learn from the wisdom and knowledge of their worldview, honoring their values, beliefs, customs, and healing practice, and respectfully acknowledging differences between personal beliefs and those of the other person. Integral to cultural humility is a life-long commitment to reflect on and challenge personal cultural viewpoints, biases, prejudices, and ethnocentrism and being comfortable in the role of a learner rather than the expert in relation to understanding the other person's culture, experience, and needs (Ackerman-Barger, 2022; ANA, 2021; Srivastava, 2023). Each theory discussed offers insights into understanding how people develop moral awareness and a grounding from which they make moral decisions. A common

CASE PRESENTATION

Three Nursing Students

Tanya, Jacob, and Kuan are discussing experiences they had in their different clinical experiences.

Tanya describes her distress about her dying patient who wanted to see her dog, her close companion since her husband died 10 years prior. Tanya sensed how important the dog was to her patient and thought this would be therapeutic. Her preceptor, however, said absolutely not because there were strict rules against bringing animals into that unit. Tanya talked about trying to find a way to sneak the dog in even if she got into trouble.

Jacob notes that he was assigned to a patient in isolation. He took a photo of himself in the mask and gown on his cell phone and showed it to others in his clinical group at lunch. They thought it was a great Halloween photo and pressed him to post it on Facebook, which he did. They told him that you could not really see the patient so it was not really a Health Insurance Portability and Accountability Act violation. He is now rethinking his decision to post the photo and wishes he had not given in to the pressure from the other students. His big worry is that an instructor might see the post before he takes it down, which could have serious consequences for him.

Kuan says she got really behind because she had to spend so much time looking things up related to her patient's condition and medications. Even though the nurse on the unit told her she could leave and that the staff would finish the care for the patient, she did not want to risk having her instructor mark her down. She decided that she had better get everything done the right way so she would get a good grade, saying that her parents would expect her to do what is right and she wants them to be proud of her.

Think About It
Indicators of Values Development
- What insights into the moral perspectives of each of these students can you glean from this discussion?
- How does each theory discussed in this chapter give you an insight into the moral reasoning of each of the students? Give specific examples.
- How do you think you would behave in the situations described by the students?
- How do you think you would respond to each student if they were your classmates? What values and processes of moral reasoning would guide your response?

theme among these theories is that people with higher levels of moral development demonstrate actions that move beyond moral behavior based on social conformity and the reaction of others to actions prompted by internalized universal guides. With this in mind, where do you see evidence in the world today of role models from different backgrounds who demonstrate a high level of moral development?

NURSING CONSIDERATIONS

The literature offers an ongoing deliberation about the ethic of care versus the ethic of justice. A comparison of the two perspectives reveals that, in the justice framework, choices are made primarily from a stance of separateness, based on objective rules and principles. The care perspective arises from natural relatedness with particular others. In this perspective, choices are contextually bound and require responding to others on their terms, developing strategies that maintain connections when possible, and striving to hurt no one. Moral concern within the ethic of justice is with rights and responsibilities; in the ethic of care the concern is with

competing needs and responsibilities in relationships. Fowler's model suggests that both are important factors in making moral decisions. Rather than negating each other, the perspectives of justice and care offer different foci from which to examine problems. Offering balance to each other, these perspectives broaden the view from which to see the situation as a whole and collectively constitute a more comprehensive moral perspective (Collins, 2015, 2017; Held, 2006). The *cultural-developmental* perspective illustrates the need for a paradigm shift that requires a reconceptualization of morality and moral language away from the notion of universal morality toward the recognition of a plurality of moral voices. This perspective reflects elements of each of the other theories: justice (autonomy), care (community), and faith (divinity).

Because of nursing's concern for relational caring, an ethic of care more faithfully reflects nursing's experience than a primary focus on justice. A moral commitment to care for all persons seeking care is fundamental to nursing practice and clearly delineated in nursing standards of care and codes of ethics (e.g., ANA, 2021; ANA, 2015, Provision 1.2, 2.1;

CNA, 2017, Part 1.A.2,1.A.3,1.D.3; ICN, 2021, Element 1.1, 1.2). One of the lessons the ethic of care offers to healthcare professionals is the directive to address the needs of particular others within the circles of their relationships. Caring takes place as nurse and patient explore and address these needs within the context of a reciprocal relationship (ANA, 2021; Collins, 2015, 2017; Fowler, 2015; Held, 2006; Lachman, 2012; Lee et al., 2017; Watson, 2012; 2018). Caring requires moving beyond personal prejudices and being willing to be open to another's perspective. Part of this process is developing a caring heart, and recognizing that emotions are a constitutive part of the moral life. Considering the politics of caring, the authors noted above speak to the need to restructure our healthcare systems to value caring, which includes supporting and justly compensating those who do the sometimes emotional and taxing work of caring.

Research supports an understanding that ethical decision making is a socially and culturally mediated process that involves emotion as well as reason (Doutrich et al., 2014; Jensen, 2015; Johnstone, 2012; Ortiz & Casey, 2017). Findings from transcultural research illustrate the limitation of using assessment approaches based on a Western developmental paradigm of moral development to measure moral judgment in different cultures. Outcomes of these and other studies indicate that transcultural assessment of moral development needs to include examples of moral dilemmas and principles that are culturally specific and to include various factors that influence moral judgment such as religion and sociocultural environment.

To have an accurate understanding of a person's moral development and decision making, we need to try to understand the person's sociocultural perspective. Understanding that there are different perspectives from which moral decisions are made enables us to better appreciate our own and our patients' approaches to ethical dilemmas. We need to honestly identify our own ethical perspectives, biases, and moral development to better understand our personal responses to situations. This enables us to recognize more effectively how our approaches may differ from those of colleagues or patients. Acknowledging differences and similarities may prevent making inappropriate judgments about another's moral capabilities, and thus make possible better communication and collaboration in care.

CASE PRESENTATION

A Difficult Decision

Reba's 82-year-old father has been hospitalized with a stroke that has left him severely incapacitated, requiring total care. She has been informed that her father is ready for discharge, and the physician is suggesting that he go to a nursing home. Reba feels that she should take him home with her because her culture and faith tell her that caring for her parents is the right thing to do. She notes that her grandmother was cared for in her parents' home when she was frail and that she feels ashamed that she is even considering not bringing her father to her house. However, the house is small and would need renovations, including a bathroom added to the first floor and a ramp to the front door. She also has concerns about performing her father's care because he is "of the old school" and very modest. She works full time and has three small children. She worries that caring for her father in her house would mean she might not be able to give her children and husband the attention they need. She has considered quitting her job, but the family needs her income because her husband's work is seasonal. When visiting her father, she tells the nurse, Janae, that she does not know what is best for him, noting that her sister in another state told her it is her duty to care for their father. Her husband, who comes from a different cultural background, says it is too much to take on with all her other family responsibilities. She asks Janae what she should do.

Think About It
Moral Development and Moral Decisions
- What factors and values do you think weigh most heavily in this situation?
- What sociocultural factors are evident here?
- How would you approach this situation from the perspective of justice? From the perspective of care? From a cultural-developmental perspective? Do you think one approach is more compelling than the other? Explain.
- How do your own ethical perspective and sense of values development and moral reasoning influence your reaction to this situation?
- If you were Janae, what would you explore more before you responded?

SUMMARY

This chapter presented an overview of theoretical perspectives related to values development, the importance of recognizing that values and beliefs are culturally relative, and nursing considerations related to moral development. Students are encouraged to explore and critique each model of values development to formulate a personal knowledge base to guide their own processes of development. Each perspective provides insight into what is true.

CHAPTER HIGHLIGHTS

- Human values development, which is a product of our sociocultural environment, reflects the content and process of learning what is considered right and wrong within the culture.
- Values development moves from a focus on self, through responding to external forces, toward being guided by universal considerations.
- Moral values need to be viewed from a cultural perspective.
- Current models of values development need continued transcultural validation.
- Kohlberg's model, often referred to as an ethic of justice, suggests that choices are based on objective rules and principles and are made from a stance of separateness.
- In Gilligan's model, often referred to as an ethic of care, the moral imperative is grounded in relationship and mutual responsibility. Choices are contextually bound, requiring strategies that maintain connections and a striving to hurt no one.
- The notion of a plurality of moral voices, which is embedded in a cultural-developmental approach to values development, is an important consideration for nursing.
- Understanding varying perspectives from which moral decisions are made enables nurses to appreciate their own and their patients' approaches to ethical dilemmas and to avoid making inappropriate judgments about another's moral capabilities.

DISCUSSION QUESTIONS AND ACTIVITIES

1. What does it mean to say that moral values need to be viewed within a cultural perspective?

2. What factors would you consider in determining a person's phase of moral development? What about a society's phase of moral development?
3. Describe what you perceive to be the stages of values development of three patients or persons you know of different ages.
4. Compare and contrast the models of values development discussed in this chapter. Discuss with classmates how each theory contributes to your understanding of your personal values development. How does each perspective offer insight into the ethical practice of nursing?
5. Why is it important for nurses to be aware of cultural perspectives regarding moral reasoning and phases of values development for themselves, patients, and colleagues?
6. Identify two contemporary individuals or groups that you believe base their moral actions and decisions on internalized universal guides. Support with specific examples.

REFERENCES

Ackerman-Berger, P. (2022, June 6–11). The intersection of cultural humility and health equity [plenary presentation]. In: *American Holistic Nurses Association annual conference*. Albuquerque, NM, United States

ANA. (2015). *Code of ethics for nurses with interpretive statements*. http://nursingworld.org/DocumentVault/Ethics-1/Code-of-Ethics-for-Nurses.html

American Nurses Association (ANA), (2021). *Nursing: Scope and standards of practice* (4th ed.). Author.

Andrews, M. M., Boyle, J. S., & Collins, J. W. (2020). *Transcultural concepts in nursing care* (8th ed.). Wolters Kluwer.

CNA. (2017). *Code of ethics for registered nurses*. https://cdn1.nscn.ca/sites/default/files/documents/resources/code-of-ethics-for-registered-nurses.pdf#:~:text=The%20Canadian%20Nurses%20Association%20%28CNA%29%20Code%20of%20Ethics,receiving%20care.%20The%20Codeis%20both%20aspirational%20and%20regulatory

Colby, A., & Kohlberg, L. (1987). *The measurement of moral judgment: Theoretical foundations and research validation* (Vol. I). Cambridge University Press.

Collins, S. (2015). *The core of care ethics*. Palgrave Macmillan.

Collins, S. (2017). Care ethics: The four key claims In D. Morrow (Ed.), *Moral reasoning: A text and reader on ethics and contemporary moral issues* (pp. 192–204). Oxford University Press.

Doutrich, D., Dekker, L., Spuck, J., & Hoeksel, R. (2014). Identity, ethics and cultural safety: Strategies for change. *Whitireia Nursing Health Journal, 21*, 15–21.

Engebretson, J. C., & Ahn, H. (2022). Cultural Engagement In M. A. B. Helming, D. Shields, K. A. Avino, & W. E. Rosa (Eds.), *Dossey & Keegan's holistic nursing: A handbook for practice* (8th ed., pp. 417–426). Jones & Bartlett.

Fowler, J. W. (1995). *Stages of faith: The psychology of human development and the quest for meaning.* Palgrave MacMillan.

Fowler, D. M. (2015). *Guide to the code of ethics for nurses with interpretive statements.* American Nurses Association.

Gilligan, C. (1982). *In a different voice: Psychological theory and women's development.* Harvard University Press.

Gilligan, C. (1987). Moral orientation and moral development In E. F. Kittay & D. T. Meyers (Eds.), *Women and moral theory* (pp. 19–33). Rowman & Littlefield.

Gilligan, C., Ward, J. V., & Taylor, J. M. (Eds.), (1994). *Mapping the moral domain.* Harvard University Press.

Guerra, V. M., & Giner-Sorolla, R. S. (2015). Investigating the three ethics in emerging adulthood: A study in five countries In L. A. Jensen (Ed.), *Moral development in a global world: Research from a cultural-developmental perspective* (pp. 117–140). Cambridge University Press.

Hadian Shirazi, Z., & Sabetasrvestani, R. (2021). Moral intelligence: An evolutionary concept analysis. *Nursing Practice Today, 8*(4), 293–302.

Hall, E. T. (1973). *The silent language.* Anchor Press.

Held, V. (2006). *The ethics of care: Personal, political, global.* Oxford University Press.

Hickman, J. R., & Fasoli, A. D. (2015). The dynamics of ethical co-occurrence in Hmong and American evangelical families: New direction for three ethics research In L. A. Jensen (Ed.), *Moral development in a global world: Research from a cultural-developmental perspective* (pp. 141–169). Cambridge University Press.

Houser, N., & Kloesel, C. (Eds.). (1992). *The essential Peirce: Selected philosophical writings (Vol. 1).* Indiana University Press.

ICN. (2021). *The ICN code of ethics for nurses.* https://www.icn.ch/system/files/2021-10/ICN_Code-of-Ethics_EN_Web_0.pdf

Jensen, L. A. (Ed.), (2015). *Moral development in a global world: Research from a cultural-developmental perspective.* Cambridge University Press.

Johnstone, M. J. (2012). Bioethics, cultural differences and the problems of moral disagreements in end-of-life care: A terror management theory. *Journal of Medicine and Philosophy, 37*, 181–200.

Kloesel, C. J. W. (Ed.), (1986). *Writings of Charles S. Peirce: A chronological edition.* Indiana University Press.

Kohlberg, L. (1981). *The philosophy of moral development.* Harper & Row.

Lachman, V. D. (2012). Applying the ethics of care to your nursing practice. *MEDSURG Nursing, 21*(2), 112–116.

Lao Tsu. (1972). *Tao Te Ching* (Gia-fu Feng & Jane English, Trans.). Vintage Books.

Lee, S., Palmieri, P., & Watson, J. (2017). *Global advances in human caring literacy.* Springer Publishing.

McFarland, M. R., & Wehbe-Alamah, H. B. (Eds.). (2015). *Leininger's culture care diversity and universality: A worldwide nursing theory* (3rd ed.). Jones & Bartlett.

Ortiz, J., & Casey, D. (2017). Dead wrong! The ethics of culturally competent care. *MEDSURG Nursing, 26*(4), 279–282.

Peirce, C. S. (1877). The fixation of belief. *Popular Science Monthly, 12*, 1–15.

Piaget, J. (1963). *The origins of intelligence in children* (M. Cook, Trans.). Norton.

Plato. (1997). The republic (G. M. A. Grube, C. D. C. Reeve, Trans.). In M. Cooper & D. Hutchinson (Eds.), Plato: Complete works. Hackett (Original work written ca. 375 B.C.E.).

Ray, M. A. (2016). *Transcultural caring dynamics in nursing and health care* (2nd ed.). F. A. Davis.

Shabib Asl, N., Ghorbani, M., Mirzaei Fandakht, O., & Alinaghi Lou, S. (2022). Moral intelligence of nursing students during Covid-19 pandemic: The role of demographic characteristics. *Health, Spirituality and Medical Ethics Journal, 8*(4), 219–226. https://doi.org/10.32598/hsmej.8.4.3.

Spector, R. (2017). *Cultural diversity in health and illness* (9th ed.). Pearson.

Srivastave, R. H. (2023). *Health care professional's guide to cultural competence* (2nd ed.). Elsevier.

Watson, J. (2012). *Human caring science: A theory of nursing* (2nd ed.). Jones & Bartlett.

Watson, J. (2018). *Unitary caring science: Philosophy and praxis of nursing.* University of Colorado Press.

6

Ethics and the Professionalization of Nursing

Nursing's story is a magnificent epic of service to mankind. It is about people: how they are born, and live and die; in health and in sickness; in joy and sorrow. Its mission is the translation of knowledge into human service.

(Rogers, 1983)

OBJECTIVES

After completing this chapter, the reader should be able to:

1. Discuss the meaning of the term *professional*, including traits commonly associated with professional status and the historical debate regarding the professional status of nursing.
2. Describe the evolution of professional nursing ethics.
3. Discuss contemporary codes of nursing ethics.
4. Discuss the importance of caring to the profession of nursing.
5. Discuss the relationships among the concepts of expertise, ethics, and professional status.
6. Discuss autonomy in terms of both the individual nurse and the profession of nursing.
7. Discuss the relationship between professional autonomy and ethics.
8. Discuss the concept of accountability, including various mechanisms of nursing accountability.
9. Explain the relationship between accountability and professional status.
10. Define the concept of authority, differentiating between professional and personal authority.
11. Discuss the concept of unity and its relationship to professional status in nursing.

INTRODUCTION

The historical evolution of the professionalization of nursing and the development of formal nursing codes of ethics have been side-by-side and interrelated century-long processes correlating with other social movements of the times. Modern views about the nature of nursing evolved from the 19th century, when nursing was considered a vocation of servitude, through the mid-20th century, when nursing strived to attain professional status. Social change along with the professionalization of nursing is the context within which nursing codes of ethics were developed. Nursing codes of ethics reflect prevailing moral values and perceptions about nursing at the time in which they are developed. An examination

of current nursing codes of ethics inevitably leads us back to an examination of early efforts to establish nursing as a profession. It was through the discipline's 20th century struggles to be recognized as a profession that organized nursing seriously began to develop codes of ethics.

Today, views about the nature of nursing are changing yet again. The fierce debate about the professional status of nursing has somewhat subsided but continues to be important. Contemporary nurses propose new perspectives from which to view the discipline. Some propose that nursing is a discipline or practice rather than a profession, and some have even suggested that nursing be viewed simply as work. Each view carries with it certain implications for nursing, but to understand the evolution of nursing ethics, it is necessary to examine the debate about nursing's professional status. This chapter examines the struggle of nursing to define itself as a profession; the historical context of nursing ethics; contemporary codes of nursing ethics; and the interrelated themes common both to nursing ethics and the professional status of nursing. These themes include caring, expertise, autonomy, accountability, authority, and unity in nursing.

THE PROFESSIONAL STATUS OF NURSING

Historically, law, medicine, and the clergy were considered true professions, although in the late 19th century, nursing seemed to have gained professional status. Perhaps due to strong leaders such as Isabel Hampton Robb, American nurses were secure in their identity as professionals. Even physicians and the judicial system recognized nursing as a profession. In 1915 however, everything changed.

Abraham Flexner, an American educator, evaluated the professional status of medical schools. In 1910 he published the Flexner Report, which reformed medical education in the United States. Flexner developed a list of traits that he observed in the established professions of medicine, law, and the clergy. He proposed that an occupation must meet all of these criteria to be recognized as a profession. Flexner proposed the following:

1. Professional activities are essentially intellectual and autonomous operations.
2. Professionals derive their raw materials from science and learning.
3. The purpose of professional learning is its practical application.
4. Professions possess orderly and highly specialized education. Professionals tend to self-organize around a democratic, professional nucleus.
5. Professions are more likely than other groups to be responsive to public interest (Flexner, 1910).

Even though the nursing community did not invite his opinion, Flexner later evaluated nursing according to his criteria and declared that nursing was not a profession. In 1915 he presented a paper to the Congress of Charities and Corrections in which he referred to nursing alternately as a "vocation" and an "occupation." He described the nurse as "another arm of the physician or surgeon" (Covert, 1917). Optimistically, Flexner

proposed that occupations can alter their status by developing the traits described in his report.

Subsequently, in 1945 and 1959, two educators, Genevieve and Roy Bixler, published landmark articles evaluating the professional status of nursing. These articles utilized criteria similar to those proposed by Flexner. They listed the following seven criteria of a profession:

1. A profession utilizes in its practice a well-defined and well-organized body of specialized knowledge that is on the intellectual level of higher learning.
2. A profession constantly enlarges the body of knowledge it uses and improves its techniques of education and service by use of the scientific method.
3. A profession entrusts the education of its practitioners to institutions of higher education.
4. A profession applies its body of knowledge in practical services that are vital to human and social welfare.
5. A profession functions autonomously in the formulation of professional policy and in the control of professional activity.
6. A profession attracts individuals of intellectual and personal qualities who exalt service above personal gain and who recognize their chosen occupation as a life work.
7. A profession strives to compensate its practitioners by providing freedom of action, opportunity for continuous professional growth, and economic security (Bixler & Bixler, 1959, pp. 1142–1147).

Predictably, the Bixlers came to the same conclusion as Flexner—nursing was not a true profession.

Following the *Flexner Report* and the subsequent Bixler articles, nurses began to question their own status as professionals (Parsons, 1986). The process of examining and evaluating, though, resulted in many positive changes for nursing. Striving to meet the criteria set by Flexner and the Bixlers, nurses began to conduct research to create a unique body of knowledge for nursing, to move "professional" nursing education to the university setting, to become politically involved, to increase the autonomy of nursing, to extend practice boundaries, and to establish a code of ethics.

Professions have been described in a number of ways, most of which can be related back to the *Flexner Report*. Professional education is geared toward the acquisition of exclusive knowledge necessary to provide a service that is either essential or desired by society. These attributes lead to a monopoly that provides autonomy, public recognition, prestige, power, and authority for the practitioner. Many other distinguishing attributes of professions have been proposed over the years. These include, among others, expertise, accountability, the presence of systematic theory, ethical codes, a professional culture, an altruistic service orientation, competence testing, licensure, high income, credentialing, the description of scope of practice, and the establishment of standards.

Professions are exclusive groups that exist to meet the needs of society. *Exclusive* means that professional groups have strict criteria for membership—they exclude all people who do not meet the criteria. For example, every state in the United States allows only those who are licensed to practice nursing to call themselves nurses. Professionals are connected to each other by common experiences, language, and body of knowledge. Nurses are connected to each other and set apart from others by virtue of the prestige and mystique offered by members of a profession, and by the knowledge that comes from personal and spiritual experiences surrounding the intimacies of human suffering and the beginning and the end of life.

Professions are formed through a social process. The larger society determines its own needs and authorizes certain people to meet those needs. There is a uniform process by which professionals develop the values that lead to a type of social responsibility and a desire to meet the needs of society. Professionals contract with society by promising to meet a set of identified needs better than any other group of people. In turn, society grants the profession a monopoly over these specific services.

Historically, professions have attempted to instill in their members a somber recognition of the profound nature of their responsibility through the recitation of pledges and oaths, such as the Hippocratic Oath for physicians and the Nightingale Pledge for nurses. In fact, Jameton suggested that being a professional is similar to having a calling. He describes a calling as "something one feels called upon to do, perhaps by God, by some deep need in one's being, or by the demands of historical circumstance. A calling is central to one's life and gives it meaning" (1984, p. 18). Reed further proposed that nursing itself is a spiritual discipline. She argued that regarding a discipline as spiritual enhances the meaning of a profession. Reed writes that there is a pragmatic and normative call to action that is freely chosen by its members—one in which the person is said to be called or propelled outward (Reed, 2000).

Nursing's struggle to be identified as a profession led to the development of a substantial body of work that attempts to describe nursing, define its boundaries, clarify the ethical parameters, and distinguish the discipline within society. The profession underwent a period of growth following Bixlers' report. Begun and Lippincott (1993) adopted Bixlers' criteria of a profession and added four additional criteria including the following: a profession provides a service that can be identified by others and requires a body of knowledge and precise judgment that is so specialized that a layperson cannot practice it safely; a profession has a reciprocal trust relationship with the larger society that includes status and privilege in exchange for provision of services; a profession has a unique culture that shares common language (i.e., terminology), symbols, and norms, and expects members to treat other members with civility; and a profession procures licensure that serves as a social contract with society. In 2001 Felton reviewed Begun and Lippincott's criteria and claimed that nursing "obviously meets the definition of a profession" (2001, p. 4).

There was fervor in the debate surrounding the professional status of nursing from the 1970s through the 1990s. The debate has been quiet over the last few years, but the issue continues to be relevant to 21st century nursing and remains an undercurrent within professional and institutional social structures.

Nurses as Professionals

Nurses' perceptions of themselves as professionals vary. In an integrative review of the literature about professional identity in nursing, Rasmussen (2018) found that strong professional identity is central to quality nursing care, recruitment of nursing students, and retention of existing staff. Rasmussen also reports that professional identity begins to emerge as soon as a student enters nursing school and evolves through ongoing experience and socialization in the nursing role (Fig. 6.1). Bochatay (2018) posits that nurses' perception of their work as meaningful contributes to their sense of professional identity and that nurses' professional values and dialog set them apart from other professional groups. However, professional self-concept can be affected by nurses' individual characteristics and working conditions (Sabanciogullari & Dogan, 2017). Interestingly, patient-centered care seems to be central to enhanced professional identity (Rasmussen, 2018). Ideally, nurses as a whole view nursing as a profession rather than simply a job.

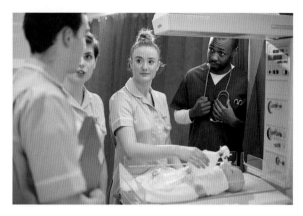

Fig. 6.1 Professional Identity Begins to Emerge as Soon as a Student Enters Nursing School. (©iStock.com/sturti.)

CODES OF NURSING ETHICS

A code of nursing ethics is an explicit, written articulation of the primary goals and values of the profession. Nearly universally accepted as one criterion of a profession, a code of ethics is a means by which a discipline articulates the values that regulate the conduct of members. Like other professions, nursing has developed and enforces specific obligations to ensure that nurses are competent and trustworthy. These obligations correlate with the rights of individual patients and society as a whole. Upon entrance into the profession, nurses make an implicit moral commitment to uphold the values and moral obligations expressed in their code. Codes of ethics direct nurses to base professional judgment on consideration of consequences and the universal moral principles of respect for persons, autonomy, beneficence, nonmaleficence, veracity, confidentiality, fidelity, and justice.

Formal codes of nursing ethics are relatively modern. In the late 19th and early to mid-20th centuries, many disciplines were struggling to develop professional codes of ethics. For nurses, this was a long struggle. Florence Nightingale set the stage for the later development of codes of ethics for nurses. In the early 19th century, there were no formal training schools and a nurse was simply a person in charge of the personal health of another (Nightingale, 1859). Hospitals that employed nurses served largely to house the dying poor. Hospital nurses were reputed to be prone to drunkenness, and nurses from religious orders were more likely to focus on spiritual matters than on healing the body. Nightingale was the first to publicly encourage nurses to be caring, to focus attention on the patient, and to follow the physical principles that promote healing. She founded the first official secular nursing school in 1860. Nursing students there were expected to be virtuous: sober, honest, truthful, and trustworthy. Nightingale's values quickly spread across the Western world.

In the early 20th century, not everyone agreed that a code of ethics was needed. The first call for a code of ethics for nurses in the United States was documented in 1897 in the founding constitution of what is now the American Nurses Association (ANA). Although it was discussed, the association did not develop a code of ethics at that time. Fifteen years later, in 1912, Isabel Hampton Robb identified a lack of uniformity among nurses and asserted that the profession needed a code of ethics. Robb authored the first ethics textbook, *Nursing Ethics: For Hospital and Private Use* (1912). For many years afterward, most nursing students used Robb's textbook.

Robb described ethics as the science that treats human actions from a standpoint of right and wrong. She suggested that a formal code of ethics, derived from the full and rich knowledge of experienced nurses, would guide young nurses. Considering the social forces of the times, it is not surprising that Robb viewed nurses' work as a ministry. She believed that nursing should be a Christian service. A contemporary of Abraham Flexner, Robb argued that nursing is a profession, but she respected those who considered nursing a religious calling or vocation (Robb, 1912).

Although members of the ANA discussed the development of a formal code of ethics through the years, the first attempt to write a code in the United States began in 1921. Five years later, an advisory committee suggested a code to the delegates of the ANA convention (Viens, 1989). The code, which was never adopted, contained a description of the nurse as obedient, trustworthy, loyal, and adept at etiquette. Renewed interest in 1940 brought revisions to the suggested code. The 1940 version began to rely more on ethical principles rather than rules of conduct but added language about nurses' loyalty to physicians (Viens, 1989). Again, the draft version of the code of ethics was not ratified by members of the organization. It was not until 1950 that the first official ANA code of ethics for nurses was finally adopted. Times were changing. The 1950 official version dropped language about nurses' loyalty to physicians. The International Council of Nurses (ICN) followed with a code of ethics in 1953, and other countries developed nursing codes of ethics in quick succession.

During the 20th century, the nursing profession established and refined an international code of ethics and codes of ethics in every Western country. These codes now serve as formal standards that have been ratified by professional nursing organizations. As made explicit by the ANA, nursing codes of ethics are the profession's nonnegotiable ethical standard that nurses are required to follow in every professional situation, regardless of other restraints such as employer policy or common practice.

Current codes of nursing ethics from around the Western world are similar in content and purpose. They all reflect a practical combination of concepts from different ethical theories and traditions. A single code of ethics may include language about ethical principles; duties and responsibilities (deontology); distributive justice (utilitarianism); beneficence, autonomy, and nonmaleficence (deontology); inherent character traits of nurses (virtue ethics); and other related concepts.

The codes of nursing from around the world are similar. Codes from the ICN and the European Union and a sample of Western countries, including the United States, Canada, Great Britain, Ireland, Australia, New Zealand, Sweden, Denmark, and Finland, include 12 strikingly similar themes. Each code of nursing ethics strongly establishes the following:

1. The nurse should respect the inherent worth, dignity, and rights of every person.
2. The nurse's primary responsibility is to the person seeking care.
3. The nurse has a duty to do good and avoid harm.
4. The nurse is responsible for the ethics of his or her own practice and must carry out daily actions with integrity.
5. The nurse must deliver care that is safe, compassionate, competent, and ethical.
6. The nurse must protect an individual when health is endangered by another person.
7. The nurse is responsible and accountable for individual nursing practice.
8. The nurse promotes justice.
9. The nurse maintains cooperative relationships with others.
10. The nurse participates in the advancement of the profession.
11. The nurse is concerned with broader societal issues that affect health.
12. The nurse must take into consideration duties to self (ANA, 2015; Australian Nursing Federation et al., 2015; CNA, 2017; Danish Council of Nursing Ethics, 2017; Finnish Nurses Association, 2021; ICN, 2021; Nursing & Midwifery Council, 2015; Nursing and Midwifery Board of Ireland, 2021; Nursing Council of New Zealand, 2012; Sasso et al., 2008; Swedish Society of Nursing, 2010).

CASE PRESENTATION

Respect for Persons

Helen is a 21-year-old registered nurse who recently graduated from nursing school. For her first nursing position, Helen began work in a federal correctional institution. John is a 21-year-old inmate who is quiet, courteous, and charming, though he often seems depressed. He comes to the prison clinic often for a variety of minor illnesses. Helen knows from media coverage that John was convicted of the brutal rape and murder of a child. Whenever she sees John, Helen is torn between her desire to be a good nurse and deliver respectful, patient-centered care versus thoughts of the terrible crimes John was convicted of committing. She wonders what her role truly is.

Think About It

How Can a Nursing Code of Ethics Guide in This Case?

- Look at the codes of nursing ethics from the ANA (2015, Provisions 1.1, 1.2, and 1.3) or CNA (2017, Parts D.1, D.2, and D.3) and the ICN (2021, Element 1.8).
- Taking nursing codes of ethics into consideration, should Helen demonstrate respect for John?
- What type of care should Helen deliver to John?
- Should Helen's approach to John be related to his punishment?
- Contrast how Helen's situation differs from non-Nazi nurses who were forced to care for victims of atrocities in Nazi concentration camps.

THEMES COMMON TO THE PROFESSIONALIZATION OF NURSING AND NURSING ETHICS

As you study the various codes of nursing ethics, you will notice the ethical principles discussed in Chapter 3. You will also notice other strong and consistent themes. These themes depict a number of important facets of ethically appropriate nursing care. The following section discusses the themes of caring, expertise, nursing autonomy, accountability, authority, and unity that appear in nursing codes of ethics.

Caring

It has been proposed that care is the root of ethics (May, 1960). The notion of caring developed throughout history in various forms—mythological, religious, philosophical, psychological, theological, and moral (Reich, 2003). We can trace the origins of caring in nursing to the work and writings of Florence Nightingale. However, the connection between nursing and caring strongly emerged during the advent of feminist ethics in the 1980s.

Historically, caring has been a major theme in nursing literature and an essential facet of nursing ethics. Rogers (1983) famously said, "Nursing is the compassionate concern for human beings. It is the heart that understands and the hand that soothes. It is the intellect that synthesizes many learnings into meaningful administrations." Curtin (1980) claimed that the distinctiveness of nursing is located in the "moral art of nursing" in which nurses are committed to caring for other human beings. The first nursing theorist to explicitly write about the process caring was Leninger, who wrote "care is the essence and the central, unifying, and dominant domain to characterize nursing" (1984, p. 3). Newman et al. defined nursing as the "study of caring in the human health experience" (1991, p. 298). Watson (2010) contends that caring is a professional and ethical covenant that nursing has with society. Clearly, caring is part of the moral essence of nursing (Fig. 6.2).

In terms of healthcare ethics, there are two distinctly different aspects of care: "caring about" and "taking care of" (Reich, 2003). Nursing codes of ethics guide nurses to practice both types of caring. Many contend that caring about others goes to the heart of nursing. This suggests a virtue of concern for the other person. Caring about another leads a person to *be with* the other person in his or her world (Mayeroff, 1971; Swanson,

1991). It is mindful and reflective, delivered with conscious intentionality (Watson, 2002) and compassionate concern. A nurse who cares about a patient is authentically committed to alleviating vulnerabilities, centering attention and concern on the person, and preserving dignity and humanity (Smith, 1999). Moral virtues and principles come naturally to the nurse who genuinely cares about the patient. The second type of care, "taking care of," encompasses competence in the technical aspects of delivering care. This type of care focuses more on knowledge of the scientific aspects of health care and on skillful practice. As you will see in the section that follows, giving expert technical nursing care is also a moral imperative.

Expertise

Expertise relates to the characteristic of having a high level of specialized skill and knowledge. It is a composite of knowledge gained through long years of study in an academic setting and superior skill. Expertise is an essential characteristic of professionals and is required by nursing codes of ethics. Professionals must have the knowledge, judgment, and technical and interpersonal competencies required to meet the needs of society and thereby fulfill the purpose of the profession. Expertise also helps ensure that the nurse's actions are beneficent and nonmaleficent. Expertise allows professions to maintain autonomy because society trusts that professionals are the only ones who fully understand the work of the profession.

Nurses must maintain competence. Each nurse must recognize and not exceed his or her own boundaries of

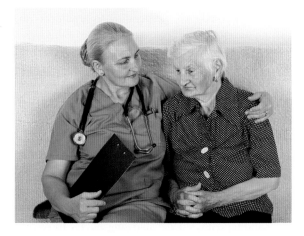

Fig. 6.2 Caring Is the Moral Essence of Nursing. (©iStock. com/Ocskaymark.)

competent practice. A review of codes of nursing ethics from a sample of Western countries (listed above) found that all nurses are expected to utilize the best available evidence base for practice and maintain knowledge and skills.

Nurses gain expertise in a variety of ways. Florence Nightingale recognized the importance of an education consisting of depth and breadth of general knowledge, combined with a specific nursing focus. Extensive educational requirements, intense guided practice, examination for licensure, certification, and mandatory continuing education are ways that nurses attain, maintain, or assert expertise. Having completed basic nursing education and successfully demonstrated a minimum level of competence through licensure examination, nurses are further required (either ethically or legally) to continue the learning process and maintain up-to-date knowledge and technical proficiency. Continuing education programs assist in this process. Nursing expertise is also advanced through graduate nursing education, specialty preparation, and the certification process. Today the discipline of nursing has a knowledge base that continually expands through research.

Aligned with expertise, a frequently cited characteristic of professions is a practice based upon a unique body of knowledge derived from research. Recall that Genevieve and Roy Bixler's (1959) first two characteristics of a profession relate to a unique body of knowledge. The Bixlers' second characteristic actually calls for professions to constantly enlarge the body of knowledge by use of the scientific method. In the past, authorities debated whether nursing's body of knowledge was unique to the profession or was borrowed from the behavioral and physical sciences and medicine. Responding to arguments that nursing was not a true profession because of this lack of a clearly unique body of knowledge, nurses in academic and clinical settings began gathering data and conducting legitimate research. Today the profession acknowledges the importance of nursing research—research that can be purely nursing or can be in collaboration with other disciplines. Most doctoral, some master's, and a few bachelor's programs in nursing require some type of research project and dissemination of results. Nursing journals are filled with research articles written by academic nurses, nursing students, and practicing nurses. Thus, the body of unique and shared nursing knowledge is expanding daily, further allowing nurses to respond more knowledgeably, skillfully, and with expertise to the needs of society.

Moving beyond the idea of competence, the Institute of Medicine (IOM) report *The Future of Nursing* (2010) suggested that to correct many problems of the current healthcare environment, nurses must practice to the full extent of their education and training. This means that nurses must practice competently, and they must unapologetically practice to the full extent of the nursing role. Further, to maintain expertise, nurses must dedicate themselves to life-long learning as they engage in new professional roles and adapt to new technologies (National Academy of Medicine, 2021). Recognizing society's faith in the profession, merely claiming expertise is not enough. Through the various mechanisms of accountability, nurses must prove that they are faithful to the promise the profession makes to the broader society. In response, society grants nurses the authority to practice with a certain measure of autonomy—as illustrated in the IOM report. Thus, the professional realms of expertise, accountability, autonomy, and authority are closely interrelated.

Autonomy

Autonomy, as described in Chapter 3, is usually discussed in terms of respect for the autonomy of others, especially patients. But to maintain integrity and fully exercise ethical practice, nurses must also be autonomous. The concept of nursing autonomy can be discussed on two levels: autonomy of the profession and autonomy of the individual practitioner. Self-regulation is the mark of collective professional autonomy. Individual autonomy involves self-determination, responsibility, accountability, independence, and a willingness to take risks and is necessary for nurses to practice ethically. Autonomy is generally considered an important criterion of professional status. People who are considered professionals have the power and authority to control various aspects of their work, including goals toward which to work, whether to work and with whom, details of how the work is to be done, choice of clientele, and so forth (Jameton, 1984). As you will learn in Chapter 7, nurses who perceive themselves as autonomous professionals are less likely to experience distress when encountering patient care situations in which their personal values are challenged.

Because the profession of nursing is self-regulating, it can be said to be autonomous. Unlike in the early years of this century, most state boards of nursing are now predominately made up of nurses. Given the authority granted by statutory law, boards of nursing enforce the individual states' nurse practice acts. This ensures the autonomy of the profession in each state. Among other tasks, boards of nursing oversee the schools of nursing within their states, control licensure, and discipline nurses.

The profession of nursing maintains autonomy through the combination of a claim to maximal competence and a continuing monopoly over nursing work so that other people are prohibited by law from practicing nursing. Credentialing such as licensure, educational requirements, certification, and so forth is the means by which nurses restrict others from doing the same work. Just as it is illegal for a nonphysician to practice

medicine, it is likewise illegal for nonnurses to practice nursing or to call themselves nurses. This legally sanctioned monopoly helps establish autonomy.

Nurses are legally and ethically required to practice autonomously. Autonomous practice serves as a safeguard for the patient, nurse, physician, and institution. Nursing codes of ethics support the nurse's responsibility to make autonomous decisions. The ANA *Code of Ethics for Nurses* (2015) explicitly calls for nurses to be autonomous, particularly in relation to their responsibility and accountability for nursing judgments and actions that protect the safety of patients. Similarly, the codes of ethics from the ICN and other Western countries implicitly and explicitly reflect nursing autonomy and responsibility. The purpose of autonomy as described in these codes is to protect the patient from harm and allow for the full benefit of professional nursing care.

Are nurses truly autonomous? We often hear questions about the autonomy of individual nurses. Can you say that you are autonomous, even though you are required to follow physicians' orders? Are you autonomous, even though you cannot get to know the patients because you have too many patients and too much work to do? Nurses are autonomous because they have the authority to make decisions about the care they provide that is within the boundaries of nursing practice. Confusion occurs because the work of nurses overlaps the domain of physicians. Some nursing actions require physician authorization and others require no authorization because they fall within the scope of autonomous nursing. This role confusion is a result of business practices.

Hospitals are businesses. They cultivate a population of physicians who bring patients, and thus profits, to their facilities. To prosper, hospitals must attract and retain a strong physician staff. So as a practical necessity, they provide qualified staff to carry out physicians' orders—an essential service. Although we, as nurses, are autonomous professionals, we are also employees. When we accept employment, we implicitly agree to perform the tasks that our employers desire (except those that may be illegal, unethical, or immoral). Even so, ethics and law require us to use autonomous judgment in our practice. Institutions and physicians should welcome independent nursing judgment because of the safeguards it provides. We commonly hear about nurses who refuse to carry out unsafe orders. Such actions protect patients from physician error and thus prevent litigation against nurses,

CASE PRESENTATION

Lewis Blackman Revisited

Recall the case presentation of Lewis Blackman in Chapter 3. Lewis was a 15-year-old healthy student athlete who died from an easily recognized and preventable adverse effect of a common analgesic drug administered after elective surgery. Even though he demonstrated dramatic signs of an impending emergency and nurses were diligently recording his signs and symptoms, none recognized the crisis until it was too late. Lewis died 31 hours after experiencing the first signs, even though his mother had repeatedly asked the nurses for help. In a series of short videos, Lewis's mother, Helen Haskell, talks about her experience. She says, "Most of Lewis's nurses were very young. They were sweet. They were articulate. They were well intentioned. They very clearly knew very little" (Haskell, 2009, video 2). Having dedicated herself to patient advocacy since her son's death, Ms. Haskell says that many nurses have shared stories about their feelings of helplessness when their own family members suffered because of medical or nursing errors.

Think About It

Nursing Errors and Patient Helplessness

- Lewis and his mother trusted the physicians and nurses to provide competent care. How would you feel if you found yourself in a similar situation?
- Helen Haskell says that Lewis's nurses were task oriented rather than goal oriented. What do you think nurses' responsibilities were regarding their ability to competently care for Lewis?
- Discuss your beliefs concerning an ethical requirement to maintain expertise in practice.
- Does the profession have an obligation to society in this regard?
- What do codes of nursing ethics have to say in regard to competent practice?

physicians, and institutions. Courts not only recognize but also expect nursing autonomy, ruling against nurses who follow questionable orders or fail to alert the hierarchical chain of command when problems arise.

Autonomy does not mean that nurses have absolute control of every facet of practice. Although accepted as one of the three prototype professions, medicine, for example, is no longer totally autonomous. Government regulations now guide many facets of medical care such as reimbursement levels and length of hospital stays. In many cases today, third-party insurance limits expensive procedures, referral networks, prescription medications, and the length of hospital stay. There are far fewer distinctions between the degrees of autonomy of the two professions than there were when Flexner made his comparison in 1915.

ASK YOURSELF

Judgments About Physicians' Orders

Nurses are frequently asked to give medications with which they are not familiar or to administer a familiar drug in an excessive dose or uncustomary route of administration. Unable to quickly determine its appropriateness or safety, a nurse might trust the physician's order and hurriedly administer the drug without fully understanding the implications or might refuse to administer the drug.

- What feelings, emotions, and values might be involved in the nurse's decision to refuse to follow a physician's order?
- What are some predictable reactions of the nurse's coworkers, supervisors, and physicians when a nurse refuses to follow a physician's order?
- What ethical principles can be used to guide such decisions?
- What type of nurse would be empowered in these types of situations? What type of nurse would not be empowered?
- How would it affect the nurse if the drug in question is later found to be safe and appropriate? How should this affect future decisions?
- How would it affect the nurse if the physician's order is later found to be a dangerous medical error? How would this affect the nurse's future decisions?
- How might a nurse gain authoritative information on the safety of the order?
- What provisions, parts, or elements of codes of nursing ethics apply to this situation?

Nurses do not always feel autonomous, and, in fact, some may not practice autonomously. Certainly, there are nurses who spend each workday following physicians' orders and completing various nonautonomous tasks, never exercising independent nursing functions, making nursing diagnoses, initiating self-directed treatment, or engaging in critical thinking. Recall the case of Lewis Blackman in which nurses were busy taking and recording alarming vital signs yet were oblivious to clear indications of Lewis's deteriorating condition. In the truest sense, these nurses were only marginally practicing professional nursing. When nurses practice in this manner, they fail the ethical duty to make autonomous nursing judgments.

Accountability

Accountability means that a person has an obligation to accept responsibility and to account for his or her actions. Accountability in nursing is tied to the moral principles of fidelity and respect for the dignity, worth, and self-determination of patients. Safe, autonomous practice is ensured through various processes of nursing accountability. Because society places trust in nurses (gained through recognition of nurses' expertise), and because society gives the profession the right to regulate practice (professional autonomy), individual practitioners and the profession itself must be accountable.

Accountability is an inherent part of everyday nursing practice. Each nurse is responsible for all individual actions and omissions. Codes of nursing ethics make it clear that each nurse has the accountability for judgments made and actions taken in the course of nursing practice, regardless of circumstances and irrespective of the healthcare organization's policies or provider's orders. As has been previously noted, the courts consistently support this claim.

Accountability has two interrelated properties: responsibility and answerability. **Responsibility** means that one is reliable and trustworthy in fulfilling obligations or duties. **Accountability** involves a reciprocal relationship in which one is responsible and therefore answerable to others for judgment and action taken in fulfilling that duty. Accepting a position means that the nurse has agreed to do the work he or she was hired to do in exchange for a salary. The nurse is responsible for doing assigned work carefully and seriously according to professional standards, the employer's instructions, policies, and procedures—with the caveat that neither nurses nor patients will be harmed, and nurses will work to improve the employment environment when necessary—and answerable to the employer and larger society for judgments and actions taken.

Accountability and Delegation of Nursing Tasks

Nurses also bear the primary responsibility and accountability for the nursing care patients receive, even when they delegate nursing activities to other registered nurses, licensed practical nurses, nursing assistants, or other licensed or nonlicensed staff (Fig. 6.3). Upholding the ethical principles of respect for persons, respect for autonomy, beneficence, nonmaleficence, fidelity, veracity, confidentiality, and justice is the responsibility of the nurse and carries through to persons who report to the nurse. Delegation of nursing tasks must be consistent with nurse practice acts, organizational policy, and standards of practice. When making judgments about delegation, nurses must consider the complexity of the patient and the knowledge, competence, and experience of the person accepting the delegation (NCSBN & ANA, 2019). In addition, the nurse must monitor and evaluate the quality and outcomes of the care provided. Organizational policies do not relieve nurses of this responsibility. Further, nurses

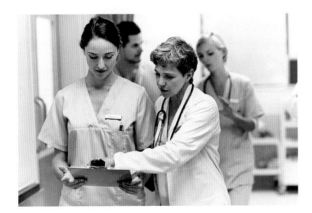

Fig. 6.3 Nurses Bear the Primary Responsibility for the Nursing Care When They Delegate Nursing Tasks. (©iStock.com/kupicoo.)

must not delegate to nonnurses complex nursing tasks that require in-depth nursing knowledge and judgment such as assessment and evaluation.

Mechanisms of Accountability: Nursing Standards of Practice

The profession of nursing has developed several mechanisms through which this relationship between nursing and society is made explicit. Standards of nursing practice, which include professional, institutional, and regulatory statements, policies, and laws, are the major mechanisms of accountability. Some other mechanisms, not discussed here, include educational requirements for practice, advanced or specialty certification, and methods for evaluating the effectiveness of nurses' performance. In both a professional and a legal sense, it is necessary that nurses are familiar with various mechanisms of accountability.

Standards of nursing practice describe the minimum expectations for safe nursing care. Standards may describe in detail specific acts performed by nurses or may outline the expected process of nursing care. Nurses are obligated to follow standards, which may be developed within the profession or within larger organizations, to guide and evaluate nursing care. Nurses are professionally, legally, and ethically accountable to meet standards. Criminal and civil courts rely on nursing standards to guide deliberations during malpractice cases and nurses involved in legal disputes may find their action and documentation judged against those standards.

Some standards of nursing are developed within the profession to describe practice and to establish the minimum level of safe practice. They help ensure that nurses are competent and safe practitioners. These documents, which are developed by nurses, guide nursing care and can be used as a yardstick to measure the practice of individual nurses. They can also be used to determine whether the actions of nurses accused of malpractice are consistent with reasonable minimum expectations. For example, in 2021, ANA published the fourth edition of *Nursing: Scope and Standards of Practice*. These comprehensive standards utilize the nursing process. All licensed professional nurses in the United States are accountable for following these standards. Specialty nursing organizations publish more focused standards of care for nurses in advanced or specialty roles such as critical care nurses, nurse practitioners, clinical nurse specialists, nurse midwives, and nurse anesthetists. Nurses in these roles must adhere to both the basic standards of care and standards established for their specialties.

Codes of nursing ethics establish standards of ethical care. They are nonnegotiable in all settings and prescriptive. Except in extreme crisis situations in which impossible decisions must be made, the nurse has no choice but to follow codes of ethics. The nurse is responsible for following codes of ethics and is answerable to others for actions that defy ethical standards. For example, the ANA (2015) establishes that the nurse must act to protect patients when their safety is threatened by "incompetent, unethical, illegal, or impaired practice or actions" (p. 12) that put a patient in jeopardy. The nurse, therefore, who smells alcohol on a physician's breath or witnesses another nurse stealing medication must follow the actions prescribed in the code. To do otherwise makes the witness nurse a liable accomplice.

Other standards of nursing practice may be developed by nonnurses, the government, or institutions. These standards, which are developed outside the profession of nursing, nevertheless describe the specific expectations of agencies or groups that utilize the services of nurses. Among others, examples include the nurse practice acts of each state, Joint Commission guidelines, and formal policies of individual agencies. Nurses are responsible and accountable to know and follow the standards of care for the profession, the specialty (if applicable), the geographic area (i.e., the state nurse practice act), and the institution.

Institutions, such as hospitals, develop standards of care in the form of policies and procedures. While ensuring safe patient care, institutional standards for nurses should be practical and reasonable. Nurses in administrative or advisory capacities are often responsible for developing institutional standards. Nurse leaders within institutions sometimes develop standards that describe in detail the highest ideal of nursing care. This type of standard may actually create risk by placing both practicing nurses and the employing institution in jeopardy of malpractice litigation because direct care nurses could be held responsible to maintain unattainable standards. Because standards are used to judge nursing actions, they should reflect reasonable expectations for safe nursing care rather than optimal or ideal care.

Nurse practice acts are considered a form of nursing standards. As the foremost legal statute regulating nursing, the nurse practice act of each state protects the public, defines nursing practice, describes the boundaries of practice, establishes standards for nurses, and protects the domain of nursing. Courts use nurse practice acts to determine the appropriateness of accused nurses' actions. Violations can result in civil or criminal prosecution.

State boards of nursing interpret and carry out the provisions of the various states' nurse practice acts. Their goal is to promote and protect public health, safety, and welfare by ensuring the safe practice of nursing. Boards accomplish this by establishing standards for safe nursing care, issuing licenses to practice nursing, monitoring the practice of nurses, and disciplining nurses as needed. Board membership varies from state to state, but commonly includes a mix of registered nurses, licensed practical/vocational nurses, advanced practice registered nurses, and consumers.

Each of the 50 US states independently develops, updates, and interprets its own nurse practice act. Though both the ANA and the National Council of State Boards of Nursing have developed model nurse practice acts in the past, the laws continue to be different in each state. Some nurse practice acts are very general and are somewhat vague in describing the boundaries of the professional role. These laws are considered permissive, allowing nursing practice to evolve dynamically. Others list each act that nurses are permitted to perform. As nursing continues to evolve, the very specific nurse practice acts, once applauded as recognizing nurses' legitimate authority to perform certain advanced tasks, have become restrictive. With nurses continually expanding the boundaries of nursing, particularly during crisis situations, these very specific and restrictive nurse practice acts have become a barrier to advanced nursing practice.

Because nurses are legally accountable to follow the standards set by the states' nurse practice acts, they must be particularly attentive to the language describing the definition of nursing and the scope of nursing practice. Because legislatures meet and pass laws regularly, nurse practice acts can be changed unexpectedly. Nurses must know even the most recent changes in their states' nurse practice acts and implement necessary changes in practice.

Evolving healthcare delivery systems, financing mechanisms, expanded roles of other healthcare professionals, and problems unearthed during the COVID-19

CASE PRESENTATION

When Standards Are Difficult to Meet

Markko is a registered nurse in charge of a large inpatient psychiatric unit. His unit houses an average of 22 patients with a variety of diagnoses, ranging from drug dependence to acute psychoses. The unit is usually staffed by one registered nurse, two licensed practical nurses, and two attendants. Hospital policy requires that the registered nurse evaluate each patient's physical and mental status at least twice per shift, supervise the administration of all psychotropic medication, participate in group activities, supervise the implementation of each patient's plan of care, and be available to individual patients for one-to-one interaction. There are additional policies and procedures that describe the appropriate care for patients who are potentially suicidal: "Patients who are identified as suicidal will be isolated in private rooms and continuously monitored by a registered nurse." When Marrko receives the report from the night nurse, he learns that two of the patients are identified as potentially suicidal, six geriatric patients with dementia need to be fed and ambulated, one patient exhibits violent behavior, all the patients need individual assessment, and one of the two licensed practical nurses called in sick. Markko calls the supervisor for assistance but is told that there is no one available to help. The reader will no doubt have noticed that in addition to the other duties, Markko is required to monitor two patients simultaneously and continuously in separate rooms—a physical impossibility. Markko tries to meet all obligations under these very strict standards, yet while he is on the phone asking his supervisor for help, one of the suicidal patients manages to seriously injure herself attempting to jump from the fourth-floor window in her room.

Think About It
Problems Posed by Unreasonable Institutional Standards

- What is the purpose of the standards that Markko is required to follow?
- What do you see as the legal liability created by the standards?
- Do you think the institution shares the legal blame for the situation?
- What is the effect of the standards on Markko's practice?
- Is there any way that Markko can meet the standards?
- What do you think you would do in similar circumstances?
- What are the ethical implications for the institution and for Markko?
- Codes of nursing ethics are the standards by which nurses' actions are judged. Once the current situation is resolved, how would codes of ethics from the ANA (2015, Provision 6.3) or CNA (2017, Parts I.A.4-5 and I.A.7) and ICN (2021, Elements 1.9 and 2.10-2.11) guide Markko's future actions?

---

pandemic require careful study of existing nurse practice acts and judicious implementation of well-considered changes. Codes of nursing ethics call on nurses to participate in the profession's efforts to implement and improve nursing standards. Thus, nurses, particularly those working in direct patient care, have an ethical responsibility to become active in evaluating and revising outdated laws and policies.

Authority

The term *authority* means that a person or group has legitimate power and sovereignty. The authority to practice nursing is granted by legal statute, based on the contract the profession has with society. The granting of authority acknowledges the professional's rights and responsibilities and requires mechanisms for public accountability (ANA, 2010). Authority assumes a certain measure of autonomy.

Society acknowledges the authority of a profession by recognizing its existence in statute and granting its members the elite privilege of membership. Thus, like autonomy, authority is two-tiered—professional and individual. State legislatures create laws designed to protect the public's health and safety. The establishment of nurse practice acts is the exercise of this type of power. Nurse practice acts define nursing, describe the scope of practice, and grant the state boards of nursing the power to oversee the licensure of nurses and the practice of nursing in the states. Thus, the state boards of nursing have the legitimate authority to regulate the practice of nursing within each state.

Like the profession of nursing itself, individual nurses also have authority. Nurse practice acts empower state boards of nursing to grant individual nurses the authority to practice through the process of examination and licensure. Licensure benefits both the public and the professional. It protects the public from those who are unqualified, and it protects professionals' job territory by establishing a monopoly. The authority given to each nurse to practice is contingent on the nurse continuing to uphold the established standards of nursing. State boards of nursing have the authority and responsibility to discipline nurses who do not follow established standards or who violate provisions of licensure law.

Unity

There is a general agreement that one of the defining characteristics of a profession is a sense of unity among its members. Unity is multifaceted and based on what Aydelotte and Chaska (1990) calls moral uniformity and class ideology among its practitioners. Unity relates to the ability of nurses to organize for the purpose of fulfilling the profession's promises and the relationships that nurses have with one another.

Unity enables nursing to coherently standardize the professional characteristics of competence, autonomy, authority, and accountability. Through political and policy processes, nurses work together to meet the healthcare needs of society and to improve the status of the profession. The structural component of a *professional* community is realized through a professional association. The professional association provides a collective identity and serves as the voice of the profession. Unity within the profession helps standardize the services provided by its members and provides a professional hub for members that assists with the educational and professional needs of members and performs political, advisory, and policy functions. Membership is an expectation within a profession.

Although systematic organization of professional groups is necessary to fulfill the profession's responsibilities, nurses also need unity among individual members. Unity involves showing sympathy, care, and reciprocity to those with whom one appropriately identifies; working closely with others toward shared goals; keeping promises; making mutual concerns a priority; sacrificing personal interests to the relationship; and attending to these over time (Jameton, 1984). Nurses are members of a special group. They share language, educational background, mysteries of practice, clothing, and other symbols of the profession. Membership in the group is restricted. Nurses are connected with the group and set apart from others.

Though loyalty is a virtue, there are certain risks when nurses experience an overly strong sense of loyalty to each other. Jameton (1984) warns that nurses must be careful that their loyalty to each other does not supersede loyalty to patients. For example, mistakes that nurses or doctors make should be reported. Because of a sense of loyalty and friendship between coworkers, there is a risk that the duty to patients will be neglected when errors occur. Nurses are required to examine and prioritize conflicting loyalties closely. Jameton identifies nurses' main priorities as patients, nurses and the nursing profession, physicians, hospitals, other health professions, and society. Questioning which of these priorities should be central and which should be peripheral, Jameton suggests that the best choices for first priority are patient, nursing, and society.

ASK YOURSELF

Are Nurses Loyal to Nursing?

Nurses who are politically active in a state nurses' association report an incident that led them to question nurses' loyalty to the profession. At the prompting of hospital and physicians' lobbying groups, a number of nurse administrators participated in writing proposed legislation that would dismantle the all-nurse board of nursing in favor of one composed of hospital administrators and physicians.

- How would you characterize the loyalty of these nurses to the profession and to other nurses?
- What circumstances could justify prioritizing employer loyalty above loyalty to patients or to other nurses?
- What are the ethical implications of the actions of the nurses described in this situation?
- What should the role of nurses' associations be in these situations?

■ SUMMARY

This chapter outlined how the historical evolution of the professionalization of nursing and the development of formal nursing codes of ethics developed side by side. An examination of current nursing codes of ethics inevitably leads us back to an examination of early efforts to establish nursing as a profession. It was through the discipline's struggles to be recognized as a profession that organized nursing seriously began to develop codes of ethics. This chapter examined the struggle of nursing to define itself as a profession; the historical context of nursing ethics; contemporary codes of nursing ethics; and the interrelated themes common both to nursing ethics and the professional status of nursing including caring, expertise, autonomy, accountability, authority, and unity in nursing.

CHAPTER HIGHLIGHTS

- Acknowledgment of professional status is dependent on meeting specific criteria that include, but are not restricted to, expertise, autonomy, authority, accountability, and unity.
- Historical and cultural influences have affected the definitions commonly used for the term professional.
- A system or code of ethics is generally accepted as one trait of professions.
- First established in the mid-20th century, nursing codes of ethics continue to evolve with sensitivity to the moral standards of society.
- Codes of nursing practice are nonnegotiable standards.
- Caring is a core value that undergirds nursing ethics.
- Because society allows professionals a monopoly over the services they provide, ethics demands that those services must be provided with expertise.
- Because it is self-regulating, the profession of nursing can be said to be autonomous.
- There are legal and ethical imperatives for individual nurses to practice autonomously.
- Autonomy does not mean full and absolute control over every aspect of practice.
- Grounded in the moral principle of fidelity, accountability refers to being answerable to someone for something one has done.
- Mechanisms of accountability include, but are not restricted to, professional guidelines and standards, codes of nursing ethics, institutional policies, and nurse practice acts.
- Authority for nurses to practice is granted through the legal processes of society.
- Nursing unity relates to the profession's ability to organize for the purpose of fulfilling the promises made to society.

DISCUSSION QUESTIONS AND ACTIVITIES

1. Write your own definition of the term professional.
2. List five different occupations and compare their common characteristics. Which occupations meet your criteria for professional status?
3. Read two current nursing codes of ethics. Find concrete examples in the codes related to the ethical principles of autonomy, beneficence, nonmaleficence, justice, and confidentiality. For example, in the ICN Code of Ethics for Nurses, the sentence "The nurse takes appropriate action to safeguard individuals, families, and communities when their health is endangered" is a practical example of the principle of beneficence.
4. Compare codes of ethics from the ANA, CNA, and ICN. What are the similarities? What are the differences?
5. Discuss the relationship between historical and cultural influences and Flexner's method of identifying professions.
6. Discuss the relationship between the concepts of fidelity, professionalism, and expertise.
7. Discuss the statement, "To be less than maximally competent is unethical."
8. Find recent examples of case law that relate to autonomy in nursing.
9. Observe a registered nurse at work. List tasks that the nurse performs and categorize them as autonomous or dependent.
10. Visit your state board of nursing website to find assistance in locating the law that regulates nursing practice. Is the code in your state vague or restrictive? Visit the websites of at least three states and compare the laws.
11. Discuss how a specific language in your state law can be used as a standard of nursing care.

REFERENCES

ANA. (2010). *Nursing's social policy statement: The essence of the profession.* Silver Springs, MD: Author.

ANA. (2015). *Code of ethics for nurses with interpretive statements.* Nursebooks.org. https://nursingworld.org/DocumentVault/Ethics-1/Code-of-Ethics-for-Nurses.html.

ANA. (2021). *Nursing: Scope and standards of practice* (4th ed.). Nursebooks.org.

Australian Nursing Federation, Australian College of Nursing, & Nursing and Midwifery Board of Australia. (2015). *Code of ethics for nurses in Australia.* https://waubrafoundation.org.au/resources/code-ethics-for-nurses-australia/

Aydelotte, M., & Chaska, N. L. (1990). The evolving profession: The role of the professional organization. *The nursing profession: A time to speak,* 9–15.

Begun, J. W., & Lippincott, R. C. (1993). *Strategic adaptation in the health professions.* Jossey-Bass.

Bixler, G. K., & Bixler, R. W. (1959). The professional status of nursing. *American Journal of Nursing, 59*(8), 1142–1147.

Bochatay, N. (2018). Individual and collective strategies in nurses' struggle for professional identity. *Health Sociology Review, 27*(3), 263–278. https://doi.org/10.1080/14461242.2018.1469096.

CNA. (2017). *Code of ethics for registered nurses.* https://cdn1.nscn.ca/sites/default/files/documents/resources/code-of-ethics-for-registered-nurses.pdf#:~:text=The%20Canadian%20Nurses%20Association%20%28CNA%29%20Code%20of%20Ethics,receiving%20care.%20The%20Codeis%20both%20aspirational%20and%20regulatory

Covert, E. C. (1917). Is nursing a profession? *American Journal of Nursing, 18*(2), 107–109.

Curtin, L. (1980).). Ethical issues in nursing practice and education: *Ethical issues in nursing and nursing education* (pp. 25–26). National Leage for Nursing.

Danish Council of Nursing Ethics. (2017). *Code of ethics for nurses.*

Felton, G. (2001). Building for the next century: Nursing's bias in its glory In N. Chaska (Ed.), *The nursing profession: Tomorrow and beyond* (pp. 3–16). SAGE. https://doi.org/10.4135/9781452232720.

Finnish Nurses Association. (2021). *Code of ethics for nurses.*

Flexner, A. (1910). *Medical education in the United States and Canada: A report to the Carnegie Foundation for the advancement of teaching.* The Merrymount Press.

Haskell, H. (2009, October 8, 2018). *The Lewis Blackman story* [Five-part video series]. QSEN. http://qsen.org/publications/videos/the-lewis-blackman-story/

ICN. (2021). *The ICN code of ethics for nurses.* https://www.icn.ch/system/files/2021-10/ICN_Code-of-Ethics_EN_Web_0.pdf

IOM. (2010). *The future of nursing: Leading change, advancing health.* N. A. Press. https://www.nap.edu/read/12956/chapter/1.

Jameton, A. (1984). *Nursing practice: The ethical issues.* Prentice-Hall.

Leininger, M. M. (Ed.). (1984). *Care, the essence of nursing and health.* Wayne State University Press.

May, R. (1960). *Love and will.* Norton.

Mayeroff, M. (1971). *On caring.* Harper & Row.

National Academy of Medicine. (2021). *The future of nursing 2020-2030: Charting a path to achieve health equity.* N. A. Press. https://nam.edu/publications/the-future-of-nursing-2020-2030/.

NCSBN & ANA. (2019). *National guidelines for nursing delegation.* ana-ncsbn-joint-statement-ondelegation.pdf.

Newman, M. A., Sime, A. M., & Corcoran-Perry, S. A. (1991). The focus of the discipline of nursing. *Advances in Nursing Science, 14*(1), 1–6.

Nightingale, F. (1859). *Notes on nursing: What it is, and what it is not.* Harrison & Sons. http://digital.library.upenn.edu/women/nightingale/nursing/nursing.html.

Nursing & Midwifery Council. (2015). *The code: Professional standards of practice and behavior for nurses, midwives, and nursing associates.* https://www.nmc.org.uk/globalassets/sitedocuments/nmc-publications/nmc-code.pdf

Nursing and Midwifery Board of Ireland. (2021). *Code of professional conduct and ethics for registered nurses and registered midwives.* https://www.nmbi.ie/NMBI/media/NMBI/Code-of-Professional-Conduct-and-Ethics.pdf?ext=.pdf

Nursing Council of New Zealand. (2012). *Code of conduct for nurses.* https://online.flippingbook.com/view/359694379/

Parsons, M. (1986). The profession in a class by itself. *Nursing Outlook, 34,* 270–275.

Rasmussen, P. (2018). Factors influencing registered nurses' perceptions of their professional identity: An integrative literature review. *Journal of Continuing Education in Nursing, 49*(5), 225.

Reed, P. G. (2000). Nursing reformation: Historical reflections and philosophic foundations. *Nursing Science Quarterly, 13*(2), 129–136.

Reich, W. R. (2003). Historical traditions of an ethic of care in healthcare In S. G. Post (Ed.), *Encyclopedia of bioethics* (pp. 349–367). Thomas Gale, Macmillan Reference.

Robb, I. H. (1912). *Nursing ethics: For hospital and private use.* E.C. Koeckert.

Rogers, M. E. (1983). *The education violet.* New York University Press. https://www.pinterest.com/pin/190628996698256687/.

Sabanciogullari, S., & Dogan, S. (2017). Professional self-concept in nurses and related factors: A sample from Turkey. *International Journal of Caring Sciences, 10*(3), 1676–1684.

Sasso, L., Stievano, A., Jurado, M., & Rocco, G. (2008). Code of ethics and conduct for European nursing. *Nursing Ethics, 15*(6), 821–836. https://doi.org/10.1177/0969733008095390.

Smith, M. C. (1999). Caring and the science of unitary human beings. *Advances in Nursing Science, 21*(4), 14–28.

Swanson, K. M. (1991). Empirical development of a middle range theory of caring. *Nursing Research, 40*(3), 161–166.

Swedish Society of Nursing. (2010). *Foundation of nursing care values.* https://swenurse.se/download/18.272cda6a1775a3fd26f4bc3d/1612192731944/foundation.of.nursing.care.values.pdf

Viens, D. C. (1989). A history of nursing's code of ethics. *Nursing Outlook, 37*(1), 45–49.

Watson, J. (2002). Intentionality and caring-healing consciousness: A practice of transpersonal nursing. *Holistic Nursing Practice, 16*(4), 12–19.

Watson, J. (2010). Caring science and the next decade of holistic healing: Transforming self and system from the inside out. *Beginnings, 30*(2), 14–16.

7

Ethical Decision Making

Peace requires that you do what in your heart you know—that your chosen values guide your actions. Peace is the means and the end, the process and the product.

(Chinn, 2004)

OBJECTIVES

After completing this chapter, the reader should be able to:

1. Describe the process of making thoughtful decisions.
2. Discuss similarities between the nursing process and ethical decision making.
3. Recognize the moral elements of everyday nursing practice.
4. Describe the role of emotions in ethical decisions.
5. Examine the process of ethical decision making.
6. Apply the ethical decision-making process to clinical cases.
7. Describe and differentiate ethical dilemmas, moral uncertainty, practical dilemmas, moral distress, moral outrage, and moral reckoning.
8. Evaluate how knowledge of the nursing code of ethics and a sense of personal empowerment help nurses avoid moral distress and moral reckoning.

INTRODUCTION

Each person makes decisions as part of everyday life. Some decisions seem routine, such as what to have for lunch or what to wear to work. Other decisions, like where to go to college, which job to accept, or whether to marry, call for more deliberation. Moral/ethical decisions such as when to discontinue life support are even more complex. Nurses constantly make decisions. We make decisions about routine matters such as patient care management and institutional policy. We also participate in decisions about moral/ethical problems. In everyday situations, we may not have a conscious awareness of our thought processes even though we have an innate sense of knowing what to do. At other times, we struggle with decisions.

Ethical decision making is not as clear-cut as decisions made in other areas of life. Moral problems are complex. They may include intricate human relationships among disparate participants who have opposing opinions and power imbalances. They incorporate a mix of values, risks, benefits, harms, and implications. The best solution is often obscure, and the ultimate outcome is unknown until the process unfolds.

Nurses are involved in patient care situations imbued with moral implications. People involved in the healthcare system make ethical decisions affecting life and death every day. Research has shown that as many as half of all nurses leave bedside nursing because of moral distress. We believe that nurses who are informed, courageous, and involved in ethical decision making are more likely to be satisfied with their work and thus stay at the bedside. Therefore, it is critical that you learn the language of ethics and have the courage to fully participate in ethical decision making. This chapter presents a discussion of moral problems, offers a guide for ethical decision making, and suggests approaches to dealing with the personal and professional consequences of difficult decisions.

PROBLEM ANALYSIS

In the context of nursing ethics, we define the term *problem* as a situation in which there is a discrepancy between the status quo (what is actually happening) and what one desires or what should be happening—that is, the situation is unwelcome, harmful, or wrong and needs to be overcome. Since subjective judgment is involved, a situation becomes a problem only if someone believes it should be different from what it is. Problems are usually unplanned and often unexpected. They may be simple or complex, routine or moral. Some can be solved, some cannot.

Before you can begin to solve a problem, you must be able to identify and categorize it. Is the problem routine, such as a minor shortage of staff for the evening shift, or is the problem complex, such as an imminent nursing strike that threatens patient care? Solutions to routine problems may involve only one decision maker and may involve how or when to do something, which item to choose, who to assign to a task, and so forth. When you closely examine a routine problem, you will find that there is a considerable focus on preference, economy, and efficiency. Although sometimes frustrating, you can usually find the resolution to routine problems once you gather the relevant information and resources. Routine problems are important from a personal or business standpoint but may have very little moral focus.

Moral problems differ from routine problems and are often complex. They have embedded human stories that we describe with value terms such as good, bad, harm, benefit, should, ought, right, and wrong. Moral problems are important, and they seem to defy easy solutions. They are complex and dynamic with elements of uncertainty and conflict. One cannot enter moral decision making capriciously because, once made, many decisions cannot be unmade, they are irreversible. Different types of problems include moral uncertainty, moral dilemmas, and practical dilemmas (Jameton, 1984). We discuss the types of moral problems and several intervening factors in the following section and throughout the chapter.

Moral Uncertainty

Moral uncertainty occurs when we sense a moral problem but are not sure of the morally correct action, when we are unsure which moral principles or values apply, or when we are unable to define the moral problems. This happens when we have a sense that something is not quite right. We are uncomfortable with a situation but can't figure out the problem. Jameton (1984) offers the example of a nurse caring for an older patient who is somewhat neglected, with little attention being given to the patient's problem. The nurse feels dissatisfied with the patient's treatment but is unable to pinpoint the nature and cause of the inadequacy.

Moral/Ethical Dilemmas

A dilemma is a problem that requires a choice between two options that are equally unfavorable and mutually exclusive. A choice must be made, but no option is desirable. A dilemma seems to defy a clear solution. The following is an example of a dilemma: An administrator has only one job opening. There are two candidates. One candidate has been with the organization for many years and is reliable and loyal. His work is consistently satisfactory but seldom excellent. The second candidate, a new employee, is brilliant but unproven on the job. The administrator cannot choose both even though each has desirable qualities. Neither choice is patently right or wrong, yet the decision will have important implications in the future for both the organization and the individuals. Because the future is unknown, the administrator will attempt to make the best choice based on the information at hand.

The previous example describes a routine problem. An ethical dilemma occurs when options include conflicting moral claims. Ethical dilemmas present in at least two ways. A person can experience a dilemma when there is evidence that a certain act is morally right and evidence to indicate that the same act is morally wrong, but no evidence is conclusive (Beauchamp & Childress, 2019). An example of this can be seen in the terminally ill patient. Although most would think it is morally right to preserve life, many would believe it is morally wrong to prolong suffering. When struggling with this problem, one would ponder whether a terminally ill person should undergo prolonged life-preserving measures even though the treatments cause extreme physical or emotional suffering, or should the person be supported toward a comfortable and peaceful death. A dilemma occurs when the decision maker believes that one or more moral claims support one course of action, and one or more moral claims support another course of action, and the two actions are mutually exclusive. Healthcare providers face this type of dilemma, for example, when they must decide who gets the critical care bed. Should they make the decision based on who is most deserving, who arrives first, who can pay, or who has the best chance of survival? Different people perceive or conceptualize conflicts in different ways. Conflicting moral claims can be said to occur, for example, between obligations, principles, duties, rights, loyalties, and so forth.

Let us examine different perceptions of conflicting moral claims. The nurse might perceive a conflict between adherence to two different principles, such as wishing to avoid the suffering a patient experiences when hearing a bad prognosis, while at the same time respecting the patient's right to know. In this instance, the nurse might perceive a direct conflict between the principles of nonmaleficence (the wish to do no harm) and autonomy (ensuring that the patient is self-governing). In another

instance, the nurse might perceive a conflict of duties. This type of conflict can occur, for example, when nurse managers must make staffing decisions. The nurse manager will recognize a duty to the institution but will also feel a duty to meet the needs of individual patients and nurses. Conflicts often arise when the needs of the institution conflict with the needs of individuals.

ASK YOURSELF

Facing Ethical Dilemmas

The situation in which a decision must be made about whether to prolong the life of a terminally ill patient who is experiencing constant, intractable suffering illustrates a conflict between the ethical principles of beneficence (do good) and nonmaleficence (avoid harm), since prolonging life can be said to be doing good while at the same time causing the harm of severe pain. Think of hypothetical patient care situations in which the following principles might conflict:

- The principle of justice versus the principle of beneficence
- The principle of veracity versus the principle of nonmaleficence
- The principle of confidentiality versus the principle of beneficence
- The principle of respect for autonomy versus the principle of justice

If you haven't had much experience in health care up to this point in your career, you may be having difficulty imagining situations that respond to these questions. Following are some extreme examples that respond to the conflicts. As you think about the examples, ask yourself the following questions: How would you respond in each of the situations? What factors would you consider in making your decision? What values and beliefs would guide your decision? As you read the following vignettes, try to think of other, less extreme examples.

- Justice versus beneficence. You are assigned to take care of a bedfast patient on a ventilator. You recognize that you have a duty to care for this patient. When a hurricane strikes, the electricity and auxiliary power systems fail, and you are required to use a handheld resuscitator to support the patient's breathing. The supervisor asks you to leave your patient to help evacuate pediatric patients on a floor that is rapidly flooding. Caring for your patient is a beneficent action, but justice may call for you to help evacuate patients for the "greater good." The two mutually exclusive, negative choices are (1) abandoning your patient who cannot breathe without assistance or (2) allowing pediatric patients to suffer or die in a flooded unit. You must make a choice—you cannot do both.

- Veracity versus nonmaleficence. A young woman is hospitalized for depression and a suicide attempt. The nurse knows that the woman's fiancé was killed in an automobile accident during her hospitalization. The patient asks why he hasn't come to visit her. The ethical principle of veracity would suggest that the nurse tell her the truth, while the principle of nonmaleficence requires the nurse to do no harm. The nurse recognizes that telling the truth (which is morally right) in this situation might result in the patient experiencing more severe depression or another suicide attempt (which is morally wrong in terms of nonmaleficence).
- Confidentiality versus beneficence. The patient in the situation above tells the nurse she is planning suicide as soon as she is discharged. She asks that the nurse keep this information confidential. To do good (beneficence), the nurse believes she must violate the patient's confidentiality.
- Autonomy versus justice. The state Medicaid program has a limited number of dollars to spend on healthcare programs, including well-child examinations, immunizations, renal dialysis, and nursing home care. An indigent, elderly woman who has out-of-control diabetes with end-stage kidney failure, which qualifies her for Medicaid, demands a pancreas transplant to treat her diabetes. The Medicaid program has never before paid for a pancreas transplant. With limited funds available and knowing that immunization programs are the most effective way to lower childhood morbidity and mortality, the program administrators deny the $400,000 surgery. Because Medicaid dollars are finite, the woman's autonomous decision to have the transplant conflicts with the distributive justice implications of providing immunization services for hundreds of children.

These vignettes portray examples of extreme situations that nurses might encounter. These moral problems offer conflicting moral claims, however conceptualized, and potential solutions that appear to be equally unfavorable. Less dramatic dilemmas occur every day. You should use the same type of deliberation when faced with a lower-magnitude ethical dilemma as you would with extreme examples.

Practical Dilemmas

One must be careful to differentiate between moral and practical dilemmas. Occasionally, situations present themselves in which moral claims compete with non-moral claims. Nonmoral claims are claims of self-interest (Beauchamp & Childress, 2019). Consider, for example, the nurse who must work overtime, caring for a gravely ill patient. The nurse might perceive a dilemma because she made a promise to take her children to the circus. Certainly, this is a dilemma. Though the nurse might say that her duty to the children conflicts with her duty to care for the patient, it can be argued that the duties are not of equal moral weight. The duty to keep the promise to her children is a practical duty that is grounded in self-interest (or the interest of her family). In decisions that involve practical dilemmas, moral claims have greater weight than nonmoral claims. When deliberating, nurses must be able to differentiate between moral and practical dilemmas.

Factors that Intervene in Ethical Decision Making

Intervening factors are elements that appear in a situation in such a way as to interfere with, alter, or obstruct action. Intervening factors create a sense of mystery and add to the complexity of ethical problems. The skillful decision maker will anticipate and recognize intervening factors and attempt to gather as much data as possible. As more data are gathered, there is a greater likelihood that a rational decision will lead to the most desirable outcome. In addition to the medical condition of the patient, the following section describes the anticipated intervening factors of uncertainty, context, stakeholders, power imbalance, extraneous variables, and urgency.

Uncertainty

Uncertainty refers to a lack of predictability because of insufficient evidence. Ethical decisions are more difficult because we can seldom accurately predict the outcome of a given act. Take, for example, a case in which an adult Jehovah's Witness sustains life-threatening injuries. She has decision-making capacity and refuses blood or blood products but agrees to surgery. During the surgery, she hemorrhages profoundly. The hemorrhage is an unexpected, intervening variable. Because she is unconscious, the patient no longer has decision-making capacity. Her husband, who is not a Jehovah's Witness, demands that the physicians administer blood transfusions. The physicians and nurses respect the patient's autonomous decision; nevertheless, they are tempted to order the transfusion based on the principle of beneficence. The decision would be easier if they knew that she would ultimately survive without the transfusion, but they cannot foresee the future. They can reduce uncertainty by gathering information about similar situations in the past. One of the goals of data gathering is to reduce uncertainty as much as possible.

Context

Context may present intervening factors. It includes a person's unique life circumstances. Context describes the world in which the person lives—his or her culture, income, home, relationships, transportation, religion, and everything else. As you gather information about the context of a person's life, you discover the patient as a person. You learn about the patient's life and find out who the patient was before the illness. Context is often the intervening factor that points toward one choice rather than another. For example, a 28-year-old man collapsed near a homeless center on Los Angeles's Skid Row. A staff member called an ambulance as the man began having a seizure. Just a couple of hours later, and still disoriented from the medication he'd been given in the emergency room, the man was back on Skid Row. He reported that the hospital had given him bus tokens and sent him "home" to his tent amid human feces, discarded syringes, and garbage (Green, 2018). The decision to discharge this man in this way was inappropriate and newsworthy because it ignored the context of his life.

Multiple Stakeholders

Stakeholders are persons with an interest in a given situation. Stakeholders can constitute intervening factors in many situations because they can affect or be affected by proposed actions. In health care, the patient is always the major stakeholder, and full consideration should be given to the patient's goals, desires, and intentions. Other stakeholders may include family members, close friends, and others. In some cultures, the family is involved in making any major decisions, even about an individual's health choices. State laws may regulate who makes decisions in the event the patient does not have decision-making capacity. However, informal rules about stakeholders' input in ethical decision making are sometimes unclear. Occasionally, when making choices about an ethical problem, we are bewildered by multiple stakeholders with strong preferences. When this happens, key information might have been obscured or distorted—especially if each stakeholder lobbies for his or her own interest. Consider this hypothetical example: An elderly woman lived for many years in the home of her daughter, who was kind and attentive. When the woman suffered a massive stroke, her son arrived and began arguing about what should be done. Before her illness, the son rarely spoke to his mother, yet because he was the oldest sibling, he believed that he was the best person to make decisions for her. Because no one had medical power of attorney and there was no advance directive, the staff was unsure who should make decisions. They wondered if hidden motives were affecting the decision-making process. The major stakeholder was, of course, the patient herself. But in this case, she could not speak for her own interests. The major challenge in a case like this is to create a safe forum that encourages people to discuss their interests candidly and search jointly for solutions.

CASE PRESENTATION

Parental Authority
Some of the most frustrating situations in pediatric care involve decisions about what is in the best interest of the child and is there a limit of parental authority. Central Elementary School is experiencing a record-breaking number of children with β-hemolytic streptococcus pharyngitis (strep throat). The third-grade classroom has eight children diagnosed with the disease. Tommie, a student in class, comes to see Harley, the school nurse, complaining of a severe sore throat. Tommie looks sick and has a high fever, enlarged lymph nodes in the neck, a sandpaper rash over the body, petechia in the throat, and a positive strep test, which Harley administered in the school clinic. Harley knows that untreated β-hemolytic streptococcal infection can result in severe complications, including rheumatic fever, glomerulonephritis, meningitis, pneumonia, and toxic shock syndrome. On the other hand, strep throat treated with antibiotics has few complications.

Harley telephones Tommie's mother, who is divorced from Harley's father, and recommends that she take Tommie to her pediatrician for treatment. Tommie's mother responds that their family relies on natural remedies such as prayer and herbal tea. She is adamant that she will not take Tommie to a pediatrician—she distrusts all physicians. Harley is frustrated and highly concerned that Tommie could experience the serious consequences of strep throat if it is not treated.

Think About It
Deciding a Child's Best Interest
- What action seems to be in Tommie's best interest?
- Do you think Tommie's mother should have the parental authority to make this decision, even though the outcomes could be serious, or even life-threatening?
- What are the important contextual factors?
- How do you think Harley should proceed in the situation?

Although we think in terms of patients' families, we might also find that healthcare professionals become stakeholders. This usually happens when a person with a strong bias seizes power. For example, a woman was pregnant with a seriously malformed fetus whose chances for survival were slim. Before the birth, the couple made the difficult decision to forego lifesaving treatments. Hospital policy required that a pediatrician attend the birth of all high-risk neonates. Immediately after the child was born, the on-call pediatrician picked up the baby, carried it to the newborn intensive care unit, and began resuscitation efforts. She ordered the nurses to continue resuscitation and she limited the parents' access to the child. The baby survived for a short time (Nathaniel, 2003). Because of a strong religious bias and sense of accountability, the physician claimed a position as stakeholder. This situation created tensions among the healthcare providers, as well as between the physician and parents. Each person had strong beliefs about which option was right and which was wrong. Decisions had to be made quickly and stakeholders in this case lacked a safe forum that would have allowed them to discuss their interests candidly and search jointly for solutions.

Power Imbalance

The preceding case is an example of power imbalance. The intervening factor of power imbalance, either real or perceived, sometimes affects the decision-making process by inhibiting honest and open discourse. A number of mechanisms are in place that maintain power imbalance within the healthcare institution. Even though nurses may sometimes be in the best position to know patients' wishes, physicians may have explicit power. Implicit social and institutional mechanisms may also disempower patients and nurses. Timid patients and their families may blindly accept the advice of physicians. Afraid to make waves, nurses may feel constrained from expressing their opinions, even if they disagree.

Physicians also feel the stress of power imbalance. Oberle and Hughes published the results of a study that compared physicians' and nurses' perceptions of ethical problems (2001). Nurses and doctors experienced problems around decision making, but their perspectives were different (Fig. 7.1). Physicians bore the burden of having to make the decisions and write the orders, whereas the nurses' burden entailed living with the decisions made by someone else. Physicians questioned themselves, and nurses questioned physicians. Nurses expected physicians to make the "right" decision, even when right was unclear, while physicians sometimes blamed themselves for poor outcomes. This study demonstrates that power imbalance can be stressful, even for those who have power.

Extraneous Variables

Intervening factors that influence decisions often include variables outside the direct patient care setting. Decision makers must consider institutional policy, professional standards, third-party payers, and public policy when making ethical decisions. For example, even if you believe that euthanasia is the best choice for a terminally ill person, legal, professional, and institutional standards in the United States prohibit it. Sometimes, the court will intercede in healthcare decisions—especially if there is disagreement on the course of action. Intervention of the court presents a strong intervening factor. For example, in the classic case of Baby K, the court favored the mother's request and ordered physicians and nurses to repeatedly resuscitate the anencephalic infant, even though all agreed that resuscitation was painful and futile and there was no chance of recovery (Perkin et al., 1997).

Other Relevant Cases

Even though each situation may seem unique, there are few truly novel moral problems. Known as casuistry, the use of well-settled cases published in the legal and ethics literature can serve as intervening factors when they influence the ethical decision-making process (Veatch & Guidry-Grimes, 2020). Comparing the present situation with others in the past may help clarify the situation and move toward a rational decision. For example, Terri Schiavo lay in a persistent vegetative state in 2005 as her husband and parents fought a highly publicized legal battle over whether to discontinue tube feedings. As you will read in Chapters 10 and 11, this case was similar to the historical cases of Nancy Cruzan and

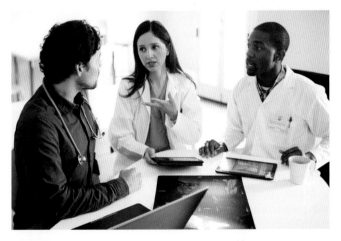

Fig. 7.1 Nurses and Physicians Experience Problems Around Decision Making, but Their Perspectives Are Different. (iStock photo ID: 655821120.)

Karen Ann Quinlan in which the courts supported the families' wishes to discontinue tube feedings. Although the media treated the Schiavo case as if it were the first of its kind, the Cruzan and Quinlan cases were among others that offered relevant information for the Schiavo case. The salient difference between this case and the others was that Schiavo's parents and husband were stakeholders with opposite and incompatible goals.

Urgency

Time itself may be an intervening factor. In certain urgent situations, you must make decisions before you have a chance to deliberate as much as you would like. This may occur when death is rapidly imminent. In these cases, failure to decide quickly is essentially the same as making a choice, because it directly affects the outcome. When you encounter an urgent situation, quickly gather as many stakeholders as possible and discuss known factors. Decisions are hard to make when pertinent data are unavailable and the future is uncertain. Because most ethicists now agree that withdrawal of life support is no different from forgoing it in the first place, you might decide to preserve life until such time that a more rational decision is possible. Recognize that the option you choose is the best one at that point in time.

ETHICAL DECISION MAKING

Four basic features constitute every type of decision. First, a problem must exist—otherwise, a decision is unnecessary. A clear statement of the problem is critical to finding a rational solution. A statement of the problem has two parts: the current situation and the desired state. When it is well articulated, an attainable desired state becomes the goal of the decision-making process. Second, there must be at least two alternative solutions from which to choose. If no course of action will affect the outcome, there is no need to engage in decision making—the outcome is inevitable. Third, every action implies uncertainty. Uncertainties are elements that we can neither control nor predict absolutely. They are important because they affect the outcome. Uncertainties create angst among decision makers. Anticipating, controlling, and predicting uncertainties to the extent possible assists with rational decision making. Fourth, every implemented decision, combined with the uncertainties, brings about an outcome. The goal of decision making is to move from the current situation to

a reasonable desired state. When the goal and outcomes are the same, people applaud the decision, even though uncertainties might have altered the outcome.

Making Decisions

As humans, we make decisions many times each day. Most decisions follow a similar pattern, whether they involve routine day-to-day problems or complex professional ones. Depending on the situation, the decision-making process ranges from a subconscious one used for minor routine problems to a sophisticated one based on scientific principles, knowledge, and experience. The pattern for most types of decision making includes five separate steps as follows: articulating the problem and rational goals, gathering data, comparing options, using some criteria for weighing the merits of each option, and making a choice. Follow-up evaluation of outcomes or circumstances surrounding the choice provides subsequent data regarding the *rightness* of the choice and may influence future decisions. A simple example of this process is how you choose what clothes to wear each day. The data you gather includes such things as where you are going, what you will be doing, the weather, what is clean or handy, your mood, the colors you prefer, and the style of clothing you anticipate others will be wearing. You may narrow choices down to several options that would be acceptable or appropriate, and you compare these based on some criteria. The criteria may be what is least wrinkled, or feels most comfortable, or makes you look or feel more confident, or is more appropriate for weather conditions, or a combination of considerations. Using the criteria, you narrow down options and make a choice. As you move through the day, you gather more data about the rightness of your decision. For example, are you comfortable? Did your friend cringe when she saw you? Do you feel dressed appropriately for the meeting? Are you warm enough? Does the color seem to make you stand out? Your evaluation of whether you made the right decision provides information about the strength or validity of the criteria you used to guide your decision and whether to use these same criteria to guide similar decisions in the future.

The Nursing Process and Ethical Decision Making

Knowledge of social rules, ethical principles, and professional standards is as important to making ethical decisions as knowledge of physical, psychological, social, and human science is to other nursing judgments. However, because of the nature of moral problems, the ability to make consistent ethical decisions requires a formal decision-making structure. When decision making follows an established procedure, the moral justification for an ethical decision can be as powerful as a scientific explanation for a medical decision. Ethical decision-making models are related to nursing care in the ethical realm in the same way that the *nursing process* is related to nursing care in the physical realm. If you understand the steps of the nursing process, the ethical decision-making model will be clearer to you.

As nurses, we commonly use the nursing process model for decision making. Utilizing logical thinking and intuitive knowing, the nursing process is a deliberate activity that provides a systematic method for nursing practice. The nursing process is a logical system that directs nursing practice and standardizes nursing care. Familiar to most nurses, the nursing process generally includes the following interactive and sequential steps: problem identification based on the assessment of subjective and objective data, development of a plan for care guided by desired outcomes, implementation of interventions, evaluation of the outcomes, and revision of the plan over time. Criteria used in making nursing care decisions derive from areas such as knowledge of anatomy, physiology, psychology, pathophysiology, therapeutic communication, sociocultural and family dynamics, pharmacology, microbiology, nursing, and other theories; familiarity with standards of care and protocols; and experience related to what has worked in similar situations. The process is systematic and involves both logical thinking and intuitive knowing. As you will see, the ethical decision-making model is similar to the nursing process. It is a necessary tool that helps nurses make consistent decisions that are grounded in knowledge, yet sensitive to each individual case.

Approaching Ethical Decisions

We believe that nurses who effectively engage in ethical decision making are less likely to experience moral distress and leave the bedside. Sadly, our research has shown that many nurses are unprepared to be equal participants in ethical decision making (Nathaniel, 2006). Jameton (1984) suggests that one takes the perspective of the responsible actor, rather than the victim, dealing actively with morally troubling patient situations and working toward solutions to the larger problems. In an

effort to make cogent and consistent moral judgments, you should familiarize yourself with the sociology and history of healthcare decision making and the basics of moral philosophy. You should articulate and examine your core values and their relationship to nursing and institutional standards. To join decision-making groups, you should become fluent in the language of nursing and bioethics and learn to appreciate the diverse moral perspectives of patients and colleagues.

Attributes of an Effective Ethical Decision Maker

In addition to the actions described previously, a nurse can cultivate a number of attributes that will help with ethical decision making. These attributes include moral integrity; sensitivity, compassion, and caring; a sense of responsibility; empowerment; and patience and willingness to deliberate (Fig. 7.2).

Moral Integrity

Moral integrity binds a person's moral virtues into a coherent package—it creates a wholeness and stability of character that lead to trustworthiness. Moral integrity involves a unified integration of different parts of the person, such as emotions, goals, hopes, knowledge, and values, in a way that is consistent, sound, and reliable. Moral integrity is integral to effective ethical decision making. A person with moral integrity does not hold stubbornly to one position, but rather encourages a climate of mutual respect and reasoned discourse. However, a person with moral integrity will not compromise beyond a certain point.

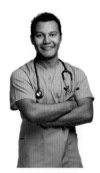

Attributes of an Effective
Ethical Decision Maker

- Moral Integrity
- Sensitivity, Compassion, and Caring
- Sense of Responsibility
- Empowerment
- Patience and Willingness to Deliberate

Fig. 7.2 Attributes of an Effective Ethical Decision Maker. (©iStock.com/aldomurillo.)

Sensitivity, Compassion, and Caring

Sensitivity, compassion, and caring are highly related human attributes. Sensitivity is a character trait that includes a delicate and profound awareness of other people's feelings and the social complexities of a situation. A nurse who is sensitive innately recognizes the suffering of others. Compassion, on the other hand, involves the feeling or emotion that one has when recognizing the suffering of another and adds a desire to prevent or relieve the suffering. Therefore, compassion can be recognized by positive or helpful acts. Compassionate nurses go out of their way to relieve the physical, mental, or emotional pains of others. They take action. When combined with an understanding of biopsychosocial and ethical principles, nurses base compassionate care on sound judgment. Many philosophers recognize compassion as one of the greatest virtues. Caring integrates the attributes of sensitivity with the motivation to act derived from compassion. Sensitive, compassionate, and caring nurses work intimately with patients—they hear what patients say and understand the meaning. They perceive the circumstances, attitudes, and feelings of others. They intimately know about suffering—from touch, sight, smell, and sound. Interests of patients become their own.

Sense of Responsibility

The nurse with a sense of responsibility recognizes a duty to the patient—an obligation to do whatever is necessary, within reason, to care for the patient or solve a problem. A nurse with a sense of responsibility, sensitivity, compassion, and caring will recognize moral problems, understand them from a human perspective, and embrace the duty to work actively toward their solution. Responsibility also includes a duty to understand ethics in a way that informs the consistent and fair application of ethics at the bedside.

Empowerment

Empowerment is the capacity of people to be active participants in matters that affect them. Empowerment is an interpersonal process by which one gains mastery over his or her life using the proper tools, resources, and environment. It allows the person to effectively work toward individual and social goals. Empowerment suggests that a person has self-confidence that he or she can effect change. It includes courage and an exercise of power. Empowerment is an essential attribute for those making ethical decisions. It creates positive action flowing from sensitivity, compassion, caring, and responsibility.

Patience and Willingness to Deliberate

During a crisis, people struggle to understand the situation and their feelings. They work to clarify and articulate their views and relate them to a framework of values. Whereas impatience is marked by a rush to get answers before really thinking through problems, patience involves a quiet willingness to tolerate negative circumstances. It requires a calm response to situations and people who might be perceived as burdensome, frustrating, or unpleasant. Patience buffers against negative emotions (Schnitker et al., 2017). The nurse must embrace respect for persons, listen, and be patient while tolerating vagueness, confusion, uncertainty, and paradox. The nurse should provide a safe environment and gently assist patients, families, and colleagues as they work through the ethical decision-making process.

Emotions and Ethical Decisions

Many approaches to ethical decision making recommend a cognitive process in which emotions are subordinated to reason. In a holistic view of people, however, both thinking and feeling are credible ways of knowing, each having a legitimate role in ethical decision making. Callahan (2000) suggested that heart and mind should not be viewed as antagonistic in the moral arena; rather, both reason and emotion should be active and in accord as we come to an ethical decision. Noting that emotions should influence reason while reason is monitoring emotions, Callahan described emotions as personal signals providing information regarding both inner processes and interactions with the environment.

It is important to appreciate not only what you *think* about what is right or wrong in a situation but also what you *feel* in relation to the circumstances and decision to be made. If you feel discomfort, even though reason is pointing in a particular direction, you should further explore both the arguments posed through reason and your reactions to them. Recognizing our healthcare culture's emphasis on technology and a tendency to devalue feelings and moral emotions, Callahan (2000) writes, "Numbness, apathy, isolated disassociations between thinking and feeling are also moral warning signals. the absence of emotional responses of empathy and sympathy become critical bioethical issues" (p. 29). The goal is to have head and heart in harmony as the decision is made.

In the same way that different people may approach an issue with various methods of moral reasoning, their emotional responses might be quite legitimate, yet different from your own. In such situations, you might broaden your own compassionate view so that you can appreciate the validity of the other person's emotional response. On the other hand, you may recognize that the chasm between the two is too deep to bridge. Callahan suggests that such social conflicts and challenges present new ethical problems that may require dealing with the consequences of an ethical decision by repeating the decision-making process.

ASK YOURSELF

The Role of Emotions in Decision Making

Consider your emotional response to the following situations and how they would affect your dealing with and caring for the people involved.

- You work in a clinic primarily serving an immigrant population, and you hear one of your coworkers comment that "Health education is a waste of time because these people don't want to learn. They are just a drain on our system."
- You just started working for a group of obstetric physicians, and you discover that the physician you are assigned to work with refuses to accept patients who drink alcohol.
- You are working in an emergency department at the local hospital where a two-year-old child dies of injuries sustained while being "disciplined" by the mother's boyfriend. The child had previously been placed in foster care due to neglect and had been returned to the mother's care only a week before this event.

Ethical Decisions at the Bedside

Nurses at the bedside make decisions related to issues of moral importance every day. In the next few pages, we introduce a formal decision-making model for you to use throughout your career to make those important, life-altering ethical decisions. We acknowledge, however, that nurses make important, but less formal, decisions many times each day. These day-to-day decisions at the bedside require a consciousness of the moral nuances in each situation. Different from ethics, we use the term **ethic** to refer to a personal consciousness of the moral importance that guides personal action in particular situations. An ethic is derived from an individual's innate values. The term *ethic* can be combined with any morally important quality or virtue. For instance, nurses might be said to have an ethic of care, an ethic of responsiveness, an ethic of attentiveness, or an ethic of respect. As nurses seek to do that which is *good*, they call on an innate consciousness of the moral value of day-to-day nursing actions. In a discussion of everyday ethics, Benner (1994) suggests that an ethic of responsiveness is central to the caring practice of nurses. A nurse's ethic of responsiveness demonstrates respect for persons and a desire to do good for this particular patient on this particular day. The nurse with this quality responds with sensitivity to the concerns, needs, and preferences of each patient.

As we have suggested in previous chapters, a nurse with a highly tuned consciousness of the moral importance of nursing actions engages with patients on a personal level and remains acutely vigilant to status changes. The expert nurse uses different ways of knowing to interpret all aspects of the patient and responds with sensitivity and caring (Benner, 1994). We mention everyday ethics at this point because we want to be clear that ethics and ethical decision making imbue every aspect of nursing—not just the newsworthy extreme examples. Ethical decisions are not limited to dramatic, life-altering issues. They surround us all the time. Standing quietly at the bedside of a dying patient, for example, is an act of moral integrity. We ask you to seek to do good, recognize moral nuances, be conscious of the ethic that guides your comportment at the bedside, and employ the best qualities in yourself as you also attend to the ethical principles and theories that guide nursing practice. For those occasions when the larger dilemmas emerge, we offer a formal guide to ethical decision making on the following pages.

ETHICAL DECISION-MAKING MODEL

We approach ethical decision making with a problem-solving frame of reference and sensitivity to the human story. Like the nursing process, ethical problem-solving includes a number of steps. As you see them here in writing, the steps may seem linear; however, we believe they must remain nonlinear and iterative—moving back and forth as needed. Ethical decision making is a process that overlays other dynamic biological, psychological, and sociocultural processes, layer upon layer. Physical conditions change, opinions change, stakeholders come and go, knowledge evolves, and time passes. Nothing in the human sphere is static.

The nature of the ethical problem requires a decision-making process by which key facets are revisited from evolving perspectives, even as you move toward a decision or resolution. Other models for decision making describe linear step-by-step processes that do not reflect the potential for an evolving perspective. The guidelines presented here provide a framework for entering a decision-making process that requires an ongoing evaluation and assimilation of information. This decision-making process is spiral in nature, with each step being revisited as often as is required and molded by the dynamics of changing facts, evolving beliefs, unexpected consequences, and participants who move in and out of the process. The following text describes a five-step process of ethical decision making.

Step 1: Articulate the Problem and Determine a Realistic Goal

The first step in the decision-making process is to clearly articulate the problem. Since a problem is defined as a discrepancy between the current situation and a desired state (goal), your next step is to clarify the goal. Ethical decision making begins when someone recognizes that there is a moral problem. If the problem is serious enough that it requires a decision, it is intolerable and should be relatively easy to identify. Once you name the current situation, there is a logical flow toward describing one or more desired states (goals). For example, if a terminally ill patient experiences intractable pain, one might describe the problem as "experiencing severe pain." Because a return to the previous way of life or absence of disease is not possible, it logically follows that the desired state (or goal) would most likely be "to be free from pain." Clearly articulating the problem and the desired goal will clear up confusion and streamline the decision-making process.

Identifying the problem serves other purposes as well. You will notice that in the previous example, the goal "to be free from pain" is a *state*, rather than a strategy. You must clearly identify the goal before you move toward strategies—step three of this model. Because strategies are often dramatic, establishing goals early will diminish conflict later in the process. In this case, the strategy might include increased analgesics, conscious sedation, or discontinuation of life support. When you clearly define the problem, you will be in a better position to judge whether the problem is an ethical dilemma or a practical dilemma. If you are a member of an ethics committee, you will likely eliminate all practical dilemmas at this point in the process.

Step 2: Gather Data and Identify Conflicting Moral Claims

When an ethical problem occurs, gather information or facts to clarify the issues. Identifying the conflicting moral claims that constitute the ethical dilemma is the first part of the process. You should examine the situation for evidence of conflicting obligations, principles, duties, rights, loyalties, values, or beliefs. Additionally, data provide an understanding of the ethical components, principles of concern, and various perceptions of issues and principles by those involved in the situation. You must pay attention to social, religious, and cultural values and beliefs. Often, a situation you initially think constitutes an ethical dilemma will actually turn out to be a practical dilemma once all conflicting moral claims are discussed. This allows the participants to appropriately weigh choices and expedite decision making.

Identify the key persons involved in the decision-making process and delineate each person's role. Teasing out the rights, duties, authority, context, and capabilities of the stakeholders is a critical component of the process. The focal question is, "Whose decision is this to make?" Identification of the principal decision maker is sometimes all that is needed to facilitate the process. Recognition that a specific person has the legitimate authority to make an important decision is an empowering event. Once the principal decision maker is identified, the roles of the other participants can be more clearly defined. For example, nurses often feel the burden of difficult ethical decisions, even though the responsibility for the decision lies with the patient or the nearest relative. In these instances, the nurse serves as an advocate, a resource for information, a source of emotional support for those making the difficult decision, and a facilitator of the decision-making process.

Knowledge of moral development and ethical theory may provide a helpful framework for understanding participants and their perspectives and responses in the process. You should assess how those involved fit into paradigms of moral development. It is valuable to recognize, for instance, whether the principal decision maker is at a developmental level in which choices reflect a desire to please others and is thus susceptible to choosing an alternative solely based on seeking approval. Refer to Chapter 5 for an in-depth discussion of moral development.

It is also crucial to identify the participants' ethical perspectives. For example, if one of the major participants involved in discussions relative to discontinuing life support believes that it is always, in all circumstances, wrong to take a life (see the discussion of deontology in Chapter 2), the process of negotiation with those who believe differently will likely be frustrating. It would be more beneficial under those circumstances to begin the discussion by defining the point at which death actually occurs, thus finding common ground. When those involved hold diverse values, your role may be to facilitate their coming to a consensus around goals and understanding principles.

Step 3: Explore Potential Strategies

Once they have come to a consensus on the desired outcomes, participants in the decision-making process should identify possible alternative strategies. Various options begin to emerge through the assessment process. Participants must consider legal and other consequences. They must also determine which alternatives best meet the identified goals and fit their basic beliefs, lifestyles, and values. This process helps narrow the list of acceptable alternatives. It is critical to eliminate all unacceptable alternatives and begin the process of listing, weighing, ranking, and prioritizing those that are found to be acceptable. Participants must make a choice among options with both head and heart, taking time to dwell on remaining alternatives and recognizing that there is rarely a good solution. Once the selection is made, the decision makers must be willing to act on the choice.

Step 4: Select and Implement a Strategy

A major turning point in the process occurs when the strategy is chosen and implemented. Although this step embodies the purpose of the decision-making process, it can stir emotions laced with both certainty and doubt about the rightness of the decision. Participants should be empowered to finalize the difficult decision at this point, setting aside less acceptable alternatives and moving forward with courage. Nurses must be attentive to the emotions involved at this point of the process.

Step 5: Evaluate Outcomes and Revise the Plan if Needed

After acting on the decision, participants begin a process of response and evaluation. As in all decision making, reflective evaluation sheds light on the effectiveness and validity of the process. Evaluate the action in terms of the effects on those involved. Ask, "Has the original ethical problem been resolved?" and "Have other problems emerged related to the action?" As the situation changes and new data emerge, participants must identify subsequent moral problems and adjust the course of action based on both new information and responses to the previous decision.

Box 7.1 offers a concise guide for ethical decision making. Remember that even though the process is listed as steps, ethical decision making is a nonlinear, iterative process. Questions may need to be revisited several times and may emerge at various points as the process unfolds and new data are presented. For example, information about options may come to light before all the parties involved are identified, and data regarding the ethical perspectives of the various parties may be clarified only at the point when options are being discussed. No matter how much information the participants gather, they may make the decision with an awareness that they would like to have still more data. Keep in mind, though, that a long list of options may actually cause confusion and make the decision process more difficult.

CASE PRESENTATION

Facing a Difficult Choice

A couple in their mid-30s is 10 weeks' pregnant with their first child after numerous unsuccessful attempts with artificial insemination. While on vacation, the mother contracted the Zika virus. During a routine ultrasound, the physician discovers that the fetus is anencephalic, a rare complication of Zika. The physician explains that anencephaly is a terrible condition for which there is no cure and no standard treatment. She informs them that the baby's prognosis is extremely poor, and death will probably occur within a few hours to days after birth. She explains that large portions of the baby's brain, skull, and scalp will be missing. The baby will have no forebrain or cerebrum (the thinking and coordinating part of the brain). The baby will be disfigured, parts of the skull will be missing, and the brain tissue that remains may be exposed to view. The baby will probably be blind, deaf, and unconscious. The couple struggles with the choice to terminate the pregnancy or to carry the baby to term. They know that if they decide to carry the baby to term, they will need to make future decisions about the level of aggressiveness of treatment such as resuscitation, life support, and artificial nutrition.

Think About It
Applying the Ethical Decision-Making Model to This Case

- *Articulate the problem.* The family must clarify the problem in terms of the present situation and the desired state. Of course, the couple would have liked to be pregnant with a normal child, but this is not a reasonable goal, so you encourage them to think about a rational goal that fits within the framework of their values. How can you assist the parents to sift through their emotions and articulate the problem? If you help them to write down the problem, how do you describe the problem in a few words? If the mother says, "I don't want my baby to struggle to live when there is no hope," would this help you clarify the problem? What is the present situation? Could you say that the present situation is a "terrible condition that leads to death"? What is the desired state? Do you think it might be "no futile struggle"? Think of other problem statements that apply to the parents, rather than the baby.

- *Gather data.* You will gather data about every facet of the case. You will discuss the biological implications of the disorder and the risks, harms, and benefits of possible treatments. For example, the parents may ask if life-sustaining measures are painful or if experimental treatments are an option. You will gather data on the context of the family's life. What are their religious and cultural beliefs? What is their living circumstance? You will also discuss the moral/ethical aspects of the case. For example, one moral conflict relates to the principle of nonmaleficence (the wish to do no harm). Terminating the pregnancy can be perceived as harmful to the baby, whereas carrying it to term may result in emotional or physical harm to both the mother and the baby. Another conflict relates to the duty to preserve life, allowing the pregnancy, birth, and death of the baby to take its natural course, versus the duty to alleviate the suffering that carrying the pregnancy to term might impose on the mother. You will want to clarify the key participants and their relationship. Do they agree or disagree on the problem? What if the mother indicates that she will "go crazy" if she carries the pregnancy to term, and the father says, "No one is going to kill my child"? What legal considerations would you need to review during the data-gathering phase?

- *Explore strategies.* Once the parents clarify the goal and identify possible strategies, how will you assist them to explore, weigh, and prioritize their strategies? In this situation, the parents might describe the desired outcome as the prevention of unnecessary suffering for the mother and baby. Further exploration might reveal the sense that carrying the baby to term would create such anguish for the mother that her emotional health, even family integrity, would be threatened. In this instance, terminating the pregnancy would be more compassionate than prolonging the suffering of the mother and allowing the inevitable, yet slow, natural death of the baby. Abortion is one strategy. Think about other possible strategies in this case. Write a problem statement and list four different strategies. Which strategies are congruent with the goal statement? Among those that are congruent, which do you think will have a higher priority for this couple?

- *Implement the strategy.* Whether deciding to terminate the pregnancy or prepare for the baby's birth, the parents move toward action. It is important at this point to attend to the parents' emotional response and ensure that they have other needed support. What if the parents feel that terminating the pregnancy is the better decision, but the local hospital has a religious affiliation that does not permit abortions, or the state has made abortion illegal? Imagine that they have no transportation to another hospital where the procedure can be done. What is the present hospital's role? What is your role? How would you assist the parents? What are the ethical implications? What costs are involved and who will pay?

- *Evaluate outcomes.* The parents resolved the dilemma of whether to terminate the pregnancy or carry it to term by choosing to proceed with termination. Reactions to the choice may emerge in the form of guilt, depression, acceptance, or always wondering how things might have been different if they had chosen the other path. If the parents have long-term reactions, such as deep guilt or depression, they may determine that, faced with the situation again, they would decide to carry the pregnancy to term. On the other hand, they may examine the emotional issues brought about by the decision to terminate and, despite the pain, they may recognize that they made the best decision at the time. What possible outcomes can you imagine for the nurses and physicians involved? What are the implications for nurses who oppose abortion because of personal beliefs?

BOX 7.1   Ethical Decision-Making Model

Step 1: Articulate the Problem and a Realistic Goal
- What is the current undesirable situation?
- What is the desired state (goal) that is possible or reasonable in this situation?

Step 2: Gather Data and Identify Conflicting Moral Claims
- What makes this situation a moral problem? Are there conflicting obligations, principles, duties, rights, loyalties, values, or beliefs?
- Who is legitimately empowered to make this decision, and who are the other key participants?
- Who is affected and how? What is most important to each?
- What is the level of competence of the person most affected?
- What are the rights, duties, authority, context, and capabilities of participants?
- What are the moral perspectives and level of moral development of the participants?
- What are the issues of conflict and agreement among participants?
- What facts seem most important?
- What emotional and cultural factors are important?
- What information is missing?

Step 3: Explore Potential Strategies
- What potential realistic strategies emerge from discussions?
- What are the risks and benefits of each identified strategy?
- How does each strategy fit the lifestyles and values of the people affected?
- What are the professional, institutional, and legal considerations of each strategy?
- How are alternative strategies weighed and prioritized?
- What alternatives are unacceptable to one or all involved?

Step 4: Select and Implement a Strategy
- Choose the strategy that seems the best.
- Give oneself permission to set aside less acceptable alternatives, remaining attentive to the emotions involved in the process.
- Implement the chosen strategy.

Step 5: Evaluate Outcomes and Revise the Plan if Needed
- Has the ethical dilemma been resolved?
- Have other dilemmas emerged related to the action?
- How has the process and outcome affected those involved?
- Are further actions required?

REACTIONS TO UNRESOLVED MORAL PROBLEMS: MORAL DISTRESS, MORAL OUTRAGE, AND MORAL RECKONING

Throughout this text, we saw that moral problems in the workplace are common. We examined moral uncertainty and moral dilemmas at the beginning of this chapter. Ethicist Andrew Jameton also described a third type of moral problem: moral distress. Nursing ethicists further clarified moral distress in the intervening years and discovered other complex processes, including moral outrage and moral reckoning, which are examined in the following sections. Moral distress and moral reckoning are not inevitable outcomes for nurses, and this section of the chapter is meant to be cautionary. With strategies presented here, nurses are more likely to move through morally troubling situations with a sense of power and integrity.

Moral Distress

Moral distress is a well-publicized phenomenon that was first observed in nurses. As you recall, an ethical dilemma is a moral problem for which two or more choices carry equal weight, thus making decisions very difficult. In the early 1980s Jameton (1984) asked a group of nurses to talk about the moral dilemmas they had faced during their careers. Jameton noticed that the nurses did not identify "dilemmas" according to the common definition, but they consistently described situations with compelling moral problems for which the nurses believed they knew the morally correct action, yet each felt constrained from following personal convictions (Jameton, 1993). Jameton concluded that nurses were compelled to tell these stories because of their profound suffering and their belief about the moral importance of the situations. Identifying this new category of moral problem, Jameton wrote, "Moral distress arises when one knows the right thing to do, but institutional constraints make it nearly impossible to pursue the right course of action" (Jameton, 1984, p. 6). Jameton later added that in cases of moral distress, nurses participated in the action that they judged to be morally wrong (1993). In other words, these nurses were unable to preserve their moral integrity. Based on Jameton's work, Judith Wilkinson defined moral distress as "the psychological disequilibrium and negative feeling state experienced when a person makes a moral decision but does not follow through by performing the moral behavior indicated by that decision" (Wilkinson, 1987, p. 16). Further refining the definitions or offering examples for clarification, nearly every subsequent source relies on either Jameton's or Wilkinson's definitions of moral distress. Since Jameton first described nurses' moral distress in 1984, hundreds of research studies have been conducted in the United States and across the globe, and other professions have embraced the concept.

Moral distress occurs when a person is aware of a moral problem, acknowledges moral responsibility, and makes a moral judgment about the correct action, yet is constrained from the self-determined morally correct action. Different people vary in their moral judgment. Moral distress is not a response to violation of what is unquestionably right, but rather a violation of what the individual judges to be right. For example, nurses in the hurried atmosphere of a particular hospital's same-day surgery department report that managers expect them to have sedated patients sign consent forms, even though they know that the physicians have not fully explained the scheduled procedures. The nurses know that this does not respect patients' rights to informed consent, yet feel they are powerless to make the necessary changes. Complicating matters, nurses know that it can be personally risky to criticize a practice that helps the hospital make ends meet (Jameton, 1984).

Nurses' moral distress is more likely to occur in highly stressful situations or with vulnerable patients. Evidence-based studies have shown that nurses who work in high-stress areas such as critical care may end up with a higher level of moral distress. Moral distress has been documented in the following specific situations: prolonging the suffering of dying patients through the use of aggressive/heroic measures; performing unnecessary tests and treatments; lying to patients or failing to involve nurses, patients, or family in decisions; and witnessing incompetent or inadequate treatment by a physician. Moral distress continues to be studied by nursing researchers focusing on its effect during COVID-19 with nearly 200 research papers written within the first three years of the pandemic. A new trigger of moral distress emerged during the COVID-19 pandemic when clinicians began to experience moral tensions when caring for willfully unvaccinated patients. Many physicians and nurses who were overworked during the pandemic experienced moral distress caring for these patients, who sometimes occupied scarce intensive care beds, believing they were risking their own health and that of their families to care for people who chose to remain unvaccinated (Kidzman, 2022). A survey of 6500 critical care nurses revealed that 76 percent of critical care nurses believe patients who choose not to be vaccinated undermine nurses' well-being and 67 percent fear taking care of COVID-19 patients put their families' health at risk (American Association of Critical Care Nurses, 2022). Ongoing longitudinal studies will provide more information on the long-term effects of the pandemic on nurses.

Certain nurse characteristics may influence the frequency and severity of moral distress. Older nurses are less likely to experience moral distress than young nurses, and Black nurses are more likely than White nurses to experience moral distress (Corley et al., 2005). Marital status, scheduling, and the number of children a nurse has can also predict which nurses are more likely to experience moral distress. Nurses who are single and those who work rotating shifts are more likely to experience moral distress than those who are married or those who work the same shift every day (Asadi et al., 2022). The number of children a nurse has can also affect the presence and severity of moral distress (Almasri & Rimawi, 2022).

The ethical climate in a healthcare facility may also contribute to moral distress. Most healthcare institutions are high-tech and fast paced, and patients are older and sicker. Many nurses view themselves as powerless within rigid and highly structured healthcare systems. They perceive little support from nursing and hospital administration. Many research studies have shown that nurses may experience moral distress as a result of being socialized to follow orders with which they disagree, having experienced the futility of past actions, and having fear of losing a job. Other organizational factors that contribute to nurses' moral distress include the quality of care, organizational ethics resources, nurses' satisfaction with the practice environment, and the law or lawsuits. Relationships with physicians constitute a type of institutional constraint. Nurses experience moral distress when physicians and nurses have different moral orientations, different decision-making perspectives, and adversarial physician–nurse relationships.

Moral distress results in unfavorable outcomes for both nurses and patients. It can lead to physical and psychological problems. Some nurses lose their capacity for caring, avoid patient contact, and fail to give good physical care because of moral distress. Individuals may cope with moral distress in a variety of ways, including avoiding patient interaction, acting in secret, working fewer hours, leaving the unit in search of better conditions, or dropping out of nursing altogether (Nathaniel, 2006). Some nurses may have stopped listening to the calls of their patients, having chosen to avoid engagement altogether (Austin et al., 2003).

Decades of research have shown that nurses experience psychosocial, physical, and emotional consequences of moral distress, including blaming others, excusing their own actions, self-criticism, self-blame, self-doubt, anger, sarcasm, guilt, remorse, frustration, sadness, withdrawal, avoidance behavior, powerlessness, burnout, and effects on spirituality. Nurses may also choose to desensitize themselves by adapting or acquiescing to cultural pressures or by rationalizing, denying, trivializing, or distancing themselves from moral problems (Deady & McCarthy, 2010). In addition, evidence suggests that prolonged or repeated moral distress leads to the loss of nurses' moral integrity (Kelly, 1998; Rushton, 2006; Wilkinson, 1987). Numerous researchers over the years have found that nurses' physical reactions to moral distress include weeping, sweating, palpitations, headaches, diarrhea, and sleep disturbances. Emotional reactions include anger, frustration, depression, shame, embarrassment, grief, sadness, and a sense of ineffectiveness (Austin et al., 2003). An increase in moral distress during the COVID-19 pandemic has been associated with a significant increase in mental health issues among nurses, particularly depression (Nemati et al., 2021).

Studies indicated that up to half of all nurses leave their units or nursing altogether because of morally troubling situations (Millette, 1994; Nathaniel, 2006; Wilkinson, 1987). The exodus of experienced nurses is compounded by a nursing shortage, which has increased during the COVID-19 pandemic. The American Association of Colleges of Nursing (2022) reports that the United States is projected to experience an increasingly severe shortage of nurses as Baby Boomers retire and the need for health care grows. The nursing shortage is an indirect but strong threat that may perpetuate moral distress. In 2022, 52 percent of nurses overall and 66 percent of critical care nurses considered leaving their current position and 92 percent believed the pandemic would cut their careers

short (American Association of Critical Care Nurses, 2022; American Nurses Foundation, 2022). Nurses believe the nursing shortage diminishes the quality of their work life and the quality of patient care, and they predict that the continuing nursing shortage will increase stress on nurses, lower patient care quality, and cause nurses to leave the profession (Buerhaus et al., 2005). The situation creates a self-perpetuating downward spiral, in that the nursing shortage leads to moral distress, which causes more nurses to leave the workforce.

Researchers have been busy for the past four decades examining the phenomenon of moral distress. Qualitative and quantitative research sheds light on the process and products of this troubling condition and suggests implications for practice. This is one facet of ethics that offers an opportunity for evidence-based practice.

ASK YOURSELF

Have You Experienced Moral Distress?
Moral distress occurs when moral problems seem to have clear solutions, yet institutional or other restraints prohibit morally correct action. This may occur in everyday life. For example, think about a used car salesperson who is encouraged to sell high-priced cars that are in poor condition. Think about a situation in which you or someone you know experienced moral distress.
- What were the circumstances?
- How did the person feel?
- How did the person resolve the distress?

Moral Outrage

Moral outrage is defined as anger that occurs when one person perceives that another has violated a moral standard or principle such as justice, respect, or beneficence (O'Mara et al., 2011; Rushton, 2013). Moral outrage is distinguished by energy-draining frustration, anger, and powerlessness (Pike, 1991).

Moral outrage occurs when someone else in the healthcare setting performs an act the nurse believes to be immoral. Unlike moral distress, nurses do not participate in the act, and therefore do not believe they are responsible, but perceive that they are powerless to prevent it. The nurse is more likely to be on the fringes of the situation rather than directly involved. For example, the charge nurse on a medical/surgical floor on the evening shift is working at the desk when the nursing supervisor comes to the floor to use the telephone to call a hospital administrator. The charge nurse overhears the supervisor describing a situation in which a physician endangered a patient when he insisted on performing a surgical procedure in the hospital room. The surgeon was in a hurry and felt the patient would be safe, even though there were violations of patient privacy, informed consent, and safety. The charge nurse is uninvolved in the situation but recognizes a grave moral problem.

Moral Reckoning

Moral distress is a triggering component of a more complex process of moral reckoning that spans some nurses' careers (Nathaniel, 2006). Moral reckoning is a three-stage process that includes a critical juncture (Fig. 7.3). After the initial novice period, the nurse begins professional life in a stage of ease in which there is comfort with rules and expectations. The work of nursing is fulfilling. The nurse knows what is expected and has technical skill and a sense of at-homeness in the workplace. Internal and external values and expectations are congruent. Core values, professional norms, and institutional norms complement each other, or at least do not conflict. Unexpectedly, a dramatic situational bind with moral implications occurs in a patient care situation. The nurse's core beliefs come into irreconcilable conflict with social or institutional norms. This constitutes a critical juncture

that forces the nurse out of the stage of ease and into the stage of resolution. At this point, the nurse attempts to resolve the conflict by choosing among conflicting values. Immediate and long-term resolution includes either giving up or making a stand. The nurse then moves into the stage of reflection, during which time he or she repeatedly examines past beliefs, values, and actions. At this point, the nurse tries to make sense of his or her experiences through remembering, telling the story, examining conflicts, and living with the consequences.

Stage of Ease

As illustrated in Fig. 7.3, certain conditions are foundational to the stage of ease, the initial stage of moral reckoning. Conditions integral to the stage of ease include the properties of (1) becoming, which signifies ongoing maturation of core beliefs and values of the individual; (2) professionalizing, which relates to internalization of professional norms; (3) institutionalizing, which signifies the process of internalizing institutional social norms; and (4) working, the unique and fulfilling experience of the work of nursing. Conflicts between and among the conditions work together during a critical incident to produce a situational bind.

As Strauss once wrote, "The human experience of time is one of process: the present is always a becoming"

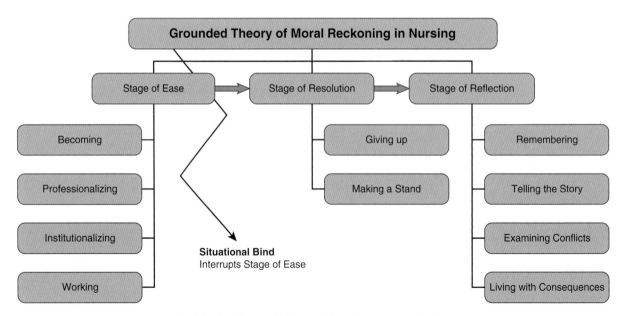

Model of the Grounded Theory of Moral Reckoning in Nursing

Fig. 7.3 Moral Reckoning in Nursing. From Nathaniel, A. K. (2006). Moral reckoning in nursing. *Western Journal of Nursing Research, 28*, 419–438.

(Strauss, 1959, p. 31). Through the process of becoming every person evolves a set of core beliefs and values, which are a product of lifelong learning about what is important and how to behave in society. Core beliefs evolve through experience and from the modeling of parents, teachers, ministers, peers, and so forth.

In nursing school and in early practice, young nurses learn certain behavioral norms—they are professionalized. These professional norms include ideals about what a good nurse should be or do. For the most part, professional norms complement core beliefs. Nursing's moral norms include "the protection and enhancement of human dignity, the alleviation of vulnerability, the promotion of growth and health, and the enhancement of coping and comfort in the face of hardship" (Penticuff, 1997, p. 51). For some, professional norms might also include implicit rules, such as follow physicians' orders, complete assigned work with expert skill, and remain altruistic. Other implicit norms include "do not cry while on duty; be strong for the patient and for other nurses, do not let emotions interfere with the tasks to be done; [and] refrain from getting emotionally involved with your patients and their families" (Davies et al., 1996, p. 502).

When they begin their first nursing job, young nurses start to become institutionalized—they learn implicit and explicit institutional rules. Sometimes institutional norms are congruent with nurses' core beliefs and professional norms, and sometimes they are not. Explicit institutional norms include completing a job according to institutional standards and respecting lines of authority. Implicit institutional norms might include assuring that the business makes a profit, following orders, and handling crises without making waves.

The work of nursing is varied, challenging, and rewarding. Nurses' descriptions of the work of nursing include vivid sensual descriptions and heart-wrenching stories. The work of nursing requires technical skill and attendance to many facets of patients' lives. The work of nursing includes knowing the patients, witnessing their suffering, accepting the responsibility to care, desiring to do the work well, and knowing what to do. The conditions of becoming, professionalizing, institutionalizing, and the work of nursing are held in fragile balance as nurses enjoy the stage of ease.

During the stage of ease, core beliefs and values motivate nurses to uphold congruent professional and institutional norms. Nurses gain technical skills and feel rewarded. They know what their managers expect, and

they feel a sense of confidence. During this stage, nurses have high standards and are proud of their abilities. The stage of ease may continue indefinitely, but for some, a morally troubling event will challenge the integration of core beliefs with professional and institutional norms. In those cases, nurses find themselves in situational binds that lead to changes in their professional lives.

Situational Binds

Sometimes, a morally troubling patient situation arises that places the nurse in a situational bind. The situational bind interrupts the stage of ease and throws a nurse into turmoil when core beliefs and other claims conflict. The turmoil may meet or exceed the traditional definitions of moral distress. Binds involve serious and complex conflicts involving professional relationships, divergent values, workplace demands, and other forces with moral overtones. Research over the past three decades has shown that the types of situational binds include causing needless suffering by prolonging the life of dying patients or performing unnecessary tests and treatments, especially on terminal patients; legally hastening the death of patients; lying to patients; witnessing incompetent or inadequate treatment by a physician; and coercing consent from poorly informed patients. When situational binds occur, nurses must make critical decisions—choosing one value or belief over another.

Often nurses' ability to follow through with their moral convictions is constrained. Wilkinson (1987) found that the external constraints nurses mentioned most often were physicians, the law or lawsuits, nursing administration, and hospital administration and policies. Nurses also experience internal constraints such as socialization to follow orders, self-doubt, and lack of courage (Nathaniel, 2006). Wilkinson (1987) also found that nurses identified the constraints of futility of past actions and fear of job loss, particularly in nonresponsive or defensive organizations.

Sometimes professional or institutional expectations challenge core beliefs. Consider the following example: A mentally competent patient had a "no code" order. Because he experienced extreme discomfort when the nurses suctioned his nasotracheal tube, he refused the procedure. When he attempted to protect himself from the pain of suctioning, the nurse followed physicians' orders and tied his arms before suctioning him. In this case, the nurse was in a bind when actions prescribed by the profession and institution (restraining the patient's hands and suctioning excess respiratory secretions) conflicted with respecting the patient's wishes, which seemed to her to be the morally correct action (Nathaniel, 2003).

Nurses perceive themselves to be in binds when they recognize a problem but cannot convince anyone about the problem or its solution. They may believe they are not part of the decision-making process. Some nurses feel that they do not have a voice as they struggle against authorities. For example, Andrews and Waterman (2005) described situations in which nurses recognized that patients' conditions were deteriorating but encountered difficulty convincing physicians.

In some instances, nurses know the professional and institutional standards and are aware of their own core beliefs yet are unable to uphold them because of workplace deficiencies. Workplace deficiencies might include chronic staff shortages, substandard equipment, and shortages of equipment or medication.

The Stage of Resolution

Nurses tell stories about how moral reckoning changes their lives. The move to set things right signifies the beginning of the stage of resolution. For many, this stage changes their professional futures. During this stage, nurses will either make a stand or give up. Making a stand takes a variety of forms—all of which include professional risk. They may refuse to follow physicians' orders, initiate negotiations, break the rules, whistle-blow, and so forth. Sometimes nurses resolve a situational bind by giving up. In general, nurses give up because they recognize the futility of making a stand. They are unwilling to sacrifice themselves to no avail. They may also give up to protect themselves or to find a place where they can work with better integration of their beliefs and professional norms. Giving up includes participating with regret in an activity they consider to be morally wrong, leaving the unit or resigning, or leaving the profession altogether. Sometimes nurses seem to give up in the short term but move toward preparing themselves for more advanced or autonomous roles or toward leadership positions—all of which prepare them to make a stand in the future.

Stage of Reflection

Afterwards, nurses spend time thinking about their actions. The stage of reflection may last a lifetime and includes remembering, telling the story, examining conflicts, and living with consequences. These are interrelated and seem to occur in every instance of moral reckoning. Nurses retain vivid mental pictures. These

indelible memories evoke emotions many years later. As one nurse said, "I don't let go of it." Nurses invariably describe the sights, sounds, and smells. Even after 15 or 20 years, they remember patients' faces, the exact locations of the patients' beds, and sometimes a patient's position in bed. They remember particulars about patients, such as their names, ages, and diagnoses (Nathaniel, 2006). Nurses also experience evoked emotions after many years, including feelings of guilt and self-blame, lingering sadness, anger, and anxiety.

Nurses continue the process of moral reckoning over time—telling and retelling the story as they try to make sense of it. As they tell their stories, they examine conflicts in the situation. They examine their values and ask themselves questions about what actually happened, who was to blame, and how they might avoid similar situations in the future. As they think about the conflicts, some set limits or make decisions about future actions. Some identify new boundaries. Moral reckoning continues for a prolonged period. Nurses may move from one institution to another or from one specialty area to another. They may seek further education, many times intending to correct the type of moral wrongs they experienced in the past. Many leave the bedside.

COVID-19 and Moral Reckoning in Nursing

The years of the COVID-19 pandemic confirm both the explanatory power of the theory of moral reckoning in nursing and its usefulness in nursing practice. Challenging moral problems during the COVID-19 pandemic seemed to cluster around three basic moral situational binds: circumstances that forced nurses to choose between their duty of care and the safety of themselves and their families; constraints that made it impossible to meet professional and personal standards; and heart-breaking distributive justice choices (Nathaniel, 2023b).

Situational Binds

During the pandemic, nurses struggled with balancing nursing duties in the face of the pandemic against promoting their own health and the health of their families. When many hospitals were unable to provide adequate personal protection (Morley et al., 2020), nurses feared they could become sick or expose their families. Nevertheless, the duty to care and a prohibition from abandoning patients is ingrained in nurses. The conflict between the duty to care and personal safety placed many nurses in painful situational binds. One faced whether or not to even continue to provide inpatient care with an immunosuppressed child at home, (personal communication, 2021) while another worried because she was, herself, immunocompromised as a triple-negative breast cancer survivor (Antelo, 2020).

Even when they continued to provide nursing care, many nurses experienced distress when they believed their care did not meet professional standards. Nurses sometimes believed they had neglected patient rights, insufficiently responded to the urgency requirements of the situation, and failed to provide patients with necessary support (Jia et al., 2021). When families were forbidden to visit, nurses could not give proper instruction to them on the care of drains, tubes, ostomies, and medication administration. Consequently, nurses believed that patients were unprepared for discharge. One nurse commented that when providing what seemed like futile care, nurses reach a point when "we feel as though we are doing things to the patient, instead of for the patient" (personal communication, 2021).

Triage decisions may have presented the most difficult situational binds during the pandemic. Decisions were forced upon the healthcare team when resources such as intensive care beds, respirators, medications, or oxygen were in short supply. Distress was most acute when beds, ventilators, or other resources were withheld or removed from some patients and given to others who were thought to have better chances of survival. Nurses were especially distressed when they believed the treatment was keeping the first patient alive (Morley et al., 2020). Swazo et al. (2020) found that faced with extreme scarcity of resources, the theoretical risk of "sacrificing the most vulnerable patients" shook professionals' ethical convictions.

Resolution

During COVID-19, nurses found ways to resolve the situational binds. Some nurses resigned from their positions in the face of pandemic stressors (Antelo, 2020; Bustan et al., 2020; Swazo et al., 2020; WSBTV.com News Staff, 2020). Tragically, two Italian nurses took their own lives as an expression of giving up (McKenna, 2020). Some nurses made a stand through extraordinary measures to deliver care. For example, one nurse supported a family member who had difficulty accepting her mother's impending death. According to another nurse who witnessed the exchange, the nurse "put on her PPE, entered the room, and dialed the daughter's number [for a video call]. She … then laid down on the floor and slid under the patient's bed so the woman could see her

mother's face one last time" (personal communication). This nurse made a stand to give the best care possible, even in the worst of circumstances.

Reflection

Stories of nurses during the COVID-19 pandemic include feelings of defeat, sorrow, guilt, regret, sleeplessness, anxiety, fear, irritability, outrage, powerlessness, and depression (Evans, 2020; Jia et al., 2021; Nemati et al., 2021; Swazo et al., 2020). Some experienced frustrations that overflowed at home as well as problems with mental and physical health (Jia et al., 2021). Nurses ruminate about what happened to them and what they should have done. Nathaniel (2023b) reported that one nurse said, "It was like we were stuck in time, grieving for some sort of normal, but the world kept moving around us. This experience has changed us" (personal communication, 2021).

Ways to Anticipate, Minimize, and Control Moral Reckoning

Nursing ethics should bind participants in shared symbolism, meaning, and purpose. It should bring together men and women, physicians and nurses, patients and providers. This leads us to wonder, why some nurses are less susceptible to moral distress and moral reckoning. Surely there are many factors. Experience, age, knowledge of the code of ethics, personal empowerment, and other personal attributes have been found to be helpful.

Nathaniel (2023a) reflects on comparisons between nurses who experience moral reckoning and professionals from other disciplines who report less, if any, struggle. A study was designed to elevate the middle range theory of moral reckoning in nursing to a formal theory by integrating data from other disciplines. Social workers and prosecuting attorneys were chosen because, like nurses, their positions placed them in the middle between their employing institutions with their powerful leaders and their clients or the victims of crimes. Surprisingly, neither the social workers nor the attorneys in the study seemed to experience moral distress or moral reckoning. Whereas no nurses in the original moral reckoning study quoted a code of ethics, the social workers almost unanimously quoted their code of ethics when asked how they made ethical decisions. Likewise, the prosecuting attorneys knew their codes of ethics. Both social workers and attorneys exercised the freedom to make autonomous decisions. Each of the nonnurse study participants avoided moral reckoning by (1) knowing the right action based upon their professional codes of ethics and (2) moving forward autonomously with their decisions.

With this in mind, we strongly believe that nurses must do a better job of learning and internalizing their nursing codes of ethics. They must think about the codes with each challenging patient care situation. Nurses should exercise personal empowerment when making decisions about their role in morally difficult patient care situations. This is not to suggest that a well-informed nurse will never experience a situational bind. Certainly, nurses have little power to change some unfortunate situations, such as those encountered during the pandemic. However, nurses who are firmly in touch with their own values and have internalized their professional code of ethics are better prepared to make informed decisions on which they can later reflect with pride, and can say, "I made the right decision. I did my best."

CASE PRESENTATION

Nurses Recognize Subtle Changes in Patients

Joanna is an experienced nurse (Fig. 7.4). She has worked on the same medical-surgical unit for the past 15 years. During a Saturday night shift, Mrs. Kelly, an 82-year-old patient diagnosed with chronic pulmonary obstructive disease (COPD), complains of abdominal pain. Joanna assesses Mrs. Kelly, who has been a patient on the unit many times in the past. The patient's vital signs are within normal limits, and there is no significant change from past readings. However, Joanna still feels uneasy. Not only does Mrs. Kelly complain of pain but she also looks sick to Joanna, who senses there is something seriously wrong. Joanna calls the medical resident, who tells her to call back if there are any changes in the vital signs. As the shift progresses, Joanna becomes more convinced that Mrs. Kelly is seriously ill. Although there are no changes in Mrs. Kelly's vital signs, Joanna can visualize her condition deteriorating. Joanna calls the resident a second time. The resident yells at Joanna and tells her to stop bothering him. After a couple of hours, Joanna decides to call her supervisor, who checks Mrs. Kelly and encourages Joanna to "get a grip." Joanna repeatedly checks on Mrs. Kelly, who remains awake throughout the night. The next morning, Joanna reports her assessment to the charge nurse and asks her to make sure someone evaluates Mrs. Kelly's abdominal pain. The charge nurse responds, "Don't worry about her. If there is anything seriously wrong, she will let us know." When Joanna returns after two days off, she learns that Mrs. Kelly died on Sunday evening of a ruptured abdominal aortic aneurysm. Joanna spends that evening crying at the nurses' station, barely able to take care of her patients.

Think About It
Reacting to Subtle Changes in a Patient's Condition

- What is the ethical problem in this case? Is this a case of moral distress, moral uncertainty, moral outrage, or moral reckoning?
- Were Joanna's actions sufficient? Did she correctly apply codes of ethics from ANA (2015, Provision 4) or CNA (2017, Part I.A.) and ICN (2021, Elements 2.1 and 2.11) to this situation?
- What institutional and professional constraints prohibited Joanna from acting?
- How could Joanna have responded to the situation in a way that would result in a better outcome?
- How might Joanna prevent a similar situation in the future?

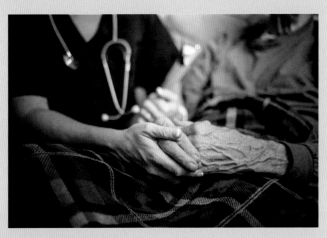

Fig. 7.4 Nurses Recognize Subtle Changes in Patients. (©iStock.com/LPETTET.)

With sufficient preparation, you should develop strategies to become more self-aware and to establish effective intraprofessional and interprofessional relationships. Anticipating moral problems that can occur, you should closely examine implicit professional and institutional messages that inhibit meaningful dialogue and sustain conflict and power imbalance. You should learn strategies and language that prepare you to participate in ethical dialogue with other professionals and to deal with the realities of day-to-day practice.

To help anticipate sources of moral problems, you should uncover potential sources of conflict between core beliefs, professional traditions, and institutional expectations. You should prepare yourself to deal with situational binds related to asymmetrical power relationships, loyalty conflicts, and workplace deficiencies. If you can imagine solutions to moral problems in hypothetical situations, you may find better ways to avoid them or deal with them when they occur in the workplace. You might also prepare for the moral reckoning stage of resolution and its properties: giving up or making a stand. If you anticipate ways to resolve moral conflicts, you may be better prepared to follow integrity-preserving courses of action when situations arise.

Nursing leaders should institute programs that encourage autonomy and collaboration in ethical decision making and implement strategies to support nurses who experience moral distress. Effective strategies include facilitating dialogue; encouraging nurses to be active participants in clinical and ethical decision making; developing support systems; providing opportunities for professional development; strengthening collaborative teamwork; and identifying and eliminating systematic patterns of dominance and subordination based on gender, race, and ethnicity. Additionally, you should budget nursing time for interpersonal care and facilitate dialogue in which nurses and physicians learn to understand and appreciate the other discipline's jobs and ethical perspectives.

SUMMARY

Ethical decision making requires knowledge and attention to many factors. Defining the problem is the beginning step in the process. Is the problem moral uncertainty, a moral dilemma, or a practical dilemma? Solving the moral problem includes defining the problem, identifying the desired objectives, listing and evaluating alternatives, choosing the best course of action based on one's knowledge and the current circumstances, and evaluating the outcomes of the action taken. One must consider both reason and emotion in making ethical decisions. Nurses are encouraged to utilize the decision-making process described in this chapter as a guide in dealing with dilemmas encountered in clinical settings. As with every other nursing skill, comfort and competency with ethical decision making comes with repeated practice, which can help the nurse avoid the undesirable outcomes of moral distress, moral outrage, and moral reckoning. Internalizing nursing codes of ethics and becoming emboldened to act autonomously are important strategies to avoid moral problems.

CHAPTER HIGHLIGHTS

- Dilemmas exist when difficult problems have no satisfactory solutions or when all the solutions appear equally unfavorable.
- In decisions involving practical dilemmas, moral claims hold greater weight than nonmoral claims.
- Making thoughtful decisions in any arena follows a pattern that includes gathering data, comparing options based on particular criteria, making and acting on a choice, and evaluating outcomes or circumstances surrounding the choice.
- One's value system affects how one defines and deals with an ethical issue; thus, the resolution of ethical dilemmas requires determining the ethical issue at hand and identifying the value systems of those involved.
- Both emotion and reason have legitimate roles in ethical decision making.
- Ethical decision making requires ongoing evaluation and assimilation of information, with revisiting of various steps in the process as often as required by the dynamics of changing facts, evolving beliefs, unexpected consequences, and participants moving in and out of the process.
- Familiarity with and practice in applying ethical decision making enables the nurse to develop competence and confidence in the process.
- Moral distress, moral outrage, and moral reckoning are responses to moral problems that have negative outcomes for nurses.

- Internalizing nursing codes of ethics and becoming emboldened to act autonomously are important strategies to avoid moral distress and moral reckoning.

DISCUSSION QUESTIONS AND ACTIVITIES

1. Working in small groups, discuss ethical and practical dilemmas that you have experienced, then choose an example of each type of dilemma to illustrate for the class.
2. Describe a situation in which you or someone you know experienced moral distress, noting moral and nonmoral claims in the situation.
3. Talk with practicing nurses about their experiences of ethical dilemmas. Identify their approaches to dealing with such dilemmas, including their processes of ethical decision making.
4. Debate with classmates how knowledge and internalization of a nursing code of ethics will help with autonomous ethical decision making.
5. Use the ethical decision-making process presented in this chapter to revisit an ethical dilemma that you have encountered in the past or to guide you through a current dilemma. Examine your sense of comfort with each part of the process, noting areas of strength and areas needing more practice.
6. Discuss the interaction among moral development, moral perspective, and ethical decision making.
7. How would you approach an ethical dilemma in which the people involved have different moral perspectives?
8. Review the chapter and discuss how specific elements of the ANA, or CNA and ICN code of nursing ethics apply to ethical problems embedded in the different cases that are presented.

REFERENCES

Almasri, H., & Rimawi, O. (2022). An evaluation of moral distress among healthcare workers during COVID-19 pandemic in Palestine. *Nursing Forum, 57*(6), 1220–1226. https://doi.org/10.1111/nuf.12829.

American Association of Colleges of Nursing. (2022). *Fact sheet: Nursing shortage.* https://www.aacnnursing.org/Portals/42/News/Factsheets/Nursing-Shortage-Factsheet.pdf

American Association of Critical Care Nurses. (2022). *A hospital without nurses can't save your life: Without enough nurses, our healthcare system ceases to function.* https://www.hearusout.com/

American Nurses Foundation. (2022). *Pulse on the nation's nurses survey series: COVID-19 two-year impact assessment survey.* https://www.nursingworld.org/~4a2260/contentassets/872ebb13c63f44f6b11a1bd0c74907c9/covid-19-two-year-impact-assessment-written-report-final.pdf

Andrews, T., & Waterman, H. (2005). Visualizing deteriorating conditions. *Grounded Theory Review, 4*(2), 63–94.

Antelo, P. U. (2020). Nurse quits in emotional video after being sent to an active coronavirus testing floor. *Talentrecap.* https://talentrecap.com/nurse-quits-in-emotional-video-after-being-sent-to-an-active-coronavirus-testing-floor/

Asadi, N., Salmani, F., Asgari, N., & Salmani, M. (2022). Alarm fatigue and moral distress in ICU nurses in COVID-19 pandemic. *BMC Nursing, 21*(1), 1–7. https://doi.org/10.1186/s12912-022-00909-y.

Austin, W. J., Bergum, V., & Goldberg, L. (2003). Unable to answer the call of our patients: Mental health nurses' experience of moral distress. *Nursing Inquiry, 10*(3), 177–183.

Beauchamp, T. L., & Childress, J. (2019). *Principles of biomedical ethics* (8th ed.). Oxford University Press.

Benner, P. (1994). Discovering challenges to ethical theory in experience-based narratives of nurses' everyday ethical comportment In J. F. Monagle & D. C. Thomasma (Eds.), *Health care ethics: Critical issues* (pp. 401–411). Aspen Publishers.

Buerhaus, P. I., Donelan, K., Ulrich, B. T., Norman, L., Williams, M., & Dittus, R. (2005). Hospital RNs' and CNOs' perceptions of the impact of the nursing shortage on the quality of care. *Nursing Economics, 23*(5), 214–221. 211.

Bustan, S., Nacoti, M., Botbol-Baum, M., Fischkoff, K., Charon, R., Made, L., Simon, J. R., & Kritzinger, M. (2020). COVID 19: Ethical dilemmas in human lives. *Journal of Evaluation in Clinical Practice.* https://doi.org/10.1111/jep.13453.

Callahan, S. (2000). The role of emotions in ethical decision making In J. H. Howell & W. F. Sale (Eds.), *Life choices: A Hastings Center introduction to bioetthics* (2nd ed.). Georgetown University Press.

Chinn, P. L. (2004). *Peace and power: Building communities for the future* (6th ed.). Jones & Bartlett.

Corley, M. C., Minick, P., Elswick, R. K., & Jacobs, M. (2005). Nurse moral distress and ethical work environment. *Nursing Ethics, 12*(4), 381–390. https://doi.org/10.1191/0969733005ne809oa.

Davies, B., Clarke, D., Connaughty, S., Cook, K., MacKenzie, B., McCormick, J., O'Loane, M., & Stutzer, C. (1996). Caring for dying children: Nurses' experiences. *Pediatric Nursing, 22*, 500–507.

Deady, R., & McCarthy, J. (2010). A study of the situations, features, and coping mechanisms experienced by Irish psychiatric nurses experiencing moral distress. *Perspectives in Psychiatric Care, 46*(3), 209–220.

Evans, M. (2020). 'It's killing us': Doctors, nurses resigned on Christmas morning as COVID cases continue to rise. *Long Beach Post News.* https://lbpost.com/news/covid-19-christmas-cases-deaths-hospitalizations

Green, C. (2018). Are LA hospitals really dumping homeless patients on the streets? *The Guardian.* https://www.theguardian.com/us-news/2018/may/04/los-angeles-hospitals-homeless-patients-skid-row

Jameton, A. (1984). *Nursing practice: The ethical issues.* Prentice-Hall.

Jameton, A. (1993). Dilemmas of moral distress: Moral responsibility and nursing practice. *Clinical Issues in Perinatal and Women's Health Nursing, 4,* 542–551.

Jia, Y., Chen, O., Xiao, Z., Xiao, J., Bian, J., & Jia, H. (2021). Nurses' ethical challenges caring for people with COVID-19: A qualitative study. *Nursing Ethics, 28*(1), 33–45. https://doi.org/10.1177/0969733020944453.

Kelly, B. (1998). Preserving moral integrity: A follow-up study with new graduate nurses. *Journal of Advanced Nursing, 28,* 1134–1145.

Kidzman, R. (2022). Need to address clinicians' moral distress in treating unvaccinated COVID-19 patients. *BMC Medical Ethics, 23*(1), 1–9.

McKenna, H. (2020). Covid-19: Ethical issues for nurses. *International Journal of Nursing Studies, 110,* 1–2. https://doi.org/10.1016/j.ijnurstu.2020.103673.

Millette, B. E. (1994). Using Gilligan's framework to analyze nurses' stories of moral choices. *Western Journal of Nursing Research, 16*(6), 660–674.

Morley, G., Grady, C., McCarthy, J., & Ulrich, C. M. (2020). Covid-19: Ethical challenges for nurses. *Hastings Center Report, 50*(3), 35–39. https://doi.org/10.1002/hast.1110.

Nathaniel, A. K. (2003). *A grounded theory of moral reckoning in nursing (Publication Number 3142913) [Dissertation, West Virginia University].* ProQuest Dissertations Publishing.

Nathaniel, A. K. (2006). Moral reckoning in nursing. *Western Journal of Nursing Research, 28*(4), 419–438.

Nathaniel, A. K. (2023a). *A formal theory of moral reckoning.* Grounded Theory Institute. [Unpublished manuscript].

Nathaniel, A. K. (2023b). Theory of moral reckoning In M. J. Smith, P. Liehr, & R. Carpenter (Eds.), *Middle range theory for nurses* (5th ed). Springer.

Nemati, R., Moradi, A., Marzban, M., & Farhadi, A. (2021). The association between moral distress and mental health among nurses working at selected hospitals in Iran during the COVID-19 pandemic. *Work, 70*(4), 1039–1046. https://doi.org/10.3233/WOR-210558.

O'Mara, E. M., Jackson, L. E., Batson, C. D., & Gaertner, L. (2011). Will moral outrage stand up?: Distinguishing among emotional reactions to a moral violation. *European Journal of Social Psychology, 41*(2), 173–179. https://doi.org/10.1002/ejsp.754.

Oberle, K., & Hughes, D. (2001). Doctors' and nurses' perceptions of ethical problems in end-of-life decisions. *Journal of Advanced Nursing, 33*(6), 707–715. http://www.ncbi.nlm.nih.gov/entrez/query.fcgi?cmd=Retrieve&db=PubMed&dopt=Citation&list_uids=11298208.

Penticuff, J. H. (1997). Nursing perspectives in bioethics In K. Hoshino (Ed.), *Japanese and Western bioethics* (pp. 49–60). Khower Academic Publishers.

Perkin, R. M., Young, T., Freier, M. C., Allen, J., & Orr, R. D. (1997). Stress and distress in pediatric nurses: Lessons from Baby K. *American Journal of Critical Care, 6*(3), 225–232. http://www.ncbi.nlm.nih.gov/entrez/query.fcgi?cmd=Retrieve&db=PubMed&dopt=Citation&list_uids=9131202.

Pike, A. W. (1991). Moral outrage and moral discourse in nurse-physician collaboration. *Journal of Professional Nursing, 7*(6), 351–363.

Rushton, C. H. (2006). Defining and addressing moral distress: Tools for critical care nursing leaders. *AACN Advances in Critical Care, 17*(2), 161–168.

Rushton, C. H. (2013). Principled moral outrage: An antidote to moral distress? *AACN Advanced Critical Care, 24*(1), 82–89. https://doi.org/10.1097/NCI.0b013e31827b7746.

Schnitker, S. A., Houltberg, B., Dyrness, W., & Redmond, N. (2017). The virtue of patience, spirituality, and suffering: Integrating lessons from positive psychology, psychology of religion, and Christian theology. *Psychology of Religion and Spirituality, 9*(3), 264–275. https://doi.org/10.1037/rel0000099.

Strauss, A. L. (1959). *Mirrors and masks: The search for identity.* Free Press.

Swazo, N. K., Talukder, M. M. H., & Ahsan, M. K. (2020). A Duty to treat? A Right to refrain? Bangladeshi physicians in moral dilemma during COVID-19. *Philosophy Ethics and Humanities in Medicine, 15*(1), 23. https://doi.org/10.1186/s13010-020-00091-6.

Veatch, R. M., & Guidry-Grimes, L. K. (2020). *The basics of bioethics* (4th ed.). Routledge.

Wilkinson, J. M. (1987). Moral distress in nursing practice: Experience and effect. *Nursing Forum, 14*(3), 344–359.

WSBTV.com News Staff. (2020). Former Paulding County school nurse resigns over COVID-19 fears. *WSB-TV.* https://www.wsbtv.com/news/former-paulding-county-school-nurse-resigns-over-covid-19-fears/W7N6ZZ2MG-BALNHZZG6BLEEHTGE/

PART III

Principled Behavior in the Professional Domain

Part III examines various categories of issues that affect the profession of nursing and the everyday practice of individual nurses. Recognizing nursing as a profession, the chapters describe nurses' responsibilities related to ethical, legal, professional, and practice issues. These issues are examined in light of ethics and contemporary nursing. This part includes chapters discussing legal issues affecting nurses; professional issues such as autonomy, authority, and accountability; issues related to the relationship between nurses and the health care system; issues related to technology and self-determination; and scholarship issues.

8

Nursing Ethics and the Law

We are caught in an inescapable network of mutuality, tied in a single garment of destiny.
Whatever affects one directly, affects all indirectly.

(King Jr., 1996/1963)

OBJECTIVES

After completing this chapter, the reader should be able to:

1. Recognize the difference between ethics and the law and discuss the relationship of each to the other.
2. Describe sources of law.
3. Distinguish between constitutional law, statutory law, administrative law, and common law.
4. Describe the difference between public and private law.
5. Discuss instances in which nurses might be accused of breaches of public law.
6. Define *tort* and distinguish between unintentional and intentional torts.
7. Discuss methods that nurses can use to limit liability.
8. Describe the role of the expert nurse witness.

INTRODUCTION

Up to this point, the focus of this book has been on values, morals, and ethics. You will recall from Chapter 2 that the prevailing cultural traditions influence individuals' moral values. Groups of people rely on values to help guide the formulation of formal and informal rules of action, usually referred to as ethics. Professional organizations, such as the American Nurses Association (ANA), the Canadian Nurses Association (CNA), and the International Council of Nurses (ICN), provide documents outlining a formal set of ethical guidelines. These guidelines offer some general rules that are intended for use as a tool to guide professional behavior but are not, in themselves, fully enforceable. Laws, on the other hand, consist of enforceable rules by which a society is governed. Many laws either directly or indirectly affect the practice of nursing. Highly publicized issues, such as termination of life support and "no code" status, indicate a recent trend toward involving the legal system in issues that were previously thought to be ethical in nature. This chapter discusses the relationship between

ethics and the law, general legal concepts, legal regulation of nursing, areas of potential liability for nurses, and legal trends. Laws and statutes vary somewhat from state to state, so content in this chapter should be viewed as a general overview of basic concepts.

RELATIONSHIP BETWEEN ETHICS AND THE LAW

The **law** is a system of rules developed to regulate the civil behavior of citizens. Laws are binding rules of conduct that are formally recognized and enforced to ensure that individuals adhere to the collective will of society. The purpose of the law is to enforce moral beliefs, promote social justice, and protect individual rights. As Oliver Wendell Holmes famously wrote, "law is not a brooding omnipresence in the sky" (Southern Pacific Company v. Jensen, 1917). Rather, it is a reflection of the evolving values of society. The law has three basic functions as follows: (1) to maintain order and regulate human interaction through the establishment of formal standards that identify what types of behavior are and are not permitted; (2) to establish the penalties that may be applied to redress wrongs; and (3) to resolve disputes that arise between people or groups with different wants, needs, views, or values.

The law establishes rules that define rights and obligations and sets penalties for people who violate them. Laws also describe how the government will enforce the rules and penalties. In the United States and Canada, there are thousands of local, state, provincial, and federal laws. Among other functions, laws ensure the safety of citizens, protect property, promote nondiscrimination, regulate the professions, provide for the distribution of public goods and services, and protect the economic and environmental interests of society.

How are ethics and laws related? Laws are intended to reflect popular belief about the "rightness or wrongness" of particular acts as established by collective society. Like ethics, laws are built on a moral foundation. In most countries, laws represent an attempt to codify ethics. The law can serve as the public's instrument for converting morality into clear-cut social guidelines and for stipulating punishments for offenses (Beauchamp, 2001). Laws are generally consistent with the prevailing moral values of a society. For example, most people would agree that the murder of an innocent person is an immoral act. Therefore, laws that prohibit murder reflect this ethical standard. Murder of the innocent is both ethically and legally prohibited in every culture, though definitions of "innocence" vary from culture to culture. As society's needs and attitudes evolve, laws emerge to reflect these changes. Occasionally, however, governments create and enforce laws that are supported by some but not by others who view specific laws to be unjust or immoral. For example, laws on abortion, physician-assisted suicide, and capital punishment have changed over time even though people's opinions continue to be polarized on these issues. In a democratic society, constitutional law provides mechanisms to change or abolish unjust or unpopular laws.

Some authors of nursing ethics texts take the view that professional ethical standards are congruent with the law—that is, that which is legal is also ethical, and vice versa. These authors imply that following a set of ethical guidelines, such as those provided by ANA, CNA, and ICN, provides nurses with a legal safety net. This, is usually, but not necessarily, true. For example, most people today would agree that overt racism is unethical. However in 1896, the Supreme Court decided by a 7–1 vote in the case of *Plessy v. Ferguson* that segregation by race was not a violation of the US Constitution (National Archives, 2022). As a consequence, during the Jim Crow era, some hospitals excluded African Americans from their premises completely, whereas others had separate wards for Black patients. Another more recent example is with illegal immigrants. Uninsured, undocumented immigrants are not eligible to enroll in Medicaid or Children's Health Insurance Plan or to purchase healthcare coverage through the Affordable Care Act (Kaiser Family Foundation, 2022). If they are indigent, undocumented immigrants have no resources to obtain health care—even for children. When undocumented immigrants seek necessary healthcare, some nurses and physicians may believe that it is immoral to deny it, even though national policy does not assist these immigrants to secure the needed resources. Thus, established laws in these two examples might be considered unethical by some people in society. These cases are examples of distributive justice policies. You can read more about distributive justice in Chapter 14.

The cases mentioned above are examples of acts that are legal, but groups of people believe are unethical. The converse is sometimes true: Some illegal acts are considered ethical by some people. For example, some might consider physician-assisted suicide a humanitarian kindness when a person requesting assistance has a terminal illness with intractable pain. However, physician-assisted suicide is illegal in most places. Thus, what is illegal in this situation is considered ethical by some people.

ASK YOURSELF

Can Legal Actions and Moral Actions Conflict?
The following examples may be considered illegal. Can you argue that they are morally permissible?
- Breaking traffic laws to rush a severely injured child to the hospital
- Breaking and entering a school and taking food to save 20 people from a blizzard (Paget & Wolfe, 2022)
- Stealing a life preserver from someone else's boat to throw to a drowning person

The following examples are legal. Can you argue that they are immoral or unethical?
- Lying in social situations
- Habitually breaking promises and disappointing your children
- Telling a child she is ugly or fat
- Turning your back on elderly parents

What are some reasons for the possible discrepancy between what is legal and what is ethical? First, there are differences between ethical points of view. Deontology and utilitarianism, for example, offer quite opposite answers to some basic ethical questions. Whereas the utilitarian perspective would allow consideration of abortion or euthanasia, for example, to provide for the good of many, deontological views might require that life be protected, regardless of circumstances. Thus, a law thought to be ethical by the utilitarian might be considered unethical by the deontologist. Second, human behavior and motivation are more complex than can be fairly reflected in law. Think back to Chapter 5. Individuals may consider the same act either right or wrong, depending to some extent on their stage of moral development. For example, acts of civil disobedience, such as those committed by Mahatma Gandhi and Martin Luther King Jr., although unquestionably illegal, are generally considered to be motivated by high ethical standards. In his 1963 letter from the Birmingham jail, Martin Luther King, Jr. wrote, "[T]here are two types of laws: just and unjust. I would be the first to advocate obeying just laws. One has not only a legal but a moral responsibility to obey just laws. Conversely, one has a moral responsibility to disobey unjust laws" (King Jr., 1996/1963). Third, the legal system judges action rather than motivation. For example, nurses following personal moral convictions or professional ethical codes can find themselves at odds with the policies or practices of their employer. In certain instances, the legal system may determine that an employer has the right to dismiss or discipline a nurse for laying aside institutional policy in favor of ethical considerations. Fourth, depending on the political climate and other variables, laws change. Examples of modern laws that have changed include those related to expanded roles of nurses, abortion, fetal tissue use, organ transplantation, self-determination, confidentiality for patients with AIDS, informed consent, and legal definitions of death. As defined in Chapter 2, integrity is fidelity in adherence to moral norms sustained over time. One should be able to predict that nurses with integrity will not alter their basic moral beliefs in response to changes in the law. Thus, there are several valid circumstances in which there may be a discrepancy between that which is legal and that which is considered ethical.

ASK YOURSELF

What Would You Do During a Disaster?

An example of the struggle of ethical versus legal received national attention during the Hurricane Katrina aftermath. A New Orleans nurse described the appalling conditions she experienced in the wake of the hurricane. The hospital where she worked was the last one to remain open during the crisis. Conditions were horrific. There was no running water, no air conditioning, no food, no sanitation, and dwindling medical supplies. Temperatures exceeded 100 degrees, the staff grabbed naps on stretchers, and people were "dying like flies." With the hospital filled to capacity, exhausted staff raided a hospital that was already evacuated for essential medicines such as insulin (Burnham, 2005).

- Stealing medications was illegal, yet it surely saved lives. Was stealing the medications justified in this circumstance?
- What are the determining factors?
- Apparently, many of the staff in this hospital remained to care for patients, even in the face of personal disaster and uncertainty. Television newscasts reported that some facilities were found to be without staff during the disaster. What are your thoughts about staying with patients versus fleeing danger to assure the safety of yourself or your loved ones?

GENERAL LEGAL CONCEPTS

Nurses need to familiarize themselves with the law and legal system for several reasons. First, the law authorizes and regulates nursing practice. Nurse practice acts of the individual states describe both the activity of nurses and the boundaries of nursing. Chapter 6 discusses the legal regulation of nursing in greater depth. Second, knowledge of legal principles is a necessary component of ethical decision making. To make informed choices, nurses, physicians, patients, and families must be able to identify potential or real legal implications. Third, the legal system scrutinizes nursing actions and omissions. The profession is in a dynamic state of change: advanced practice nurses expand the traditional boundaries, critical care nurses perform complex and vital tasks, staff nurses care for older and sicker patients, and many nurses practice in newly emerging settings. As we work in this demanding and quickly evolving healthcare environment, we must stay current with relevant laws, policies, and legal processes. This knowledge will help ensure that our actions are consistent with legal principles and will help protect us from liability.

Sources of Law

At least four different sources of law affect the practice of nursing: constitutional law, statutory (legislative) law, administrative law, and common law. Additionally, law can be divided into two main branches: private law and public law. Some laws are made by legislation, some by rule-making bodies, and some by judicial precedent. Adding to an already confusing mix, there is frequent overlap between the sources and branches of the law.

Constitutional Law

A constitution is a formal set of rules and principles that describe the powers of a government and the rights of the people. The principles laid out in a constitution, coupled with a description of how these principles are to be interpreted and carried out, form the basis of constitutional law. The Constitution of the United States is the preeminent source of US law. Ensuring the legal rights and responsibilities of citizens and establishing the general organization of the federal government, constitutional law in the United States supersedes all other laws.

The Bill of Rights of the US Constitution and subsequent amendments guarantee each citizen the rights, among others, of equal protection, due process, freedom of speech, and freedom of religion. Nursing actions must take into account these basic rights. Rights guaranteed in the Bill of Rights are consistent with the ethical principles of autonomy, confidentiality, respect for persons, and veracity. The same rights that apply to patients also apply to nurses. As participants in the healthcare system, nurses cannot be forced to forfeit any constitutionally guaranteed rights.

Statutory/Legislative Law

Formal laws (or statutes) that are written and enacted by federal, state, or local legislatures are known as statutory or legislative laws. Congress and the state legislatures pass thousands of laws each year. These are added to the hundreds of volumes of federal and state statutes already in force. Because many people think every problem in society can be solved by passing a law, legislatures make more and more laws to satisfy the demands of society and special-interest groups. Changes in Medicare and Medicaid laws, statutory recognition of nurses in advanced practice (including prescriptive authority), and healthcare reform legislation are all examples of statutory or legislative law.

Administrative Law

Administrative law involves the operation of government agencies. National, state, and local governments set up administrative agencies to do the work of government. These agencies regulate such activities as education, public health, social welfare programs, and the professions. Administrative law consists mainly of the legal powers granted to administrative agencies by legislative bodies and the rules that the agencies make to carry out their powers. State boards of nursing are examples of administrative government agencies. These boards are granted the authority to execute the intent of state statutes by creating, implementing, and enforcing comprehensive and appropriate rules and regulations. As administrative bodies, the role of boards of nursing is to protect the public rather than advocate for nurses. Rules promulgated by the individual states' boards of nursing carry the same weight as other laws.

Common Law

The United States (except Louisiana), Canada (except Quebec), Great Britain, and some other English-speaking countries have a common law system, also known as case law. In the common law system, there is no overarching set of written laws. Decisions are based on earlier court rulings in similar cases. These are also known as precedents. In the common law tradition, case law strengthens and perpetuates itself when lower courts make decisions consistent with previous rulings of higher courts. The common law system is also self-correcting because the appeal process allows higher courts to revisit and overturn unfair or unworkable decisions. Over time, precedents take on the force of law.

Types of Law

Law is a system of enforceable principles and processes that govern the behavior of people with respect to relationships with others and with the government. Law can be divided into two different types: public and private. In general, legal problems related to the relationship between people and the government are the domain of public law, and problems occurring as a result of relationships between people are the domain of private law.

Public Law

Public law defines a person's rights and obligations in relation to the government and describes the various divisions of government and their powers. One important branch of public law is criminal law. Criminal law deals with actions considered harmful to society. Even though a crime might be committed against a particular person, the government considers the commission of a serious act, such as murder, to be harmful to all of society. In the United States, each state, as well as the federal government, has its own set of criminal laws. Nevertheless, the criminal laws of each state must protect the rights and freedoms guaranteed by the federal constitution. Crimes range in seriousness from public drunkenness to murder. Criminal law defines these offenses and sets the rules for the arrest, the appropriate procedures to ensure due process, and the punishment of offenders.

In the course of practice, nurses can be accused of a variety of criminal offenses. For example, nurses can be accused of intentionally or unintentionally injuring a patient, either through errors or willful negligence. They can be charged with the criminal offenses of theft, assault, battery, and sexual abuse of patients. Nurses can also be accused of crimes related to their actual relationship with the government. These include such actions as falsifying narcotic records, forging prescriptions, drug diversion, failure to renew licenses, and fraudulent billing. Crimes are delineated according to seriousness as either felonies or misdemeanors.

Felonies are serious crimes that carry significant fines and jail sentences. Examples of felonies include first- and second-degree murder, arson, burglary, extortion, kidnapping, rape, and robbery. These crimes are punishable by jail terms. Nurses are rarely accused of felonies in the course of practice. However, this can occur. For example, it is possible that those participating in the unauthorized removal of life support from a terminally ill patient could be accused of first-degree murder because of the intentional nature of the act that resulted in death. This could occur even though the act might be viewed as beneficent by a majority of people. A nurse who unintentionally causes the death of a patient by administering a medication to which a patient is allergic could be charged with a lesser crime such as manslaughter, particularly if the patient's allergy was well documented beforehand.

Misdemeanors are less serious crimes, usually punishable by fines, short jail sentences, or both. Examples of misdemeanors include disturbing the peace, solicitation, assault, and battery (assault and battery are also considered intentional torts and can be decided by private or civil law). For example, a nurse who slaps a patient or gives an injection without consent can be accused of the misdemeanor of battery.

ASK YOURSELF

Institutional Versus Individual Negligence

Occasionally, nurses find themselves in situations in which employer standards are inconsistent with public law. In these instances nurses and other staff members can be accused of crimes. In 1986 members of the administrative staff of a nursing home in Louisiana, including the chief nursing officer, were charged with cruelty, neglect, and mistreatment of the infirm. In *The State of Lousiana v. Brenner* (1986), the staff was charged for the following reasons:

1. Failure to feed and care for the patients adequately
2. Failure to train the staff properly
3. Failure to provide adequate medical supplies
4. Failure to supply adequate staff
5. Failure to maintain a sanitary nursing home
6. Failure to maintain patients' records
7. Failure to see that the appropriate and necessary health services were performed

- Ethics and the law are usually, but not always, consistent. Think about each of the seven accusations listed here in terms of breaches of ethical principles. What is the relationship between the accusations and ethical principles?
- Imagine that you live in a small community and are employed by a nursing home with similar problems. How do you think you would deal with the problems in a manner that is both legal and ethical? How would your answer change if you couldn't afford to lose your job at the nursing home?
- Do you believe that individual nurses should be punished for actions that are clearly caused by institutional negligence? Substantiate your answer with ethical arguments.

Private Law

Private law, also called civil law, is different from public law, in that it generally involves relationships between individuals rather than between the government and individuals. Private law determines a person's legal rights and obligations in many kinds of activities that involve other people. These activities include everything from borrowing or lending money to buying a home or signing a job contract. More than a million civil suits are tried in the US courts each year. The six branches of private law include contract and commercial law, tort law, property law, inheritance law, family law, and corporation law. The branches of private law that are most applicable to nursing practice are contract law and tort law. When private laws are violated, individuals who are harmed (plaintiffs) bring lawsuits against violators (defendants). The government does not prosecute violations, and a person cannot be sent to jail for violating private laws. In general, the penalties associated with violation of private laws are monetary. The courts grant monetary awards to the plaintiffs. Malpractice lawsuits are examples of private law.

Contract law. Contract law deals with the rights and obligations of people who make contracts. A contract is a legally enforceable agreement between two or more people. Contracts may be either written or oral; however, in the presence of both a written and an oral contract, the written contract takes precedence. In health care, contracts may be either expressed or implied. Expressed contracts occur when the two parties agree explicitly to its terms, as in an employment contract. Implied contracts occur when there has been no discussion between the parties, but the law considers that a contract exists. The nurse–patient relationship is essentially an implied contract in which the nurse agrees to give competent care.

Tort law. A tort involves a wrong or injury that a person suffers because of someone else's action, either intentional or unintentional. The action may cause bodily harm; invade another's privacy; damage a person's property, business, or reputation; or make unauthorized use of a person's property. The victim (plaintiff) may sue the person or persons responsible. Tort law deals with the rights and obligations of the persons involved in such cases. Many torts are unintentional, such as damages that occur as a result of accidents. If a tort is deliberate and involves serious harm, it may also be treated as a crime. The purpose of tort law is to make the victim whole again, primarily through the award of monetary damages. Because it includes negligence and malpractice, tort law is the branch of law with which nurses are most familiar.

Unintentional torts. Unintentional torts occur when an act or omission causes unintended injury or harm to another person. Nurses are familiar with the unintentional torts of negligence and malpractice. You might hear these terms used interchangeably, but each has a technical meaning that is distinctly different from the other. As a nurse, you should understand the difference between negligence and malpractice and the relevance of each to safe and effective nursing practice.

The term *negligence* is derived from the Latin term *negligentia* and literally means "not to pick up," thus to neglect. Negligence denotes failure to do something that a reasonable person would do in similar circumstances or doing something careless that a reasonable and prudent person would avoid doing. Negligence refers to conduct that fails to use reasonable care.

As part of ensuring the safety of citizens, the law requires every person to be accountable for behaving in a reasonable way, particularly if the welfare of others is jeopardized. For example, there is no law against throwing rocks into the air. However, within a crowd of people, this is not the act of a reasonable person. Although the person throwing rocks may enjoy the beauty of the arc or the distance of the throw and has no intention of harming others, a resultant injury would be the outcome of negligence. A nurse who pours liquid on the floor in a patient's room would be held to the same standard; a reasonable person would recognize that wet floors often cause falls and would immediately clean the floor and warn people who may be walking in the vicinity.

Negligence can also occur because of an omission. The nurse in the previous situation may have walked into the room and found that the patient had spilled water. Even though the nurse did not cause the spill, if he or she ignores it, the nurse will be responsible for the results. Acts of negligence in nursing can be judged on the criteria of the knowledge and abilities expected of a reasonable and prudent nurse. Because the knowledge base of nursing is broad, technical, and specific to the profession, these criteria go far beyond those required of the ordinary person. *Malpractice* is the legal term that refers to negligence committed by a person in a professional capacity, such as a physician, nurse, or lawyer. Professional misconduct, unreasonable lack of professional skill, or failure to adhere to the accepted standard of care that causes injury to a patient constitutes malpractice. To be held liable for malpractice, the nurse's actions must fall below what reasonable and prudent professional nurses with the same knowledge and education would do under similar circumstances. Most sources recognize four components of malpractice. The plaintiff must prove each of the elements to establish liability on the part of the defendant nurse as follows:

1. The nurse had a duty to the patient.
2. There was a breach of that duty.
3. Injury, harm, or damage occurred to the patient.
4. The harm or damage was caused by the breach of duty.

Closely related to the ethical principles of beneficence, nonmaleficence, and fidelity, the duty of care is an overarching legal principle that calls for the nurse to act in the same way that an ordinary, prudent, reasonable nurse would act in similar circumstances. The duty of care exists when there is a nurse–patient relationship. The relationship is formalized when the nurse is employed by a healthcare facility, is assigned to the specific patient care setting, and has direct or supervisory care over the patient. Duty of care carries with it an obligation to adhere to a standard of reasonable care while performing acts that have the potential to harm another person. For nurses, the duty of care is measured in terms of standards that define an acceptable level of nursing care. In determining the extent of the duty of care, the court asks what a reasonable, prudent nurse with like experience and education would do under similar circumstances. The duty of care requires the nurse to (1) possess the knowledge and skills that would be required of a competent nurse engaged in the same specialty, (2) apply that knowledge and skill at or above the level that a reasonably competent nurse in the same specialty would, and (3) exercise informed nursing judgment in the delivery of that care.

The second element of malpractice is breach of duty. When a breach of duty is claimed, the patient must be able to establish that the nurse actually owed a duty of care—that is, that there was an implicit or explicit nurse–patient relationship. If such a duty is found to exist, the nurse may be found to be in breach of duty if his or her conduct falls short of the expected standard of care. Standards of care are "yardsticks" by which the legal system measures the actions of a nurse in a malpractice suit. Standards include state and federal laws, rules, and regulations; statements of professional organizations; professional practice guidelines; current professional literature; job descriptions; facility policies; procedures; bylaws; and so forth. An example of a well-known standard of care by which all registered nurses are judged is the ANA *Scope and Standards of Practice* (2021). In a court of law, a nurse's actions may be compared with all pertinent standards.

Standards of care require specialized nursing knowledge that prepares nurses to predict potential benefits, harms, and risks of specific actions and omissions. A court might ask, "Should the nurse have reasonably foreseen that his or her act could harm the patient?" Frequent legal cases concerning **foreseeability** include those involving medication errors. For example, every nursing student learns about the actions and effects of insulin. So, a reasonable and prudent nurse should be able to predict that administering a large dose of short-acting insulin to a patient who has been without food for 24 hours could cause life-threatening hypoglycemia. This might happen when a patient has been held NPO for tests or surgery. A reasonable and prudent nurse would understand the action of insulin and use professional judgment when deciding how to proceed.

The third element of malpractice requires that the plaintiff sustain **injury** or damage. The plaintiff must show that physical, financial, or emotional harm occurred as a direct or proximate result of the breach of duty. If a nurse commits an error or omission that does not result in injury, the case does not possess all the elements required to demonstrate liability. For example, a nurse may discover that she had inadvertently administered the wrong medication. Although the error might have been serious, if the patient was not harmed, the case would not meet the criteria for liability.

Causation, the fourth element of malpractice, refers to a causal relationship between an action and the resulting injury. To determine causation, the "but for" test is often used. For example, you might ask whether the diabetic patient in the previous example who has had no food or drink for 24 hours would have developed life-threatening hypoglycemia but for the short-acting insulin that the nurse administered. The cause can be actual or proximate. The actual cause is straightforward—an action is the direct cause of an injury. For example, administration of insulin lowers blood glucose levels and can cause hypoglycemia. If an action is not an actual direct cause, the court may ask if the action was the proximate cause of the injury.

A proximate cause is an action sufficiently related to an injury that it can be said to have caused the injury. A court might recognize proximate cause, even if a nurse's action was not the first action in a chain of events or the last action before the injury occurred. To determine the proximate cause, the court would seek to understand if the injury was foreseeable. Could the nurse have reasonably predicted that an action could result in injury? Proximate cause is not found in cases in which injuries are caused by unpredictable chains of events. So, even if an injury can be indirectly traced back to a nurse's action, the nurse would not be found liable if the injury could not have been foreseen. For example, a nurse properly positions a wheeled intravenous (IV) pole at the head of the patient's bed. An inebriated visitor stumbles and knocks the IV pole onto the patient, causing a laceration. The nurse's action in positioning the IV pole was within the standard of care and the injury was not foreseeable, so a court should not consider the nurse's action to be a proximate cause of the injury. However, if the nurse had placed the IV pole in the direct path of visitors, the action might be considered the proximate cause, because the nurse should have been able to foresee that an IV pole in the middle of a traffic pattern might be inadvertently knocked over, causing injury.

Nurses and the tort of malpractice. Remember, malpractice is almost always a tort offense—a civil, rather than criminal, matter. The purpose of tort law is to make the person whole again, primarily through the monetary awards to the plaintiff. These monetary awards are called damages. The purpose of awarding damages is not to punish the defendants, but to compensate the plaintiff and restore his or her previous financial position. Awarded damages might include compensation for financial losses and expenses incurred as a result of the injury; emotional damages, especially if there is apparent physical harm as well; and general damages inherent to the injury itself, including compensation for pain and suffering, permanent disability, and disfigurement. Punitive damages

are awarded if the court finds that there was malicious, willful, or wanton misconduct on the part of the nurse (Guido, 2019).

Data about healthcare providers' malpractice suits in the United States are available to the public via the National Practitioner Data Bank (NPDB), an electronic database housed in the US Department of Health and Human Services (HHS). Congress created the NPDB in 1986 to restrict the ability of practitioners to move from state to state or facility to facility without disclosing malpractice payments or actions against their credentials or licenses. It includes information related to professional competence and conduct of healthcare providers. Registered nurses have been included in the data bank since 1997. State licensing boards, hospitals, healthcare entities, and professional societies are expected to identify and discipline providers who engage in unprofessional behavior and are required to report negative actions to HHS via the NPDB (U.S. Department of Health & Human Services, 2023). In addition to demographics, data collected include malpractice payments; healthcare-related civil or criminal convictions; and negative actions by employing agencies, certification boards, professional organizations, and so forth. Sharing this critical information helps ensure quality health care and a skilled healthcare workforce. The reports about individual providers are available to healthcare facilities and licensing boards but are restricted from the public. De-identified, aggregate data are available to the public for research and statistical purposes.

Analysis of the publicly available NPDB data illustrates trends in negative actions against practitioners' licenses and malpractice awards. The number of malpractice awards and the percentage of each profession against whom awards were made can be calculated from the publicly available NPDB data. The good news is that nurses are less likely to experience malpractice claims, and malpractice payout amounts are exponentially less for nurses than for physicians. Since 2017, an average of only 2.8 percent of malpractice payment reports have been for registered nurses and 3.5 percent for advanced practice nurses, whereas 73 percent of payment reports were for physicians (U.S. Department of Health & Human Services, 2023). But the number of professionals affected is proportionally very small. In 2022, for example, only 0.004 percent of registered nurses, 0.4 percent of advanced practice nurses, and 0.5 percent of physicians were required to pay malpractice claims (American Association of Colleges of Nursing, 2022; Michas, 2022; U.S. Department of Health & Human Services, 2023; Zippa, 2023).

Although the number of malpractice suits against nurses is relatively small, they do occur. Recall that for a plaintiff to show that a nurse was negligent, the nurse must have (1) a duty to care, (2) a breach of duty that violates standards of care, (3) harm or injury to the plaintiff, and (4) evidence that the injury was caused by the breach of duty. Negligence can have many root causes. The nurse may have a lack of knowledge or skill, inattention, an unreasonable workload, impairment by drugs or alcohol, or a basic lack of caring. A review of the literature and news media reveals several areas that are frequent causes for nurse malpractice claims, as depicted in Box 8.1 and described as follows:

- **Failure to properly assess and monitor**. Assessment and monitoring are key functions of nurses in the inpatient setting. The largest proportion of malpractice claims involving nurses is related to failure to monitor appropriately, with many claims involving the death of the patient (Gleason et al., 2021; Hakim et al., 2022; Myers et al., 2020). Because assessment and monitoring are basic nursing functions with a long history as standards of nursing care, the nurse must actually carry out the assessment, monitoring, and evaluation of patients, delegating only minor and routine tasks appropriate for nonnursing staff. The nurse must also recognize what he or she is seeing. To properly assess and monitor the patient, the nurse must possess the necessary knowledge and skills and be sensitive to subtle or dramatic changes in a patient's condition. The nurse must know what the patient's condition has been, what it

is now, and what it should be. The nurse should also recognize the implications of changes in a patient's status. In a recent case, a 68-year-old man underwent a total knee replacement. Postoperatively, he experienced an episode of hypotension, which was treated successfully with ephedrine. He was then transferred to a medical-surgical unit, where the nurse assessed him and determined that he was stable. After three hours the patient complained of nausea and vomiting. Ten minutes later, the nurse discovered that he was cyanotic and unresponsive. The nurse immediately called a code, and the patient was intubated and transferred to the intensive care unit. The patient subsequently died, and the eventual diagnosis was anoxic encephalopathy caused by the time that elapsed before cardiopulmonary resuscitation was initiated. In addition, the nurse had failed to document that she had taken the patient's vital signs as ordered. Experts determined that because the patient had experienced hypotension in the recovery room, the nurse should have assessed and monitored him more closely. In an out-of-court settlement the family was awarded $250,000 plus $14,139 in legal expenses (Nursing Service Organization, 2017).

Ferris v. County of Keenebec (1999) offers another example of a nurse's failure to assess that is so extreme as to be labeled deliberate indifference. When a woman was arrested, she told jail officials that she was pregnant. Two days later, she began having vaginal bleeding and pelvic pain. The woman complained to the nurse that she was having a miscarriage. The nurse took the woman's pulse, told her she was menstruating, instructed her to lie down, and refused to give her sanitary napkins. The woman was unable to continue to lie down because of her pain, but the nurse made no further attempt to assess her condition, telling her that she would be transferred to another cell if she continued to refuse to lie down and follow orders. Continuing to complain of severe pain, the woman was transferred to a smaller cell and had no further contact with the nurse. A few hours later she had a miscarriage in her jail cell. After release, the woman filed a lawsuit. Finding in favor of the woman, the court determined that it was obvious that the woman was complaining of a serious condition that was ignored and untreated by the nurse. The nurse made no effort to assess or treat the woman beyond taking her pulse.

BOX 8.1 Frequent Sources of Malpractice Claims Against Nurses

- Failure to properly assess and monitor
- Failure to administer medications properly
- Failure to communicate
- Failure to act
- Failure to use medical equipment properly
- Failure to properly plan and administer nursing care
- Failure to exercise ordinary care to avoid causing emotional harm

CASE PRESENTATION

Failure to Monitor

Imagine that James was the registered nurse assigned to provide nursing care to 76-year-old Mr. White, who was admitted to the ICU with pneumonia. When James went to a mandatory meeting in the hospital, he transferred responsibility for his patients to Jordan, another registered nurse. Mr. White's pulse oximeter began to alarm while James was at the meeting. Mr. White's wife saw that the pulse oximeter reading was 60 mm Hg. The alarm, which was audible at the nurses' station, sounded for five minutes before Mr. White's daughter walked to the nurses' station and asked Jordan for help. Because she was busy attending to other duties, Jordan failed to check on Mr. White. After the family activated the call button a second time, Jordan entered the room, reset the alarm, and said, "That noise is so annoying! Hopefully, it won't bother you anymore." One minute later, the alarm began to sound again. Noticing the oximeter reading was 55 mm Hg, the family activated the nurses' call button two more times, but no one responded. The pulse oximeter alarm sounded nearly continuously for 45 minutes. When James returned to the unit, he immediately responded to the alarm, began oxygen administration, and called for assistance. Mr. White sustained brain damage that was determined to have been caused by oxygen deprivation.

Think About It

- Think about two ethical principles that apply to this hypothetical situation.
- Do the ethical principles correlate with the law in this instance?
- Did Jordan have a duty to care for Mr. White?
- Does this situation meet the "but for" test of causation?
- With extended lack of oxygenation, was Mr. White's brain injury foreseeable?
- Do you think James, Jordan, or both would be liable if a malpractice lawsuit were initiated?
- "Alarm fatigue" is a well-documented problem in ICU nurses who are overwhelmed with a variety of alarms going off simultaneously. Do you think this is an appropriate defense for Jordan?

- **Failure to administer medications properly**. Accounting for thousands of deaths each year, medication errors are the second most common type of adverse event (Hakim et al., 2022). Medication errors are preventable events that include administering the wrong medication, in the wrong dose, via the wrong route, at the wrong time, or to the wrong patient. Medication errors also include a failure to foresee the adverse effects of medications in particular situations. For example, even though there is a physician's order for the medication, a nurse should know to withhold an IV dose of potassium chloride from a patient whose recent laboratory results show elevated serum potassium. Nurses are responsible for the safe and appropriate administration of medication, regardless of physician orders, medications dispensed, workload, unusual circumstances, or institutional policy. Nurses face legal liability even if they administer medication that is ordered in error via a dangerous route or in an excessive dose or dispensed in error by a pharmacist. For example, a nurse must recognize when an adult dose of medication is dispensed for an infant and must act to avoid harm to the child. In one highly publicized case, a nurse administered 1000 times the intended dosage of heparin to the newborn twins of actor Dennis Quaid (Pozgar, 2018; Fig. 8.1). Some nurses hesitate to speak up when they have a concern, fearing physician anger or retribution for questioning authority or reporting an error. Failure to confront a physician or pharmacist can affect everyone involved. So institutions should empower their nurses to speak up when they notice potential errors in medications that are ordered or dispensed.

- **Failure to communicate**. Healthcare delivery must be a team effort. As coordinators of care, nurses are in close contact with patients and have immediate access to the results of diagnostic testing. They must be alert for clues to a patient's deteriorating condition and must swiftly notify physicians when the patient's condition changes substantially. Communication with physicians includes electronic communication, telephone communication, face-to-face communication, and complete and timely written documentation. Problems with written documentation occur when nurses fail to document altogether, document inaccurately, fail to update changes in a timely manner, or use incorrect words and abbreviations in their documentation. Failure to communicate also includes failing to properly obtain informed consent and failing to properly inform patients or families of important instructions on discharge. In a recent study, Gleason et al. (2021) found that failure to communicate among providers was the most frequent contributing factor in diagnosis-related malpractice suits against nurses.

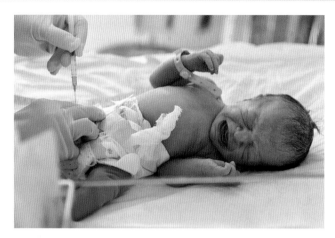

Fig. 8.1 Careful Medication Administration to a Newborn. (©iStock. com/Coral222.)

- **Failure to act**. The nurse must act as an advocate for the patient. Focused on patient safety, advocacy is an integral element of the nurse–patient relationship. When an urgent or emergent patient situation arises, the nurse must swiftly take appropriate steps. Advocacy involves assessing a patient, forming a nursing diagnosis, and then communicating that assessment. This can involve actions such as calling for help, administering medication or oxygen, or notifying the physician. In unusual situations, the nurse may need to take the issue up the chain of command. Recall the case of Lewis Blackman in Chapter 3. After an elective surgery, 15-year-old Lewis experienced clear signs of acute distress, yet the nurses failed to adequately assess him, failed to effectively communicate with the physician, and failed to act on Lewis's behalf. After his death, Lewis's family settled out of court with the hospital for nearly one million dollars (Monk, June 16, 2002).

- **Failure to use medical equipment properly**. The nurse must be proficient in the use of medical equipment, be alert for medical equipment that is not in proper working order, take steps to remedy the situation, and record their actions. Failure to use medical equipment properly can range from routine to complex nursing acts. Sources of injury from routine acts, for instance, can be from improper or clumsy insertion of urinary or IV catheters, forceful insertion of rectal thermometers, flawed intramuscular or subcutaneous injection techniques, injection of an air bubble through an IV catheter, infiltration of an IV, failure to

reposition tubes and lines, and administration of dangerously excessive oxygen flow. Other injuries can include any manner of trauma such as hitting a patient with a heavy piece of equipment, burning a patient, leaving a tourniquet on an arm after a procedure, injuring a patient on a hoist, leaving a bed elevated after a procedure, using contaminated needles or equipment, or leaving a medical instrument in the patient's body.

- **Preventable pressure injuries are sometimes caused by medical devices such as oxygen and IV tubes and cervical collars**. A review of more than 300 studies revealed an incidence of device-related pressure injuries in up to 38 percent of the general acute care population. Seventy-four percent of pressure injuries were not identified until they were stages III, IV, or unstageable, and 63 percent had no documentation of device removal, pressure relief, or skin inspections (Apold & Rydrych, 2012). This is a special liability risk in ICU settings. Nurses must recognize the potential for preventable medical device injury, assess patients properly, and act to prevent injury.

- **Burns can occur when nurses improperly use medical devices**. In one case a three-month-old infant suffered second- and third-degree burns on his buttocks after an operating room nurse placed him on a heating pad at the instruction of the anesthesiologist. The purpose of the heating pad was to help the child maintain body temperature during surgery. Though neither the nurses nor the surgeon noted anything unusual after surgery, arriving at home, the parents found blisters on the infant's back, which were so severe that the baby required skin grafts. The heating pad came with a manufacturer's warning to avoid the use of the heating pad on an infant, invalid, or sleeping, or unconscious person (Smelko v. Brinton, 1987).

- **Failure to properly plan and administer nursing care.** The nurse must skillfully plan and carry out appropriate nursing and medical interventions. Because it is an integral part of the nursing process, a recognized standard of care, and a requirement of many federal program regulations, failure to plan may result in accusations of malpractice. In *Smith v. Juneau* (1997), for instance, nurses were found negligent for failing to develop a plan of care to protect an orthopedic patient's skin. There was no plan to reposition the patient or to assess the patient's skin under a traction sling. The court awarded $500,000 to the plaintiff and held that the nurses' negligence resulted in serious ulcers.

CASE PRESENTATION

"Please Don't Let Me Die!"

In May 2006 a jury awarded $20 million to the family of Loren Richards, an 84-year-old Kentucky man. In addition to the nursing home corporation, two nurses were found culpable in Mr. Richards' death. In the final hours of his life, Richards screamed in pain as he pleaded for help, "I need a doctor. I need a nurse . . . . Please don't let me die." He died about 10 hours after he first complained of pain caused by an untreated bowel obstruction. Thirteen staff, three of whom were nurses, took care of 100 patients on that day. At one point, 10 of the 13 were on break, including all three nurses. The jury heard testimony that the nurses failed to monitor Richards' condition or respond to symptoms including pain and vomiting. The family alleged that there was an acute shortage of staff at the facility, owned by the nation's largest nursing home chain. Defendants' attorneys responded that the case was really about the family's greed (Richards v. Beverly Health & Rehabilitation of Frankfort, 2006).

Think About It

- If the nursing home was understaffed, why were the nurses found to be culpable?
- Why were the nurses judged responsible, rather than the nursing assistants?
- How did the nurses violate the code of nursing ethics?
- What other standards did the nurses violate?
- What would you have done in that situation?

- **Failure to exercise ordinary care to avoid causing emotional harm.** Because nursing care focuses on the psychosocial-spiritual realms as well as the physical, failure to implement care in these areas may result in nursing malpractice. Intentional infliction of emotional distress is an extreme example of this. There are certain contractual relationships, such as in the transmission and delivery of telegrams announcing the death of a close relative and services incident to a funeral and burial, that carry with them deeply emotional responses. Legal claims have been recognized that require a duty to exercise ordinary care to avoid causing emotional harm in such situations.

Criminal charges for malpractice. The combination of an evolving healthcare delivery system, increased public awareness, and a vigorous legal system has led to changes in the delivery of care, exposure to potential sources of liability, and changing legal trends. The public has begun to subject both the individual provider and the healthcare system to intense legal scrutiny. Traditionally, nurses who made errors that caused harm to patients were charged with the unintentional tort of malpractice. Either heard in civil court or settled out of court, charges of negligence against nurses have seldom resulted in criminal prosecution. It appears, however, that there may be a trend toward charging nurses with criminal negligence in particularly dramatic cases.

Until recently, the risk of criminal prosecution for nursing practice was nonexistent unless nursing action arose to the level of criminal intent, such as the case of euthanasia leading to murder charges. However, in a landmark 1997 case, three nurses were indicted by a Colorado grand jury for criminally negligent homicide in the death of a newborn. Public records show that a mother/baby nurse was assigned to care for the baby. A second nurse offered to assist her colleague in caring for the baby, so the mother/baby nurse transferred the baby's care to her. A neonatal nurse practitioner (NNP) was also working in the hospital nursery. Because the baby was at risk for congenital syphilis, the physician ordered 150,000 units of intramuscular penicillin—which would have required five separate injections. Earlier in the day, the baby had been subjected to a lumbar puncture that required six painful attempts. To avoid inflicting further pain, the nurse asked the NNP if was possible to administer the penicillin by a less painful route. The nurse and NNP searched recognized pharmacology references and determined that IV administration would be acceptable. The NNP had the authority to change the route and directed the nurse to administer the medication intravenously. The nurses failed to catch an error made by the pharmacist, who dispensed a dose 10 times greater than was ordered—1.5 million units. The baby suddenly died as the nurse was administering the penicillin. The Colorado Board of Nursing initiated disciplinary proceedings against the nurse and NNP but not against the mother/baby nurse. The grand jury indicted all three nurses on charges of criminally negligent homicide but did not indict the pharmacist (Cady, 2009). The NNP and nursery nurse accepted a plea bargain. They pled guilty, and their sentences were deferred and there was no prison sentence or fine. The mother/baby nurse went to trial and was acquitted by a jury after a short deliberation. This case is a frightening example of the devastating consequences that can occur when a nurse makes a serious error.

A more recent Tennessee case attracted national attention in the United States. A nurse was convicted of criminally negligent homicide and gross neglect of an impaired adult for the death of a 75-year-old patient. The patient became paralyzed and died when the nurse inadvertently administered a fatal dose of vecuronium, a powerful paralytic agent, rather than Versed (generic name midazolam), a sedative (Kelman, 2022). The case against the nurse hinged on the use of an electronic medication cabinet. According to documents filed in the case, the nurse initially tried to withdraw Versed from a cabinet by typing "VE" into its search function, whereas she should have used the code for the generic name of the drug. When the cabinet did not produce Versed, she engaged an override that unlocked a group of medications and searched for "VE" again. This time, the cabinet produced vecuronium. Although institutional and systemic problems were noted in the case, prosecutors argued that the nurse made several errors when she chose the wrong drug, failed to check the name of the medication, and failed to read the warning notices on the packaging. The nurse admitted that she accidentally selected vecuronium from an automatic dispensing cabinet override mode and administered the drug to the patient. She also admitted other serious errors including failing to monitor the patient after administration of the drug. The nurse was sentenced to three years' probation. In addition, the Tennessee Board of Nursing revoked her nursing license indefinitely, fined her $3000, and stipulated that she pay up to $60,000 in prosecution costs. Although it happens rarely, the Colorado and Tennessee

ASK YOURSELF

Criminal Negligence Versus Malpractice
- What feelings are evoked as you consider the Colorado and Tennessee nurses' criminal convictions of nurses who committed serious errors?
- What ethical principles apply to the case of the Tennessee nurse?
- Can you think of other occupations in which the consequences of unintentional errors have greater legal implications? Discuss your answer with classmates.
- How could adherence to the ANA *Code of Ethics for Nurses with Interpretive Statements*, the ICN *Code of Ethics for Nurses*, or the *Canadian Code of Ethics for Registered Nurses* have affected the nurses' actions in these cases?
- How should the profession respond to this type of legal threat?

CASE PRESENTATION

Emotional Harm
Just before her five-month prenatal checkup, Susan Oswald began experiencing bleeding and painful cramping. Her physician, Dr. Smith, ordered an ultrasound, after which she was examined by Dr. Smith's associate, Dr. LeGrand. Dr. LeGrand found no explanation for the problem, so he instructed Susan to go home and stay off her feet. Later the same day, she began bleeding heavily and was taken by ambulance to Mercy Health Center. The bleeding stopped, so Dr. Smith discharged Susan with instructions to take it easy. The following day, her symptoms worsened, so her husband, Larry Oswald, drove her to the Mercy emergency room. Another associate of Smith and LeGrand, Dr. Clark, examined Susan and advised her that there was nothing to be done and she should go home. Larry insisted, so Dr. Clark admitted her to the labor and delivery ward, where her first contact was with a nurse who said, "What are you doing here? The doctor told you to stay home and rest." Later, another nurse told Susan that if she miscarried there would not be a baby, but rather a "big blob of blood" (Furrow et al., 2004). Susan reported that she was scared. The next morning Susan overheard a loud argument outside her door, in which Dr. Clark was heard yelling, "I don't want to take that patient. She's not my patient and I am sick and tired of Dr. Smith dumping his case load on me" (Furrow et al., 2004, p. 166). Urged by

Larry, Dr. Clark apologized and assured Susan that he would care for her until he left for vacation at noon that day, at which time Dr. LeGrand would take over. Susan began experiencing a great deal of pain at around 9:00 a.m., and Dr. Clark instructed the staff to schedule her for an ultrasound and amniocentesis. After viewing the ultrasound, Dr. Clark told the Oswalds that the situation was unusual. He left the hospital without explaining the situation further. Confused, distressed, and in extreme pain, Susan began giving birth in the hallway outside the x-ray laboratory. Larry summoned two nurses, who delivered a one-pound baby girl. The nurses determined that the baby was not alive. They wrapped the baby in a towel, placed her on an instrument tray, and told the parents she was stillborn. After calling relatives to break the sad news, Larry touched the baby's hand and was startled when his grasp was returned. The nurses rushed the infant to the neonatal intensive care unit, where she died several hours later (Oswald v. LeGrand, 1990).

Think About It
Emotional Harm

- Was there negligence on the part of any of Susan Oswald's healthcare providers?
- Larry and Susan contend that they suffered severe emotional distress because of breaches of professional conduct. Think about the several instances in which either the physicians or nurses may have contributed to the Oswalds' emotional distress.
- Do you believe there should be a duty to exercise ordinary care to avoid causing emotional harm? Was that duty breached in this instance?
- What elements of the nurses' code of ethics from the ANA, CNA, or ICN could have affected the nurses' actions toward a more positive conclusion to this case?

---

cases serve as a warning to nurses that serious errors can lead to serious consequences.

Intentional torts. Intentional torts occur when someone intentionally injures another person or interferes with the person's property. The perpetrator intends to bring about a specific result or consequence. A tort must include three elements to be considered intentional: the act must be intended to interfere with the plaintiff or his or her property, there must be intent to bring about the consequences of the act, and the act must substantially cause the consequences (Box 8.2). Examples of intentional torts include fraud, invasion of privacy, assault, battery, false imprisonment, slander, and libel. Damages

---

BOX 8.2 Components of Intentional Torts

1. The defendant's act must be intended to interfere with the plaintiff or his or her property.
2. The defendant must intend to bring about the consequences of the act.
3. The act must substantially cause the consequences.
4. There is no legal requirement that the act causes damages or injury—proof of intention is sufficient.

---

awarded for intentional torts tend to be more generous than those awarded for unintentional negligence.

An intentional tort, or fraud, consists of deliberate deception for the purpose of securing an unfair or unlawful gain. Examples of potential areas of nurses' fraud include falsification of information on employment applications, untruthful billing procedures, false representation of a patient's physical condition to induce contracts for services, drug diversion, and falsification of patient records to cover up an error or avoid legal action. Healthcare fraud statutes are outlined in the US False Claims Act, the Anti-Kickback Statute, the Physician Self-Referral Law, the Social Security Act, the US Criminal Code, and other state and federal statutes (Center for Medicare & Medicaid Services, 2021). As is true with some other intentional torts, fraud can lead to both civil and criminal proceedings.

One of the main sources of healthcare fraud and abuse involves the Medicare program. Medicare is a federal health insurance program designed to pay a large percentage of healthcare costs for most individuals 65 years of age and older. Medicare also pays healthcare costs for people under age 65 who receive disability benefits from Social Security or the Railroad Retirement Board and those with end-stage renal disease. Exceeding 15 percent of the total US federal budget, Medicare pays hundreds of billions each year (U.S. Department of Health & Human Services, 2022). Medicare officials recognize that improper payments can result from a spectrum of intentional or unintentional billing practices. Improper payments can result from common mistakes such as incorrect coding, inefficiencies such as ordering excessive diagnostic tests, bending the rules with improper billing practices such as "upcoding," or intentional deceptions resulting in fraud such as billing for services or supplies that were not provided or appointments that patients failed to keep (Center for Medicare & Medicaid Services, 2021). Because of the deliberate nature and potential harm of fraudulent acts, court decisions tend to be harsh. Penalties for Medicare fraud and abuse can include civil monetary penalties, criminal sanctions, and exclusion from future participation in federal programs. Civil monetary penalties can be up to $50,000 per violation and can include three times the amount that was fraudulently received. Criminal convictions, which fall under federal sentencing guidelines, can include years of imprisonment. In addition, mandatory exclusion from participation in all federal healthcare programs is imposed if a provider is convicted of Medicare fraud; patient abuse or neglect or the felonies of other healthcare-related fraud, theft, or other financial misconduct; or unlawful manufacture, distribution, prescription, or dispensing of controlled substances (Office of Inspector General, 2023).

Healthcare fraud costs US taxpayers tens of billions of dollars each year. As the primary agency responsible for investigating this crime, the Federal Bureau of Investigation considers healthcare fraud a high priority. The bureau partners with other government entities such as HHS, the Food and Drug Administration, the Drug Enforcement Administration, and the Internal Revenue Service Criminal Investigation Unit. Together these agencies seek to identify and pursue investigations against healthcare fraud offenders (U.S. Federal Bureau of Investigation, 2019). Although nurses compose a small percentage of those who are investigated and convicted of fraud, some nurses have been sentenced to prison, many have been charged with fraud, and hundreds have been charged with opioid diversion and abuse (U.S. Department of Health & Human Services and U. S. Department of Justice, 2022).

Invasion of privacy can be an intentional tort offense. The right to privacy is the right to be left alone or to be free from unwanted publicity. Individuals have the right to withhold themselves and their lives from public scrutiny. The intentional tort of invasion of privacy occurs when a person's privacy is violated. In terms of tort law, there are four basic types of invasions of privacy related to patient care: (1) intrusion on the patient's physical and mental solitude or seclusion, (2) public disclosure of private facts about the patient, (3) publicity that places the patient in a false light in the public eye, and (4) appropriation of the patient's name or likeness for the defendant's benefit or advantage. Many legal cases involve invasions of privacy. A recent case of invasion of privacy involved a plaintiff who used the pseudonym

John Smith. John Smith's physician was treating him for acute kidney failure. During an emergent bedside consultation in the patient's private hospital room, the physician mentioned his HIV-positive status. A third person was also in the room. The patient claimed that the physician thereby revealed his HIV-positive status to the third party without his consent. The patient said the physician was negligent, careless, reckless, willful, and wanton. He stated that the disclosure caused him pain and suffering, emotional distress, and permanent injury with physiological consequences. The courts upheld the patient's right to file the lawsuit (*John Smith, a fictitious person, Plaintiff-Respondent, v. Arvind R. Dalta, M.D. and Consultants in Kidney diseases, P.A., Defendants-Appellants*, 2017).

In a classic invasion of privacy case against nurses, Earl Spring, a 78-year-old man with dementia, resided in a nursing home where he was undergoing kidney dialysis. In an attempt to discontinue dialysis treatments, his legal guardians, his wife and son, were involved in a prolonged court battle. In opposition to the family's position, and without their consent, the nursing home staff permitted right-to-life advocates to interview the man. Interviews with the patient and four nurses were published. After winning a Superior Court ruling regarding discontinuing the dialysis, Mrs. Spring sued the nursing home and the four nurses for $80 million in damages. She claimed that her husband's right to privacy had been violated. Although the attorney for the nursing home maintained that the patient had become a "public figure," the jury found in favor of Mrs. Spring, awarding her a total of $2,771,728 (*Blanche Spring, individually and as executrix, v. Geriatric Authority of Holyoke & Others*, 1985).

In this age of electronic communication, nurses have plenty of opportunities to intentionally or unintentionally invade patients' privacy. Nurses discuss patient care over telephones, send records via fax or e-mail, participate in video conferencing, and record protected patient data via smartphones and tablets. Because of the pervasive use of electronic media, we have a duty to be especially vigilant against invasions of privacy and confidentiality. Interception of electronic confidential material can occur in a variety of ways. For example, unauthorized personnel may have access to electronic information on an institution's computer network, wireless and mobile telephone communications may be intercepted, online communications pass through a number of nonsecure computers, and portable devices such as laptops and smartphones can be lost or stolen. See Chapter 10 for an in-depth discussion of the ethical and legal implications of electronic communication devices and methods.

Federal legislation made the delicate balance between ethical principles more complex when confidentiality of patient information became a legal mandate. In 1996 Congress enacted Public Health Law 104–199, the Health Insurance Portability and Accountability Act (HIPAA). In the early 1990s people were becoming more mobile, healthcare costs were rising, and it became apparent to some that the healthcare industry would be more efficient if medical records were computerized. It also became apparent that there was a need for new standards for the management of healthcare data. Because of a growing number of criminal violations of electronic records, Congress required HHS to create medical privacy rules. Effective since 2003, the HIPAA Privacy Rule made confidentiality of medical records a legal requirement. Whereas other ethical principles do not carry the weight of law per se, confidentiality stands alone. Today, a breach of confidentiality may result in criminal conviction or other penalties. The HIPAA Privacy Rule protects all information that can be used to identify an individual and relates to an individual's past, present, or future physical or mental health or condition; the provision of health care to the individual; and the past, present, or future payment for the provision of health care to the individual (HIPAA Privacy Rule, 1996). If protected health information is used for teaching, research, or quality improvement, it must be deidentified. This means that any personal information that can reasonably be used to identify a specific person must be removed. HIPAA stipulates the removal of 18 specific identifiers such as identifiable photographs; names; dates; phone numbers; e-mail addresses; Social Security numbers; and geographic identifiers such as address, zip code, and city.

Assault and **battery** are also intentional tort offenses. The terms *assault* and *battery*, though usually used together, have different legal meanings. Assault is defined as the unjustifiable, intentional attempt or threat to touch a person without consent that causes the person to fear imminent harm. Assault includes a threat of harm plus an apparent ability to cause the harm. Assault does not require that the offensive contact actually occur. Battery is the unlawful, harmful, or unwarranted

touching of another or the carrying out of threatened physical harm. Battery includes any intentional, nonconsented, angry, violent, or harmful touching of a person's body or clothes, or anything held by or attached to the person (such as a scarf or purse). Battery can be either an intentional tort or a criminal offense. Surgical procedures performed without informed consent are the most common example of battery occurring in the hospital setting. In the course of everyday activities, nurses have been accused of both assault and battery. For example, actionable assault occurs when a nurse threatens to give an injection to an unruly or noncompliant adult patient without consent. Battery is often thought of as such actions as slapping, shoving, or pinching, but the courts have upheld battery charges in actions that were much less dramatic. Regardless of intent or outcome, touching without consent is considered battery. Even when the intention is beneficent and the outcome is positive, if the act is committed without permission, the nurse can be charged with battery.

Necessity and consent are two defenses that nurses can use when accused of battery in the course of administering care. Necessity refers to touching a person without consent in an emergency. It may be necessary to touch a person without consent to provide direct medical aid in an emergency or to protect oneself or others from a combative or violent person. In its most basic form, consent refers to approval or assent, particularly after thoughtful consideration. Consent may be explicitly expressed in verbal, nonverbal, or written form, or it may be implied. Because most nursing acts do not require a formal consent process, consent is often considered to be implied. For example, if a nurse enters the room and asks, "May I change your dressing?" and the patient removes his blankets and positions himself for a dressing change, he can be considered to have given implied consent. For this reason, asking permission for even the simplest procedure is a good idea because it elicits implied consent and may constitute a good defense against a charge of battery. The informed consent process for invasive procedures is a common type of explicitly expressed consent.

The case of *Robertson v. Provident House* (1991) illustrates an example of battery involving nurses. Although having an order for an "as needed" indwelling catheter, a quadriplegic patient objected when nurses tried to insert one. He had experienced pain and complications with indwelling catheters in the past. The nurse reportedly told the patient to "shut up" and then proceeded to insert the catheter. The catheter was removed after repeated requests from the patient and family. Subsequently, ignoring the patient's objections, the nurse reinserted the catheter. An injury occurred when a nurse forcefully pulled the catheter out. The family eventually sued for damages and recovered $25,000. The Louisiana Supreme Court found that battery occurs when a nurse ignores the objections of the patient and performs an invasive procedure, such as the insertion of an indwelling catheter.

A patient's refusal to consent is more complex in some cases. An exception to the requirement of consent from competent adults may be made for prisoners. Some states permit nurses to obtain blood and other specimens without consent from persons under arrest if police request the tests as part of a criminal investigation. Institutions should provide nurses with very clear guidelines for cases such as this. Police can obtain a court order to get a blood sample if a patient refuses, but the nurse should not have to decide the issue without administrative support. Two cases illustrate this issue. In the case of *O'Brien v. Synnott* (2013), a patient was brought to the emergency room in the middle of the night by police. The patient was reportedly driving erratically when he ran into a police officer who was on foot. The police shot the man in the lower back, arrested him, and brought him to the hospital. A nurse caring for the patient was approached by a policeman who gave her a vial and quietly asked her to draw a sample for blood alcohol analysis. The nurse was new to the emergency department, there were no supervisors within sight, and there was no court order for the blood draw. The nurse entered the patient's room, proceeded with other nursing care acts, and then drew the patient's blood. He allowed her to draw the blood but later contended that she did not inform him that the blood sample was to be tested for alcohol. The nurse was convicted of battery. In contrast, an experienced Utah nurse was awarded $500,000 in an out-of-court settlement after she was arrested because she refused to draw blood without a court order on a patient who was not under arrest. As the encounter was occurring, the nurse consulted hospital protocols and contacted hospital administration for guidance. She advocated for the patient when she refused to allow the police officer himself to collect the patient's blood sample. In a highly publicized scuffle, the nurse was arrested and handcuffed after her refusal

but was later released without charges (Stevens, 2017). The two cases offer a clear contrast between the nurses' actions and legal outcomes.

False imprisonment is defined as the unjustifiable restraint of a person within fixed boundaries, or an act intended to result in such confinement, without consent and without authority of law. False imprisonment can include physical restraint of the person or acts intended to accomplish confinement, such as refusing to release clothing or car keys. If a patient is competent, even blocking a doorway or delaying or coercing a patient can lead to claims of false imprisonment. If false imprisonment is accompanied by forcible restraint or the threat of restraint, assault and battery may also be charged. However, the states have different legal rules and procedures granting authorization to detain, for a limited period, specific categories of persons who are disoriented, mentally ill, or impaired by drugs or alcohol. Although it rarely occurs, people may also be confined without their consent in the United States for the purpose of isolation and quarantine if they have the communicable diseases of cholera, diphtheria, infectious tuberculosis, plague, smallpox, yellow fever, viral hemorrhagic fevers (such as Ebola), severe acute respiratory syndromes, or influenza that can cause a pandemic (CDC, 2019). Generally, persons can be held without consent for a short time while the hospital reports them to authorities and obtains commitment or custody orders.

Nurses have been accused of false imprisonment for restraining patients, locking patients in rooms, and detaining patients for payment of bills. An example of false imprisonment is seen in the case of *Big Town Nursing Home, Inc. v. Newman* (1970), in which a 67-year-old man was kept against his will for nearly two months. Having been brought to the nursing home by his nephew, the man attempted to leave several times. The staff of the nursing home forcibly detained him when he walked away, restrained him with tape in a chair, and denied him the use of a telephone and his clothing. The court found that the staff of the nursing home acted recklessly, willfully, and maliciously in unlawfully detaining him. In another case, *Blackman for Blackman v. Rifkin* (1988), the court held that some circumstances justify detainment. In this instance, the court upheld the hospital's duty to prevent further harm by detaining a highly intoxicated patient with a head injury, even though she insisted that she wanted to leave.

The court ruled that the hospital could assume that the patient would have consented to the treatment had she not been intoxicated.

Defamation occurs when one harms a person's reputation and good name; diminishes others' value or esteem; or arouses negative feelings toward the person in others by the communication of false, malicious, unprivileged, or harmful words. The only remarks or statements that constitute defamation are those that might arouse negative opinions about a person. Additionally, defamation only occurs when the words are communicated to a third person—that is, two persons directing remarks and insults to each other are not liable for defamation. In most states, there are two distinct forms of defamation: slander and libel.

Slander occurs when one person defames or damages the reputation of another by speaking unprivileged or false words. Slander can occur in nursing practice when nurses make cruel, false, or unsubstantiated claims against patients. By making value judgments or voicing the opinion that a patient is uncooperative, malingering, unintelligent, or drug-seeking, a nurse may be committing actionable slander. Nurses may also be accused of slander as a result of inappropriate defamatory remarks voiced against another professional.

Libel consists of defamation by written words and images that injure a person's reputation or cause others to avoid, ridicule, or view the person with contempt. Nurses risk accusations of libel, for example, when writing information in patients' charts that can be damaging. Judgmental, critical, or speculative statements made in patients' charts such as "The patient is drug-seeking" or "The patient is rude" can lead to charges of libel, particularly if the patient has reason to believe that the words adversely affect the care given by others. Even when lawsuits end in verdicts in favor of the defendant, the process can be anxiety provoking. In the case of *Chapman v. Maxwell* (2014) a nurse practitioner was accused of libel because of remarks she wrote in a patient's chart. The nurse saw the patient, who complained of back pain after a fall. Imaging tests were negative. The nurse practitioner ordered a limited number of analgesic tablets and recommended that the patient rest. The patient returned several times, each time complaining of back pain, which was not corroborated by any physical evidence. The patient asked for specific opioid analgesics by name. The nurse wrote in the chart that in her opinion, the patient might be malingering and/or drug-seeking. The patient requested that her medical records be shared with her employer and other medical practitioners as she applied for compensation. Release of information forms were properly signed. The nurse was surprised when she learned that the patient was suing her for defamation. The plaintiff claimed that the nurse's remarks on the chart harmed her employment and caused other medical practitioners to refuse to see her. The case involved a court battle and appeal to the Supreme Court. Both courts found in favor of the nurse because her notes expressed her opinion rather than a statement of fact.

If the defamatory remarks have the potential to harm the business prospects of the person, proof of damage is not needed. An example of this can be seen in the case of *Schessler v. Keck* (1956). In this case, an unmarried female caterer had a false-positive test for syphilis. Though the patient had never had the disease, a nurse seeing her catering at a party told the hostess that the woman was being treated for syphilis. This resulted in destroying the patient's business. The appeals court found that there was a valid basis for her claim of slander.

Nurses, themselves, have been harmed by defamation. A physician accused his office nurse of having mixed up reports on a patient's chart and lying about it. He fired her the next day and called a meeting of his office employees. He told his staff that he could not work with anyone who was a liar, untrustworthy, and disloyal. A jury awarded the nurse $125,000 in damages (Creighton, 1986). In 2018 the Ohio Supreme Court affirmed a lower court decision in favor of a nurse in another defamation lawsuit. The nurse, who had an excellent employment record in the hospital, was active in a union with which the hospital had refused to bargain. Against the recommendation of the hospital's human resources department, the hospital administration fired the nurse for neglect of duties and falsifying a medical record. The hospital reported her to the Ohio Board of Nursing. After she was fired, the nurse applied for multiple nursing positions. She was granted only two interviews and could not find a permanent nursing position. In the court's opinion, the hospital's accusations against the nurse were unsubstantiated, the firing was the direct result of her union activities, and the report to the Ohio Board of Nursing harmed her professional employment (Wayt, Appellee, v. DHSC, L.L. C., D.B.B. Affinity Medical Center, Appellant, 2018).

In certain instances, derogatory remarks may not constitute defamation. Two defenses to defamation include truth and privilege. In fact, there may be a legal or moral duty to pass on defamatory information in certain circumstances. For instance, a nurse has the duty to report suspected child abuse; a director of nursing services has a duty to report truthfully the character and qualifications of nurses to potential employers; and peer review groups are required to discuss privileged information for the purpose of improving services, disciplining providers, and so forth. Additionally, nurses are ethically obligated to report the illegal or incompetent practice of others. To avoid charges of defamation, prudent nurses will take care to observe appropriate channels of communication when making reports of this nature. In the absence of privileged communication, truth is a good defense for defamation.

Legal Jeopardy for Personal Conduct Outside of Work

Nurses can confront one additional type of legal jeopardy: career-ending loss of nursing license. Remember that state boards of nursing function to protect the public through regulation of the profession. Rules promulgated by a board of nursing carry the same weight as other laws. Because maintaining a state license in good standing is key to remaining employed in nursing, nurses must know the laws that apply to nursing practice. Nursing boards can take action against licensed nurses for unprofessional conduct in their private lives (Fig. 8.2). Boards of nursing have the power to investigate and prosecute a nurse in virtually all areas of a nurse's life, especially behaviors that suggest a nurse's judgment or moral character is questionable or indicate that the nurse poses a threat to the health, safety, or welfare of the public. Chronic drug or alcohol abuse are common causes of nurse discipline in this regard. Other events, such as a criminal conviction or a no-contest plea to a criminal charge, can trigger a board investigation. Criminal convictions can indicate that a nurse's conduct is in opposition to the moral and ethical codes of the profession or that the nurse is likely to defraud, deceive, or generally pose a danger to the public. The types of criminal violations that can trigger an investigation include public intoxication; failing to pay child support; domestic violence; child or elder abuse; harassment; stalking; violation of a restraining order; indecent exposure or other lewd acts; assault and battery; theft; fraud; firearms charges; failure to file tax returns; and the possession, sale, or distribution of controlled substances without legitimate prescription purposes. A board of nursing can also discipline a nurse for knowingly or inadvertently disclosing patients' private information or photographs, such as on social media; knowingly falsifying an application for employment, such as leaving out information from an employer who may give a bad reference; lying about or exaggerating licensure status, education, clinical experience, or skill level; or submitting other false information to the board. A board may also consider acts of misappropriating medications, supplies, or personal items belonging to either a patient or an employer to be misconduct, even if criminal charges are not filed (Lilly, 2015).

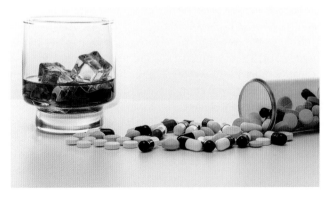

Fig. 8.2 Conduct in Personal Life Can Affect Professional Licensure. (©iStock.com/Giselleflissak.)

REDUCING RISK

The government, healthcare institutions, and individuals have increased their focus on reducing risk in health care. In addition to adherence to codes of nursing ethics and other standards of care, nurses can reduce their risk of liability through maintaining good communication, clinical competence, autonomy, and sufficient liability insurance.

In an effort to improve health care and reduce risk to patients, in 1999 the Institute of Medicine (IOM) published its landmark report, *To Err Is Human: Building a Safer Health System*. The eye-opening report noted that between 44,000 and 98,000 people were dying in hospitals each year because of preventable medical errors. In addition to the human cost, the IOM estimated that the total cost at that time included the expenses of additional care, lost income and productivity, and disability which amounted to between $17 billion and $29 billion per year. In the decades since *To Err Is Human* was disseminated, government and private organizations have begun to adopt initiatives to reduce errors. One such program is the "never events" initiative developed by the National Quality Forum (NQF). Following is a discussion of **serious reportable events** (SREs) and strategies that individual nurses can use to reduce risk in their own practices.

Serious Reportable Events

SREs, often referred to as "**never events**," and **hospital-acquired conditions** are phrases used to identify clusters of negative patient conditions that are almost universally avoidable with proper care. In 2002 the NQF identified 28 SREs that are so unambiguous, serious, and preventable that they should never happen. The list has been updated multiple times and now consists of nearly 30 SREs grouped into seven categories. In addition, the Centers for Medicare and Medicaid Services (CMS) lists a number of hospital-acquired patient conditions that overlap significantly with NQF's list of SREs and have a strong implication for healthcare insurance. Some of CMS's hospital-acquired conditions are not caused by errors per se but could reasonably have been prevented through the application of evidence-based guidelines and good care. In addition to liability lawsuits against nurses, hospitals, and physicians, SREs and hospital-acquired conditions account for millions of dollars in insurance payouts or tremendous losses for hospitals. These events and conditions must be reported in many states. CMS and other third-party payers may either decline to pay hospital costs for them or reduce payments to the worst-performing hospitals (Agency for Healthcare Research and Quality, 2019; Centers for Medicare & Medicaid Services, 2022a). Below is the ever-evolving integrated list of serious reportable never events and hospital-acquired conditions:

1. Surgical Events
   - Surgery or other invasive procedures performed on the wrong site or the wrong patient
   - Wrong surgical or other invasive procedures performed on a patient
   - Unintended retention of a foreign object in a patient after surgery
   - Intraoperative or immediately postoperative/postprocedure death in an American Society of Anesthesiologists Class I patient
   - Surgical site infection following coronary artery bypass graft, bariatric surgery, implantation of a cardiac implantable electronic device, or certain orthopedic procedures of the spine, neck, shoulder, and elbow

2. Product or Device Events
   - Patient death or serious injury associated with the use of contaminated drugs, devices, or biologics provided by the healthcare setting
   - Patient death or serious injury associated with the use or function of a device in patient care when the device is used or functions other than as intended
   - Patient death or serious injury associated with intravascular air embolism that occurs while being cared for in a healthcare setting
   - Patient death or serious injury associated with iatrogenic pneumothorax with venous catheterization

3. Patient Protection Events
   - Discharge or release of a patient/resident of any age who is unable to make decisions to other than an authorized person
   - Patient death or serious injury associated with patient elopement (disappearance)
   - Patient suicide, or attempted suicide, or self-harm that results in serious injury while being cared for in a healthcare setting

4. Care Management Events
   - Patient death or serious injury associated with a medication error

- Patient death or serious injury associated with unsafe administration of blood products
- Maternal or fetal death or serious injury associated with labor or delivery in a low-risk pregnancy
- Patient death or serious injury associated with a fall in a healthcare setting
- Any stage III, stage IV, or unstageable pressure ulcers acquired after admission/presentation to a healthcare setting
- Artificial insemination with the wrong donor sperm or wrong egg
- Patient death or serious injury resulting from the irretrievable loss of an irreplaceable biological specimen
- Patient death or serious injury from failure to follow up or communicate laboratory, pathology, or radiology test results
- Patient death or serious injury as a manifestation of poor glycemic control
- Catheter-associated urinary tract infection
- Deep vein thrombosis or pulmonary embolism following certain orthopedic procedures, including total knee replacement and hip replacement
- Patient death or serious injury resulting from an air embolism

5. Environmental Events
   - Patient or staff death or serious injury associated with an electric shock in the course of a patient care process in a healthcare setting
   - Any incident in which systems designated for oxygen or other gas to be delivered to a patient contains no gas, the wrong gas, or is contaminated by toxic substances
   - Patient or staff death or serious injury associated with a burn incurred from any source in the course of a patient care process in a healthcare setting
   - Patient death or serious injury associated with the use of physical restraints or bedrails while being cared for in a healthcare setting

6. Radiological Events
   - Death or serious injury of a patient or staff associated with the introduction of a metallic object into the magnetic resonance imaging area

7. Criminal Events
   - Any instance of care ordered by or provided by someone impersonating a physician, nurse, pharmacist, or other licensed healthcare provider

- Abduction of a patient/resident of any age
- Sexual assault/abuse of a patient or staff member within or on the grounds of a healthcare setting
- Death or significant injury of a patient or staff member resulting from a physical assault (i.e., battery) that occurs within or on the grounds of a healthcare setting (Centers for Medicare & Medicaid Services, 2022b; National Quality Forum, 2019).

Reducing Liability Risks

How can nurses limit the risk of lawsuits? Much of today's litigation occurs as a result of events over which nurses have little control. Unfortunate outcomes can result from institutional circumstances, errors or incompetence of other professionals, or unpredictable or intractable physical phenomena. Other litigation occurs because of thoughtless or negligent actions on the part of nurses or other professionals. Though it is impossible to eliminate the risk of litigation, attention to a number of critical factors may reduce the threat of malpractice suits. Critical factors include maintaining good communication, clinical competence, autonomy, and sufficient liability insurance (Box 8.3).

Maintain Good Communication

One of the most important nurse characteristics that reduces the risk of lawsuits is a genuine regard for others. This quality produces nurses who are courteous, honest, and caring. They maintain open lines of communication, spend the time that is required to show respect, have genuine interest and patience, listen to understand, and advocate for their patients. Poor communication is the source of many malpractice lawsuits. Patients tend to become hostile if they believe they are not being taken seriously, are not being listened to, are being belittled, or are denied involvement in the decision-making process. Hostile or angry patients are more likely to file lawsuits.

Anecdotal information reveals that a professional's lack of listening is a key element for patients who are inclined to file lawsuits. Good communicators listen objectively, avoid making value judgments, and include patients in healthcare decisions. The value of good listening skills cannot be overemphasized. Nurses with good listening skills are more likely to involve patients in decision making. In addition to the psychosocial benefits, attentive listening can provide important information that might otherwise have gone undetected.

BOX 8.3   Reducing Liability Risks

- Maintain good communication
  - Be courteous, show respect, and take time to listen attentively.
  - Do not belittle patients or make value judgments.
  - Involve patients in decision making.
  - Assess patients' level of understanding.
  - Explain in language that patients can understand.
  - Enlist qualified interpreters.
  - Utilize extreme caution with telephone communication.
  - Document:
  - Patient assessment and monitoring
  - Changes in the condition of patients
  - Results of diagnostic tests and procedures
  - Relevant discussions with patients and physicians
- Maintain clinical competence
  - Follow documented nursing standards.
  - Be familiar with and follow institutional and professional standards of care.
  - Keep up to date in both knowledge and skills.
  - Do not attempt any task or give any medication that is unfamiliar.
  - Practice within the professional and statutory scope of practice.
  - Complete proper patient assessment and monitoring.
  - Pay close attention to detail, avoiding distraction.
- Maintain autonomy and empowerment
  - Challenge questionable physician orders.
  - Seek attention for patients with changing health status.
  - Challenge bureaucratic structures that threaten patient welfare.
  - Avoid institutional settings that produce systematic and persistent threats to patient welfare.
- Maintain sufficient liability insurance

Good communication strategies include assessing patients' level of understanding and finding ways to help patients understand important information. Nurses can be charged with malpractice when injury occurs because patients fail to understand treatment options, potential outcomes of treatments, side effects of drugs, self-care, discharge instructions, and so forth. Nurses should check and recheck patients' understanding and involve other family members when appropriate. They should teach and explain in common language, avoiding confusing medical terms and jargon. Qualified professional interpreters should be used for all patients who have limited proficiency in the English language. The use of patients' families for interpretation is risky because nonmedical interpreters may not truly understand what is being said. Because lawsuits are frequent and it is particularly difficult to assess patients' level of understanding, nurses need to be especially careful about giving advice or patient teaching over the telephone.

The risk of lawsuits can be reduced with good two-way communication with physicians and coworkers. Patient care teams are composed of professionals who must communicate with one another. Healthcare delivery is complex and poses many communication challenges. Coordination of care between individuals and disciplines is critical for patient safety and requires effort and skill in inter- and intra-professional communication. Multiple research studies over the years have shown that communication between nurses and physicians is a significant factor associated with patient mortality (Ellison, 2015; Knaus et al., 1986; Kramer & Schmalenberg, 2003; Manojlovich & DeCicco, 2007; O'Daniel, 2008; Seago, 2008). And, as was seen in the legal cases cited in this chapter, negative patient outcomes are more likely to trigger malpractice lawsuits. Nurses should take the lead and cultivate positive relationships with physicians and colleagues. As patient advocates, nurses must be comfortable communicating with physicians and must speak up when they identify a problem or potential error. When speaking with physicians, nurses' communication should be powerful, clear, organized, logical, precise, and concise.

Written communication is equally important in reducing the risk of malpractice lawsuits. Documentation is crucial for effective communication among nurses and with other disciplines. In addition to ensuring continuity of care, good written documentation can highlight the quality of nursing care that was delivered if a nurse is charged with malpractice. Documentation should be legible, accurate, complete, contemporaneous, concise, thorough, organized, and confidential (ANA, 2010). As alluded to in many of the cases noted in this chapter, good written communication includes careful documentation of care plans, patient assessment and monitoring, changes in the condition of patients, results of diagnostic tests and procedures, and relevant discussions with patients and physicians.

Maintain Clinical Competence

One of the most effective ways to reduce liability risk is to maintain a broad level of knowledge and skills. Competent practice is not only one hallmark of a professional but is also a legal and ethical imperative. There have been monumental advances in knowledge and technology in the past several years. With the advent of health insurance in the post–World War II era and malpractice litigation in recent years, standards of care have become very stringent. Society's expectations of nurses' knowledge and abilities are high. Consequently, nurses must strive to maintain up-to-date knowledge and technical skills. Lack of knowledge is no defense in a court of law. It is, in fact, tantamount to an admission of negligence. It is important that nurses know and uphold institutional, professional, and legal standards of practice and work within their scope of practice, never attempting to perform any task or administer any medication that is unfamiliar. Nurses' actions are examined in light of current information, professional or statutory scope of practice, and institutional and professional practice standards. Statements such as "Everyone does it that way," "That is what I learned in school 20 years ago," or "I did the best I could" will not protect a nurse from being found negligent. Advances in the body of nursing knowledge are never ending, so nurses should continuously improve and update knowledge throughout their professional lives.

Maintain Autonomy and Empowerment

Autonomy is an essential component of professional nursing practice and has been shown to be a core factor in the delivery of quality nursing care. Studies consistently demonstrate that the value and contribution of nurse autonomy increase the quality of patient outcomes (Aiken et al., 2009; Lake & Friese, 2006; Rao et al., 2017). As the examples in this chapter have illustrated, the courts demand that nurses practice autonomously. Time and again, court decisions indicate that society expects nurses to be courageous in questioning physicians' orders (particularly those given over the telephone), vigorous in seeking attention for patients with changing health status, and active in challenging bureaucratic structures that threaten patient welfare. The courts know that nurses have in-depth knowledge in areas such as pharmacology and pathophysiology and expect nurses to protect patients from harm. Facing institutional situations that systematically present threats to patient safety and welfare and being unable to bring about change, nurses may find they can protect themselves from liability only by leaving the situation.

Maintain Sufficient Liability Insurance

Despite efforts to reduce the risk of liability, nurses are increasingly vulnerable to claims of malpractice. Regardless of nurses' level of expertise, patients can be injured. Even if a claim has no merit, the process of defense is time consuming, emotionally exhausting, and costly. Liability insurance is an important risk management strategy that protects assets and income and affords nurses peace of mind. Professional liability insurance provides for payment of lawyer fees and settlement or jury awards. No practicing nurse should ever be without liability coverage.

There are two basic types of liability insurance coverage. **Occurrence-based** policies provide broad coverage. These policies cover the nurse for claims arising from incidents that occur during the period that the policy is in effect. Occurrence-based policies protect the nurse when lawsuits are filed after the policy has expired, even if the policy was not renewed. Nurses who work with children or infants run the risk of lawsuits being filed many years after an injury occurs, so occurrence-based policies may be more appropriate for these nurses. All states have different laws regarding their statutes of limitations which define how long after an incident the injured person has to make a claim. Depending upon state law, if the injured person was a minor child when the injury occurred, the statute of limitations might begin when the child reaches majority, often at the age of 18 years. This means a nurse could conceivably be sued for liability up to 20 years after an incident with a child occurred—potentially well into retirement. Occurrence-based policies cover any claims made during the time the policy was in effect, even after the policy is discontinued. **Claims-made** policies, on the other hand, provide coverage only when both the injury and the claim are made during the time in which the policy is in effect. Claims-made coverage is adequate if the nurse maintains continuous coverage and purchases **tail coverage** to provide an uninterrupted extension for a period after the policy period. Tail coverage is less expensive special liability coverage that permits an insured person to report claims that are made after a claims-made policy has expired or been canceled. Occurrence-based policies are preferable for most nurses.

Another distinction is made between malpractice policies and professional liability policies. Generally speaking, malpractice policies offer coverage exclusively for claims of malpractice. Though specific coverage differs from policy to policy, professional liability insurance offers protection against various injuries that are not directly related to malpractice.

Nurses also question whether they need individual coverage if their group or employer provides insurance. Individual coverage is purchased by the individual and offers the policyholder 24-hour protection against liability claims for actions that fall within the scope of professional nursing practice, either paid or volunteer (Guido, 2019). Individual coverage pays lawyer fees and monetary damages (in relation to limits of the specific policy) and offers the nurse some control over the details of the defense strategy. Infrequently used by nurses, group coverage is purchased by professionals who have essentially the same job descriptions and covers only those activities performed during office hours. This is particularly attractive as a less expensive choice for nurse practitioners in group practice. On the other hand, employer-sponsored coverage is purchased by the employing agency for the purpose of protecting business concerns. Coverage under employer-sponsored policies limits the protection to activities performed within the scope of employment while the nurse is on duty. Though employers may claim that employer-sponsored coverage is adequate, it is actually the most limited type of liability insurance. In fact, if found negligent, nurses may be required to repay the employer a portion of the loss. Nurses who rely solely on hospital policies have a greater chance of inadequate monetary protection and inadequate legal counsel (Guido, 2019).

NURSES AS EXPERT WITNESSES

Because of the complex and highly technical nature of nursing, attorneys require the assistance of knowledgeable and experienced expert witnesses. Nurses, as expert witnesses, may be hired by either the plaintiff or the defendant. Serving the legal system, expert witnesses are neither parties to the dispute nor patient advocates. Ideally, they remain neutral and honest when they offer objective opinions to the court.

Until recently, most courts accepted physicians as expert witnesses in cases involving nurses.

Historically, court rulings tended to reflect society's confusion about the relationship between nursing and medicine. There has been a slow evolution in the courts. In 1958 a California judge accepted a physician's testimony about nursing standards of care, saying, "Surely a qualified doctor would know what was standard procedure of nurses to follow" (Goff v. Doctor's General Hospital of San Jose, 1958). More recently, a 1972 judicial opinion acknowledged that a physician might not be the best expert on nursing standards but admitted physicians' testimony because "all areas of medical expertise within the knowledge of nurses are also within the knowledge of medical doctors" (*Taylor v. Spencer Hospital*, 1972). A 2004 Illinois Supreme Court decision became a landmark case for nurses. In this case, the Supreme Court upheld a lower court ruling that the doctor who testified as an expert was not competent to give testimony as to the standard of care for nurses (*Sullivan v. Edward Hospital*, 2004).

Serving as an expert witness involves a complex and extensive process of examining evidence, reviewing pertinent nursing literature, giving depositions, and testifying in court. The expert witness is expected to become familiar with all medical records of the patient during the time of the incident; pertinent written policies and procedures of the institution; nursing assessment, diagnosis, plan, interventions, and evaluation; the state nurse practice act; applicable nursing standards; current professional literature outlining accepted practice at the time of the incident; and opinions from the state board of nursing. The expert witness must describe the standards of care to the court, evaluate the nurse's actions against the standards, and discuss conclusions relative to the accusation of malpractice. The effectiveness of the expert witness is influenced by the breadth of experience, degree of preparation, depth of knowledge, and confident delivery.

The use of expert witnesses gives strength to the argument that nursing is a true profession. It supports the autonomy of nursing, in that no other professional can appropriately judge the practice of nurses. Advertisements for educational courses and organizations for nurse expert witnesses are now common in nursing periodicals and websites. The profession is taking seriously this newly acquired judicial recognition.

SUMMARY

As the enforceable system of principles and processes that govern the behavior of people, laws reflect moral and ethical traditions. Though there is sometimes disagreement regarding the rightness or wrongness of certain laws, the laws are generally consistent with popular beliefs.

Laws in the United States are constitutional, statutory, or administrative and are divided into public and private realms. Public law deals with the relationship between persons and the government, and private law deals with the relationship between people. Nurses and other healthcare providers are more likely to be involved in liability cases related to tort law, a division of private law. Tort law includes unintentional torts, such as negligence and malpractice, and intentional torts, such as fraud, invasion of privacy, assault, battery, false imprisonment, and defamation.

With the increase in malpractice litigation, nurses are wise to take certain precautions to limit the risk of lawsuits. Critical factors include maintaining open lines of communication with patients through the use of good listening techniques, an accepting demeanor, and attention to patient's level of understanding; maintaining clinical competence, including retaining expertise and ensuring attention to detail; maintaining autonomy through courageous and vigorous patient advocacy; practicing effective communication; and maintaining continuous professional liability insurance. When patients accuse nurses of malpractice, expert nurse witnesses can serve the court by describing standards of care, evaluating the nurse's action against standards, and discussing conclusions relative to the accusation of malpractice.

CHAPTER HIGHLIGHTS

- Ethics is the foundation of law; however, because laws are created by individuals and there are differences in beliefs among people, ethics and the law are not always congruent.
- Constitutional law supersedes all other laws.
- Statutory law is created through the lawmaking process in state or federal legislatures; it is also called *legislative law*.
- Administrative law consists mainly of the legal powers granted to administrative agencies by the legislature and the rules that the agencies make to carry out their powers.
- Common law, also known as *case law*, is a system of law based largely on previous court decisions.
- Public law defines a person's rights and obligations in relation to government and describes the various divisions of government and their powers.
- Private law, also called *civil law*, determines a person's legal rights and obligations in many kinds of activities that involve other people.
- A tort is a wrong or injury that a person suffers because of someone else's action, either intentional (willful or intentional acts that violate another person's rights or property) or unintentional (an act or omission that causes unintended injury or harm to another person).
- Changes in healthcare financing and delivery have caused litigation related to corporate liability.
- Nurses can limit the risk of liability through maintaining open communication with patients, expertise in practice, attention to detail, and autonomy.
- Supporting the autonomous nature of nursing, expert nurse witnesses serve the court through the process of examining evidence, applying nursing standards, reviewing pertinent nursing literature, and explaining conclusions.

DISCUSSION QUESTIONS AND ACTIVITIES

1. Search the Internet for references to recent court decisions. You may begin by visiting Google and searching for "recent malpractice cases." Find examples of recent court cases related to issues such as termination of life support, fetal tissue use, genetic engineering, and patient self-determination. Discuss your beliefs related to the court decisions. What ethical principles apply?
2. Discuss with classmates opinions about the criminal courts becoming involved in issues that have traditionally been considered ethical in nature.
3. Locate and read the Bill of Rights of the US Constitution. How do the rights guaranteed in the Bill of Rights relate to patient care? How do they relate to nurses' employment?
4. To gain a better understanding of the difference between actual and proximal cause of injury, search the Internet for the interesting 1928 case, *Palsgraf v.*

Long Island Railroad Co. What was the actual cause of the injury? Were the railroad employees liable for the injury?

5. There are many recent examples of controversial and historic state and federal legislation that have created changes in the healthcare delivery system or in the practice of nursing. Discuss with classmates recent examples, making sure to listen thoughtfully to classmates with opinions that are different from yours.

6. In the common law system, how do previous court decisions affect the outcome of current cases?

7. Discuss instances in which nurses can be charged with crimes of public law, even though acts were committed without malice in the process of giving nursing care.

8. Discuss specific examples of unintentional torts of which nurses have been accused.

9. How can you protect yourself from being accused of an unintentional tort?

10. In what instances can nurses be charged with intentional torts, even though they follow a professional code of ethics?

11. Discuss new areas of potential liability for nurses and the present healthcare delivery system.

12. Review the ANA ethics and human rights position statements page and examine at least three of the official position statements at http://www.nursingworld.org/positionstatements.

REFERENCES

Agency for Healthcare Research and Quality. (2019). *Never events.* https://psnet.ahrq.gov/primer/never-events

Aiken, L. H., Clarke, S. P., Sloane, D. M., Lake, E. T., & Cheney, T. (2009). Effects of hospital care environment on patient mortality and nurse outcomes. *The Journal of Nursing Administration*, *39*(7-8 Suppl), S45–S51. https://doi.org/10.1097/NNA.0b013e3181aeb4cf.

American Association of Colleges of Nursing. (2022). *Nursing fact sheet.* https://www.aacnnursing.org/news-Information/fact-sheets/nursing-fact-sheet#:~:text=Nursing%20is%20the%20nation%27s%20largest,84.1%25%25%20are%20employed%20in%20nursing.&text=The%20federal%20government%20projects%20that,each%20year%20from%202021%2D2031.

ANA, (2010). *Principles for nursing documentation.* Nursebooks.org. https://www.nursingworld.org/~4af4f2/globalassets/docs/ana/ethics/principles-of-nursing-documentation.pdf.

ANA, (2021). *Nursing: Scope and standards of practice* (4th ed.). Nursebooks.org.

Apold, J., & Rydrych, D. (2012). Preventing device-related pressure ulcers: Using data to guide statewide change. *Journal of Nursing Care Quality*, *27*(1), 28–34.

Beauchamp, T. L. (2001). *Philosophical ethics: An introduction to moral philosophy* (3rd ed.). McGraw Hill.

Big Town Nursing Home, Inc. v. Newman (Tex. Civ. App. 1970). https://casetext.com/case/big-town-nursing-home-v-newman

Blackman for Blackman v. Rifkin(1988). https://law.justia.com/cases/colorado/court-of-appeals/1988/85ca1272-0.html

Blanche Spring, individually and as executrix, v. Geriatric Authority of Holyoke & Others (Franklin County, MA 1985). http://masscases.com/cases/sjc/394/394mass274.html

Burnham, H. (2005). New Orleans medical staff raid empty hospital for vital supplies. *Nursing Standard*, *20*(1), 12.

Cady, R. F. (2009). Criminal prosecution for nursing errors. *JONA's Healthcare Law, Ethics & Regulation*, *11*(1), 10–18. https://doi.org/10.1097/NHL.0b013e31819acb0d.

CDC. (2019). *Legal authorities for isolation and quarantine.* https://www.cdc.gov/quarantine/aboutlawsregulationsquarantineisolation.html

Center for Medicare & Medicaid Services. (2021). *Medicare fraud & abuse: Prevent, detect, report.* https://www.cms.gov/Outreach-and-Education/Medicare-Learning-Network-MLN/MLNProducts/Downloads/Fraud-Abuse-MLN4649244.pdf

Centers for Medicare & Medicaid Services. (2022a). *Hospital-acquired condition reduction program.* https://www.cms.gov/Medicare/Medicare-Fee-for-Service-Payment/AcuteInpatientPPS/HAC-Reduction-Program#:~:text=The%20Hospital%2DAcquired%20Condition%20(HAC,in%20the%20inpatient%20hospital%20setting.

Centers for Medicare & Medicaid Services. (2022b). *Hospital-acquired conditions.* https://www.cms.gov/Medicare/Medicare-Fee-for-Service-Payment/HospitalAcqCond/Hospital-Acquired_Conditions

Chapman v. Maxwell (Montana 2014), Affirmed. https://law.justia.com/cases/montana/supreme-court/2014/da-13-0428.html

Creighton, H. (1986). *Law every nurse should know* (5th ed.). Saunders.

Ellison, D. (2015). Communication skills. *Nursing Clinics of North America*, *50*(1), 45–57.

Ferris v. County of Kennebec, 44 F. Supp. 2d 62 (Dist. Court, D. Maine 1999).

Furrow, R. R., Greaney, T. L., Johnson, S. H., Jost, T. S., & Schwartz, R. L. (2004). *Liability and quality issues in health care* (6th ed.). West Group.

Gleason, K. T., Jones, R., Rhodes, C., Greenberg, P., Harkless, G., Goeschel, C., Cahill, M., & Graber, M. (2021). Evidence that nurses need to participate in diagnosis: Lessons from malpractice claims. *Journal of Patient Safety*, 959–963. https://doi.org/10.1097/PTS.0000000000000621.

Goff v. Doctor's General Hospital of San Jose (District Court of Appeal, Third District, CA 1958). https://caselaw.findlaw.com/ca-court-of-appeal/1764514.html

Guido, G. W. (2019). *Legal & ethical issues in nursing* (7th ed.). Pearson.

Hakim, M. J., Hanscom, R., Icenhower, M., Miller, S., Montminy, S., Ricci, B., & Small, M. (2022). *A dose of insight: A nurse's crucial role in patient safety*. https://www.coverys.com/knowledge-center/a-dose-of-insight-nurses-patient-safety

HIPAA Privacy Rule, § 160.103 (1996). https://www.hhs.gov/hipaa/for-professionals/privacy/index.html

IOM, (1999). *To err is human: Building a safer health system*. N. A. Press. https://www.nap.edu/download/9728.

John Smith, a fictitious person, Plaintiff-Respondent, v. Arvind R. Dalta, M.D. and Consultants in Kidney diseases, P.A., Defendants-Appellants (Superior Court of New Jersey, Appellate Division 2017). https://caselaw.findlaw.com/nj-superior-court-appellate-division/1867635.html

Kaiser Family Foundation. (2022). *Health coverage of immigrants*. https://www.kff.org/racial-equity-and-health-policy/fact-sheet/health-coverage-of-immigrants/

Kelman, B. (2022). Tennessee nurse convicted in lethal drug error sentenced to three years probation. *Kaiser Health News*. https://www.npr.org/sections/health-shots/2022/05/13/1098867553/nurse-sentenced-probation.

King Jr, M. L. (1996/1963). Letter from the Birmingham jail In J. Feinberg (Ed.), *Reason and responsibility: Readings in some basic problems of philosophy* (9th ed., pp. 572–580). Wadsworth.

Knaus, W. A., Draper, E. A., Wagner, D. P., & Zimmerman, J. E. (1986). An evaluation of outcomes from intensive care in major medical centers. *Annals of Internal Medicine*, *104*(3), 410–418.

Kramer, M., & Schmalenberg, C. (2003). Securing 'good' nurse physician relationships. *Nursing Management*, *34*(7), 34–38.

Lake, E. T., & Friese, C. R. (2006). Variations in nursing practice environments: Relation to staffing and hospital characteristics. *Nursing Research*, *55*(1), 1–9.

Lilly, L. L. (2015). Your personal conduct outside of work can lead to discipline from the nursing boards. *West Virginia Nurse*, *18*(1), 7.

Manojlovich, M., & DeCicco, B. (2007). Healthy work environments, nurse-physician communication, and patients' outcomes. *American Journal of Critical Care*, *16*(6), 536–543.

Michas, F. (2022). *Total number of active physicians in the U.S., as of May 2022, by state*. https://www.statista.com/statistics/186269/total-active-physicians-in-the-us/#:~:text=As%20of%20May%202022%2C%20the,physicians%2C%20followed%20by%20New%20York.

Monk, J. (June 16, 2002). Special report: How a hospital failed a boy who didn't have to die. *The State*, 8-9http://www.lewisblackman.net/

Myers, L. C., Heard, L., & Mort, E. (2020). Lessons learned from medical malpractice claims involving critical care nurses. *American Journal of Critical Care*, *29*(3), 174–181. https://doi.org/10.4037/ajcc2020341.

National Archives. (2022). *Plessy v. Ferguson*. https://www.archives.gov/milestone-documents/plessy-v-ferguson

National Quality Forum. (2019). *List of SREs*. http://www.qualityforum.org/Topics/SREs/List_of_SREs.aspx

Nursing Service Organization. (2017). *Failure to adequately assess and monitor*. https://www.nso.com/Learning/Artifacts/Legal-Cases/Nurse-Case-Study-Failure-to-adequately-assess-and-monitor-the-patient-post-operatively-resulting-in

O'Brien v. Synnott (Superior Court, Chittenden Unit, VT 2013). https://law.justia.com/cases/vermont/supreme-court/2013/2012-164.html

O'Daniel, M. (2008). *Professional communication and team collaboration*. Agency for Healthcare Research and Quality.

Office of Inspector General. (2023). *Fraud & abuse laws*. https://oig.hhs.gov/compliance/physician-education/fraud-abuse-laws/#:~:text=The%20five%20most%20important%20Federal,Monetary%20Penalties%20Law%20(CMPL).

Oswald v. LeGrand (Iowa Supreme Court 1990). https://law.justia.com/cases/iowa/supreme-court/1990/89-166-0.html

Paget, S., & Wolfe, E. (2022). *Man breaks into school and shelters more than 20 people from blizzard*. https://www.cnn.com/2022/12/30/us/blizzard-new-york-rescue-school-break-in/index.html

Palsgraf v. The Long Is. R.R. Co. (Court of Appeals of NY 1928). http://www.courts.state.ny.us/reporter/archives/palsgraf_lirr.htm

Pozgar, G. D. (2018). *Legal aspects of health care administration* (13th ed.). Jones & Bartlett.

Rao, A. D., Kumar, A., & McHugh, M. (2017). Better nurse autonomy decreases the odds of 30-day mortality and failure to rescue. *Journal of Nursing Scholarship*, *49*(1), 73–79. https://doi.org/10.1111/jnu.12267.

Richards v. Beverly Health & Rehabilitation of Frankfort (Franklin, County 2006). http://www.juryverdicts.net/KY6-06.pdf

Roberson v. Provident House (Lousiana 1991). https://law.justia.com/cases/louisiana/supreme-court/1991/90-c-1388-2.html

Schessler v. Keck (Second Dist., Div. Two, CA 1956). https://law.justia.com/cases/california/court-of-appeal/2d/138/663.html

Seago, J. A. (2008). *Professional communication*. Agency for Healthcare Research and Quality.

Smelko v. Brinton (Kansas 1987). https://law.justia.com/cases/kansas/supreme-court/1987/59-850-2.html

Smith v. Juneau (Court of Appeal of Lousiana, Fourth Circuit 1997), Affirmed. https://caselaw.findlaw.com/la-court-of-appeal/1466688.html

Southern Pacific Company v. Jensen, 205 (U.S. 1917), (Oliver Wendell Holmes, Jr. dissenting opinion).

The State of Lousiana v. Brenner (Lousiana 1986). https://law.justia.com/cases/louisiana/supreme-court/1986/85-kk-1624-1.html

Stevens, M. (2017). Arrested nurse settles with Salt Lake City and university for $500,000. *New York Times*. https://www.nytimes.com/2017/11/02/us/utah-nurse-settlement.html

Sullivan v. Edward Hospital (IL 2004). https://law.justia.com/cases/illinois/court-of-appeals-second-appellate-district/2002/2010518.html

Taylor et vir v. Spencer Hospital (PA Superior 1972). https://casetext.com/case/taylor-et-vir-v-spencer-hospital

U.S. Department of Health & Human Services. (2022). *HHS FY 2022 Budget in Brief*. https://www.hhs.gov/about/budget/fy2022/index.html

U.S. Department of Health & Human Services. (2023). *National Practitioner Data Bank*. https://www.npdb.hrsa.gov/

U.S. Department of Health & Human Services and U. S. Department of Justice. (2022). *Health Care Fraud and Abuse Control Program FY 2021*. https://oig.hhs.gov/publications/docs/hcfac/FY2021-hcfac.pdf

U.S. Federal Bureau of Investigation. (2019). *Health care fraud*. https://www.fbi.gov/investigate/white-collar-crime/health-care-fraud

Wayt, Appellee, v. DHSC, L.L. C., D.B.B. Affinity Medical Center, Appellant (Ohio 2018). https://casetext.com/case/wayt-v-dhsc-llc

Zippa. (2023). *Advanced practice registered nurse demographics in the U.S.* https://www.zippia.com/advanced-practice-registered-nurse-jobs/demographics/

9

Ethics and Professional Relationships

These virtues we acquire by first exercising them. ... Whatever we learn to do, we learn by actually doing it. ... By doing just acts we come to be just; by doing self-controlled acts, we come to be self-controlled; and by doing brave acts, we become brave.

(Aristotle, ca. 350 B.C.E./2000)

OBJECTIVES

After completing this chapter, the reader should be able to:

1. Clarify personal values and professional codes of ethics as they relate to professional relationships.
2. Describe constructive strategies to solve professional relationship problems in the workplace.
3. Discuss ethical issues embedded in nurses' professional relationships with institutions, other nurses, physicians, and subordinates.
4. Examine how ethics relates to the workplace issues of racial discrimination, sexual harassment, and discrimination against people with disabilities.
5. Describe how nursing codes of ethics address violence in the workplace including incivility and bullying.

INTRODUCTION

Creating and sustaining an ethical practice environment is the duty of all nurses. A positive practice environment depends upon the quality of professional relationships. Therefore, it is incumbent upon nurses to know the code of nursing ethics, which informs all professional relationships. "An ethical professional practice environment facilitates nursing care that prioritizes ethical reflection and inquiry, allows for expression of varying viewpoints without fear of reprisal, and promotes professional and ethical values and trust" (ANA Center for Ethics and Human Rights, 2021, p. 1). An ethical work environment has both individual and institutional perspectives. An ethical environment is one in which each person understands the meaning of an *ethical culture*, identifies the existing culture as one that maintains an ethical climate, and accepts the responsibility to voice ethical concerns (ANA Center for Ethics and Human Rights, 2021). The institution's responsibility is to create and uphold policies and procedures that address ethical

principles, furnish a safe forum where purposeful discussions of ethical concerns can take place, and provide specific behavioral expectations (2021).

Solutions to problems in the workplace should consistently honor the uniqueness and value of each person and faithfully adhere to the general principles of ethics. This process requires us to critically examine our personal values, determine an ethically sound method of conflict resolution, even before conflict arises, and to create and sustain an institutional climate in which this can occur. We must enter professional relationships with attentiveness and skill. This chapter provides the opportunity to critically examine selected problems related to nurses' relationships within the healthcare delivery system.

PROBLEM SOLVING IN THE PROFESSIONAL REALM

Nurses face practical and ethical dilemmas in everyday nursing practice. Though many moral problems involve patients, nurses can encounter troubling moral questions related to other facets of work. There are layers of meanings, expectations, and relationships in the workplace. Each person has unique perspectives and values; each profession has certain values and expectations; each facility has explicit and implicit mandates; and each relationship has meaningful overtones of loyalty, power, and influence. These strata constitute a confusing, often contradictory arrangement. For example, you have a duty to your patient, yet the institutional budget may not provide the best equipment and staffing. You expect that others will respect your autonomy yet feel that you are unheard. You may be friendly with a colleague yet be concerned about his or her substance use. Professional relationship problems are often more troubling than problems directly involving patients but can nevertheless affect patient well-being. Therefore, workplace problems are important on the level of professional ethics and deserve serious exploration.

Nurses must try to anticipate problems with workplace relationships and devise strategies to prevent or deal with them when they occur, relying always on professional codes of nursing ethics. Although there is no absolute formula with which to solve conflicts, the following general guidelines can be helpful:

1. Maintain moral integrity
2. Clarify obligations
3. Determine the nature of the problem
4. Choose from alternative solutions thoughtfully

The following section includes a brief discussion of these steps as they specifically relate to professional relationships and the workplace.

Maintain Moral Integrity

Recall from Chapter 2 the discussion of moral integrity, which is perhaps a nurse's most important virtue. Moral integrity refers to a sound, whole, and integrated moral character. A person with integrity has a consistency of convictions, actions, and emotions. Integrity is compromised when the nurse acts inconsistently or in a way that is not supported by professed moral beliefs. Integrity ultimately leads to trustworthiness and the respect of others. Often doing the right thing boils down to listening to one's conscience and paying attention to personal values. Because the nursing profession expects nurses to accept personal responsibility, institutions should recognize and encourage moral integrity coupled with professional autonomy.

Reciprocal respect between the institution and nurse or the nurse and other professionals allows the nurse to act rationally, free from coercion or manipulation, and in ways that are consistent with personally held values and principles. In addition to enhancing professional relationships, nurses' integrity contributes to patient well-being. Gadow (1980) asserts that only nurses who act out of self-unity can truly assist patients in reaching decisions that express their complex totality as individuals. Integrity is required of us because the welfare of patients is our primary obligation.

Clarify Obligations

The terms *obligation* and *loyalty* have very different meanings but are often confused in day-to-day life. An obligation signifies a commitment to do something because of a moral rule, a duty, or some other binding demand. Loyalty refers to faithfulness to a person, an ideal, or a duty. Unlike obligation, loyalty is a choice, not a requirement. Obligations and loyalty generally occur together but may sometimes conflict.

Some obligations derive from a particular role or relationship. For example, parents have an obligation to feed and clothe their children. When you accept a position and a paycheck, you have an obligation to fulfill the requirements of your employer. However, even nurses who possess a high level of integrity experience conflicting obligations or loyalties on occasion. There is a certain mix of obligations and loyalty owed to any of the following: the patient, the employer, peers and other coworkers, physicians, the broader society, family, and self. Before workplace problems arise, you should articulate and thereafter consistently follow a morally derived hierarchy of obligation and loyalty. Keep personal moral values and professional ethics in mind as you examine to whom you owe primary and secondary obligations. Recognize that obligations may sometimes override some loyalties, such as loyalty to a friend or coworker.

Obligation to Patients

As a part of professional nursing practice, nurses' first obligation is to patients. Because nurses are professionals, we have a moral obligation to give priority to meeting the needs of our patients. All Western codes of nursing ethics are clear that the nurse's primary responsibility is to the patient. This obligation is nonnegotiable. By following established professional codes of ethics and maintaining integrity and duty to care for patients, we also fulfill related obligations to broader society, the profession, and ourselves.

In the midst of the COVID-19 pandemic, Rushton (2021) wrote about maintaining integrity in the face of unfathomable circumstances when nurses were facing a chasm between what they felt they ought to be doing and what they were actually doing. Rather than abandon their integrity or quit the profession altogether during the worst days of the pandemic, Rushton (2021) suggested that nurses must "accept the reality of what has happened without abandoning what matters most" (p. 68) by expanding the focus from individual patients to the needs of the larger society to bring about the greatest good for the greatest number of people. With this utilitarian ideal in mind, nurses were not being asked to abandon core values, but rather to "recalibrate our expectations, and perhaps to arrive at a new understanding of integrity within the current constraints" (p. 68). Rushton's suggestions offer a means to maintain integrity, even when circumstances are horrific.

Obligation to the Employer

Nurses have a second-order obligation to their employers. By accepting and maintaining terms of employment and payment for services, we have both a legal and moral obligation to the institution. This obligation, however strong, does not suggest that we should jeopardize personal integrity or subordinate loyalty to the patient. To succeed in the age of technological advancement, competition, and litigation, institutions desperately need the services of nurses who express the professional characteristics of autonomy, integrity, and ethically based practice.

CASE PRESENTATION

When Economy Replaces Excellence

Community Hospital is a large metropolitan hospital that boasted the reputation of maintaining excellent nursing care services for many years. Because of fierce competition and increasing financial strain, the hospital board of trustees decided to affiliate with a large hospital corporation. Television and radio advertisements describing the hospital corporation as having state-of-the-art equipment and services were far from reality. Immediately after the official affiliation was finalized, the hospital began dismissing nurses, cutting back supplies, eliminating unprofitable patient care services, and increasing patient charges. It was soon clear to nurses that patients would no longer receive the excellent nursing care that had been the hallmark of that hospital for many years. Nurses who remained on staff were faced with a changing environment that was no longer patient centered, discouraged autonomous nursing practice, and led to ethical and practical dilemmas directly caused by an explicit focus on profit. Many felt trapped because of a shrinking job market and years of investment in the hospital retirement program. They also felt powerless to change impersonal policies that were created by faceless bureaucrats hundreds of miles away.

Think About It

How Do Nurses Respond to Bottom-Line Economics?
- What kinds of dilemmas are likely to occur in this situation?
- Recognizing that a nurse's primary responsibility is to patients, how does the new hospital arrangement affect nurse–patient relationships?
- Can nursing practice maintain a patient-centered, ethically sensitive focus in this type of setting?
- What solutions can you suggest that will help solve potential problems faced by nurses at Community Hospital?
- How does the situation at Community Hospital differ from the circumstances that evolved during the worst of the COVID-19 pandemic?
- What implications for nurses do codes of nursing ethics from the ANA (2015b, Provisions 5.4 and 8.4) or the CNA (2017, Part B. 5 and Appendix B, p. 38), and the ICN (2021, Elements 1.9 and 3.7) have on the situations in Community Hospital and hospitals during the height of the COVID-19 pandemic?

Determine the Nature of the Problem

When a difficult situation arises, the nurse should clarify the nature of the problem. Is this a problem of a practical or ethical nature? Is this a problem of moral uncertainty, moral distress, moral dilemma, or moral outrage? It is important to know the answer to these questions because a problem that seems immense on an emotional level may be insignificant when the nurse considers the bigger picture. Ethical considerations should carry more weight than matters of self-interest—although, clearly, we owe some consideration to our own needs. For example, with changing patient demographics and increasing hospital bed vacancies, we are sometimes asked to "float" to unfamiliar settings. This practice redistributes the workload and offers the promise of improved nursing care. However, nurses frequently object to the prospect of being asked to float. Some nurses complain, "I've never worked there; I would be unsafe to practice in that setting!" These nurses are faced with a moral dilemma. Recall that the nurse has obligations to both ensure the welfare of the patient and meet the needs of the institution. The actions the nurse is expected to perform must be relatively certain to do good and do no harm. In that regard, neither the nurse, the patient, nor the institution will benefit from requiring a nurse to perform beyond his or her ability. To do so would be unethical. On the other hand, to leave a patient unit critically understaffed would also be unethical. When faced with situations of this sort, we should look to our codes of ethics for help. Regarding this particular situation, the nurse must either accept or reject role demands and assignments based on their educational preparation, knowledge, competence, and experience, taking into consideration their assessment of the level of risk to the patient (ANA, 2015b). Further, registered nurses have the "professional right to accept, reject or object in writing to any patient assignment that puts patients or themselves at serious risk of harm" (ANA, 2009). The position of the Canadian Nurses Association is the same as the ANA, adding that nurses remain with the patient until another nurse is available (CNA, 2017). It is clear that codes of ethics support nurses who recognize their own limitations.

Paradoxically, it could also be said that to refuse an assignment is unethical on a number of levels. Nurses must not abandon patients in need of care. If there is no one else available to care for the patients, we are obligated to give care, but only the type of care for which we are prepared and competent. For example, nurses temporarily assigned to specialty units can be asked to give basic, supportive nursing care, but should not be asked to perform technical tasks for which they are unprepared. To do so is both ethically wrong and legally risky. We should not refuse to accept assignments simply because we fear the unknown, or familiarity is comfortable, or for other self-interested reasons.

CASE PRESENTATION

Facing a Dilemma in the Newborn Nursery
Angela is an experienced registered nurse employed in the newborn nursery of a small rural hospital. The only registered nurse on the day shift in the nursery, she is scheduled to leave work at 3:00 p.m. This gives her time to get home and prepare for her son's wedding rehearsal dinner, which she is hosting at 7:00 p.m. By 4:00 p.m. the nurse from the next shift has not yet arrived. A licensed practical nurse (LPN) experienced in the newborn nursery is also on duty. Hospital policy requires the presence of a registered nurse (RN) in the unit at all times. There is no nursing supervisor on duty, and the hospital is otherwise short of staff. All the babies are quiet. Angela expects the evening-shift RN to arrive soon and feels the LPN can handle the nursery for a short time. Angela is torn between honoring her duty to the babies versus leaving for her son's rehearsal dinner.

Think About It
What Should the Nurse Do?
- Is this a practical or an ethical dilemma? What factors make this either a practical or an ethical dilemma?
- Do you think Angela's duty to stay outweighs her obligation to her family?
- What is the harm that could occur if she leaves before the evening-shift RN arrives?
- What is the harm that could occur if Angela misses the wedding rehearsal dinner?
- What specific guidance would a code of nursing ethics (ANA, CNA, or ICN) give Angela in this case?

The situation in the Case Presentation, *Facing a Dilemma in the Newborn Nursery*, constitutes a practical dilemma. Moral and nonmoral claims are in conflict. Based on the principles of beneficence, nonmaleficence, and fidelity, Angela has a moral obligation to the patients committed to her care and she also has an obligation to the institution. On the other hand, her family obligation is a powerful force since the occasion is fundamental to an important family life transition. Nevertheless, her family obligation is a matter of self-interest—it is not based on moral principles. There is the potential for harm to the newborns if she leaves the unit inappropriately staffed. An emergency could arise that the LPN is not prepared to handle. Possibly the evening-shift RN will not arrive at all. Based on a comparison of moral versus practical considerations and the potential harm that could result if Angela left the unit improperly attended, it is clear that she should not leave. This is not meant to imply that nurses should always subjugate personal needs to patient or institutional ones. Staying at work later than scheduled as a result of an occasional, unpredictable circumstance is one thing; being required to stay frequently is something entirely different.

Choose From Alternative Solutions Thoughtfully

Nurses encounter problems involving professional relationships on occasion. These problems present implicit layers of meanings, expectations, and relationships in the workplace. To solve professional relationship problems, nurses must choose solutions thoughtfully, keeping in mind overriding goals and anticipating the potential for good and harm that each alternative might produce. Ideal solutions will diminish harm, engender good, preserve the integrity of each person involved, and maintain positive relationships. Nurses should try to anticipate the long-term consequences of their actions, since some alternatives may seem attractive initially, yet lead to unintended and undesirable long-term effects.

NURSES' RELATIONSHIPS WITH INSTITUTIONS

We enter the workforce with very different perceptions than our employing institutions. Having learned that autonomy and accountability are valuable components of the nursing role, we understand that we owe primary loyalty to patients. We expect that our beliefs will be honored and that our opinions and knowledge will be respected. Hospitals and other healthcare facilities, on the other hand, tend to be sharply hierarchical and bureaucratic institutions that expect nurses' and other subordinates' primary loyalty to be toward the institution. Moreover, institutions expect nurses' actions to be directed toward attaining the goals of the system—goals that focus on ensuring the well-being of the institution itself and sustaining patterns of power and control. Difficulties emerge when there is a conflict between the goals of patient-centered nurses and the goals of the institution.

Problems arise, in part, because the institution's demands for loyalty are often inequitable. Though requiring employees to respond to certain requests, institutions rarely reciprocate with similar loyalty to nurses. For example, due to budget constraints, most institutions

are rigid about nurses' work hours. Nurses are expected to arrive ready to begin and complete work according to a set schedule. Nurses are sometimes directed to complete more work than can reasonably be done in the given amount of time. Nurses loyal to the institution and to the duty that they feel toward the patients in their care, are often willing to skip meals and breaks and complete work after "clocking out." In essence, these practices—though very stressful for nurses—are financially appealing to institutions (Jameton, 1984).

It becomes a real balancing act when nurses must consider personal commitments along with professional obligation and the ideal of compassionate service. The ANA *Code of Ethics for Nurses* (2015b) supports the nurse's professional role, which may include working overtime and attending meetings at one's own expense, to improve patient care or to establish and maintain conditions of employment conducive to high-quality nursing care. However, habitual self-sacrificing, altruistic behavior on the part of nurses is self-defeating and does not establish conditions of employment conducive to high-quality nursing care. It tends to support and perpetuate a flawed system: as long as nurses continue to work selflessly, the system (rather than the patient) benefits. Nurses willing to work for free devalue the work of all nurses and perpetuate the expectation that this type of one-sided self-sacrifice will continue. Of course, crisis situations can occur in any institution, but when nurses repeatedly accept workloads that are unreasonable, they become complicit in continuing the wrongs. On the surface, consistently working extra hours or assuming an unreasonable workload may appear to fulfill professional obligations and the ideal of compassionate service, yet ultimately it is harmful to nurses, the profession, and patients.

CASE PRESENTATION

When Patients Suffer From Lack of Nursing Care
Tim, an RN, works weekends on the skilled nursing unit of a small rural hospital. Recently purchased by a large corporation, the hospital was forced to dismiss nearly one-third of the staff of the skilled nursing unit. Lately, when Tim comes to work, he feels totally overwhelmed. Although he always considered himself efficient, Tim is distressed because he rarely has enough time to complete his work. He knows that many of the patients suffer because of lack of attention. Those who are bedfast are not turned on a regular schedule, they often wait for

assistance with eating until their food is cold, and medications are rarely given on time.

Suffering from expressive aphasia and hemiplegia secondary to a stroke, Mrs. Wallace was admitted to the skilled nursing unit after two weeks in the intensive care unit. After three weeks, her daughter, Helen, notices a large, reddened area surrounding a small gray ulcer over her mother's coccyx. Concerned, Helen asks Tim what caused this problem. Even though Mrs. Wallace's nursing care plan calls for frequent turning and sitting in a chair twice daily, Tim suspects that this was not consistently done the previous week. He determines that the reddened area is the beginning of a large pressure ulcer, a problem that might have been prevented with proper attention to activity and good nutrition. Tim hesitates to tell Helen that the problem is a potentially serious one that might have been prevented by good nursing care measures. He believes she has a right to know, but he is hesitant to implicate himself or the other nurses, and he is afraid that he will lose his job if he complains.

Think About It
How Do Nurses Make Decisions When Loyalties Conflict?
- What are the ethical principles implicit in this situation?
- What are Tim's conflicting loyalties?
- The staff on the unit is efficient and hardworking—often skipping lunch and staying overtime to complete their work. Do you believe the staff is responsible for the apparently poor nursing care that Mrs. Wallace is getting?
- Do you believe Tim should tell Helen the truth about the pressure sore?
- Should Tim risk losing his job by whistle-blowing?
- Is this an ethical or a practical dilemma?
- What would you do?

The Case Presentation, *When Patients Suffer from Lack of Nursing Care*, presents another example of a practical dilemma. The conflict that Tim is experiencing is between the principle of beneficence (the desire to do good for the patient) and a sense of loyalty to the institution or the other nurses with whom he works. There may also be an element of self-interest—Tim may not want to be implicated in the harm that the patients are experiencing as a result of the staff cutbacks. Tim's primary loyalty is owed to the patients—Mrs. Wallace, other patients suffering from the shortage of staff, and

future patients who could be harmed by perpetuation of the problem. There are strong arguments that he should act to correct the situation. He may choose to take any number of actions: He can work through the administrative hierarchy to improve staffing; he can answer Helen's questions honestly; and, if other solutions are unsuccessful, he can inform the media of the problems that were created by the drastic staffing shortages. In any case, if Tim fails to act to solve the problem, he will be complicit in its perpetuation and the subsequent harm to patients.

In some instances, nurses demonstrate **altruism** on misguided beliefs about duty. Altruism is a motivation for action which is displayed as a selfless concern for the well-being of others. Some nurses seem to believe that altruism is necessary to fulfill their duty to patients. Though many philosophers consider altruism and sacrifice a virtue, Ayn Rand (1966) suggested that altruism has a dehumanizing effect. Rand viewed a persistent willingness to sacrifice as flowing from poor self-esteem and inappropriate priority-setting. Moreover, she believed that those with poor self-esteem have difficulty valuing others. Because genuine regard is partially a product of sympathy (imagining oneself in the situation of another), according to Rand, one must value oneself to value others. This suggests that nurses who repeatedly sacrifice for the good of an institutional system fail to assume the power to change the wrongs that are committed.

Another example related to institutions' inequitable demands for loyalty is seen in the customary practice of requiring nurses to complete incident reports. To prevent litigation, institutions discourage nurses from talking to patients about medical or nursing errors. Hospitals much prefer nurses to file incident reports. Designed to meet institutional goals, incident reports are filed and kept for use in the event the hospital needs a legal defense, intends to fire or discipline workers, or reorganizes services to prevent future incidents (Jameton, 1984). Thus, patient-centered goals based on the principles of autonomy, fidelity, veracity, and respect for persons are subordinated to the institutional subgoals of employee control and risk management.

Nurses' loyalty to the institution is an important mode of control. Without loyalty, administrators cannot manage institutions. For this reason, supervisors and administrators sometimes react negatively when nurses support and cooperate with each other to make changes.

The ensuing perception of nonsupportive supervisors is a contributing factor for job stress and dissatisfaction. In the end, this can be harmful to nurses and patients alike because it can interfere with nurses' expressions of loyalty to patients.

NURSES' RELATIONSHIPS WITH OTHER NURSES

Nurses work together in close proximity day in and day out. No other profession is so intimately connected with the essence of life. The knowledge gained from the intimate experiences of birth, illness, life, and death are both powerful and mysterious. Nurses are connected to each other and set apart from others—connected by common experience, language, and knowledge and set apart through professional mystique. Nurses work together closely, identify with each other, and supervise or are supervised by other nurses. The practice of one affects that of others.

Loyalty among nurses is a natural product of long-term acquaintance and close working relationships. Some view loyalty among members as a distinguishing characteristic of a profession. Loyalty is a social, interpersonal phenomenon in which a person chooses devotion to another person. People who are loyal show sympathy and care toward those to whom they are loyal. Loyalty unites people together in their service. It is freely given, not coerced. Loyalty is actively practiced by words and deeds. People who are loyal keep promises and sacrifice personal interests to the relationship. They share common goals.

In most practical matters, loyalty is a productive virtue. It enhances unity, strength, and power. Facing bureaucratic, economic, and political forces, nurses' loyalty to each other and to the profession adds strength to the call for improved patient care, public welfare, nursing autonomy, and optimum employment conditions.

Though normally viewed as admirable, loyalty is seldom regarded as a virtue because there is a potential for misplaced loyalty, fanaticism, and blind injustice. Misguided or fanatical loyalty can lead to a confused sense of obligation. Though nurses' primary obligation is to patients, those who are overly loyal to other nurses might act in ways that harm patients. For example, a nurse who is loyal to a coworker might pretend not to see the coworker's incompetent practice, illegal drug use, or other actions that have the potential to harm patients. For this reason, nurses must maintain objectivity in balancing loyalty to other nurses against the obligation owed to patients.

CASE PRESENTATION

Nurses' Loyalty to the Profession
Several years ago, politically active nurses in a small state lobbied for a bill mandating nurse representation in government bodies that regulated healthcare facilities and services. Positions included membership on committees, task forces, advisory panels, and so forth. The bill included a stipulation that every public hospital should include one nurse on its governing board. As the largest group of healthcare professionals, nurses believed their knowledge and experience would be a welcome addition. Though there was confident and unified nursing support, the bill was fiercely opposed by both the state hospital association and individual hospitals. When public hearings were held, nurses in favor of the bill were surprised that commanding and articulate nurse administrators testified against the bill. Representing individual hospitals, nurse administrators cited nurses' ignorance of healthcare finance and a gossipy tendency to spill industry secrets as reasons to defeat the bill.

Think About It
Examining Differences in Loyalty
- Can you think of a moral justification for the diverse positions of nurses?
- To whom is each group of nurses loyal?
- How would you characterize each group's stance in relation to the professionalization of nursing?
- What accounts for the diverse positions of the nurses?

NURSES' RELATIONSHIPS WITH PHYSICIANS

The work of nurses and physicians should be complementary, synergistic, and productive. Because both professions' primary goal is to improve patient health, one would expect a sense of collegiality and collaboration between them. A positive nurse–physician relationship is rewarding and productive for both the nurse and physician, and patient care is improved. Studies have shown that good nurse–physician relationships lower overall patient mortality, lower transfers to critical care, decrease patients' length of stay, decrease overall healthcare costs, and increase satisfaction among nurses and physicians (Schmalenberg & Kramer, 2009). When there is conflict between nurses and physicians, the relationship is stressful and damaging to nurses, physicians, and patients alike.

Nurse–physician relationships have historically reflected the prevailing gender roles in society. These roles were well defined for centuries. The traditional nurse was expected to obey the physician, much as the wife was expected to obey her husband. Physicians demanded obedience, and nurses hesitated to disagree with physicians, even if there was good reason to do so. The good news is that times are changing. Today, the vast majority of nurse–physician relationships are positive. In two large multisite studies, researchers explored nurses' perceptions of nurse–physician relationships. Five types of relationships were identified: collegial, collaborative, student–teacher, friendly stranger, and hostile/adversarial (Schmalenberg & Kramer, 2009). When describing collegial relationships, nurses and physicians use words like *peers* and *equals*. The collegial relationship entails equal trust, power, and respect. Collaborative relationships include mutual (rather than equal) trust, power, respect, and cooperation. In the student–teacher relationship, either the nurse or the physician can be the student. In the friendly stranger relationship, information is exchanged formally, but there is a neutral tone. The only negative relationship, hostile/adversarial, is marked by anger, verbal abuse, and real or implied threats (Schmalenberg & Kramer, 2009). Nurses reported that only a very small percentage of relationships fall into the hostile/adversarial type. Although hostile/adversarial relationships are relatively rare, they do matter.

Given the bureaucratic nature of most healthcare institutions, particularly hospitals, the hierarchical relationship between physicians and nurses is complex and peculiar. Most hospitals require nurses to implement physicians' orders. Nevertheless, nurses are autonomous professionals. Nursing autonomy does not suggest that the nurse is in charge of all aspects of patient care, but rather that the nurse must use independent judgment and advocate for patients in all instances. Questioning a physician or refusing to carry out an order or administer a medication that will harm a patient is the duty of the autonomous nurse. The outdated tradition of the nurse who blindly obeys the physician conflicts with the concept of the autonomous nurse who thinks independently and rationally.

Because relationships evolve over time, the nurse can develop strategies to nurture positive nurse–physician relationships. Strategies should be geared toward creating mutual respect and trust. Following are five strategies that will help the nurse cultivate long-term positive relationships with physicians:

- Practice with skill. Physicians are more likely to show respect and remember nurses who demonstrate knowledge and skill. Most physicians understand that excellent nurses are an asset to their own practice.
- Communicate clearly. Physicians respond to communication that is well articulated, important, organized, clear, concise, complete, and based upon objective data.
- Project confidence. Nurses command respect when they project a sense of confidence, grounded in self-assured knowledge.
- Avoid negative behaviors. Negative behavior such as angry outbursts, sniping, blaming, and complaining are unprofessional and counterproductive and will erode physicians' respect.
- Reciprocate respect. Reciprocal relationships engender a spirit of cooperation and interdependence (Fig. 9.1).

Most nurse–physician interactions are productive, but sometimes that is not the case. On occasion, a nurse must question the appropriateness of a physician's order. The nurse must remember that the primary obligation is owed to the patient, not the physician. As autonomous practitioners, nurses have the knowledge and experience and the legal and ethical responsibility to make independent judgments, even when carrying out physicians' orders. If medical care constitutes incompetent, unethical, or illegal practice, the nurse is clearly obligated to disobey orders (ANA, 2015b). When deciding what course to take in situations in which nurses disagree with physicians' orders, nurses can apply the test of urgency. Low-urgency problems are minor and may be solved at a leisurely pace. With low-urgency problems, there is little risk of serious harm, or there is significant time available to examine all aspects of the situation. Very urgent problems require quick solutions and immediate actions. High-urgency situations consist of emergencies in which lifesaving actions must be carried out quickly. Nurses may have time to discuss and negotiate satisfactory solutions to problems at the low-urgency end of the spectrum, but problems at the high-urgency end of the spectrum require immediate, sometimes drastic action.

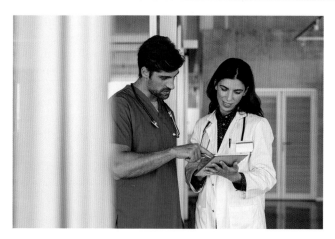

Fig. 9.1 The Work of Nurses and Physicians Should be Complementary, Synergistic, and Productive. (iStock photo ID: 655821120.)

CASE PRESENTATION

Making a Decision in an Urgent Situation

Marta, a night-shift charge nurse in the emergency department, is well liked among staff and hospital leadership and has been noted for her expertise. She has advanced certification and 25 years of experience. Marta works well with other members of the emergency room staff and is comfortable and efficient in situations of extreme urgency. The emergency department is usually staffed by board-certified emergency physicians. But recently physicians with various degrees of preparation and ability have been assigned to the department, particularly on the night shift. During an unusually busy shift, an ambulance arrives with a middle-aged man having severe chest pain and dyspnea. His condition quickly deteriorates, and after a few minutes, he experiences respiratory arrest. The physician on duty, Dr. Andrews, is a first-year family practice resident physician moonlighting in the emergency room after his regular shift at a local community health center. Dr. Andrews seems nervous and hesitant. During the first phase of the "code," Dr. Andrews seems uncertain of every detail. As the nurse in charge, Marta begins instituting a seldom-used protocol that was developed for use in the event that the nurses are faced with a respiratory or cardiac arrest when no physician is present. All the nurses are advanced cardiac life support certified and trained in intubation techniques. It quickly becomes apparent that the patient needs to be intubated, but hospital policy requires that a physician, not a nurse, intubate patients.

Marta asks Dr. Andrews to intubate the patient. After several clumsy attempts, Dr. Andrews angrily orders Marta to call an anesthesiologist at home to come and intubate the patient. Marta has been trained to intubate and realizes that the patient's chances of survival are very low if he is not intubated quickly. She asks the unit clerk to call the anesthesiologist. Over Dr. Andrews's angry objections, Marta picks up the laryngoscope and intubates the patient quickly and successfully. Although the patient responds to resuscitation attempts and is discharged five days later, Dr. Andrews complains to the nursing administrator that Marta was insubordinate during the resuscitation.

Think About It

Was Marta's Decision Correct?

- What is your immediate response to the situation in which Marta finds herself?
- Where would you place this situation on the "spectrum of urgency"?
- What are the arguments in favor of Marta's actions?
- What are the arguments in favor of Marta following Dr. Andrews' orders?
- Do you consider Marta's actions to be based on ethical principles?
- Did Marta place herself at risk of reprisal or legal action?
- Would you define Dr. Andrews' behavior as bullying?
- Which of Marta's characteristics make her a target for bullying?

Nurses must make thoughtful, fair, and knowledgeable decisions in relation to physicians' orders, while also being careful to consider the overall harm that can result from any given action. Recognizing that the physician's goal, like that of the nurse, is the welfare of the patient, nurses must be mature and objective when questioning orders. Nurses have an ethical obligation to protect the patient from medical incompetence. Nevertheless, they must be careful, keeping in mind the overall harm that can result from the practice of constantly and inappropriately questioning insignificant aspects of physicians' orders.

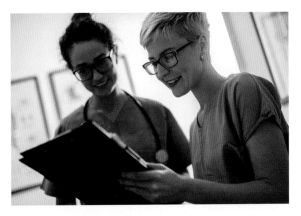

Fig. 9.2 Good Nurse Leaders Inspire and Motivate Others. (iStock photo ID: 912401464.)

NURSES' RELATIONSHIPS WITH SUBORDINATES

As the coordinator of patient care, the professional nurse is morally and legally accountable for the quality of nursing care rendered to patients. This accountability includes supervision, delegation of nursing care functions, and disciplining of other healthcare providers. The inherent practical, moral, and legal implications of these functions are facets of the role of the professional nurse that must be undertaken with sensitivity and respect. Nurses must be sensitive to those who work beside them, recognizing that each person is a moral agent, worthy of dignity and respect.

Most nurses are leaders. They may be informal leaders of a small number of assistive personnel, or they may be leaders of large organizations. The actions of a leader send value messages. The quality of a nurse's leadership is reflected in the quality of the work of subordinates. Good leaders are those who inspire, motivate, and pay attention to individuals. They inspire others to work toward a common goal. Poor leaders may be abusive bullies who degrade, ridicule, and otherwise terrorize; or they may be passive and ineffective to the point that problems become so serious that they demand attention and invite bullying among coworkers. Because nurses work toward the goal of improving patients' health, the quality of nurses' leadership carries moral weight (Fig. 9.2).

Delegating

The structure of healthcare delivery in some institutional settings makes the professional nurse responsible for delegating a number of nursing functions to subordinate staff members. **Delegation** occurs when a nurse assigns the responsibilities of certain nursing duties to another person. The nurse has a moral obligation to

ensure that each patient receives proper nursing care, to respect the value of each individual, and to make sure the situation is conducive to high-quality nursing care. As the coordinator of patient care, the nurse is accountable for all nursing care that patients receive, whether from the nurse or subordinates. The ANA *Code of Ethics for Nurses* specifies that delegation of nursing tasks is a role function that nurses must take very seriously. According to a joint statement by the ANA and the National Council of State Boards of Nursing (2015), the nurse is accountable to determine the appropriate utilization of nursing and assistive staff involved in providing direct patient care. The nurse may delegate certain components of care but cannot delegate the higher functions of nursing such as assessment, planning, evaluation, and nursing judgment. When deciding whether to delegate, the nurse must use well-informed judgment. The nurse must assess the other worker's competence, knowledge, and skill, taking into consideration the person's training and experience, and determine the appropriate tasks to be delegated and the degree of supervision that will be needed. When delegating tasks, the nurse's communication must be clear, concise, and complete, and the nurse must give assistive personnel the opportunity to ask questions and clarify expectations (ANA & National Council of State Boards of Nursing, 2015).

Disciplining

In addition to delegation, the supervisory role of professional nurses occasionally includes disciplining subordinates. In the workplace, *disciplining* means to punish or reprimand a subordinate with the intention of correcting or altering their subsequent behavior. Disciplining is a difficult task that must be done with insight, respect, compassion, and logic. The nurse must be keenly aware of the effect of disciplinary action on others and must focus on the intended goal. The traditional methods of discipline, such as punishment and chastisement, are damaging to the spirit and counterproductive in practice. A nurse manager's method of disciplining may set the tone for the entire nursing unit. Discussing poor leadership, Dilley (2000, p. 9) wrote, "Nurse managers from hell can be easily identified. They use coercion—as in, 'do as I say, or you'll find yourself on the night shift.' They belittle their employees in front of patients or other staff. They communicate by memo rather than face-to-face. They change policies without input from others. They are rude and thoughtless." It has been our experience that nurse managers "from hell" do exist, but are rare—most nurses are good leaders.

A good nurse leader will set the tone of the unit through the style of discipline. The great teacher Maria Montessori wrote, "Our aim is to discipline for activity, for work, for good; not for immobility, not for passivity, not for obedience" (Montessori, 1912, p. 93). Leah Curtin (1996) suggested that the most meaningful method is through encouraging self-discipline, which corrects the problem, strengthens the character of the worker, and improves performance. This process is possible only if the person knows the rules, understands their purpose, and agrees that they deserve compliance. To achieve this result, the nurse must model the expected standard daily and have a few rules—all of which are applied consistently, change infrequently, and apply to all personnel equally. The nurse has a moral obligation, to both patients and personnel, to uphold rules that protect the health or safety of patients, other employees, the institution, and self.

VIOLENCE IN THE WORKPLACE: INCIVILITY AND BULLYING

The incidence of violence in the healthcare workplace, demonstrated through incivility and bullying, is rising. *Incivility* is a term for damaging social behavior. Incivility, which may be unintentional, consists of rude, inconsiderate, discourteous, disrespectful, impolite, and offensive actions such as gossiping, spreading rumors, eye-rolling, refusing to assist a coworker, name calling, using a condescending tone, or publicly criticizing others. *Bullying* is more frequent and intense than incivility.

The term *bullying* refers to more fierce and intentional repeated "health-harming" mistreatment that can take the form of verbal abuse; behaviors perceived as threatening, intimidating, or humiliating; repeated abuse of power that reveals itself in actions intended to humiliate, offend, and cause distress; character assassination; or work sabotage (ANA, 2015a; Workplace Bullying Institute, 2021). Bullying occurs in every workplace. It occurs in clinical settings, in the policy arena, and in educational settings. It occurs between coworkers, students, and staff nurses, or between leaders and subordinates, or faculty and students. Examples of bullying actions include threats, taunts, hostile remarks, persistent criticism, verbal attacks, work sabotage, scapegoating, ostracism, and intimidation (Sharma et al., 2021; Workplace Bullying Institute, 2021). Incivility and bullying have been studied and extensively reported among nurses around the globe.

Incivility and bullying can either be horizontal or lateral. **Horizontal violence** can occur top down in which supervisors, professors, and so forth address harmful actions such as oppressive supervision, constant criticism, or unrealistic demands toward those who report to them. A 2021 survey found that 65 percent of bullying occurs from the top down (Workplace Bullying Institute, 2022). Horizontal violence can also occur from bottom up in which workers or students bully or are uncivil to those who supervise or teach them through such as actions as public criticism, social media bashing, overt rudeness, and threatening or vindictive remarks. Fourteen percent of bullying reported in 2021 was from the bottom up (Workplace Bullying Institute, 2022). **Lateral violence**, on the other hand, occurs when a person is uncivil to or bullies another person who is otherwise an equal (ANA, 2015a). Common workplace violence includes nonverbal innuendo, verbal affront, undermining, withholding information, scapegoating, backstabbing, breaking confidences, gossip, putdowns, blaming, impatience, angry outbursts, condescending language, and aggressive competitiveness. Unfortunately, incivility and bullying are common in the workplace and in schools of nursing. Often directed toward new, inexperienced nurses and nursing students, incivility warrants attention because of its prevalence in the nursing workplace and its potential to lead to serious consequences.

The consequences of incivility are immense, including physical and psychological effects on victims, decreased productivity, threats to patient safety, and loss of nurses from the workforce. Uncivil behavior and bullying make the recipient feel upset, threatened, humiliated, or vulnerable. This harms the person's sense of self-worth and undermines self-confidence. Nurses who have experienced incivility or bullying in the workplace complain of physical symptoms such as headaches, tachycardia, gastrointestinal problems, sleep disturbances, fatigue, increased blood pressure, and anorexia. Psychological consequences include heightened levels of stress, sleep disorders, loss of libido, fear, depression, sadness, anxiety, nervousness, irritability, mistrust, suicide ideation, and suicide (ANA, 2015a; Goh et al., 2022; Vessey et al., 2010). As a result of the physical and psychological consequences of bullying, nurses who are victims are more likely to report being sick than those who are not affected by workplace bullying. However, the effects of incivility extend beyond individual nurses.

CASE PRESENTATION

Incivility in the Classroom

Mary Dupont is a 55-year-old, PhD-prepared professor of nursing. She has practiced nursing part-time and taught simultaneously for 25 years and is considered an international expert in pediatric nursing education. Professor Dupont has conducted research, contributed chapters to pediatric nursing textbooks, and received university awards for teaching excellence. Heather is a 23-year-old nursing student enrolled in Professor Dupont's pediatrics course. Heather is inattentive, unprepared, and often late to class. She openly makes rude, disrespectful, and sarcastic comments toward her teacher. Professor Dupont learns that Heather maintains a social media page for nursing students. The page is private, but another student tells the professor that Heather's comments are very critical of her and the school. When Heather makes a C grade on the midterm examination, she rudely challenges Professor Dupont about every question in front of other students. Even though other students in the class are motivated and pleasant, interactions with Heather take a toll on Professor Dupont.

Think About It

- Do you consider nursing students to be part of the profession of nursing? If so, how do Heather's actions reflect on the profession?
- Can you predict how Heather will interact with coworkers, physicians, and patients when she becomes a nurse?
- Is Heather's behavior an example of horizontal or lateral violence?
- What is Professor Dupont's best response to Heather's behavior?

Who are the targets of bullies? Although they do target those they dislike because of differences or vulnerabilities, adult bullies are more likely to target people who make them feel insecure or threatened. They want to eliminate their competition or make their own work seem better than the work of others, so they target people who are good at their jobs—those who impress coworkers and leaders. Especially if they are unpopular, bullies target social people who are popular and well liked. Bullies also target coworkers or subordinates with high moral integrity and those with new and independent ideas (The Bully Project, n.d.; Workplace Bullying Institute, 2021). The goal is to tear down the reputation of others to heighten their own reputation.

Bullying disrupts the critical components of nursing work, including communication, the exchange of crucial health information, and collaborative decision making. Nurses who experience bullying have poor morale, decreased productivity, increased errors, impaired clinical judgment, and significantly lower levels of job satisfaction. They may avoid or delay effective communication, experience poor concentration, which prevents them from providing safe and effective care, fail to raise safety concerns, and begin to demonstrate bullying behaviors themselves (Hutchinson & Jackson, 2013). Many nurses who are bullied leave work complaining of illness, and others leave the workforce altogether. This affects the healthcare economy because the cost of registered nurse turnover has a profound effect on the already diminishing hospital profit margin, particularly since the beginning of the pandemic with nurses resigning at a significantly increased rate (Advisory Board, October 17, 2022). The cost to a hospital when one registered nurse leaves averages $40,000. The average hospital loses over seven million dollars every year replacing and retraining nurses who have left their jobs (Nursing Solutions, 2022). The high cost to the individual, profession, and healthcare industry calls for solutions to the problem.

The ethical implications of workplace bullying on patient care are immense since nurses are expected to do good and avoid harm. Nurses who report that they have been bullied are less likely to report that they provide good or excellent quality of nursing care (Pogue et al., 2022). Creating a barrier to effective communication, bullying is associated with increased errors and poorer patient outcomes (ANA, 2015a; Vessey et al., 2010). Indirect outcomes that occur when nurses are bullied include patient falls, treatment or medication errors, increased patient mortality, surgical errors, and delayed care (Goh et al., 2022). In addition, public displays of workplace bullying have the potential to erode patients' confidence in nurses, decrease patient satisfaction, and increase nurses' hostile behaviors toward patients (Hutchinson & Jackson, 2013).

Prevention or elimination of violence in the workplace requires multi-faceted solutions and dedicated leaders but is the responsibility of all involved. The ANA's *Code of Ethics for Nurses with Interpretive Statements* states that nurses are required to "create an ethical environment and culture of civility and kindness, treating colleagues, coworkers, employees, students, and others with dignity and respect" (2015b, p. 4). Codes of ethics and position statements from the ICN and CNA also consider bullying and workplace violence a matter of ethics (CNA, 2017, Parts A.13 and F.5; CNA & CFNU, 2008; ICN, 2021, pp. 14, 17). In addition to condemning workplace violence, the CNA enjoins nurses to "take action to minimize risk and to protect others and themselves" when violence cannot be anticipated or prevented (CNA, 2017, p. 9). So the fight against bullying is an ethical imperative that requires action. Promoting a positive workplace culture with authentic leaders is a key to eliminating bullying. Authentic leadership significantly reduces workplace bullying (Trépanier et al., 2016). Authentic leaders as those who are self-assured and self-aware, reveal their genuine selves to subordinates, analyze information objectively, recognize their own internal values, and purposely offer themselves as role models when their actions are consistent with both personal and professional values.

The best way to avoid bullying in the workplace is to prevent it from happening. Primary prevention strategies include individual nurses becoming familiar with their employer's incivility and bullying prevention policies, professional and institutional codes of conduct, and nursing codes of ethics. Nurses must engender trust and commit to promoting positive interpersonal relationships with each other and with other members of the healthcare team. In addition, nurses should anticipate bullying behaviors and practice responses to deflect incivility and bullying when they occur. Above all, nurses should demonstrate professional behavior by treating others with respect, using clear communication, being sensitive to how words and actions affect others, avoiding gossip, offering assistance when needed, demonstrating openness to other points of view, and mentoring others (ANA, 2015a). If bullying does occur, nurses should create a detailed written account of the incident and report the event as soon as possible. A nurse who observes bullying or incivility should provide support to the colleague who was the target. Support can take the form of acknowledging that the behavior was unprofessional and inappropriate or assisting the victim to report the event (ANA, 2015a).

Improving leadership is a key to reducing bullying in the workplace. Whereas autocratic, nonsupportive, and disengaged leadership increases bullying behaviors in the workplace, positive leadership promotes a climate of trust, congenial professional relationships, and reduced workplace bullying (Karatuna et al., 2020). What can leaders do to curb workplace bullying? They should be encouraged to recognize the signs of horizontal or lateral violence in the workplace and institute education programs and strategies to reduce bullying. Organizations should eliminate behaviors such as finger-pointing, which can itself be a bullying behavior, and view mistakes as opportunities for learning and improvement. Because significant bullying is perpetrated by poor nursing leaders, heightened awareness of the problem through leadership education and training is essential. Education should focus on increasing trust and developing authentic leadership. Specific strategies to avoid or eliminate bullying in the workplace have been suggested by the ANA (2015a) and other organizations and include the following:

- Maintaining open lines of communication
- Taking all reports of bullying seriously
- Creating and enforcing formal zero-tolerance policies
- Being aware of potential targets of bullying
- Holding everyone accountable for reporting bullying
- Leading by example
- Implementing training including improved communication skills and recognition of bullying behavior
- Engendering respect among staff and leadership

Leadership sets the standards for behavior, but the responsibility to stop bullying in the workplace rests on the shoulders of all nurses.

DISCRIMINATION IN THE WORKPLACE

Discrimination is a well-documented problem in the workplace. Discrimination is defined as unjust prejudicial treatment of a person or group, especially based on personal characteristics such as race, gender, sexual orientation, disabilities, or other traits. Psychological and physical health are affected when people believe they have been victims of discrimination or harassment in the workplace. Victims of discrimination experience psychological distress, depression, loneliness, low self-esteem, and anxiety (Kim, 2015; Obrien et al., 2016). They are more likely to report higher levels of poor health days, perceived poor health, lifetime disease, weight gain, and generally poorer health (Anderson, 2013; Kim, 2015). The impact of discrimination on physical and mental health also affects the workplace. Those who perceive that they are discriminated against withdraw from the organization and have decreased organizational commitment. Their productivity is lower, their performance is comparatively poor, and their turnover rate is high—thus creating a self-perpetuating downward spiral. The effects of discrimination begin at the individual level and cascade through the organization and society.

Because discrimination is harmful, it is a violation of ethical principles, professional values, and federal law. Discrimination violates several principles of ethics but particularly the principle of justice. Justice requires that resources, benefits, rewards, opportunities, and so forth are fairly distributed. Discrimination violates this principle because it excludes certain groups of people from benefits available to other groups. Discrimination also violates professional values. Most professional nursing organizations have explicit statements in opposition to discrimination. Because the effects can be egregious, discrimination is also legally prohibited in the United States. The Bill of Rights of the US Constitution (U.S. Const. Amend. I_X), the Civil Rights Act of 1964, the Americans with Disabilities Act of 1990 (ADA), and the Civil Rights Act of 1991 provide legal protection against discrimination in the workplace.

As the professional organization of nursing in the United States, the ANA condemns discrimination in all forms, stating that "discriminatory practices must not be tolerated and must be immediately addressed" (ANA Center for Ethics and Human Rights, 2018, p. 1). Recommendations for combatting discrimination, include personal introspection and resolution of conflicts between personal and professional values surrounding mutual respect, civility, and inclusiveness. Citing a need for mutual respect, caring, justice, inclusiveness, and diversity, the ANA recommends that

nurses advocate for each organization to adopt aggressive policies that contribute to human rights for all employees, patients, and others within the community to combat discrimination (ANA Center for Ethics and Human Rights, 2018).

Millions of Americans have experienced employment discrimination. Recent literature points to evidence of continuing discrimination in nursing related to gender, age, race, disability, and sexual orientation. The US Equal Employment Opportunity Commission (EEOC) enforces federal laws that make it illegal to discriminate against an employee or job applicant because of the person's race, color, religion, sex (including pregnancy, gender identity, and sexual orientation), national origin, age, disability, or genetic information. The EEOC also considers it illegal to retaliate against a person who complained about discrimination, filed a charge of discrimination, or participated in an investigation or lawsuit pertaining to employment discrimination (EEOC, n.d.-b). Retaliation is the most frequent discrimination claim, followed in descending order of frequency by disability, race, sex, age, national origin, color, and religion (EEOC, 2022).

Racial Discrimination

The Civil Rights Act of 1964 made it unlawful for an employer to fail or refuse to hire or to discharge any individual, or to otherwise discriminate against any individual, because of the person's race, color, religion, sex, or national origin. Unlawful acts include discrimination in terms of compensation or payment, conditions of employment, or privileges of employment. Considered one of America's strongest civil rights laws, the Civil Rights Act of 1964 primarily protects the rights of African Americans and other minorities. Attempting to correct a long tradition of racial discrimination, this act ensures that minorities receive fair and equal treatment from the government, other persons, and private groups, including schools and employers. It also specifically forbids discrimination within any program that receives money from the federal government. The act is enforced by the EEOC.

The Civil Rights Act of 1964 enjoins employers to provide equal employment opportunities to individuals from the initial recruitment or application process through termination of employment. When considering claims of discriminatory practices, the legal system looks at two discriminatory outcomes: disparate treatment and disparate impact. **Disparate treatment** occurs when an individual is treated differently by a superior or by organizational policy. For example, if a supervisor passes over all Hispanic nurses who apply for promotion, regardless of their qualifications or abilities, disparate treatment exists. Workplace bullying can signify a type of discrimination. For example, among school nurses, minorities are bullied at a higher rate than White nurses (Sharma et al., 2021) and Hispanics are bullied significantly more often than other groups (Workplace Bullying Institute, 2022). **Disparate impact** occurs when employers unintentionally, but consistently apply policies that appear to be fair to all employees but actually adversely affect one group. For example, 346 men received a five million dollars settlement in a disparate impact claim. The men were denied medical and dental insurance coverage for their children because of a former requirement that children of employees and pensioners live with them full time (EEOC, 2001). Denial of coverage for these men was considered disparate impact because the court found that certain social and ethnic groups are less likely to have intact families living together in one home.

Nursing codes of ethics identify racial discrimination as an ethical issue. Racism is prohibited by all. The ANA is active in identifying and eradicating racism in the profession. For many years, the American Nurses Association recognized progress that has been made in reducing discrimination related to race, gender, and socioeconomic status, including improving access to quality health care (ANA Center for Ethics and Human Rights, 2018). To further clarify their position, in 2022 the ANA Center for Ethics and Human Rights released a position statement entitled *The Nurse's Role and Responsibility in Unveiling and Dismantling Racism in Nursing*. The purpose of the position statement was twofold: (1) to publicly address the nursing profession's historic complicity in White ethnocentrism and racially unjust systems and (2) to recommend strategies aimed toward social justice. We encourage all nurses to read the position statement, particularly the recommendations, which are condensed and paraphrased as follows:

All nurses must:

- Intentionally educate themselves about the history of racism and its role in perpetuating health disparities.
- Move beyond a focus on patient behaviors regarding established interventions and attend to socially constructed disparities experienced and propagated by the nursing profession.
- Take action when any level of aggression is witnessed or experienced.
- Avoid terms such as *noncompliant* when patients are experiencing disproportionate suffering.
- Recognize that identifying people or groups by their race leads to inequality in healthcare access and treatment and affects outcomes.
- Engage in learning about the profession's history of racist practices and begin the process of unlearning practices that sustain inequality and harm (ANA Center for Ethics and Human Rights, 2022).

Like the ANA, the CNA condemns racism in nursing. Recognizing that Black, Indigenous, and other people of color have been subjected to racism since the inception of Canada, CNA acknowledges the impact of anti-Black racism on Black Canadians. This sentiment extends to nursing itself since prospective Black students were refused admission into nursing schools until the 1940s. The purpose of CNA's position statement on racism is to call on nurses to participate in individual and systemic action to "de-colonize the nursing profession and ensure the profession can continue to provide safe, compassionate and ethical care to Black and racialized clients and communities" (CNA, 2020).

Discrimination Against Persons With Disabilities

The Americans with Disabilities Act of 1990 (ADA) was signed into law on July 26, 1990. Considered the most significant piece of legislation since the Civil Rights Act of 1964, this act provides comprehensive protection to Americans with disabilities. The aim of Congress in drafting this legislation was to ensure equality for the disabled without creating undue hardships for employers (Americans with Disabilities Act of 1990). The ADA recognizes a covered disability if there is a record of physical or mental disability that causes an impairment substantially limiting one or more of the major life enjoyments of the person and if the person actually has such an impairment. Major life enjoyments include activities that the average person can perform with little or no difficulty, such as caring for oneself, performing manual tasks, walking, seeing, hearing, speaking, learning, and working. A physical impairment includes any physiological disorder or condition, cosmetic disfigurement, or anatomic loss affecting any body system. A mental impairment includes any mental or psychological disorder, such as mental retardation, organic brain syndrome, emotional or mental illness, and learning disabilities. Mental or psychological conditions that result from such conditions as diabetes, cancer, AIDS, alcoholism, and drug abuse qualify under this definition.

Related to the Civil Rights Act of 1964, the ADA has several provisions. The act ensures that people with disabilities are not excluded from job opportunities or adversely affected in other aspects of employment unless they are unqualified or unable to perform the job. This protection extends to application, salary, promotion, discharge, transfer, and all other aspects of work. The ADA prohibits employers from requiring medical examinations before employment except for drug testing, which may be performed. Medical examinations may be done only after a job offer has been extended. Employers may question individuals about their educational qualifications, experience, and ability to perform the job safely with or without accommodation. To avoid the suggestion of discrimination, the prospective employer may not ask questions about disabilities, past medical problems, or previous workers' compensation claims. Upon request from employees with disabilities, employers must make necessary physical accommodations to the workplace, such as wheelchair accessibility, telephone systems for the hearing impaired, and so forth, but may be exempted from hiring persons with disabilities if the necessary accommodations cause undue hardship because they are extremely expensive or difficult to implement. Undue hardship is based on cost, number of employees, and the type of business (Americans with Disabilities Act of 1990). The ADA does not require employers to hire individuals with disabilities. It demands, however, that employers base employment decisions solely on job qualifications and ability, without regard to physical or mental disabilities. It also protects employers from financial ruin in the case of undue hardship related to making workplace accommodations for persons with disabilities.

SEXUAL HARASSMENT AND DISCRIMINATION

Sexual harassment is a widespread problem for which the WHO has developed a worldwide initiative proposing that sexual exploitation, abuse, and harassment violate the dictum to do no harm and to protect the vulnerable (WHO, n.d.). The EEOC defines sexual harassment as unwelcome sexual advances, requests for sexual favors, and other verbal or physical conduct of a sexual nature that makes a person feel offended, humiliated, and/or intimidated (Fig. 9.3). No current studies have determined the prevalence of sexual harassment and discrimination against nurses in the United States; however, international studies suggest the problem occurs to 13 percent of all nurses (Lu et al., 2020). Sexual harassment is a form of sex discrimination that violates the Civil Rights Act of 1964. Sexual harassment is illegal when it is so severe and frequent that it affects an individual's employment; interferes with work performance; or creates an intimidating, hostile, or offensive environment in the workplace (EEOC, n.d.-c). Recognizing sexual harassment as a significant problem, federal and state courts have struggled with the issue for the past several decades. The problem was brought to the attention of the public with the highly publicized Senate confirmation hearings of Supreme

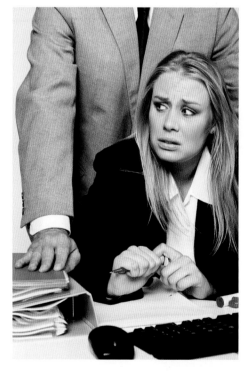

Fig. 9.3 Sexual Harassment Is Unwelcome Conduct of a Sexual Nature That Makes a Person Feel Offended, Humiliated and/or Intimidated. (iStock photo ID: 168639331.)

Court nominee Clarence Thomas. As a direct result of these hearings, the Civil Rights Act of 1991 was signed into law on November 21, 1991.

Sexual harassment can occur in many different circumstances; however, the harasser's conduct must be unwelcome. The sex of the harasser and victim does not matter, and the victim does not need to be of the opposite sex (EEOC, n.d.-a). There are two categories of sexual harassment: *quid pro quo* and hostile work environment. The phrase quid pro quo is literally translated as "something for something." Quid pro quo sexual harassment occurs when an employee is asked for sexual favors in exchange for benefits in the workplace. Quid pro quo occurs in the workplace when a person with power over another suggests that he or she will give the employee (or job applicant) something such as a raise or promotion in return for sexual favors. It also occurs when the person with power threatens negative action such as firing or demotion if the employee or applicant refuses sexual advances. Sexual harassment can also lead to an employee's claim that the action created a hostile work environment. A hostile work environment can be claimed with such behavior as posting pornographic pictures, repeated offensive jokes, sexual innuendo, offensive gestures, and so forth. The employee who claims to have been subject to the hostile work environment does not need to be the direct target of the offenses. The two factors that must be shown in claims of a hostile work environment are that the harassment unreasonably interfered with work and that the harassment would affect a reasonable person's work. The harasser can be the victim's supervisor, a supervisor in another area, coworker, or a nonemployee (EEOC, n.d.-a). It is not necessary to prove that terms of employment are attached to a hostile work environment and sexual harassment.

Prevention of sexual harassment in the workplace is challenging. Sexual harassment is difficult to identify and difficult to prove, and many nurses are afraid to report incidents, fearing reprisal. The EEOC suggests some guidelines for sexual harassment policies. A good policy should provide a clear definition of prohibited conduct, explain how employees can report harassment, assure confidentiality for anyone who reports sexual harassment, assure employees who file complaints that they will be protected from retaliation, assure confidentiality to the greatest extent possible, identify reporting and investigative procedures that are free of chain-of-command entanglements, guarantee prompt investigations, assure immediate and appropriate action when sexual harassment is found to have occurred, and identify consequences of violating harassment policies (EEOC, 2019).

Students have special protection against sexual discrimination, harassment, and assault. Title IX of the Educational Amendments of 1972 is a federal civil rights law that states, "No person in the United States shall, on the basis of sex, be excluded from participation in, be denied the benefits of, or be subjected to discrimination under any education program or activity receiving federal financial assistance" (Education Amendments of 1972). Title IX applies to all educational programs that receive federal financial assistance from the US Department of Education, including approximately 7000 colleges and universities. The law requires all programs to operate in a nondiscriminatory manner. Key areas covered by the law include student recruitment, admissions, and counseling; financial assistance; athletics; sex-based harassment; treatment of pregnant and parenting students; discipline; single-sex education; and employment (Title IX and sex discrimination, 2019). Since the law was enacted, the US Supreme Court has issued decisions that clarify that Title IX requires schools to respond appropriately to reports of sexual harassment or sexual violence against students (Office of Civil Rights, 1997), reasoning that students who suffer sexual assault or harassment are deprived of equal access to education.

SUMMARY

In the professional realm, nurses are faced with the dichotomy of striving to meet their primary obligation to patients while dealing with problems among providers and within the institutional system. Nurses must be prepared to examine personal beliefs, prioritize obligations, and utilize professional codes of nursing ethics as they choose morally sound solutions to problems. Solutions must reflect an overall respect for persons and recognize the moral agency of individuals. Nurses are guided in this endeavor by personal values, professional codes of ethics, and laws.

CHAPTER HIGHLIGHTS

- As a moral agent, each person has the duty to pursue solutions to moral problems.

- Solutions to practical and ethical problems in the professional realm must be sensitive to personal values and beliefs.
- Nurses must be able to identify and prioritize conflicting obligations.
- It is important for nurses to determine the nature of conflicts in the professional realm.
- Problem resolution requires thoughtful consideration and weighing of alternative solutions.
- In solving problems, nurses must recognize that each person is an autonomous being, worthy of respect.
- Nurses must seek solutions to moral problems related to conflicting role expectations in the institutional setting.
- Nurses must seek solutions to moral and practical problems related to relationships among nurses, physicians, and subordinates.
- Discrimination is prohibited by the ethical principle of justice because it entails claims related to fair and equitable treatment of persons.

DISCUSSION QUESTIONS AND ACTIVITIES

1. Explore the EEOC Newsroom website at https://www.eeoc.gov/newsroom/search. Identify three recent court cases involving discrimination or harassment. Report the court decisions to the class.
2. Explore the ANA policy statements at https://www.nursingworld.org/practice-policy/nursing-excellence/official-position-statements/ or the CNA policy statement at https://www.cna-aiic.ca/en/policy-advocacy/policy-support-tools/position-statements. Entire ANA position statements are available online only to members. However, you can read a synopsis of two position statements on discrimination or harassment. How do these position statements, or those of the CNA, fit with your experience in the health care system?
3. Describe potential problems in the professional realm that fall into each of the following categories: conflicts of obligation, conflicts of principle, practical dilemmas, and conflicts of loyalty.
4. Discuss with your classmates situations involving professional relationships in the workplace that would constitute an appeal to conscience.
5. Review your nursing code of ethics. List statements that apply to problems related to nurses'

relationships with other professionals. Discuss the practical application of each of these statements.
6. Interview nurses who have been in practice for one year or less. Ask them to compare their expectations of the work environment with the reality that they faced on graduation.
7. Discuss the conflict that results as shrinking institutional budgets require cutbacks in nursing staff.
8. List the positive and negative aspects of loyalty. Do you feel loyalty is a virtue?
9. Describe experiences that you've seen or heard about in which nurses experienced bullying or lateral violence.
10. Describe the ideal professional relationship between nurses and physicians.
11. Role-play a situation in which a nurse is sensitive and respectful in disciplining a subordinate—focusing on the goal of improving performance rather than punishing.
12. How do nursing codes of ethics inform nurses' reactions to racial discrimination, discrimination against persons with disabilities, and sexual harassment.
13. Visit websites for impaired nurses. Discuss sensitive yet effective ways to approach an impaired nurse with these resources. Which resources would be most helpful to the nurse who is impaired?

REFERENCES

Americans with Disabilities Act (1990). *Americans With Disabilities Act of 1990.* https://www.ada.gov/pubs/adastatute08.htm#12102

Advisory Board. (October 17, 2022). *The impact of nurse turnover in 2 charts.* https://www.advisory.com/daily-briefing/2022/10/17/nurse-turnover

ANA, (2009). *Patient safety: Rights of registered nurses when considering a patient assignment.* Nursebooks.org. ANA position statement. Issue.. https://www.nursingworld.org/practice-policy/nursing-excellence/official-position-statements/id/patient-safety-rights-of-registered-nurses-when-considering-a-patient-assignment/

ANA, (2015a). *Position statement on incivility, bullying, and workplace violence.* Nursebooks.org. https://www.nursingworld.org/~49d6e3/globalassets/practiceandpolicy/nursing-excellence/incivility-bullying-and-workplace-violence--ana-position-statement.pdf.

ANA, (2015b). *Code of ethics for nurses with interpretive statements.* Nursebooks.org. http://nursingworld.org/DocumentVault/Ethics-1/Code-of-Ethics-for-Nurses.html.

ANA, & National Council of State Boards of Nursing. (2015). *Joint statement on delegation: American Nurses Association (ANA) and the National Council of State Boards of Nursing (NCSBN)*. https://www.nursingworld.org/practice-policy/nursing-excellence/official-position-statements/id/joint-statement-on-delegation-by-ANA-and-NCSBN/

ANA Center for Ethics and Human Rights. (2018). *The nurse's role in addressing discrimination: Protecting and promoting inclusive strategies in practice settings, policy, and advocacy.* https://www.nursingworld.org/~4ab207/globalassets/practiceandpolicy/nursing-excellence/ana-position-statements/social-causes-and-health-care/the-nurses-role-in-addressing-discrimination.pdf

ANA Center for Ethics and Human Rights. (2021). *Nurses' professional responsibility to promote ethical practice environments.* Nursingworld.org. https://www.nursingworld.org/~4ab6e6/globalassets/practiceandpolicy/nursing-excellence/ana-position-statements/nursing-practice/nurses-professional-responsibility-to-promote-ethical-practice-environments-2021-final.pdf.

ANA Center for Ethics and Human Rights. (2022). *The nurse's role and responsibility in unveiling and dismantling racism in nursing.* https://www.nursingworld.org/~48e2dd/globalassets/practiceandpolicy/nursing-excellence/ana-position-statements/ana-the-nurses-role-and-responsibility-in-unveiling-and-dismantling-racism-in-nursing_bod-approved-formatted.pdf

Anderson, K. F. (2013). Diagnosing discrimination: Stress from perceived racism and the mental and physical health effects. *Sociological Inquiry, 83*(1), 55–81. https://doi.org/10.1111/j.1475-682X.2012.00433.x.

Aristotle. (2000). *Nicomachean ethics* (R. Crisp, Trans.). Cambridge University Press (Original work published ca. 350 BCE)

Civil Rights Act of 1964, Pub. L. No. 88-352, 78 Stat. 241 (1964). https://www.govinfo.gov/content/pkg/STATUTE-78-Pg241.pdf (govinfo.gov)

Civil Rights Act of 1991, Pub. L. No. 102-166 (1991). https://www.govinfo.gov/conent/pkg/COMPS-344.pdf

CNA. (2017). *Code of ethics for registered nurses.* https://cdn1.nscn.ca/sites/default/files/documents/resources/code-of-ethics-for-registered-nurses.pdf#:~:text=The%20Canadian%20Nurses%20Association%20%28CNA%29%20Code%20of%20Ethics,receiving%20care.%20The%20Codeis%20both%20aspirational%20and%20regulatory.

CNA. (2020). *CNAs key messages on anti-Black racism in nursing and health.* https://hl-prod-ca-oc-download.s3-ca-central-1.amazonaws.com/CNA/2f975e7e-4a40-45ca-863c-5ebf0a138d5e/UploadedImages/documents/Anti-Racism-key-messages_e.pdf

CNA, & CFNU. (2008). *Joint position statement: Workplace violence and bullying.* Workplace-Violence-and-Bullying_jointposition-statement.pdf (nursesunions.ca)

Curtin, L. (1996). Ethics, discipline and discharge. *Nursing Management, 27*(3), 51–52.

Dilley, K. B. (2000). Out from under their thumbs. *American Journal of Nursing, 100*(5), 9.

Education Amendments of 1972, Public Law No. 92-318 (1972). STATUTE-86-Pg235.pdf (govinfo.gov)

EEOC. (2001). *EEOC, private plaintiffs and American Cast Iron Pipe Company settle lawsuit.* https://www.eeoc.gov/eeoc/newsroom/release/1-4-01.cfm

EEOC. (2019). *Harassment policy tips.* https://www.eeoc.gov/employers/smallbusiness/checklists/harassment_policy_tips.cfm

EEOC. (2022). *Charge statistics (charges filed with EEOC) FY 1997 through FY 2021.* https://www.eeoc.gov/data/charge-statistics-charges-filed-eeoc-fy-1997-through-fy-2021

EEOC. (n.d.-a). *Facts sheet: Sexual harassment discrimination.* https://www.eeoc.gov/laws/guidance/fact-sheet-sexual-harassment-discrimination

EEOC. (n.d.-b). *Retaliation: Considerations for federal agency managers.* https://www.eeoc.gov/laws/types/sexual_harassment.cfm.

EEOC. (n.d.-c). *Sexual harassment.* https://www.eeoc.gov/laws/types/sexual_harassment.cfm

Gadow, S. (1980). Existential advocacy: Philosophical foundation of nursing In S. F. Spicker & S. Gadow (Eds.), *Nursing: Images and ideals, opening dialogue with the humanities.* Springer.

Goh, H. S., Hosier, S., & Zhang, H. (2022). Prevalence, antecedents, and consequences of workplace bullying among nurses: A summery of reviews. *International Journal of Environmental Research and Public Health, 19.* https://doi.org/10.3390/ijerph19148256.

Hutchinson, M., & Jackson, D. (2013). Hostile clinician behaviours in the nursing work environment and implications for patient care: a mixed-methods systematic review. *BMC Nursing, 12*(1), 25–44. https://doi.org/10.1186/1472-6955-12-25.

ICN. (2021). *The ICN code of ethics for nurses.* https://www.icn.ch/system/files/2021-10/ICN_Code-of-Ethics_EN_Web_0.pdf

Jameton, A. (1984). *Nursing practice: The ethical issues.* Prentice-Hall.

Karatuna, I., Jönsson, S., & Muhonen, T. (2020). Workplace bullying in the nursing profession: A cross-cultural scoping review. *International Journal of Nursing Studies, 111* https://doi.org/10.1016/j.ijnurstu.2020.103628.

Kim, S. (2015). The effect of gender discrimination in organization. *International Review of Public Administration, 20*(1), 51–69. https://doi.org/10.1080/12294659.2014.983216.

Lu, L., Dong, M., Lok, G., Feng, Y., Wang, G., Ng, C. H., Ungvari, G. S., & Xiang, Y. (2020). Worldwide prevalence of sexual harassment towards nurses: A comprehensive meta-analysis of observational studies. *Journal of Advanced Nursing, 76*(4), 980–990.

Montessori, M. (1912). *The Montessori Method* (A. E. George, Trans.). Frederick A. Stokes Co. http://digital.library.upenn.edu/women/montessori/method/method-V.html

Nursing Solutions (2022). *2022 National health care retention & RN staffing report*. https://www.nsinursingsolutions.com/Documents/Library/NSI_National_Health_Care_Retention_Report.pdf

Obrien, K. R., McAbee, S. T., Hebl, M. R., & Rodgers, J. R. (2016). The impact of interpersonal discrimination and stress on health performance for early career STEM academicians. *Frontiers in Psychology, 7*, 615. https://doi.org/10.3389/fpsyg.2016.00615.

Office of Civil Rights. (1997). *Sexual harassment guidance.* https://www2.ed.gov/about/offices/list/ocr/docs/sexhar00.html

Pogue, C. A., Li, P., Swiger, P., Gillespie, G., Ivankova, N., & Patrician, P. A. (2022). Associations among the nursing work environment, nurse-reported workplace bullying, and patient outcomes. *Nursing Forum, 57*(6), 1059–1068. https://doi.org/10.1111/nuf.12781.

Rand, A. (1966). The ethics of emergencies. In J. Feinberg (Ed.), *Reason and responsibility: Readings in some basic problems of philosophy* (9th ed., pp. 541–545).

Rushton, C. H. (2021). Preserving integrity and staying power as a nurse in a pandemic. *AJN The American Journal of Nursing, 121*(3), 68–69. https://doi.org/10.1097/01.Naj.0000737332.30793.91.

Schmalenberg, C., & Kramer, M. (2009). Nurse-physician relationships in hospitals: 20,000 nurses tell their story.

Critical Care Nurse, 29(1), 74–83. https://doi.org/10.4037/ccn2009436.

Sharma, S., Scafide, K., Dalal, R. S., & Maughan, E. (2021). Individual and organizational characteristics associated with workplace bullying of school nurses in Virginia. *Journal of School Nursing, 37*(5), 343–352. https://doi.org/10.1177/1059840519871606.

The Bully Project. (n.d.). *Adult bullying: Characteristics of adult bully targets.* https://www.thebullyproject.com/adult_bullying

Title IX and Sex Discrimination. (2019). https://www2.ed.gov/about/offices/list/ocr/docs/tix_dis.html

Trépanier, S-G., Fernet, C., Austin, S., & Boudrias, V. (2016). Work environment antecedents of bullying: A review and integrative model applied to registered nurses. *International Journal of Nursing Studies, 55*, 85–97. https://doi.org/10.1016/j.ijnurstu.2015.10.001.

U.S. Const. *Amend. I-X.*

Vessey, J. A., Demarco, R., & DiFazio, R. (2010). Bullying, harassment, and horizontal violence in the nursing workforce: The state of the science. *Annual Review of Nursing Research, 28*, 133–157.

WHO. (n.d.). *Preventing and responding to sexual exploitation, abuse, and harassment.* https://www.who.int/initiatives/preventing-and-responding-to-sexual-exploitation-abuse-and-harassment

Workplace Bullying Institute. (2021). *Work shouldn't hurt.* https://workplacebullying.org/

Workplace Bullying Institute. (2022). *2021 WBI U.S. workplace bullying survey.* https://workplacebullying.org/wp-content/uploads/2021/04/2021-Full-Report.pdf

10

Ethical Issues Related to Selected Healthcare Technologies

There is an appointed time for everything, and a time for every affair under the heavens.

(Ecclesiastes 3:1)

OBJECTIVES

After completing this chapter, the reader should be able to:

1. Discuss the impact on nursing and healthcare of technologies that support patient care and modify or prolong life.
2. Apply beneficence and nonmaleficence to decisions about the use of healthcare technology.
3. Discuss potential ethical issues and dilemmas related to healthcare technologies that are integral to nursing practice.
4. Relate the concept of medical futility to healthcare decisions at the end of life.
5. Relate economics to decisions regarding the use and availability of healthcare technologies.
6. Discuss ethical considerations related to end-of-life care decisions.
7. Describe legal issues associated with the use of healthcare technology.
8. Discuss issues and dilemmas associated with technologies affecting reproduction, genetics, genomics, and organ transplantation.
9. Identify issues and dilemmas associated with research into controversial technologies.
10. Discuss issues related to the use of healthcare information technology and social media in nursing and healthcare.
11. Discuss the impact of healthcare technologies on patient care and on nursing health and well-being.
12. Discuss elements of codes of nursing ethics that guide nursing practice and response to issues related to healthcare technologies and patient care.

INTRODUCTION

Contemporary nursing practice is inextricably intertwined with healthcare technology that is integral to many aspects of patient care. Technology as discussed in this chapter refers to both routine patient care and safety aids and to medical interventions that support healing, sustain life, and may have the potential to modify life. Technology that is a routine part of nursing care includes such things as electronic charting, medical equipment, IV infusion pumps, monitoring devices, electronic tracking of patient healthcare information, devices that facilitate correct patient identification, informatics, and

the like. Examples of technology related to medical interventions include robotic surgery, machines to enhance medical diagnostics and interventions, machines that can keep heart and lungs functioning, laser and radiation treatment, reproductive interventions, genetics and genomics, and many more. Few would deny the benefits of medical advances, often referred to in terms such as wonders or miracles. However, the many benefits brought to the healthcare arena by these advances are often accompanied by serious dilemmas for both practitioners and patients. Questions related to issues of living and dying and the changing definitions of both arise in relation to advances in healthcare technology. Dilemmas include the availability of equipment and interventions, what patient situations warrant the use of available diagnostics and interventions, who decides when to initiate and when to withdraw particular interventions, and patient values, beliefs, and preferences regarding use of various technologies. Nurses must be concerned about the amount of nursing energy and attention required to be with patients and families receiving these interventions, as well as dealing with the technology used to assess, monitor, and treat patients. Additionally, nurses must be alert to issues related to the use of healthcare information technology and social media. As much as we say that nursing focuses on holistic caring for the patient, nurses are faced with increasing demands to focus attention on patient care technology rather than on their patients.

This chapter focuses on common ethical issues related to the use of technology in today's healthcare settings. Because ethical dilemmas arise more frequently related to life-sustaining interventions, a particular emphasis is placed on issues of end-of-life care. The list of technologies included in this chapter is not meant to be all-inclusive; rather it is meant to be representative of the types of issues that involve technology. Patient self-determination as discussed in Chapter 11 is intertwined with ethical issues related to healthcare technology, and readers will note some overlap between these two chapters. Nurses who are directly involved with situations that present ethical dilemmas, as well as those who are more on the periphery, must be aware of considerations regarding the effect of healthcare technology on patient care and upon patients. These considerations include values, attitudes, beliefs, communication, and attention to the humanistic caring role. Changing technologies bring with them the challenge of dealing with new issues and ethical concerns, and nurses need to be prepared to face this challenge.

BENEFITS AND CHALLENGES OF TECHNOLOGY

Scientific advances in the past 100 years have been phenomenal. They include medications, surgical techniques, machines and equipment, diagnostic procedures, specialized treatments, expanded understanding of the causes of and progression of the disease, gene diagnosis and therapy, electronic communication and storage systems, and greater insight into what is required for people to stay healthy. New interventions have saved lives, improved the quality of life, alleviated suffering, and significantly decreased the incidence of some diseases. Before the advent of many modern health-related technologies, people experienced illness and death as an inevitable part of the cycle of their lives. Although death was not necessarily welcomed, it was expected as the natural outcome when the body could no longer ward off the effects of certain diseases or injuries. If someone was born with, or developed, a deformity, it may have been seen as a curse but was also considered part of who the person was. Life began when the infant started breathing, and life ended when the heart and breathing stopped.

Technology makes it possible to, among other things, restart arrested hearts, keep people alive with mechanical devices, correct deformities, assist in more accurate medical diagnoses, assist the body in dealing with disease through the use of various interventions, eliminate diseased parts through minimally invasive surgery, and replace malfunctioning or diseased organs or joints. The ability to prolong life, or at least to extend the functioning of the physical being, has prompted the necessity of dealing with some very important issues. One dilemma relates to questions of quality of life and whether physical existence is synonymous with living. Another issue relates to whether the availability of certain technologies and interventions means they should always be used. Many issues relate to decisions about how and for whom technologies will be used.

Quality of Life

The ability to keep people alive and physically functioning through the use of technology has led to much reflection and discussion about what constitutes life and living. Some people believe that biological life must be preserved, regardless of the effect on the person whose body is being kept alive. A frequently asked question is whether a person is truly alive in situations where there is merely physiological functioning, without awareness of oneself or others. Many suggest that living implies a quality that goes beyond physical existence. Quality of life is a subjective appraisal of factors that make life worth living and contribute to a positive experience of living, and it means different things to different people. It is difficult to find a clear and concise definition of quality of life because of the multidisciplinary usage and variable cultural understandings of the concept. Definitions of quality of life vary from global understandings of the concept, such as satisfaction with life, to focused definitions used for research—for example, health or functional ability (Boggatz, 2016; Vanleerberghe et al., 2017). Discussions of quality of life encompass physical, emotional, spiritual, and social considerations. Ideas incorporated in understandings of the concept include fulfillment; satisfaction/dissatisfaction; meaning and purpose; conditions of life; happiness/unhappiness; experiences of life; and factors such as comfort, functional status, socioeconomic status, independence, and conditions in one's environment.

Evaluating the dimensions of the concept presents challenges in defining quality of life (Boggatz, 2016; Flannery, 2017). For instance, when assessing personal quality of life, which does a person rank as more important: happiness or functional status, such as the ability to get around and care for oneself? Nurses need to understand patient perspectives of what constitutes quality in their lives to incorporate these factors into goal setting and care planning.

Quality of life is a personal perspective that is determined by each individual. Recognizing this, we should not judge the quality of another's life based on our own values. If judgments about a person's worth and quality of life are based on factors such as contributions to society, age, mental capacity, or ability to function, then discrimination against those who are judged to have a lesser quality of life may easily follow. Perceptions of quality of life often change with age and life experiences. For example, persons with debilitating health concerns may rate the quality of their lives quite positively, although others might feel that they could never live with such limitations. When patients and families are confronted with technological options, nurses need to help them clarify their perceptions regarding the quality of life and discuss not only how life might be extended but also how the quality of life may be affected by various options.

Principles of Beneficence and Nonmaleficence

When dealing with issues of technology, the principles of beneficence and nonmaleficence may be in conflict. A particular technology, which may be implemented with the intention of doing good (beneficence), may result in much suffering for the patient. Inducing such suffering is counter to the maxim of do no harm (nonmaleficence). In some circumstances, this is accepted as part of the treatment process, such as pain associated with surgery or side effects of chemotherapy. Patients are often willing to endure the discomfort because there is an expectation of recovery and that they will ultimately be or feel healthier. In circumstances in which there is little or no expectation of recovery or improved functioning, the essential question is whether the harm imposed by the intervention outweighs the good intended by its use. Suffering associated with technological interventions may include physical, spiritual, and emotional elements for both patient and family. Making decisions regarding the use of these interventions may cause pain, and there is suffering in living with the unknown results of these ongoing decisions. Relief of suffering, a goal of healing from its earliest days, needs to be addressed in all patient encounters.

HEALTHCARE TECHNOLOGY: ETHICAL ISSUES AND DILEMMAS

Healthcare interventions that rely heavily on technology such as organ and tissue transplantation, some cancer treatment, robotic surgery, genetic engineering, reproductive assistance, and life-sustaining treatments have profound potential for affecting our lives and health in positive ways. Their use also presents dilemmas for patients, families, professionals, and society. Nurses generally do not make the decisions regarding implementing or withdrawing particular interventions (except perhaps in situations such as initiating cardiopulmonary resuscitation [CPR]), yet we are involved as the caregivers of those receiving interventions and in many levels of patient care that involve the use of technological interventions. One of nursing's primary responsibilities is to help patients and families deal with the purposes, benefits, and limitations of the specific intervention.

Personal attitudes prompt different expectations and scenarios when we are faced with decisions about heroic efforts and life-sustaining technologies. We must be aware of our own attitudes concerning living and dying, as well as the beliefs and expectations of patients, families, and other healthcare providers. Such awareness alerts us to situations in which there are differing attitudes among the parties involved and provides an opportunity for opening lines of communication before a serious dilemma arises. Consider, for example, the patient who tells the nurse that he feels that his body is just giving up in spite of all the medications and treatments he is receiving, and he says he would like to go home to die peacefully, yet the physician is considering another surgery that is helpful about 30 percent of the time. In such a situation it is important for the nurse to explore this area further with the patient and either communicate his wishes to the physician or facilitate the patient's talking with the physician about his wishes.

This section focuses primarily on the issue of withdrawing or withholding treatment as a prime example of a dilemma related to technological interventions. Other issues related to technology are discussed briefly. The reader is encouraged to further explore particular areas as the need or interest arises.

Treating Patients: When to Intervene and to What End

One of the most controversial bioethical topics of recent years relates to withholding or withdrawing life-sustaining treatments when they are deemed to have poor outcomes or offer no benefit. Decisions about withholding or withdrawing medical treatment are generally made by physicians in consultation with patients and family members. Approaches to dealing with these decisions reflect varying attitudes and concerns and may be confusing for all involved. A brief look at history sheds light on current attitudes regarding dealing with contemporary medical treatment. Questions related to the ethical limitations of medical care date back to the time of Hippocrates, when physicians were taught that the goal of medicine was to relieve suffering and reduce the effects of disease by lending support to natural processes. When the body was overpowered by disease, there was a concern that using medical interventions might merely prolong the suffering. The limitations of medicine were recognized, and it was considered ethical to withhold treatments that held little potential for healing.

The scientific era that began emerging in the 17th century fostered a change in this ethical stance. Rather than revering and working with natural processes, conquering and dominating nature became the goal of science. In the 19th century, as medicine began to align more with science and as biological causes for diseases were discovered, the goal of medicine became the conquest of disease by exercising power over nature. Within the current narrow focus on curing disease, ethical issues frequently relate to aggressive medical treatments, and issues of personal quality of life and dimensions of suffering are often unrecognized and neglected. With their attention to healing and caring, nurses play an important role in calling attention to concerns that go beyond the narrow focus of curing.

Issues of Life, Death, and Dying

Ethical dilemmas faced in healthcare settings often relate to issues of, and attitudes toward, living and dying. Important questions that are deliberated by those involved include:

- When does life begin?
- When does life end?
- How can we be sure that someone has died?
- Who decides?

Technology has stretched the boundaries and clouded the waters surrounding life's beginning and ending. Perspectives range from the belief that life begins at conception to the view that it begins when an infant can survive outside the womb. Technology makes this discussion even more complex and raises questions such as "What happens when conception cannot occur 'naturally' and artificial processes are employed either in vivo or in vitro?" and "Is the laboratory embryo a life?"

Today, many low-birth-weight infants and those with certain birth defects, who would not have survived in prior eras, survive with the support of machines, medications, and surgical procedures. In the process, however, some babies are kept alive only to die after months of expensive treatment. Others survive to face chronic health problems, with their associated financial, emotional, and physical strains on families and the healthcare system. There is no definitive way to predict which infants will have problems as they grow and develop. Ethical questions arise regarding how much effort to invest in "saving" a few infants who have a high probability of living only a short time or with significant health problems.

In our society, death has become an unnatural event, frequently associated with hospitals and other institutions, surrounded by tubes, machinery, and heroic efforts (Fig. 10.1). Determining when life ends has become a critical issue related to the use of

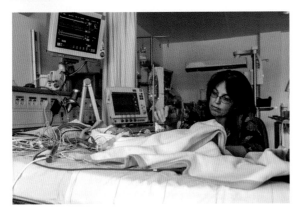

Fig. 10.1 Life-Sustaining Technology Carries With It Both Hope for Healing and the Challenge of Facing the Possibility of Death. (©iStock.com/Perboge.)

technology, prompting the involvement of courts in decision making. A pervasive attitude within our society is that death is the enemy to be overcome or kept at bay for as long as possible, regardless of the age or health condition of the person. Thus, death is often viewed as a failure on the part of the healthcare provider. It is understandable therefore that many healthcare providers have difficulty dealing with death as a possible outcome for patients and thus find it a difficult topic to discuss. Another reason that the topic of death may be avoided is that discussing death requires us to face issues of meaning in life, as well as anxieties and fears regarding our own mortality. However, lack of discussion of death as a possible outcome may lead families and patients to have unreasonable expectations and false hopes of what the system can offer. Demands for inappropriate interventions or accusations that not enough was done may arise from such situations. Patients and families need support in recognizing and honoring their own responses, beliefs, and fears regarding death. By facing our own issues about death, we are better able to facilitate this process with patients.

In many cultures, death is viewed as part of our life cycle that comes in its own time. Healthcare focused on curing is provided when there is reasonable hope of benefit, but people recognize when it is time for care to mean letting go and facilitating the transition through the dying process. In such cultures, dying often occurs at home, surrounded by family and friends.

ASK YOURSELF

What Are Your Views of Death and Dying?
What many people fear most regarding death is suffering and dying alone.
- How do available technological interventions contribute to this concern or attitude?
- What has your experience been related to death, what has shaped your attitudes regarding death, and what are your fears related to death? How does your family or culture approach death and dying?
- How can nurses temper the effects of technological interventions on patients in the dying process?
- How can nurses support patients and families in recognizing and honoring their own responses and beliefs regarding death? What guidance do codes of nursing ethics give in this regard?
- If machines and medication are keeping a body functioning, even if the person is apparently unaware, is that person still alive? Discuss your response.
- Do you think that brain wave activity in the midst of severe deterioration of major systems constitutes living? Discuss your response.

CASE PRESENTATION

A Child With Leukemia
Lindsay, a 12-year-old child with leukemia, has relapsed in spite of routine chemotherapeutic interventions. This child has suffered the side effects of the treatment, including nausea, hair loss, and frequent hospitalizations with infections, and is deteriorating physically. She says she feels as if she is being tortured with all the needles, spinal taps, and bone marrow samples; that she has no friends; and that this kind of life is not worth living. A bone marrow transplant (the only hope for a cure at this point) would mean subjecting her to intensive chemotherapy, total-body irradiation, and weeks in isolation after the transplant. The family is told that there is a 40 percent chance that the transplant will be effective. The procedure is very expensive, and the family has already had to obtain a second mortgage for their home because their insurance has not covered many of the expenses to date.

Think About It
Factors Influencing Choices Regarding Technology-Based Medical Interventions
- What factors do you think need to be considered in making the decision about having the bone marrow transplant?

- How do percentages of risk and benefit affect your decision making?
- In this situation, do you think a 40 percent chance of success is enough to go ahead with the transplant? What if it were 60 percent? What about 20 percent?
- How can you help patients and families use statistical information in thinking about their decisions? What other factors would you help them to consider, such as the impact of the intervention on Lindsey's physical and emotional well-being and quality of life?
- Who should be involved in making this decision? The parents? Lindsay? Others?

Dying is more than a medical occurrence; it is a spiritual process touching the individual, family, and community. Although medical interventions can assist and support those in the dying process, current technologies can prolong suffering by prolonging the dying process and can separate people from their families through actual physical barriers and institutionalization. Relieving suffering and supporting a dignified death are important elements of the nursing role delineated in nursing codes of ethics and standards of practice (ANA, 2015, Provision 1.3; CNA, 2017, Part I.D. 2, 8: ICN, 2021, Element 1.8; ANA, 2021, p.1). Addressing patient needs may require nurses to make decisions to stretch institutional policy regarding such things as visitors and visiting hours to ensure that the patient is not alone or to risk confrontations with physicians over pain management or other aspects of care.

Medical Futility

Ethical and legal arguments for initiating or discontinuing life-sustaining treatments are based primarily on the relative benefits and burdens for the patient. Most ethical and legal discussions regarding life-sustaining treatments make little, if any, distinction between not implementing a life-sustaining treatment and discontinuing one that has been initiated. Withholding or removing life-sustaining treatments in situations in which the burden or harm has been determined to outweigh the benefits is, in essence, allowing the person to die as a result of the natural progression of the illness. From both practical and moral perspectives this is different from euthanasia, which means actively causing the painless death of a person to end or prevent suffering. Ethicists argue that it is the deterioration of the patient's

condition that causes death, not the removal of the technology that is artificially supporting life.

In deliberations regarding withholding, initiating, or withdrawing life-sustaining interventions, medical futility related to the patient's situation is a major consideration. Medical futility refers to situations in which interventions are judged to have very little or no medical benefit or in which the chance for success is low. Futility is often discussed in relation to CPR, but it relates as well to interventions that preserve patients who are in persistent vegetative states or dependent on the technology of tertiary care settings. One difficulty associated with medical futility is that there is no set definition of the concept. Because each case is different, developing empirical guidelines regarding medical futility is very difficult (Fontugne, 2014). Thus, there are only suggested parameters that vary greatly in guiding healthcare providers. Literature on futility discusses both quantitative definitions of futility that would justify unilateral decisions by physicians to withhold or withdraw interventions and qualitative, value-laden definitions such as situations in which interventions do not lead to an acceptable quality of life for the patient (Fontugne, 2014; Jacobs, 2014; Lo, 2013; NCD, 2019; Shin, 2016). Quantitative definitions of futility include interventions that have no pathophysiological rationale, have already failed in the patient, or will not achieve the goal of care, as well as situations where maximal treatment is failing. Objective data and the clinical expertise of the physician are the basis of determining futility in these situations. Medical ethicists generally agree that physicians have no ethical duty to provide interventions that are futile in the quantitative sense and may well have an ethical obligation not to provide them even if they are requested (Lo, 2013; Shin, 2016). Organizations such as the National Council on Disability (NCD) (2019), however, raise the concern that such decisions can be affected by physician bias about quality of life and not purely based on scientific evidence.

Qualitative definitions of futility include situations that prompt variable interpretations and thus are more confusing—for example, situations in which the likelihood of success is very small, no worthwhile goals of care can be achieved, patient quality of life as determined by the patient is unacceptable, and the prospective benefit is not worth the resources required. The meaning of futility in such cases must consider perceptions of the patient and family and judgments of the healthcare team. In these situations the literature suggests that describing interventions as *potentially inappropriate* or *medically nonbeneficial* is more specific terminology than using the term *futile* (Olmstead & Dahnke, 2016). In the absence of clear external guidelines, these less clear situations require more skillful nursing care, as the persons involved draw on their own understandings and resources shaped by personal beliefs and cultural values.

ASK YOURSELF

What Constitutes Medical Futility?
- What do you think about these definitions of futility? Where would you envision potential problems or dilemmas based on these definitions?
- Who do you think should be involved in decisions about medical futility?
- Would you consider an expensive treatment that has a five percent chance of improving a patient's health situation to be futile? What if the patient wants to try everything? Explain.
- Should medical futility be an issue when treatments are not expensive? Explain.
- Do you think a decision about futile treatment should be different with children and younger adults than with the elderly? What about persons with physical or mental disabilities? Discuss your response.
- How would you see a patient's inability to pay for treatment affecting decisions about futility?

Because personal values come into play, healthcare providers, patients, and families may have differing views of what is a benefit or burden. The difficulty in defining and developing clear guidelines for medical futility or potentially inappropriate interventions has prompted healthcare practitioners to focus more on the process of working with the patient or healthcare surrogate and family to explain fully the medical circumstances and to negotiate care that is in the best interest of the patient. The process-oriented approach focuses on open communication and shared decision making. This includes early discussion with patients, family, or surrogates about both the benefits and limitations of technology and ongoing deliberation and negotiation with all stakeholders as patient status changes. If there are unresolved differences among those involved regarding the appropriateness of a treatment plan, additional steps in the process may include getting a second opinion,

having an ethics committee consultation, transferring care to another physician (or nurse), or transferring to another institution (Jacobs, 2014; Olmstead & Dahnke, 2016; Shin, 2016).

ASK YOURSELF

When Does Life Begin?
- What are your beliefs about when life begins? What shaped these beliefs?
- Consider that you are a member of a special task force called together by your hospital to establish guidelines for allocating dwindling funds for support of low-birth-weight infants in the neonatal intensive care unit. What criteria would you use to determine which of the infants who cannot survive without technology at birth will receive such interventions? Incorporate your understanding of distributive justice (see Chapter 3) into your deliberation.
- If an infant will die without a technological intervention and the intervention is withdrawn, do you consider that a natural or unnatural end of life? Why?

Views of the various parties may differ in a variety of ways. For example, a patient or family may find hope and be willing to consider a treatment that has a 5 percent likelihood of success, whereas the healthcare providers see this as a futile effort. When considering quality of life, the perspective of the patient and family is essential in any determination of what is potentially inappropriate. Deciding when it is not worth continuing life-sustaining treatment is another circumstance in which the views of the parties involved may differ. Consider, for example, a 72-year-old quadriplegic patient on a ventilator at home who has been deteriorating and having frequent infections. She had to be resuscitated when recently hospitalized for a severe respiratory infection. The physician discussed the situation with the patient and the family and suggested a do-not-resuscitate (DNR) order, which is a written directive placed in the patient's medical chart indicating that CPR is to be avoided. (See further discussion on DNR orders later in this chapter.) Even though the patient and most family members indicated agreement, the daughter, who is the caregiver, says she wants every effort made to keep her mother alive, saying that God will take her mother when He is ready. In another situation, healthcare providers might view continuing treatments that prolong a patient's life a few more days to be causing unnecessary suffering, whereas for the patient and the family this is important "saying goodbye" time.

When considering situations of medical futility or potentially inappropriate interventions, we need to be aware of the impact on all those involved. Although the primary focus is on the wishes, quality of life, and potential suffering of the patient, it is important to recognize that family, nurses, and other hospital staff, and even the institution may suffer as a consequence of treatment decisions. Family or healthcare surrogates may experience questions of faith, grief, anger, or guilt that cause emotional suffering. Nurses, who are the primary caregivers of the patient, may suffer despair, moral distress,

and burnout related to having to provide care that seems to be causing suffering for the patient. If the situation is unresolved and there is legal action or the patient has to be transferred to another facility, the institution's reputation may suffer (Mendola, 2015).

Because nurses provide continual care and presence with patients and families, they need to be alert for ethical issues related to life-sustaining technologies. Nurses should serve on institutional ethics committees and be involved with developing policies for resolving issues related to futile or potentially inappropriate interventions. It is also imperative that nurses advocate for policies and procedures within their institutions that support nurses in dealing with despair, moral distress, and burnout that such ethical issues engender.

CASE PRESENTATION

Mr. Mason and His Son

Mr. Mason is a 78-year-old retired, widowed ironworker. He has been estranged from his adult son, an only child, for many years. He was recently diagnosed with advanced lung cancer. He recognized that he needed to make some plans for his immediate future, so he contacted his son and allowed him power of attorney. Mr. Mason is admitted to your unit in severe pain and a very poor prognosis due to having no further cancer treatment options. He is somewhat confused, and you are unable to elicit information from him about his wishes regarding life-sustaining measures. You carefully begin discussing this difficult subject with his son, as it is your hospital's policy to review the advance directives of all admitted to your oncology unit. Following are three possible twists this case could take, each of which is based on a real-life situation.

Ending 1. Mr. Mason's son begins to sob uncontrollably, saying, "I was never a very good son. I left home when I was barely 19 and didn't even write or call for many years. I am just getting to know my dad, and now this happens. I want as much time with him as possible. He told me a few days ago that he was ready to die and didn't want to be kept alive on machines. But it is so unfair to me. I want him alive and more time with him. Please, do everything you can to keep him alive. I need some more time with him. I need for him to forgive me."

Ending 2. Mr. Mason's son seems impatient, continually looking at his watch as you talk to him. Finally, seeming exasperated, he says, "Look, he's going to die anyway, right? Two things: First, I'm a busy man, and the quicker we get this over with, the better; second, I have an

appointment in 20 minutes with a real estate agent, and later with Dad's stockbroker. I'd really like to start arranging to sell his house and cash in some of his stocks. My son starts college in two months, and we could use the money. I suppose you think this is cruel, but realistically, would Dad rather we spend the money he worked so hard for to keep him alive, when he's bound to die anyway, or on his grandson's education? It's pretty clear to me. I say, just let Dad go; that would be the best for everyone concerned."

Ending 3. The son quickly acknowledges that he understands the question. Without hesitation, he says, "Do all you can to keep him alive. The tyrant was mean to me all of my life. I hate him. I want him to suffer as long as possible."

Think About It

Family Reactions to Decisions About Potential Medically Inappropriate Interventions

- What is your response to the son's statement in each of these scenarios? Include both your thinking response and your feeling response.
- How would your feelings lead you to advise one option over another?
- What values and dilemmas are evident in each scenario?
- Identify your personal and professional values and biases related to each scenario.
- Who should make the decision? What conflicting loyalties do you see in these situations?
- How would you respond to the son's decision in each situation? How would codes of nursing ethics guide your response?

Economics and Medical Futility

The cost of healthcare, particularly in relation to advances in healthcare technology, has brought economic factors into discussions of futility. Some suggest that the principle of justice indicates that if a particular intervention is judged to be of limited or no benefit for one person, it should be discontinued so it is available for another patient who can make better use of the scarce resource. Political and economic developments in medicine, particularly prospective payment systems, have prompted physicians and hospitals to look more closely at futile treatments. Under prospective payment systems, physicians and institutions lose money if patients are maintained on particular treatments beyond a predetermined length of time. Because reimbursement for medical care requires justification that the care is medically indicated, the physician's responsibility to limit excessive treatments has become a kind of social mandate (Baily, 2011; NCD, 2019). Many argue that it is ethical and justifiable for physicians to limit access to treatments that are expensive while offering limited benefits and that, given limited healthcare resources, such decisions are socially responsible. Such an argument is consistent with utilitarian ethics, a perspective often used by government agencies when deciding about distribution of goods and services. Although economic issues do affect healthcare decisions, and some raise concerns that medical futility may be a subtle form of rationing, the important focus is not the cost of the therapy but whether the benefits outweigh the disadvantages for the patient from the patient's perspective. Whatever the decision regarding the therapy, nursing must focus on high-quality care and communication with the patient and family.

ASK YOURSELF

How Are Economics and Decisions About Medical Futility Related?

- Are there circumstances in which you feel physicians or institutions should be able to limit a patient's access to expensive treatments? Include ethical principles and codes in your response.
- How do you think economics affects decisions about medical futility or potentially inappropriate treatments? How might personal bias be part of such decisions?
- How might patient care be affected by these decisions?
- What are the potential legal ramifications of such decisions?

Cardiopulmonary Resuscitation, Technology, and Do-Not-Resuscitate Orders

CPR is a life-saving intervention that may be initiated by persons in various settings with or without technological assistance. CPR is often followed by the use of life-sustaining technology to help stabilize and support the person through the healing process. CPR is unique among medical interventions because it is the only intervention where a presumption to provide the intervention exists, unless there are documented physician orders or clear directives in a patient's advance directives not to do CPR. These directives are known as DNR orders and are a key part of a person's advance directives, which are discussed in Chapter 11. DNR is the most common terminology used to indicate the decision to not initiate CPR and will be used throughout this book. The acronyms **do not attempt resuscitation (DNAR), do not intubate (DNI),** and **allow natural death (AND)** are also used in the literature and in some institutions. Miscommunication may occur when patients and families are not familiar with the meaning of these acronyms. Thus, it is part of a nurse's ethical responsibility to patients to be fluent "with terminology related to resuscitation and the capacity to support patient decisions in ways that are consistent with patient preferences and values" (ANA, 2020, p. 3).

When considering the use of CPR at the end of life or in situations in which quality of life (as perceived by the patient) is seriously compromised with little to no chance of improvement, many people have concerns about being kept alive using machines or feeding tubes rather than being allowed to die a natural death. These concerns frequently lead people to request a DNR order. The legal definition of DNR is not to initiate CPR in the event of a cardiac or pulmonary arrest (Fig. 10.2). As noted previously, DNR orders are written directives placed in a patient's medical record indicating that the use of CPR is to be avoided in the event of a life-threatening emergency. Principles that inform decisions regarding resuscitation include autonomy, nonmaleficence, respect for persons, and patient self-determination. Guided by these principles, particularly patient self-determination (see Chapter 11), a DNR order is preceded by a documented discussion with the patient, family, or surrogate decision maker addressing the patient's wishes about resuscitation interventions.

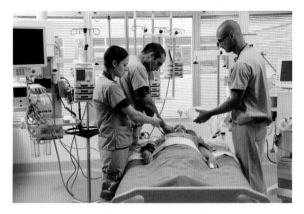

Fig. 10.2 CPR Is to be Initiated Unless There is a DNR Order. (©iStock.com/FangXiaNuo.)

In hospitals and other healthcare institutions, nurses have an active role in decisions to initiate or withhold CPR. Decisions to initiate or withhold CPR require attention to professional, ethical, legal, and institutional considerations. Nurses have the responsibility to ensure that DNR orders are documented in a patient's healthcare record, including documentation of discussion with the patient, family, or surrogate decision maker regarding the goals of care and the patient's wishes about resuscitation interventions.

Determination of whether DNR is appropriate takes into consideration the efficacy of attempting CPR, the balance of its benefits and burdens, patient wishes, and therapeutic goals (ANA, 2020). DNR decisions require open communication among the patient or surrogate, the family, and the healthcare team. This communication needs to include an explicit discussion of the efficacy and desirability of CPR, balanced with the potential harm and suffering it may cause the patient. People often overestimate the effectiveness of CPR and may not understand that CPR is not always medically indicated. To make informed decisions regarding CPR, patients and families need to understand the patient's clinical condition and prognosis. People often do not appreciate that CPR is a harsh and traumatic procedure and that patients with multiple, severe, chronic health problems who receive CPR often do not survive to be discharged (Druwe, et. al., 2020).

The relevance of considering the patient's or family's values in justifying DNR orders may vary, depending on the rationale given for the decision (ANA, 2020; Hickman et al., 2009; Jacobs, 2014). In situations in which CPR would be medically ineffective, patient autonomy and consent are considered less relevant. However, when the rationale for the decision is based on the patient's quality of life, either after or before CPR, the determination of whether the benefit of continued life outweighs the risk of harmful consequences, such as debility or suffering, must flow from the values of the patient or the patient's surrogate. Competent patients have the right to refuse CPR and may request DNR orders after they have been informed of the risks and benefits involved. Good communication is the most critical factor in ensuring that any DNR decision is acceptable to all parties involved.

DNR orders apply only to resuscitation. The fact that CPR might be considered futile does not necessarily imply that other life-sustaining interventions are futile or that other treatments will not be used. Healthcare providers often fail to make this distinction, thus causing confusion for patients as well. Many institutions require more specific instructions regarding what is and is not to be done for a patient. These interventions might include treatment of physiological abnormalities such as fever or cardiac arrhythmias, nutrition, or the use of mechanical ventilation and CPR. Plans for and parameters of DNR orders need to be discussed with all members of the healthcare team so that the goal of care is clear. **It is imperative to remember that DNR does not mean do not treat**. The presence of DNR orders requires nurses to become even more focused on providing supportive and comfort interventions and to ensure that there is no reduction in the level of care for the patient and family. A DNR order means only that in the event of cardiac or respiratory arrest, there are to be no attempts to resuscitate. Presuming there is no cardiac or respiratory arrest the patient may recover from the problem necessitating hospitalization and return home.

Many years ago Scofield suggested that decisions to not resuscitate ask us "individually and collectively, to arrive at a consensus on how to integrate death and decisions about it into the legitimating values of our moral universe. Deciding what kind of life we want involves deciding what kind of death we can face" (1995, p. 184). He noted that death, which was once considered fate, is now often a matter of a choice that we do not want to have to make. His comments are still relevant today because those involved in DNR decisions face this dilemma.

Mistaken Resuscitation

Jacob has had a chronic lung condition for the past 10 of his 32 years. The condition causes some restrictions on his life, but he has kept up with a regular job and is very involved in his church. He is currently hospitalized with a severe respiratory infection. Although his condition did not seem to be that serious, when he was admitted he made sure that there was a DNR order in his chart, noting that he has a firm religious conviction that the Creator, and not the doctor, is to decide when it is time for him to die. Because of a staff shortage, George, a registered nurse who usually works on another unit, has been assigned to Jacob's unit. Although he has been working on the other side of the unit, he is presently covering the whole unit while other staff are at lunch. As he answers a call light from Jacob's roommate, he notices that Jacob is not breathing and has no pulse. Because he is unfamiliar with Jacob's DNR request, he immediately calls a "code" and initiates CPR, figuring that there would be no question that this would be the appropriate action for someone this age. Although Jacob is successfully resuscitated and placed on a respirator for a short period of time with no serious sequelae, he is intensely angry, saying that this was interference with the Creator's plan.

Think About It

Decisions Regarding Resuscitation

- What do you think about Jacob's request for a DNR order? What ethical principles are involved in his choice?
- What do you think about George's response to the situation? Do you think he acted appropriately under the circumstances?
- How do you think you might respond in a similar situation? What principles would guide your actions?
- Describe the potential legal ramifications of this situation.
- What guidelines would your state's laws regarding DNR status offer to George? Would they support his actions?

Nursing Considerations Related to End-of-Life Decisions and DNR Orders

Although it is generally considered the domain of the physician to write a DNR order, nurses need to be aware of the parameters surrounding such orders. Some suggest that nurses are as well qualified as physicians to write DNR orders. Because nurses are professionals who are in close and continuous contact with patients, they are perhaps better able to help patients and families articulate their views regarding end-of-life care and concerns. Nursing's role and responsibilities related to end-of-life decisions include the following:

- Respecting human dignity and advocating for patient values, preferences, and right to accept, refuse, or terminate treatment
- Encouraging patients to think about end-of-life preferences in illness or a health crisis, and supporting patients/surrogates and their families in having end-of-life discussions
- Promoting informed decision making by providing patients and families with accurate and complete information about available treatment options (including choosing no treatment) in a manner that they understand; assisting them in considering risks, benefits, and potential burdens of various options; and supporting patients in reviewing and revising their end-of-life decisions as desired in response to changes in their condition or preferences
- Providing the same quality nursing care for patients with DNR orders as for any other patient, with particular attention to the patient's well-being, alleviation of suffering, and respecting and advocating for patient's preferences and values
- Ensuring that advance directives are implemented appropriately and responsibly in accordance with the patient's wishes; advocating for a patient's end-of-life preferences particularly if faced with the potential choice to not honor them by the surrogate decision maker or physician; and communicating known information that is relevant to end-of-life decisions to appropriate healthcare personnel
- Fostering discussions about end-of-life decisions that are interdisciplinary and collaborative, including the healthcare team, patient/surrogate, and family, to ensure that the patient's wishes are respected
- Being alert for emotional stress, distress, and potential moral distress associated with end-of-life decisions and patient care (for nurses as well as family), and seeking appropriate support for self and others

Ethical grounding for these roles and responsibilities is found in nursing codes of ethics and position statements. In particular, readers are encouraged to review the following:

ANA (2015) *Code of ethics for nurses with interpretive statements* Provision 1.1 – Respect for human dignity; 1.2 – Relationships with patients; 1.3 – The nature of health; 1.4 – The right to self-determination; 2.3 – Collaboration

ANA (2020) *Revised position statement: Nursing care and do not resuscitate (DNR) decisions*

CNA (2017) *Code of ethics for registered nurses* Part I C – Promoting and respecting informed decision making; D – Honoring dignity

ICN (2021). *The ICN code of ethics for nurses* Element 1 – Nurses and patients or other people requiring care or services 1.2; 1.3; 1.8; 1.11

ICN (2012). *Position Statement: Nurses' role in providing care to dying patients and their families*

In some states, persons with serious medical conditions keep a special medical order form documenting end-of-life wishes posted in a prominent place at home (or in the chart if the person is in a long-term care facility). This form specifies end-of-life wishes regarding end-of-life treatments (including DNR orders), is readily available to emergency personnel, and travels with the person to the hospital or other treatment facility as a portable medical order. A copy of the Physician Orders for Life-Sustaining Treatment form used in several states is available at https://polst.org/. Other forms of "portable" DNR orders include wallet cards, bracelets, and necklaces. Nurses need to know which patients under their care have DNR orders, and these orders need to be documented clearly in a patient's chart, and perhaps at the bedside, and reviewed periodically as the patient's condition changes. Nurses are often the bridge between patient and physician. If a patient or appropriate healthcare surrogate indicates to the nurse the desire not to be resuscitated and there is no order in the chart, the nurse should document the request in the patient's chart and bring this to the immediate attention of the physician. The nurse may wish to explore the request with the patient or surrogate and may need to facilitate a discussion of the issue between the patient and physician. Orders should specify which interventions are to be withheld and considerations regarding circumstances in which they are to be withheld. All persons involved in the care of the patient need to know about the orders. Because attitudes affect one's approach to others, nurses need to reflect on their own attitudes and biases toward decisions regarding withholding of interventions, both in general and in particular patient situations.

Artificial Sources of Nutrition and Hydration

Maintaining nutrition is a natural life-sustaining measure and a common part of the nursing role. Once a person has difficulty with functions associated with nutrition, such as chewing or swallowing, or is not conscious enough to participate in these activities, decisions about artificial sources of nutrition and hydration must be made. Ethical dilemmas arise concerning whether to classify such interventions as feeding or as medical treatments, or as ordinary or extraordinary measures. The ANA's (2017) policy on Nutrition and Hydration at the End-of-Life stresses the importance of determining whether food and fluid are more beneficial or harmful to a patient, noting that artificially provided nutrition and hydration may not be ethically justified.

Utilizing artificial sources of nutrition may present dilemmas in situations involving persons in persistent vegetative states or end-stage dying processes for whom this intervention is maintaining physical life. We know that withholding food will eventually lead to starvation and death and, under most circumstances, is not considered an ethical action. However, it is considered appropriate to withhold or discontinue life-sustaining medical interventions, including artificial sources of nutrition, when they are not benefiting the patient or are contrary to the patient's wishes. There are fewer complexities surrounding decisions to withhold artificial sources of nutrition than there are regarding decisions to withdraw medical interventions.

As with any such decision, we must consider the wishes of the patient or surrogate. Quality of life is an important factor, and if interventions contribute more to a patient's suffering, rather than relieving it, the principle of nonmaleficence may sway one toward a decision of not implementing or discontinuing such therapies. Evidence suggests that tube feeding does not improve outcomes and may have substantial risks in some patients, particularly those with dementia or multisystem illness (ANA, 2017; Geppert et al., 2010). Additionally, there is little evidence to suggest that either using or withdrawing hydration alleviates discomfort at the end of life (ANA, 2017). Healthcare providers need to ensure that patients and families understand the benefits and burdens of artificial nutrition and hydration so that they can make informed decisions. Once artificial measures have been implemented, it is often psychologically more difficult to decide on their removal. With any technological intervention, we must consider whether its use is prolonging living or prolonging dying. When competent patients refuse food or fluid, respect for persons directs nurses to honor this refusal. Nursing's role of providing high-quality care with attention to providing comfort and promoting a patient's dignity is especially important when a decision has been made to forgo artificial nutrition or hydration. Nurses need to help family and other caretakers understand that people who are dying often have a decline in appetite and that the care of keeping the person comfortable does not need to include efforts to maintain nutrition. It is often helpful to involve family in providing comfort measures, such as offering ice chips or using mouth swabs to keep the mouth moist.

Legal Issues Related to End-of-Life Technology

As noted in Chapter 8, what is considered an ethical decision by some may not be upheld as a legal action. In the area of life-sustaining technology, the courts have intervened in some decisions related to withholding or withdrawing life-sustaining treatments when there has been disagreement among the involved parties. Legal precedents regarding issues such as what constitutes clear evidence of a person's wishes related to these treatments and what is considered standard practice have been set in the process. Examples of two such cases are presented here. When one looks at dilemmas faced by families, healthcare providers, institutions, and the legal system in situations such as these, the importance of having advance directives becomes evident. **Advance directives** are instructions indicating one's wishes regarding healthcare interventions or designating someone to act as a healthcare surrogate in making such decisions in the event that one loses decision-making capacity. Advance directives are discussed in Chapter 11.

When issues arise related to technology or other aspects of care that may have an ethical component, it is appropriate for nurses to initiate an ethics consultation with the institution's ethics committee. An ethics committee is generally made up of representatives from various disciplines such as nursing, medicine, social work, and chaplains. The role of the ethics committee is to gather information about the issue from all

involved (including the patient, family, key healthcare providers, and other key persons involved in the situation); to arrange for a patient care conference, if appropriate; to develop recommendations related to resolving the issue and communicate these to the patient and healthcare team; to work with those involved as needed to come to some resolution of the issue; and to follow up on the outcome of the issue. The reader is encouraged to review the information about ethics committees and consultation found at http://www.wvnec.org/Ethics-Committee-Tools.

CASE PRESENTATION

Karen Quinlan

The seminal case of Karen Quinlan (Devettere, 1995; Pence, 1995) is the story of a 21-year-old woman who, in 1975, was found to have suffered cardiopulmonary arrest at home alone after having been drinking at a local bar. After the ambulance crew restored her heartbeat through CPR, she was admitted to the local hospital and placed on a ventilator. Within a few days, she was transferred to a larger hospital, where she was kept alive with the assistance of a respirator and feeding tube. Over months she lost weight, developed contractures, and was given no hope of regaining awareness. After much deliberation, the family asked that the respirator be discontinued, but the hospital indicated that it could not grant the request unless the father was named as her guardian. When the father asked the court to appoint him a guardian with authority to make decisions to discontinue extraordinary interventions, the court appointed him guardian of her property but not of her person and appointed a guardian ad litem to represent Karen. The guardian ad litem felt responsible for preserving Karen's life and opposed removing the respirator. The physician's lawyer argued that removing a respirator from a living person was not a standard medical procedure, and the judge sided with this view. When the family appealed the ruling to the New Jersey Supreme Court, the decision of the lower court was reversed and the father was appointed as her guardian. When the father requested that the respirator be removed, the physicians initiated a process of weaning her from it, resulting in her being able to breathe without the machine. Totally unconscious with severe contractures, she was transferred to a nursing home, where she died 10 years later.

Nancy Cruzan

In another seminal case, Nancy Cruzan was found unconscious and not breathing after her car went into a ditch in the winter of 1983 (Angell, 1990; Annas, 1990; Pence, 1995). Although emergency personnel restored her breathing, she never regained consciousness. After a year of being sustained through the use of a gastrostomy tube for artificial nutrition, it was determined that she was in a persistent vegetative state. When her parents, acting as her guardians, asked that the artificial feeding be discontinued because she had indicated previously that she would not want to be kept alive in this condition, the physicians and hospital refused. When the case went to court, the evidence supporting discontinuing the feeding was based primarily on a statement she had made to a roommate that she would not want to live if she were a vegetable. The judge ruled that the medical nutrition could be removed, but that decision was appealed to the Missouri State Supreme Court by a guardian ad litem. The Missouri Supreme Court reversed the previous decision, claiming that there was no clear and convincing evidence that this would be her wish; that she was not terminally ill or suffering; and that there was no reason to act contrary to the state's interest in preserving life, regardless of how minimal that life had become. An appeal to the US Supreme Court upheld the decision that medical nutrition could not be withdrawn because of the lack of clear and convincing evidence. In 1990, almost eight years after her accident, Nancy's parents appealed again to the local court with the evidence of three of her friends who stated that she had told them that she would not want to live in a vegetative state. At that time, the physician agreed that it was no longer in her best interests to be medically nourished, and the judge agreed that there was now clear and convincing evidence indicating that it was in her best interests to terminate artificial nutrition.

Think About It
When the Courts Intervene
- Reflect on these two cases (and the case of Terri Schiavo, presented in Chapter 11). Which position do you support, that of the family or that of the guardian ad litem?
- Which court decisions do you think are more valid? Defend your position.
- Describe the ethical principles and dilemmas evident in these situations.
- If one of your family members was in a similar situation, how do you think you would respond? Would you expect solidarity or disagreement with this position from other members of your family?
- Consider that you are a nurse caring for Karen or Nancy at various stages in her situation. How would you feel about caring for her? How would you respond to the various parties involved as decisions about her care are being discussed? How would codes of nursing ethics guide your response?
- What do you think about the role of the legal system in decisions regarding the use of technology?

End-of-Life Care—Palliative Care and Hospice

Palliative care focuses on enhancing the quality of life for patients and families living with serious illness such as cancer, heart, liver and lung diseases, Parkinson disease, and others. Patients of any age or stage of their illness are eligible for palliative care. Palliative care interventions focused on management of pain, other symptoms, and stressors related to the illness are integrated with curative and other medical interventions with a goal of helping patients to be as functional as they can in body, mind, and spirit. Palliative care is an option for end-of-life care for people who wish to continue receiving interventions focused on possible cure or limiting disease progression even to the point of death. Many health insurances pay for palliative care.

Hospice has a specialized palliative care focus. When life-sustaining interventions are no longer of benefit or are not desired by the patient, the focus of care is directed toward comfort and support. Hospice care is comprehensive, interdisciplinary, and total care, focusing primarily on the comfort and support of patients and families who face terminal illness that is no longer responsive to curative treatment (ANA, 2016; NCHPC, 2018). Hospice focuses on the best quality of life for the patient and family through meticulous control of pain and other symptoms, a personalized plan to optimize the quality of life as defined by the patient and family, and spiritual and psychosocial care. Palliative care requires the delivery of coordinated and continuous services in the home, hospice centers, skilled nursing facilities, or a hospital and includes support in bereavement. Members of the hospice care team include nurses, physicians, spiritual support persons, pharmacists, social services, mental health services, in-home caregivers, and pain services. Eligibility for hospice requires a prognosis of six months or less to live (although coverage can be extended beyond this time) and is regulated by Medicare. Further comparison of Hospice and Palliative care can be found through the websites of the National Hospice and Palliative Care Organization https://www.nhpco.org/wp-content/uploads/2019/04/PalliativeCare_VS_Hospice.pdf and the National Institute on Aging https://www.nia.nih.gov/health/what-are-palliative-care-and-hospice-care.

Primary obligations that we have to people who are dying are comfort, relief of suffering, and compassionate presence (ANA, 2016; CNA, 2017, Part I.D.11; ICN, 2012) The backbone of hospice and palliative care is good nursing care that continues to support the dignity and self-respect of the patient and family. In addition to providing care to the patient and the family, nurses often coordinate hospice and palliative care teams. When families disagree about when it is time to stop other interventions and focus on comfort care, the nurse's ability to communicate effectively with and facilitate communication among those involved is crucial. Families often need time to see what we see regarding the patient's condition and the expected outcomes of various interventions. We have to be willing to take as much time as necessary and as often as needed to explain and negotiate care decisions. Care conferences focused on end-of-life choices and decisions may be initiated by nurses or physicians as part of the plan of care or may come about after a request for an ethics committee consult. Such conferences can take different forms. Box 10.1 illustrates one approach to an end-of-life care conference.

BOX 10.1   Sample Process for Palliative/Hospice Care Conference

- Have a holistic view of the patient, including present health status, prognosis, significant relationships, living situation, family dynamics, decision-making capacity, advance directives or healthcare surrogate, and spiritual support.
- If the patient does not have decision-making capacity and there is no surrogate, seek to have a surrogate named.
- Before scheduling the conference, inform the patient or surrogate that the purpose of the meeting is to determine the best way to provide quality end-of-life care to the patient and family, and stress the need for family and significant persons, including spiritual support persons, to participate. The conference is set at a time when most people can be there. The primary nurse, physician, and palliative care, hospice, and other involved healthcare team members are included.
- In opening the meeting, the palliative/hospice care team member describes the process that will be followed to allow everyone an opportunity to speak and ask questions and to arrive at a consensus regarding what is truly best for the patient.
- The meeting is opened by introducing everyone present and their role or relationship with the patient. To prevent any confusion that can occur with the high emotions of the circumstances, those present are asked one by one, beginning with the patient/surrogate, to name things that they enjoyed in life and what is important now. This process helps the physician and other care providers step back from the clinical picture and see the patient as a person with individual values and meaning. Next, the physician is asked to discuss the current status and prognosis, allowing an opportunity for the family to ask any questions. The primary nurse is then asked to discuss daily care and interactions with the patient and to respond to any questions. The patient and family are able to ask questions as needed. Through this process, the family is often able to acknowledge that their loved one will not return to the state they once enjoyed, which leads to the beginning of acceptance and consideration of what is truly best for the patient at this time.
- When the patient does not have decision-making capacity, everyone in turn is asked what they know or believe to be the desires of their loved one regarding end-of-life care. This includes the values of the patient and what family members consider to be in the best interest. This process may prompt tears and reminiscing. Spiritual support persons may comment about the patient's spiritual values and considerations or intervene as needed to support those participating.
- Throughout this process, the hospice/palliative care team member periodically restates what the general consensus of the group seems to be. This helps clarify what is being said and provides an opportunity for anyone present to bring up concerns or issues. The meeting generally concludes with consensus regarding what is best for the patient and discussion regarding comfort measures desired by the patient/family and that the care providers feel will best suit the patient. (In some situations more than one meeting may be needed before consensus is reached.)
- Those involved may remain with the patient after the meeting for further conversation, reminiscing, silent presence, and perhaps prayer to the extent they are comfortable with this. The family usually has open visitation and is involved as much as they wish in care for the patient.
- Documentation of the process, participants, content, and outcomes is completed in the patient's record, and ongoing follow-up is initiated.

Examples of Potential Ethical Dilemmas With Other Technological Interventions

In addition to life-sustaining interventions, advances in technology affect nursing and healthcare in other arenas. Examples of selected technologies are briefly presented here. Nurses who work with patients whose care involves such technologies need to be aware of potential ethical issues associated with their use, as well as the benefits of such interventions. The intention here is to alert the reader to some of the questions and dilemmas that may be associated with these technologies. The reader is encouraged to explore these areas further, reflecting on personal values related to each technology.

Assisted Reproduction

Because the inability to conceive and bear children can be a very distressing experience for a couple, any technology that can facilitate the process may be viewed as a life-affirming gift. Such technologies include artificial insemination by donor, in vitro fertilization, and surrogate embryo transfer. Although scientists develop and refine these technologies to benefit people, ethicists and others raise questions related to the moral implications of their use. Some questions focus on the potential for changing society's concept of family and parenthood. For example, in the case of surrogacy, is the mother of the baby the woman whose ovum is joined with her husband's sperm or the woman who donates her body for the baby's development and birth? A question to ponder is whether the use of such technologies might relegate childbearing to little more than the production of a product. Other ethical questions arise regarding who has custody of frozen embryos and whether these embryos have rights. A related consideration is the potential that women may become more exploited than liberated by the use of these technologies. Because these interventions are expensive, questions arise regarding who should pay for them and for whom they should be made available. For example, there are racial and ethnic disparities regarding the availability of some of these technologies. Ethical considerations regarding these technologies include attention to societal attitudes about who should or should not have children and what kind of children should be born. Another potential ethical concern is the public availability of DNA testing for exploring one's genealogy. This technology enables people to identify and link with others who share the same DNA, which may give rise to issues of confidentiality related to the identity of sperm or egg donors.

Genetics and Genomics

The NIH National Genome Research Institute (2018) defines **genetics** as "the study of genes and their roles in inheritance" that "involves scientific studies of genes and their effects," and **genomics** as "the study of all of a person's genes (the genome), including interactions of those genes with each other and with the person's environment… [and] includes the scientific study of complex diseases such as heart disease, asthma, diabetes, and cancer." Advances in genetics and genomics offer possible remedies for many diseases and other health concerns through new technologies for screening, diagnosis, and both physical and pharmacological interventions. These can benefit patients and enhance healthcare services. Implications for nurses are that "patients now expect nurses to have an understanding of the care issues around genetics" and that "the ethical dimension is of paramount concern for nurses, who now have to take into account the ethical challenges around offering these new treatments" (ANA, 2023). In addition to the ethical challenges, there are legal and social justice questions.

Genetic diagnosis and **genetic engineering** are examples of two technologies that impact nursing practice. Genetic diagnosis, which is usually done within an in vitro fertilization program, involves a process of biopsy of embryos to determine the presence of genetic flaws and gender before implantation. Such diagnosis is generally aimed at couples who have a high risk of conceiving a child with a serious genetic disorder, with the intent that only embryos that are free of genetic flaws would be implanted.

Genetic engineering is the ability to alter organisms genetically for a variety of purposes, such as developing more disease-resistant fruits and vegetables, or eventually being able to alter embryos genetically so that the fetus and baby will be healthier. Through **genetic screening** it is possible to determine whether persons are predisposed to certain diseases and whether couples have the possibility of giving birth to a genetically impaired infant. **Good genetic counseling** is imperative before genetic screening, as well as clear discussion of results and the implications of the findings. When genetic testing reveals information about a patient's health status that could have serious health implications for that patient's relatives and the patient does not want to share the information, healthcare providers may be faced with an ethical dilemma—feeling a duty to warn the family members, while at the same time feeling bound to honor patient confidentiality (Beamer, 2017; Weaver, 2016). A trusting, respectful, and caring relationship between patient and provider is critical to working through such situations.

The implications of having technologies for **genetic modification** available include the potential for correcting some genetic defects in the embryo, eliminating some very serious genetic diseases, and producing food that is more nourishing and resilient. We must, however, make a distinction between the therapeutic use of these interventions and the possibility that these interventions may be used to modify human characteristics beyond those that are needed to sustain or restore health. The possibility of their use to enhance certain human characteristics has significant social implications. For example, such interventions could offer control over genetic inheritance, including the biological properties and personality traits of children. Ethical concerns that arise in relation to genetically engineering an embryo for implantation include who holds the copyright for the modifications, whether insurance companies have access to the DNA if they pay for the procedure, and how this practice might change us as a species (Ball, 2017).

The ability to discard "undesirable" traits and improve those that are "desirable" may lead to a form of **eugenics**, meaning "good birth." The eugenics movement of the early 20th century sought to promote traits that proponents felt were desirable for society, while weeding out what they considered undesirable. In the United States and elsewhere around the world, eugenics led to efforts to discourage procreation among people deemed to be "socially inferior" through compulsory sterilization of many people, particularly those who were poor, in prison, of nondominant races or ethnicity, or in mental institutions. Another concern that nurses need to be aware of is the potential for these technologies to lead to the imposition of a skewed or harmful definition of what is normal regarding human traits, as well as what is considered abnormal or undesirable. Because individuals and societies tend to impose their values and

standards on others, this could lead to serious transcultural implications.

Concerns related to these technologies are as varied as their potential benefits, particularly the recognition that relaxing criteria related to a person's value or rights in one arena may lead to abuses or exploitation in other circumstances. Ethicists often speak of these concerns in terms of a slippery slope where, for example, one decision based on relaxing criteria supporting the value of human life makes it easy to slide into acceptance of lower standards as ethical guides. For example, one concern is that genetic engineering might produce organisms that could be harmful to humans; another is that employers or insurers might use information gained from genetic screening to exclude people with particular traits from certain jobs or from being insured. Might genetic screening and diagnosis lead to abuses, such as forbidding people with certain traits to have children, insurers refusing to cover expenses if insured mothers give birth to genetically impaired infants, or prohibiting the birth of babies with particular genetic features deemed undesirable by those in power in a society? These areas include other broad societal implications, such as who pays for the procedures, who determines guidelines for their use, and to whom they are made available. Readers are encouraged to explore this issue further at NIH National Human Genome Research Institute: https://www.genome.gov/about-genomics/fact-sheets/Genetics-vs-Genomics and International Society of Nurses in Genetics: https://www.isong.org/.

Cloning and Stem Cell Research

In spite of their potential benefit for human health, some biotechnologies raise serious ethical concerns even in the research phase. Cloning and embryonic stem cell (ESC) research are examples of technologies that continue to engender debate among ethicists and within the public forum. Ethical concerns related to these technologies are briefly discussed here, and readers are encouraged to deepen their understanding of the scientific and ethical debate surrounding these technologies through further study.

Cloning is the process of creating a cell or an entire organism that is identical in every way to another. Types of cloning include molecular, cellular, and cloning of entire organisms. Techniques of mammalian cloning include embryo twinning and somatic cell nuclear transplantation. The prospect of using somatic cell nuclear transfer to create human beings raises the greatest ethical concern (Werner-Felmayer & Shalev, 2015). The national and international debate on the issue acknowledges that cloning can be both useful and damaging for human health and that both advantages and disadvantages need to be considered. Häyry (2018) notes that the discussion is not progressing regarding the ethical acceptability of human cloning, rather arguments have focused on similar issues such as cloning posing a threat to one's genetic identity, human dignity, and integrity for several decades. The stance of the international nursing community is that vigorous national and international analysis; monitoring; and debate of the ethical, social, legal, scientific, and health concerns related to human cloning are needed and that there must be a mandatory presence of nurses on policy boards examining these issues. Nursing's position includes support for scholarly examination of the implications of core professional nursing values for cloning in humans and ethical analysis of the possible merits of different techniques of cloning for human health.

The ethical concerns surrounding stem cell research vary depending on the origin of the stem cells. Human stem cells used in research are termed *adult, embryonic*, and *germline*, based on how they are obtained (Hyun, 2018). Adult stem cells (ASC) are cells found in adults that can replace old cells by reproducing new ones. Blood cells and liver cells are two examples. Bone marrow transplants are examples of the use of ASC in therapy. Stem cells retrieved from umbilical cord blood after birth have similar properties to ASC and are also used in the treatment for some forms of leukemia. Embryonic stem cells (ESC) are collected from the inner cell mass of an early embryo, thus destroying the embryo. These cells are unspecified (or pluripotent), meaning that they have the ability to develop into any type of cell in the body except the placenta. They also are able to renew themselves indefinitely in the laboratory. Embryonic germline stem cells are immature cells that can become sperm and egg cells. The goal of stem cell research is a relief of human suffering, which, ethically, is good. Potential benefits of interventions developed through stem cell research include therapies for Parkinson disease, regenerating various tissues that are diseased, and using ESC to develop an entire organ to be used for transplant.

The main controversy surrounding stem cell research focuses on the use of ESC, because the process of obtaining these cells results in the destruction of the embryo. There are two main objections to stem cell research (Guenin, 2008; Hyun, 2018). The first focuses on whether the destruction of the human embryo constitutes the killing of a human being. The second objection raises the concern that, if one considers that research on human embryos is not wrong in itself, would it lead to a slippery slope of treating human life as a commodity through practices that are dehumanizing, such as using fetuses for spare parts? Views about when human life begins and whether the early embryo is considered a person with moral status are at the heart of ethical deliberations related to ESC research. Those who believe that human life and personhood begin at conception hold that the destruction of a human embryo constitutes killing; thus, stem cell research using ESC is never morally allowed. Those who hold the view that the embryo is afforded personhood at the point of viability may consider use of early embryonic tissue permissible for research. Those who suggest that sentience, life history, and memory are requirements for personhood argue that the early embryo does not possess personhood; thus, it is morally acceptable to do ESC research using the early embryonic tissue if this may benefit human health.

Other ethical concerns related to stem cell research include issues of obtaining informed consent from donors, the potential of combining ESC and cloning techniques, issues of ownership of the biological materials derived from the cells, the potential development of embryo farms, and stem cell tourism. Stem cell tourism refers to *stem cell clinics* run by unscrupulous clinicians around the world who exploit patients by indicating they can provide effective stem cell therapies for conditions other than the few conditions for which stem cell therapy has become the clinical standard of care. These clinics are very expensive and lack patient protection, oversight, transparency, credible scientific rationale, and regulated research protocols (Hyun, 2018). Because outcomes of stem cell research have the potential to alter human genetics and the human life cycle, there can be social and environmental consequences of extending human life, as well as a shift in our understanding of what it means to be human (Ball, 2017; Lauritzen, 2005). The need for monitoring stem cell research is addressed by the International Society for Stem Cell Research in their *Guidelines for Stem Cell Research and Clinical Translation* (ISSCR, 2022). Among other things, these guidelines stress the need for rigor, integrity, transparency, and informed consent from donors related to both use and reuse of materials in both research and clinical applications.

Organ and Tissue Procurement and Transplantation

Organ transplantation is no longer considered as extraordinary or uncommon a healthcare event as it was in the not-too-distant past. As techniques become more refined, the possibility of a transplant becomes a hope for more and more people afflicted with the failure of a vital organ. Because the demand for organs is great and the supply limited, dilemmas related to allocation of scarce resources emerge. Questions arise regarding the eligibility of recipients for organ transplant. Should these determinations be made based on a potential recipient's expectation of survival posttransplant, or ability to pay for the procedure, or power and prestige, or some combination of these and other factors? Transplantation may involve organs from dead or living human donors, animals, or artificial appliances, and there are dilemmas associated with each. This discussion focuses on human donor issues.

Because transplantation requires well-nourished organs, procurement must occur as soon after death as possible. Thus, having criteria for determining when death occurs is imperative. Irreversible cessation of cardiopulmonary functioning is one such criterion. However, until CPR has been attempted, how is one to know if the cessation is irreversible? If CPR is initiated, organs to be donated may be damaged, raising an issue of how to deal with a person's desire to be an organ donor with consideration for CPR. Questions regarding when and how intensively to initiate CPR become important issues regarding organ donation.

If a person has been maintained on life-support technology, brain death is the most likely criteria to be used, which leads to issues regarding what constitutes death. Currently, the most commonly accepted definition of brain death is the irreversible cessation of all brain function, including the brainstem. However, there are no uniform medically accepted standards regarding criteria for determining that brain function has ceased (Pope & Okninski, 2016). Some argue that if vital functions are maintained through the use of life-sustaining technologies, death has not occurred. Others reflect that in the case of brain death, these technologies are just permitting the cells and tissues to be maintained in a living state even though the person has died. An ethical concern that arises in such circumstances is distinguishing between living human beings and living human cells when making decisions related to discontinuing life-sustaining technologies (Condic, 2016). In recent years there have been legal cases that challenge whether medical criteria used to determine brain death satisfy legal requirements for being both *medically accepted standards* and rigorous enough to accurately measure irreversible cessation of all functions in the whole brain (Pope & Okninski, 2016). Nurses providing care in the midst of such challenges and debates still need to focus on providing compassionate care for the patient and family, while also addressing their own needs for self-care related to moral distress that such care may engender.

The scarcity of available organs and the long waiting lists of potential recipients raise the possibility that people may be declared dead prematurely. This scarcity of organs also affects organ procurement from living human beings. With living donors, issues related to voluntary informed consent and the buying and selling of organs are of concern. There are places in the world where organs are taken from poor people or prisoners, without their knowledge or against their will, and sold to procurement centers in more affluent countries. Desperate straits have prompted some individuals to sell an organ to raise money for personal or family needs, raising a question about whether there can be true voluntary informed consent under such circumstances.

In cases of sudden accidental death, family members may be asked to consider donation of viable organs. Consider whether there can be true voluntary consent when the family is in the midst of crisis and shock. With the urgency for a decision due to time factors for harvesting organs, coercion could be a factor. In some settings, nurses are expected to approach patients or families about considering organ donation. In such situations, nurses need to be clear about their own feelings regarding organ procurement and transplantation, and they must remember that attention to family needs takes precedence over the time constraints of organ harvesting.

Ethics and Information Technology

The explosion of information technology related to communication and storage of healthcare information, although beneficial in many ways, poses risks to privacy and confidentiality of protected health information (PHI) unknown in the past. The use of electronic medical records (EMRs), fax machines, e-mail, texts, digital communication and other Internet transactions, patient clinical portals, cellular phones, and telehealth consultation have become commonplace in healthcare settings. Computerized medical databases, including EMRs, are standard in both private practice settings and in large organizations such as hospitals, clinics, and national systems such as the Veterans Health Administration. Patient information and images can be stored on tablets, laptops, CDs, DVDs, thumb drives, and cell phones; transmitted to cloud storage or industry platforms; or shared via e-mail. Handheld electronic devices, although convenient, are easily misplaced or stolen, and confidential patient information on these devices can be compromised.

EMR systems have many benefits, such as providing ready access to patient healthcare information by practitioners, the ability to facilitate communication and ease of sharing data about patients among healthcare team members, and ability to flag and monitor important patient health data and health promotion protocols. However, any method of electronically storing, retrieving, or transferring PHI also poses the possibility of unintentional breaches in confidentiality. Because practitioners, including nurses, cannot completely control access to computerized databases, concern arises that patients may withhold important health information or refrain from seeking care due to fear that their records will not remain private. Although the Health Insurance Portability and Accountability Act (HIPAA) regulations are designed to protect the privacy and security of any electronic transactions of PHI, data breaches do occur. Privacy breaches may occur at the level of the primary user, that is, those who collect, process, and store PHI (such as physicians, nurses, and pharmacists); at the level of the secondary user (such as third-party payers and the health information services industry); and at the level of the technology itself through lack of proper encryption techniques, security loopholes that enable hacking of stored data, or improper disposal of old equipment without purging private information. Other US federal regulations give the Department of Homeland Security the power to bypass HIPAA regulations and access health information for security reasons. See Chapter 8 for further discussion of HIPAA privacy requirements.

Nurses must be careful not to violate patients' rights to confidentiality. The ethical and legal obligation to protect the confidentiality of patient information requires that nurses implement appropriate safeguards when storing and transferring PHI electronically. Healthcare institutions, professional organizations, and other agencies have policies and procedures aimed at ensuring the privacy and confidentiality of PHI. These policies include:

- Ensuring that computer systems have security software, effective virus protection that is updated frequently, overwrite protection, password-protected screen savers, and ways to limit the visibility of information on the screen for anyone other than the person using the computer
- Using secure passwords that are changed regularly and not shared with others
- Using only agency e-mail for transmission of health information that includes a confidentiality statement and precautions to prevent misdirected e-mail
- Never using personal e-mail to discuss or transfer data pertaining to patients
- Including a confidentiality statement on the cover sheet when faxing PHI
- Only storing PHI on institution-approved electronic devices (including notebook computers and tablets) that use data encryption technology, taking care to maintain physical control of the device, using a secure password when turning on the device and a timeout to reactivate the password, and backing up any confidential information using approved back-up procedures
- Ensuring that all private information is purged from devices that are no longer used for care of the patient or when discarding the device

Nurses need to be alert to any breach of confidentiality of health records or information related to the use of electronic devices, take action to correct the situation, and be involved in developing policies and guidelines aimed at safeguarding the confidentiality of all health information and records (ANA, 2015, Provision 3.1; CNA, 2017, Part I.E; ICN, 2021, Element 1.4; 1.5).

Ethical Concerns Related to Electronic Medical Records

In addition to issues related to privacy and confidentiality, healthcare providers can experience other ethical challenges when using EMR systems. McBride et al. (2018) highlight several ethical concerns related to using EMRs in clinical practice. Documentation in EMRs can pose challenges to the quality of care and patient safety. Systems vary in their complexity of use and the number of menus and screens nurses and other providers need to "click" on to access and record patient information. This adds time to patient encounters, and practitioners may choose to "streamline" charting in various ways to meet institutional expectations regarding the number of patients seen or to be able to leave work on time. The available computerized templates may not allow the recording of patient-specific variations in physical findings and fail to fully capture the patient's story related to the health concern, resulting in the possibility that the treatment plan is developed with incomplete information. Clinicians may copy and paste patient data to speed up the time spent in documentation, leading to a risk of having outdated symptoms, assessments, diagnoses, medication lists, and treatment plans associated with a current visit. Clinician fatigue in utilizing EMRs can lead to false entries, which can follow patients for years with a possibility of afwfecting things like applying for insurance. Nurses and other providers may experience moral distress due to the overemphasis on documentation and meeting electronic quality measures at the expense of quality patient care.

Another area that raises ethical concerns described by McBride et al. (2018) relates to clinical decision support (CDS) processes embedded within the EMR. The CDS process is linked to evidence-based protocols that alert clinical providers to such things as pertinent clinical information and evidence-based guidelines for care related to patient health concerns and to electronic quality measures on which the organization can be penalized if the measures are not met. Patient safety and quality-of-care issues can arise when CDS and other information within the EMR is not aligned with the clinical judgment of the healthcare team. Nurses need to remember that technologies are meant to assist in clinical practice and are not replacements for nurses' knowledge and skills. Critical thinking and accurate clinical assessment that lead to appropriate diagnosis and interventions for the patient are essential. Relying on an EMR-suggested protocol without critical thinking regarding other possibilities based on a more complete picture of the patient can jeopardize patient safety and quality of care.

CASE PRESENTATION

EMR Protocols and Clinical Judgment

McBride et al. (2018) give an example of a patient presenting to a busy emergency department with symptoms that result in the patient scoring high on the hospital sepsis tool embedded in the EMR. The nurse, who has worked in the emergency department for 10 years, assesses the patient and finds both pitting edema and crackles in both lungs. She is aware that the afebrile patient has had a prior admission with fluid overload from heart failure and suspects that the patient's symptoms may more likely reflect an exacerbation of heart failure with possible pulmonary edema. Treatment guidelines according to the Clinical Decision Support Software sepsis alert call for fluid resuscitation, which would create a risk for fluid overload if the patient's symptoms are reflective of heart failure. The physician is ready to initiate treatment for sepsis based on the protocol and have the patient admitted to the intensive care unit. The nurse is concerned about this decision and feels the physician is paying more attention to meeting the hospital's sepsis quality metrics than to addressing the patient's full clinical picture.

Think About It

- What ethical issues are evident in this situation?
- What is the nurse's professional responsibility in this case?
- What do you think the nurse should do to address her concerns about the patient's situation?
- How would nursing codes of ethics guide the nurse's actions in this situation?
- If the physician initiates treatment for sepsis, what would be the nurse's moral duty to the patient?
- What institutional or other barriers might be present that would keep the nurse from being able to fully advocate for patient safety in this situation?
- How might this situation lead to moral distress or moral reckoning?

Ethical Issues Related to Social Media

Social media is part of the fabric of our lives, both personally and globally. Social media refers to various online and mobile tools and platforms that enable the sharing of information, images, video and audio clips; developing online content; and communicating with others who one knows and does not know. Social media include social networking sites like Facebook and LinkedIn, as well as Twitter, Instagram, TikTok, blogs (personal and professional), discussion forums, professional networks, podcasting, YouTube and other video-sharing sites, chat rooms, texts, and the like. Professional organizations acknowledge the benefits of using social media to access health promotion information and programs and in helping nurses keep a dialog with other professionals, keep up with ever-changing healthcare developments, access continuing education, and the like (ANA, 2011; ICN, 2015; NCSBN, 2018). However, the inappropriate use of social media by nurses can cause both ethical concerns and legal problems.

Ethical issues related to nurses' use of social media most frequently involve breaches of privacy and confidentiality. Examples of such breaches include posting to personal social media sites any patient-related information such as photos, descriptions of care and interactions, or derogatory comments, even if the nurse believes the patient cannot be identified. Nurses need to take care when discussing events of their work experiences and frustration online or through social media and avoid comments about patients or coworkers that may include potentially identifiable characteristics. Violation of patient confidentiality and privacy rules is contrary to professional ethics and can potentially lead to legal action and discipline by the board of nursing. Other violations of ethical principles related to inappropriate use of social media by nurses include lateral violence against colleagues through derogatory or threatening online posts, failure to report others for media posts that violate patient privacy, violation of professional boundaries by contacting patients or former patients through social media, and posts that reflect unethical or unprofessional conduct (Balestra, 2018; Lachman, 2013). Nurses need to be aware that anything posted online is discoverable, permanent, and easily public, even within "private" sites. Balestra (2018) notes that personal posts by nurses such as those related to alcohol or drug use, profanity, racially derogatory comments, inappropriate photos, and the like may negatively affect their professional life. Remember that social media posts can unintentionally become public and be discovered by employers, teachers, and the board of nursing.

Because of the impact of social media on professional practice and ethics, the American Nurses Association (ANA, 2011), the International Council of Nurses (ICN, 2015), and the National Council of State Boards of Nursing (NCSBN, 2018) have each developed principles and practices to guide nurses in their use of this technology (Fig. 10.3). They all reflect that professional codes of conduct, standards, and policies apply equally to online activities as to other activities of nurses, both personal and professional. They remind nurses to maintain patient privacy at all times and to keep the professional and personal use of social media separate (which includes not using personal social media while at work). The NCSBN (2018) social media guidelines call on the nurse to strictly safeguard all patient information gathered during the course of treatment. The following guidelines are excerpted from a more comprehensive list available on the NCSBN website: (1) nurses must not identify patients by name, post, or publish information that may lead to the patient's identification; (2) nurses must not use personal devices to take, transmit, or post any photo or video images of patients; (3) nurses must not refer to patients in a disparaging manner on social media; (4) nurses must maintain appropriate professional boundaries of the nurse–patient relationship on social media; (5) nurses must immediately report any breach of confidentiality or privacy; and (6) nurses must comply with all employer policies related to employer-owned computers, cameras and other electronic devices, and use of personal devices in the workplace (NCSBN, 2018). *The International Council of Nurses Position Statement—Nurses and Social Media is outlined in* Box 10.2. The ANA (2011) *and the* Canadian Nurse Protective Society (2023) *have published similar principles and guidelines for nurses regarding social networking.* Students are encouraged to retrieve and study the guidelines developed by each of the nursing organizations noted here, as well as the HIPAA social media policies. Websites are included with "Discussion Questions and Activities" at the end of this chapter.

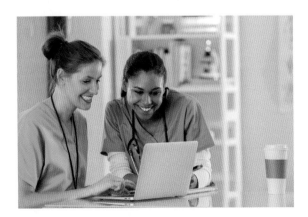

Fig. 10.3 Nurses Must Observe Standards of Patient Privacy and Confidentiality at All Times and in All Environments, Including Online. (©iStock.com/Steve Debenport.)

BOX 10.2   The International Council of Nurses Position Statement

Nurses and Social Media

Nurses need to:

- Educate themselves about both the opportunities in the use of social media in relation to enhancing knowledge and informing practice and healthcare teaching and the risks related to its use.
- Adhere to legal, regulatory, institutional, and/or organizational standards, guidelines, policies, and codes of conduct with respect to the use of social media and apply these codes, standards, guidelines, and policies equally to online activities as they do in other activities.
- Ensure they have the required competencies, are practicing within their scope of practice, and are legally authorized to do so if providing health information, advice, or services through social media.
- Be aware of the quality and reliability of information online and recognize how this information affects patients' health and illness experiences.
- Inform and educate patients regarding both the opportunities and risks related to social media in the context of their health.
- Keep personal and professional use of social media separate and refrain from using social media for personal use while at work.
- Maintain patient privacy and confidentiality at all times and not discuss issues related to their workplace online or post any information relating to patients or their families.

- Formally seek approval if they are going to record or archive interactions with patients and be aware of the legal position in terms of access to such material in conduct cases or when there are legal proceedings.
- Respect the boundaries of the therapeutic nurse–patient relationship and not connect with or accept patients or former patients as electronic "friends" on personal social media sites due to the risk of breaching therapeutic relationships.
- Refrain from posting defamatory or offensive comments about employers, educational institutions, colleagues, or patients and be aware that an unnamed patient or person may be identifiable from posted information.
- Report identified breaches of privacy or confidentiality.
- Be aware of and use privacy settings to maintain control of access to personal information.
- Be aware of copyright restrictions and the risks of breaching copyright when posting information online.
- Be aware of the rapidity of communication through social media outlets and the possibility of instant reposts or retweets and therefore the importance of being thoughtful of what is being communicated before posting.
- Recognize that everything posted online is public and permanent, even if deleted, and that using pseudonyms does not provide anonymity.
- Be aware of the image they are portraying when posting content even when not work related and help reinforce a positive global image of nursing.

(From International Council of Nurses, Geneva, Switzerland.)

CASE PRESENTATION

Patient Confidentiality and Social Media

Nurses have an ethical and legal obligation to ensure patient confidentiality. Posting any patient-related information to social media, even generalized comments without identifiers is a violation of patient confidentiality. Although the breach of confidentiality may be unintentional, there can be serious consequences. Consider the following real-life case situations:

1. A nurse posted several comments on Facebook about a child with a rare case of measles at her hospital. The nurse had previously been antivaccination and commented about her experience of seeing a boy suffering from a disease that could have been prevented through vaccination.
2. After work one night, while at home, a nurse posted on her social media page her frustrations and anger about having worked to save the life of the man accused of killing a policeman, saying she had come face-to-face

with a "cop killer." She did not discuss his condition or any identifying information.

3. Several nurses who worked in the same emergency department discussed patients on social media, taking care not to post any identifying information.
4. While contributing to a public blog, a nurse discussed a specific patient, without using the name, but included other details in the description that made it possible to identify who the patient was.
5. A nursing home employee took a cell phone photo of a resident's genitals and sent it to a friend, who posted it on a social media site.

Think About It

Dealing With Inappropriate Use of Social Media by Nurses

- Review the ANA, ICN, CNPS, NCSBN, and HIPAA principles and guidelines for use of social media by nurses.

Where is there evidence of a lack of following professional standards and guidelines in these cases?

- Do you think there is a breach of patient confidentiality when there are no patient identifiers included in a post or discussion? How might a third party know who the patient might be?
- Would you consider these situations to be intentional violations of privacy?
- Discuss how the patient in each of these situations could be harmed.
- If you were a colleague of any of these nurses and discovered their posts, how would you respond? What would be your professional responsibility?
- What do you think the consequences should be in each of these case situations? Review the actual outcomes

next and discuss whether you think they are appropriate consequences.

Outcomes of These Cases

1. The nurse was fired for violating HIPAA rules by posting PHI on a social media website.
2. The nurse was fired after this posting on social media—the patient was easily identifiable.
3. These nurses were fired for discussing patients on social media. Although no identifying information was posted, they had violated the hospital's HIPAA policy.
4. The nurse received a warning, almost lost her job, and had her reputation marred.
5. The employee was fired. Legal action was taken, and both were charged with invasion of privacy and conspiracy.

NURSING PRACTICE IN A TECHNOLOGICAL AGE

Nursing practice continues to evolve with expanding knowledge and scientific advances in many areas. As healthcare technology continues to be developed and refined, related nursing responsibilities also expand in response to the evolving technologies. In the midst of these changes, the essence of nursing remains the human focus of caring for patients and families—being attentive to the needs of persons whose lives are affected by technology. Integrating caring with attention to technology and juggling the demands of patients and families present challenges for nurses in any area of practice. As new technologies become available, they will bring with them associated issues of concern. Regardless of the technology, important considerations for nursing relate to patient safety and quality of care, attitudes and values, communication, maintaining the human focus of care, and personal well-being.

Alarm Fatigue—Unintended Consequence of Medical Technology

Computerization of healthcare technology is aimed at providing careful monitoring of patients and alerting nurses and other caregivers to significant changes in the patient's condition. However, there are unintended consequences associated with this technology. Nurses who work in hospitals, particularly in intensive care units, are inundated with alarms and alert signals associated with medical equipment, monitoring devices, patient-safety aides, electronic charting, and other technologies that are integral to patient care. The ever-present alarms

vary in significance from critical or urgent to routine, and attention to operating and monitoring the various devices along with the constancy of the alarms can cause sensory overload for nurses. This may cause nurses to feel overwhelmed and to become desensitized to the alarm sounds and their importance. This is known as **alarm fatigue** (Lewandowska et al., 2020; Gorisek et al., 2021; Asadi et al., 2022). Ethical concerns related to alarm fatigue include risks to patient safety, diminished quality of care, moral distress, and nurse burnout. When nurses become desensitized to alarm sounds, they may miss alarms of a critical or urgent nature or delay responding to them, putting patient safety at risk. The time and focus nurses need to direct to medical equipment and technology takes time away from providing the quality of care for patients they would like to give. The stress of dealing with the technology coupled with not being able to provide the quality of patient care nurses feel is necessary can lead to moral distress and nurse burnout. Ultimately moral distress has a negative impact on both the nurse's health and on patient care. The ever-present alarms can also be distressing for patients, interrupting sleep, causing too much auditory stimulation, and ultimately affecting the healing process.

Nurses need to be alert for environmental factors such as alarms that affect their patients, their ability to provide safe and quality patient care, and their own physical and mental well-being, and to take steps to minimize or control these factors as much as possible. Nursing organizations such as the American Association of Critical-Care Nurses (AACN, 2018) offer strategies for managing alarms to decrease alarm fatigue. Recognizing the need to address the issue of alarm fatigue the Joint Commission (2021) included *Improve the safety of clinical alarm systems* as a national patient safety goal for the hospital program.

Attitudes and Values

The importance of self-awareness related to values, beliefs, and reactions, as discussed in Chapter 4, is especially significant when dealing with issues related to technology. The process of being more attentive to personal perspectives regarding such issues as quality of life, living, dying, medical futility, and allocation of scarce resources may be facilitated by pondering questions such as those posed throughout this chapter. Such awareness enables the nurse to differentiate personal values from those of patients and others involved in the situation. Principles of self-determination and autonomy counsel the nurse to understand that individuals may judge the benefits of an intervention from varying perspectives. Recognizing where personal values may be different from those of the patient enables nurses to be more attentive to fostering good communication, encouraging others to make their own decisions, avoiding judgment about the rightness or wrongness of the decision based on personal values, and accepting those decisions even if they are different from what the nurse would do.

As the various examples presented in this chapter suggest, many dilemmas that emerge surrounding technology relate to differing values among the parties involved. Facilitating discussion of values among patients and families may help them clarify their own perspectives. Nurses also need to be alert to situations in which there may be differences in values among the patient, family, and physician. Encouraging timely communication may avert a major dilemma or facilitate more effective resolution of the concern. Nurses who cannot reconcile their values with a particular situation need to take the necessary steps to remove themselves from that situation to not compromise patient care or personal integrity. In so doing, it is essential to avoid abandoning the patient by ensuring that there are others who will provide the needed care for the patient (ANA, 2015, Provision 5.4; CNA, 2017, Part I.G.7; ICN, 2021, Element 2.6).

The Importance of Communication: Who Decides?

As noted above, many factors are involved in making decisions about initiating, withholding, or withdrawing life-sustaining treatments and utilizing other technologies. Nurses need to determine who is involved in making the decision and how the nurse fits into the scenario. Utilizing the decision-making process described in Chapter 7 may assist in this process. Nurses need to be aware of institutional policies and protocols regarding various technologies. Such policies should include approaches to reaching decisions about interventions for particular patients, ways of dealing with conflicts that may arise, protection of patient rights, description of roles of those involved in the decision-making process, and directions for documenting the decision in the patient's chart. In most situations the patient or the patient's healthcare surrogate has the ultimate authority to decide which interventions to use or withhold.

Because nurses are in close and continual contact with patients, they are often perceived as more available and more approachable than physicians. Patients or family members may discuss their concerns about interventions more readily with the nurse, seeking information or advice. It is important to know what patients have been told by the physician, determine the patient's and family's level of understanding about the situation, and determine whether they have the necessary information to make an informed decision. If information is needed in such areas as risks, discomforts, side effects, potential benefits, likelihood of success, treatment alternatives, or estimated costs, advocating for the patient in this regard is an expected nursing response. Nurses are in a key position to utilize conversations with patients and families to discover areas of confusion and to elicit information about patients' wishes regarding interventions.

Sometimes people just need to talk out their concerns and sort through sometimes conflicting messages coming from the head and the heart. Providing a listening presence can help people vent their emotions, speak about their fears, and clarify their concerns. At times the concern may be such that the nurse must advocate for the patient by facilitating communication with the physician, support people such as family or pastor, or other appropriate persons such as a patient representative or member of the ethics committee. Collaboration among all involved is important to ensure an informed choice. Effective communication can be facilitated by providing an environment that is not rushed, using terms and language that are understood by the other person, allowing time for and encouraging questions, practicing attentive listening, and offering a caring presence.

Caring: The Human Focus

In the context of expanding scientific and technological knowledge, nurses have the responsibility for helping patients and families benefit from what technology offers, while always remembering the human focus of care. Nursing care in its fullest meaning is most essential when medical treatments are no longer effective. This is evident especially in nursing's role in palliative care. However alert, and in whatever stage of living and dying a person is, they have a life story that continues to unfold, a story that continues to intertwine with lives of others. In the midst of the technology, nurses can encourage family and loved ones to talk with, touch, and be in touch with the patient. In this way, nurses acknowledge the primary importance of relationships, even in a healthcare setting filled with machines, noises, and other evidence of advanced technology.

Attention to the human focus includes helping patients and families become more comfortable with the sometimes formidable array of machines and equipment and make sense of the large amounts of clinical data that are generated. Incorporating family members in caring for the patient provides time for connecting and observing the patient in both good and bad moments and engenders a more realistic view of the patient's condition. Rather than engendering anxiety and mistrust by shutting the family out of the patient's life and experiences at critical moments, nurses should encourage them to share directly in the patient's journey. This provides families with more experiences on which to base hard decisions.

The nursing role of providing care and comfort is paramount in any healthcare setting and has many facets. It may take the shape of explaining, as often as necessary, the purpose and problems related to interventions. Caring requires that the nurse see the experience from another's point of view so that questions, fears, concerns, and frustrations may be addressed appropriately. Providing care and comfort also requires that the nurse support and encourage behaviors that enable patients and families to choose in accordance with their own beliefs and values. Being proficient in technical skills with the intent of doing what is best for the patient is part of human care, as is the ability to be with and wait with persons as they struggle through difficult situations.

Nursing Self-Care

Nurses need to be attentive to taking care of themselves as they deal with the impact of healthcare technology on their care of patients, interactions with colleagues, and their personal lives and values. The stress of working with technology in its various forms and being alert to ethical and other considerations related to the ever-present technology can feel overwhelming. To be of service to others, nurses need to value themselves and mobilize whatever resources are needed to promote their own well-being (AHNA, 2019). Self-care practices need to be personalized, recognizing that different people find some approaches more effective than others. Melnyk and Neale (2018) describe several practices that focus on stress and emotional wellness. These include developing cognitive-behavioral skills, journaling, regular physical activity, sleeping at least seven hours each night, focused breathing exercises, body awareness techniques, positive thinking, being in nature, meditation, disconnecting from technology, and connecting personally with important people in one's life. Many resources for self-care are available online. Information on self-care for nurses is available through the American Holistic Nurses Association (AHNA) at https://www.ahna.org/Resources and at the ANA Health Nurse Healthy Nation website https://www.healthynursehealthynation.org/.

■ SUMMARY

Many of the major ethical dilemmas encountered by nurses and other healthcare providers today are associated with advances in scientific knowledge and healthcare technology. To recognize and deal with such dilemmas, nurses need to clarify their own values and appreciate differences in values among the various people involved in making patient care decisions. The many directions that technology can take us prompt very deep questions about life and death that must be addressed on individual, professional, and societal levels. Issues of quality of life, relief of suffering, and futility of interventions are some facets of these questions. Decisions about when to intervene and reasonable goals of interventions are made more difficult because of varying perceptions of the value of such interventions, the lack of definitive outcomes, and issues related to availability of interventions. Principles of beneficence, nonmaleficence, justice, autonomy and respect for persons provide the basis for arguments on different sides of issues related to technology. Nurses must take into account their responsibilities to patients and the profession, as well as personal integrity and self-care, when dealing with ethical dilemmas engendered by technology. Nurses must remember that in the midst of the technology with its associated dilemmas are patients and families who need the human focus of care that is the essence of nursing practice.

CHAPTER HIGHLIGHTS

- The impact of healthcare technology on all aspects of patient care has prompted the need to address important ethical questions regarding life, death, and allocation of resources.
- Utilization of healthcare technology may give rise to conflicts between the principles of beneficence and nonmaleficence.
- Appropriate utilization of healthcare technologies requires that healthcare providers, patients, and families understand the purposes, benefits, and limitations of specific technologies.
- Attitudes and beliefs concerning life and death affect how healthcare providers, patients, families, and the legal system approach issues related to healthcare technology. Ethical dilemmas may arise when there are differing opinions among the parties involved related to the use of technological interventions.
- Determination of medical futility is an important consideration in decisions to withhold or withdraw life-sustaining interventions. Ethical decisions regarding these measures require consideration of whether they are prolonging living or prolonging dying.
- Economics may factor into decisions related to medical futility, availability of technology, and accessibility to many interventions.
- Withholding or withdrawing life-sustaining treatments in situations in which the burden or harm has been determined to outweigh the benefits constitutes allowing a person to die and is not euthanasia. Dilemmas may arise regarding whether to classify the use of specific interventions as ordinary or extraordinary measures. The courts have sometimes been involved in making this determination.
- Patient self-determination and distributive justice must be considered in decisions regarding technological interventions. Vigilance is required to ensure that people are not harmed, exploited, controlled, discriminated against, or excluded from care by the use of healthcare technologies.
- Nurses are in a key position to help patients and families articulate their preferences regarding technological interventions and to facilitate communication with other health team members in this regard. This role requires familiarity with patient and family decisions and institutional policies regarding life-sustaining interventions and awareness that when medical care is deemed futile, nursing care in its fullest meaning is most essential.
- Nurses need to be attentive to taking care of themselves in the midst of dealing with the impact of technology on their care of patients, interactions with colleagues, and attending to their personal lives and values.
- Social media offers benefits to nurses that include access to health promotion information and programs, ability to easily dialog with other professionals, ability to keep up with ever-changing healthcare developments, access to continuing education, and the like. However, the inappropriate use of social media by nurses can cause both ethical concerns and legal problems.

DISCUSSION QUESTIONS AND ACTIVITIES

1. Explore information and resources related to advance directives at the website http://www.wvethics.org/advance-directives-forms-and-laws/. Develop advance directives for yourself, considering interventions you would choose and parameters regarding these choices. Discuss and compare your directives with classmates. Advance directive forms for your state can be found at https://www.caringinfo.org/planning/advance-directives/.
2. Discuss your beliefs regarding determinants of the beginning and end of life.
3. Describe quality of life as it relates to healthcare decisions. Share with classmates your beliefs and feelings about what constitutes quality of life for you.
4. Discuss potential slippery slope elements related to reproductive and genetic technologies, cloning and stem cell research, and organ procurement and transplantation. Investigate issues related to stem

cell research and cloning at the following websites and discuss with classmates:

National Institutes of Health—Information on stem cells—http://stemcells.nih.gov/

Hastings Center—https://www.thehastingscenter.org/briefingbook/stem-cells/

International Society for Stem Cell Research—https://www.isscr.org/guidelines

ANA—https://www.nursingworld.org/practice-policy/nursing-excellence/ethics/genetics/

National Human Genome Research Institute—https://www.genome.gov/

International Society of Nurses in Genetics—http://www.isong.org/

5. Plan and engage in a debate in your class focused on economic and distributive justice issues related to healthcare technologies.

6. If possible observe one or two patients who are receiving technological interventions and note how the technology is affecting them and their families, issues surrounding its use, the focus of nursing care, and your reaction to the situation. Describe the strengths of the nursing care you observe and aspects that you might do differently if you were providing care. Talk to nurses and patients regarding the impact of technology on their health and care.

7. Discuss your view about nurses writing DNR orders.

8. Investigate whether your state, province, or hospital has specific policies for determining medical futility. How would you handle a situation where you feel the physician's decision regarding life-sustaining interventions is inappropriate for your patient?

9. Choose one of the topics discussed in this chapter and explore the websites of the ANA, the CNA, and the ICN regarding policies or position statements on this issue. You may include information from other disciplines as well. Compare and contrast the positions of the various organizations. Discuss your views about this issue and how they compare with the positions of professional organizations.

ANA—http://www.nursingworld.org (practice and advocacy)

CNA—https://www.cna-aiic.ca/en/ (policy-advocacy)

ICN—https://www.icn.ch/nursing-policy/position-statements

10. Explore the following websites regarding issues of confidentiality and privacy and share information with classmates:

https://www.cms.gov/Outreach-and-Education/Medicare-Learning-Network-MLN/MLNProducts/downloads/SE0726FactSheet.pdf

https://www.hipaajournal.com/hipaa-social-media/ (HIPAA rules for posting on social media)

https://www.hhs.gov/web/social-media/policies/index.html (HIPAA social media policies)

https://www.nursingworld.org/~4ad4a8/globalassets/docs/ana/position-statement-privacy-and-confidentiality.pdf

https://www.icn.ch/sites/default/files/inline-files/E10a_Nurses_Social_Media.pdf

https://www.ncsbn.org/brochures-and-posters/nurses-guide-to-the-use-of-social-media

11. Role-play a palliative/hospice care conference with students in the class, using a real or hypothetical patient case situation, or attend an ethics committee meeting at your hospital. Review and discuss the ethics committee tools available online at http://www.wvnec.org/ethics-committee-tools/

12. Explore self-care modalities offered by the AHNA (https://www.ahna.org/Resources—Self-care Modalities) and other resources related to self-care for nurses. Discuss various self-care practices with classmates and develop a personal self-care program for yourself.

REFERENCES

American Association of Critical-Care Nurses. (2018). *Practice alert outlines: Alarm management strategies.* https://www.aacn.org/newsroom/practice-alert-outlines-alarm-management-strategies.

American Holistic Nurses Association (AHNA), (2019). *Holistic nursing: Scope and standards of practice* (3rd ed.). American Nurses Association.

American Nurses Association (ANA), (2011). *ANA's principles for social networking and the nurse.* Author.

ANA. (2015). *Code of ethics for nurses with interpretive statements.* http://nursingworld.org/DocumentVault/Ethics-1/Code-of-Ethics-for-Nurses.html

American Nurses Association (ANA). (2016). *Revised position statement: Nurses' roles and responsibilities in providing care and support at the end of life.* https://www.nursingworld.org/~4af078/globalassets/docs/ana/ethics/endoflife-positionstatement.pdf

American Nurses Association (ANA). (2017). *Position statement: Nutrition and hydration at the end of life.* https://www.nursingworld.org/practice-policy/nursing-excellence/official-position-statements/id/nutrition-and-hydration-at-the-end-of-life/.

American Nurses Association (ANA). (2020). *Revised position statement: Nursing care and do not resuscitate (DNR) decisions.* https://www.nursingworld.org/~494a87/globalassets/practiceandpolicy/nursing-excellence/ana-position-statements/social-causes-and-health-care/nursing-care-and-do-not-resuscitate-dnr-decisions-final-nursingworld.pdf

American Nurses Association (ANA), (2021). *Nursing: Scope and standards of practice.* Author.

American Nurses Association (2023). *Practice policy: Genetics and personalized medicine.* https://www.nursingworld.org/practice-policy/nursing-excellence/ethics/genetics/

Angell, M. (1990). Prisoners of technology: The case of Nancy Cruzan. *New England Journal of Medicine, 322,* 1226–1228.

Annas, G. J. (1990). Nancy Cruzan and the right to die. *New England Journal of Medicine, 323,* 670–672.

Asadi, N., Salmani, F., Asgari, N., & Salmani, M. (2022). Alarm fatigue and moral distress in ICU nurses in COVID-19 pandemic. *BMC Nursing, 21,* 125. https://doi.org/10.1186/s12912-022-00909-y.

Baily, M. A. (2011). Futility, autonomy, and cost of end-of-life care. *Journal of Law, Medicine & Ethics, 39*(2), 172–182.

Balestra, M. L. (2018). Social media missteps could put your nursing license at risk. *American Nurse Today, 13*(3), 20–21. 63.

Ball, T. (2017). The ethics of genetics. *American Medical Writers Association Journal, 32*(4), 182–184.

Beamer, L. C. (2017). Ethics and genetics: Examining a crossroads in nursing through a case study. *Clinical Journal of Oncology Nursing, 21*(6), 730–737.

Boggatz, T. (2016). Quality of life in old age—A concept analysis. *International Journal of Older People Nursing, 11,* 55–69.

Canadian Nurse Protective Society. (2023). *InfoLAW: Social media.* https://cnps.ca/article/social-media/

CNA. (2017). *Code of ethics for registered nurses.* https://cdn1.nscn.ca/sites/default/files/documents/resources/code-of-ethics-for-registered-nurses.pdf#:~:text=The%20Canadian%20Nurses%20Association%20%28CNA%29%20Code%20of%20Ethics,receiving%20care.%20The%20Code%20is%20both%20aspirational%20and%20regulatory

Condic, M. L. (2016). Determination of death: A scientific perspective on biological integration. *The Journal of Medicine and Philosophy, 4*(3), 257–278.

Devettere, R. J. (1995). *Practical decision making in health care ethics: Cases and concepts.* Georgetown University Press.

Druwé, P., Benoit, D. D., Monsieurs, K. G., Gagg, J., Nakahara, S., Alpert, E. A., van Schuppen, H., Élő, G., Huybrechts, S. A., Mpotos, N., Joly, L. -M., Xanthos, T., Roessler, M., Paal, P., Cocchi, M. N., Bjørshol, C., Nurmi, J., Salmeron, P. P., Owczuk, R., … (2020). Cardiopulmonary resuscitation in adults over 80: Outcome and the perception of appropriateness by clinicians. *Journal of the American Geriatric Society, 68,* 39–45. https://doi.org/10.1111/jgs.16270.

Flannery, M. (2017). Conceptual issues surrounding quality of life in oncology nursing. *Oncology Nursing Forum, 44*(3), 285–287.

Fontugne, E. A. (2014). To treat or not to treat: End-of-life care, patient autonomy, and the responsible practice of medicine. *Journal of Legal Medicine, 35,* 529–538.

Geppert, C. M., Andrews, M. R., & Druyan, M. E. (2010). Ethical issues in artificial nutrition and hydration: a review. *Journal of Parenteral and Enteral Nutrition, 34*(1), 79–88.

Gorisek, R., Mayer, C., Hicks, W. B., & Barnes, J. (2021). An evidence-based initiative to reduce alarm fatigue in a burn intensive care unit. *Critical Care Nurse, 41*(4), 29–37. https://doi.org/10.4037/ccn2021166.

Guenin, L. (2008). *The morality of embryo use.* Cambridge University Press.

Häyry, N. (2018). Ethics and cloning. *British Medical Bulletin, 128,* 15–21. https://doi.org/10.1093/bmb/ldy031. https://academic-oup-com.wvu.idm.oclc.org/bmb/article/128/1/15/5094025.

Hickman, S. E., Nelson, C. A., Moss, A. H., Hammes, B. J., Terwilliger, A., Jackson, A., & Tolle, S. W. (2009). Use of the physician orders for life-sustaining treatment (POLST) paradigm program in the hospice setting. *Journal of Palliative Medicine, 12*(2), 133–141.

Hyun, I. (2018). *Bioethics briefings: Stem cells. Hastings Center.* https://www.thehastingscenter.org/briefing-book/stem-cells/.

International Council of Nurses (ICN). (2015). *Position statement: Nurses and social media.* https://www.icn.ch/sites/default/files/inline-files/E10a_Nurses_Social_Media.pdf

ICN. (2012). *Position Statement: Nurses' role in providing care to dying patients and their families.* https://www.icn.ch/sites/default/files/inline-files/A12_Nurses_Role_Care_Dying_Patients.pdf

ICN. (2021). *The ICN code of ethics for nurses.* https://www.icn.ch/system/files/2021-10/ICN_Code-of-Ethics_EN_Web_0.pdf

International Society for Stem Cell Research (ISSCR). (2022). *Guidelines for stem cell research and clinical translation.* https://www.isscr.org/guidelines

Jacobs, C. A. (2014). Legal issues involved in "do not resuscitate" order. *Journal of Legal Nurse Consulting, 25*(2), 30–35.

Joint Commission (2021). *National patient safety goals, Goal 6: Improve the safety of clinical alarm system.* https://www.jointcommission.org/-/media/tjc/documents/standards/national-patient-safety-goals/2021/npsg_chapter_hap_jan2021.pdf

Lachman, V. D. (2013). Social media: Managing the ethical issues. *Medsurg Nursing, 22*(5), 326–329.

Lauritzen, P. (2005). Stem cells, biotechnology, and human rights: Implications for a posthuman future. *Hastings Center Reports, 35*(2), 25–33.

Lewandowska, K., Weisbrot, M., Cieloszyk, A., Medrzycka-Dabrowska, W., Krupa, S., & Ozga, D. (2020). Impact of alarm fatigue on the work of nurses in and intensive care environment – A systematic review. *International Journal of Environmental Research and Public Health, 17,* 8409. https://doi.org/10.3390/ijerph17228409.

Lo, B. (2013). *Resolving ethical dilemmas: A guide for clinicians* (5th ed.). Lippincott Williams & Wilkins.

McBride, S., Tietze, M., Robichaux, C., Stokes, L., & Weber, E. (2018). Identifying and addressing ethical issues with use of electronic health records. *Online Journal of Issues in Nursing, 23*(1). http://ojin.nursingworld.org/MainMenu-Categories/ANAMarketplace/ANAPeriodicals/OJIN/TableofContents/Vol-23-2018/No1-Jan-2018/Identifying-and-Addressing-Ethical-Issues-EHR.html.

Mendola, A. (2015). Faith and futility in the ICU. *Hastings Center Report,* 9–10.

Melnyk, B. M., & Neale, S. (2018). Emotional wellness. *American Nurse Today, 13*(3), 61–63.

National Coalition of Hospice and Palliative Care (NCHPC), (2018). *Clinical practice guidelines for quality palliative care* (4th ed.). Author.

National Council on Disability (NCD). (2019). *Medical futility and disability bias: Part of the medical ethics and disability series.* https://ncd.gov/sites/default/files/NCD_Medical_Futility_Report_508.pdf

National Council of State Boards of Nursing (NCSBN). (2018). *A nurse's guide to the use of social media.* https://www.ncsbn.org/brochures-and-posters/nurses-guide-to-the-use-of-social-media

NIH National Human Genome Research Institute. (2018). *Genetics vs genomics fact sheet.* https://www.genome.gov/about-genomics/fact-sheets/Genetics-vs-Genomics

Olmstead, J. A., & Dahnke, M. D. (2016). The need for an effective process to resolve conflicts over medical futility: A case study and analysis. *Critical Care Nurse, 36*(6), 13–23.

Pence, G. E. (1995). *Classic cases in medical ethics.* McGraw-Hill.

Pope, T. M., & Okninski, M. E. (2016). Legal standards for brain death and undue influence in euthanasia laws. *Journal of Bioethics Inquiry, 13,* 173–178.

Scofield, G. R. (1995). Is consent useful when resuscitation isn't? In J. H. Howell & W. F. Sale (Eds.), *Life choices: A Hastings Center introduction to bioethics* (pp. 172–187). Georgetown University Press.

Shin, P. (2016). Defensible limits in critical care: An ethical analysis of a recent multisociety policy statement. *American Journal of Bioethics, 16*(1), 58–60.

Weaver, M. (2016). The double helix: Applying an ethic of care to the duty to warn genetic relatives of genetic information. *Bioethics, 30*(3), 181–187.

Werner-Felmayer, G., & Shalev, C. (2015). Human germline modification—A missing link. *American Journal of Bioethics, 15*(12), 49–51.

Vanleerberghe, P., De Witte, N., Claes, C., Schalock, R. L., & Verté, D. (2017). The quality of life of older people aging in place: A literature review. *Quality of Life Research, 26,* 2899–2907.

11

Ethical Issues Related to Patient Self-Determination

The task set before us is to find the golden mean between moral autonomy and the cooperative action necessary to contemporary life.

(Curtin, 1982)

OBJECTIVES

After completing this chapter, the reader should be able to:

1. Discuss ethical issues related to autonomy and patient self-determination.
2. Describe factors that may threaten autonomy in healthcare settings and situations in which autonomy may be limited.
3. Examine the interaction of justice and autonomy.
4. Discuss informed consent as it relates to patient self-determination.
5. Examine legal and ethical elements of informed consent.
6. Discuss the place of advance directives in healthcare decisions.

7. Describe the nursing role and responsibilities related to informed consent and advance directives.
8. Discuss patient autonomy related to choices for life and health.
9. Describe ethical concerns, nursing role, and ethical obligations related to patient lifestyle and health choices that affect personal and public health.
10. Discuss the practical application of codes of nursing ethics that guide nursing practice and response to issues related to patient self-determination and care.

INTRODUCTION

The role of the patient and that of the healer, and the implied responsibilities of each, have varied throughout history and in different cultures. In some cultures, decisions regarding "what is best" for the patient are deferred to the healer, who is presumed to know what will bring about healing. Indeed, until recently, the physician was often viewed in this light. Such paternalism has been challenged in recent years, and greater emphasis has been placed on the role and rights of patients in making healthcare decisions. This chapter focuses on ethical issues related to patient self-determination. Discussion of these issues includes both ethical and legal components and is intertwined with issues of technology and economics as discussed in Chapters 10 and 15.

AUTONOMY AND HEALTHCARE DECISIONS

Self-determination derives from the principle of autonomy. Recall that autonomy, the first ethical principle discussed in Chapter 3, denotes having the freedom to make choices about issues that affect our own lives and to make decisions about personal goals. Autonomy means self-governing and implies respect for persons, the ability to determine personal goals and decide on a plan of action, and the freedom to act on the choices made. The value placed on the primacy of the individual implicit in autonomy is primarily an Anglo-Western concept, and the sense of personal autonomy varies among cultures. Autonomy includes an appreciation for the self in relation to others, recognizing that choices are made in the context of community. Implications of this view for healthcare include viewing patients as members of a social world in which healthcare decisions affect others and are made in conjunction with trusted persons. Indeed, in many non-Western cultures, family and community are key participants in making healthcare decisions for individuals.

Factors that may threaten autonomy in healthcare settings include persisting attitudes that promote the dependent role of the patient, assumptions that a patient's values and thought processes are the same as those of the healthcare provider, failure to appreciate a difference in knowledge level regarding health matters, and a focus on technology rather than caring. Although there has been greater emphasis on supporting patient autonomy in recent years, attitudes that the healthcare provider knows what is best for the patient still exist. In healthcare, this attitude has historically been the basis for allowing physicians to make unilateral decisions about patient care without their full consent or knowledge (Will, 2011). Such attitudes contribute to situations in which patients and families struggle with healthcare providers over control of healthcare decisions. Although the principle of beneficence suggests that decisions are focused on the patient's well-being, the power inherent in such a hierarchical arrangement can be abused, and decisions made may reflect the interests of the healthcare provider more than those of the patient. Consider, for example, elderly patients in nursing homes who may be sedated "for their own protection" because of "agitation and confusion." It is worth pondering whether medication used in this way is for the benefit of the patient, or rather to make life easier for the staff.

The authoritarian approach is based on the belief that physicians and other healthcare providers possess the most appropriate skills and capacities to exercise decision-making power and that patients and families lack sufficient knowledge and background to make adequate decisions in the face of illness. What this attitude does not address, however, is the reality that decisions about health require more than scientific expertise. Such decisions need to consider factors such as the patient's values, culture, and spiritual and other beliefs; an evaluation of risks, benefits, and economic considerations; and effects on lifestyle and role in family. The principle of autonomy directs nurses and others to engage patients in the decision-making process in relationship with others

who may need to be part of the process. Respecting autonomy also means appreciating situations in which patients are asking that family and others have a prominent role in making decisions for them (Jensen, 2015; Leever, 2011; Sakalys, 2010).

CASE PRESENTATION

Determining What Is Best for the Patient

Mr. Zumma, a former butcher who is 84 years old, has had evidence of memory loss and periodic confusion for about 18 months. He has been functional at home, able to do personal care, household chores, and shopping and has been on no medication. One night he came into the bedroom with two straight razors and told his wife to stay still so he could slit her throat. She was able to escape by exiting through a nearby door and running to a neighbor's house. Reluctant to call the police because "he is not a criminal," she called her son, who came and calmed his father down. On the advice of another family member, Mrs. Zumma contacted a geriatric psychiatrist, who immediately hospitalized Mr. Zumma and started him on Haldol. When he got worse, the physician increased the dose of the medication. Although he was walking and talking when he was admitted, after one day in the hospital the patient became incontinent, could not walk, was drooling, and had to be restrained. The decline in his condition throughout the week in the hospital concerned Mrs. Zumma, and she approached the psychiatrist about taking him on a previously planned vacation. The psychiatrist indicated that this would be impossible and that the patient would need to go to a nursing home. With persistence, however, Mrs. Zumma was able to convince the psychiatrist to discontinue the medications, after which Mr. Zumma's condition improved and he walked out of the hospital and did well on the vacation trip. Although he still gets confused, he remains functional without medication at home, where his wife makes sure that all sharp or dangerous objects are kept hidden.

Think About It
When Interventions Do More Harm Than Good
- How did the physician's attitude of "knowing what is best" factor into the case of Mr. Zumma?
- What ethical issues are evident in this case?
- If you were the nurse caring for Mr. Zumma and his wife approached you with her concerns about his condition, how would you respond?
- Describe patient and family values that you believe influenced decisions about Mr. Zumma's care.

How Far Does Autonomy Go?

Although the principle of autonomy has become a key consideration in healthcare ethics, it does have limits. Practitioners are not obligated to honor requests from patients or families for interventions that, in the best judgment of the practitioner, are outside accepted standards of care or that are contrary to the practitioner's own ethical views. Autonomy may also be limited by the availability of resources and economic circumstances.

In discussions of patient self-determination, the principle of justice needs to be considered along with that of autonomy. Recall from Chapter 3 that justice implies fair, equitable, and appropriate treatment in light of what is due or owed to persons, recognizing that giving to some may deny receipt to others who might otherwise have received these things. In determining who deserves what portion of finite healthcare resources, autonomy and justice may conflict where needs or demands for healthcare by autonomous patients outweigh available resources. The rights of family members and of society must be considered in relation to the needs of individuals. Hardwig (2000) suggests that the medical and nonmedical impacts of treatment decisions on both the patient and the family need to be considered. He reflects that patient autonomy implies the responsible use of freedom, which means considering the needs of family and society as well as our own desires. He raises the question of whether it is legitimate to ask families to make sacrifices of major resources to meet the needs of one member. The limited availability and expense of many medical interventions bring such questions to the fore. Because people can be maintained on very expensive treatments for prolonged periods, justice requires us to ask not only who deserves such an intervention but also who is expected to pay for it. Although the moral relevance of considering the interests of the family is often not addressed in current ethical theory, dilemmas faced by patients, families, and practitioners include these issues, and it is well worth pondering their implications.

INFORMED CONSENT

Informed consent provides legal protection of a patient's right to personal autonomy. The concept of informed consent is one that has come to mean that patients are given the opportunity to autonomously choose a course of action in regard to plans for healthcare. The choice includes the right to refuse interventions or recommendations about care and to choose from available therapeutic alternatives. This is usually discussed in relation to surgery and complex medical procedures but also includes consent to more common interventions that may have undesirable side effects, such as immunizations and contraceptives. Exceptions to informed consent include emergencies in which there is no time to disclose the information and waivers by patients who do not want to know their prognosis or risks of treatment.

The emergence of informed consent as we know it has been affected by several factors. One factor has been the institutionalization of healthcare in hospitals, with their associated technologies and life-prolonging interventions over which people have little control and limited understanding. When healthcare providers visited the home, informed consent was not as necessary, because people had more control and a better understanding of traditional remedies (Will, 2011). The courts, however, have exerted the most significant influence on shaping the doctrine of informed consent.

The history of the concept dates back to several landmark legal cases (Leclercq et al., 2010). In *Slater v. Baker & Stapleton* (1767), a decision was made that prohibited "unauthorized touching." This decision held that a person has a right to know what is to be done to his or her body. It did not require any participation in the decision-making process. In the case of *Mohr v. Williams* (1905) and the case of *Schloendorff v. The Society of New York Hospital* (1914), separate rulings established the patient's right to know what was to be done and

---

ASK YOURSELF

Should There Be Limits to Patient Autonomy?
- Can you think of healthcare situations in which the interests of the family should take precedence over those of the patient? Upon what criteria do you base this decision?
- How would you describe nursing's role regarding patient autonomy? Are there situations in which you feel a nurse is justified in not honoring a patient's

healthcare choice? What guidance do you find in nursing codes of ethics? Give examples.
- Have you experienced situations of paternalism in nursing?
- How do you feel about the suggestion that the healthcare provider is most qualified to make healthcare decisions? Have you experienced this personally or with a family member? How did you/they respond?

the right to give or withhold consent. These decisions did not address the patient's right to be informed about the risks of treatment or nontreatment or about the existence of alternative therapies. In the case of *Salgo v. Leland Stanford, Jr.* (1957), the California Supreme Court ruled in favor of a patient who had not been informed of the risks of aortography and subsequently became paralyzed. This ruling established a patient's right to be advised of the risks involved in any proposed treatment. The requirement of including *all* risks and alternatives in informed consent was expanded by the 1972 case of *Canterbury v. Spence*. Including the risks of doing nothing or postponing intervention became standard elements in informed consent following the 1980 case of *Truman v. Thomas* in which a woman, who had refused a Pap smear, claimed she had not understood that lack of early detection of cancer might mean it was discovered too late for curative treatment.

Ethical and Legal Elements of Informed Consent

Although the informed consent doctrine has foundations in law, it is essentially an ethical imperative based on respect for persons as autonomous agents. Informed consent is more than simply a legal document and a process of having a patient sign a form. Consent is a process of shared decision making flowing from communication between patient, family (when they are part of the process), and healthcare provider that is based on mutual respect and participation. The two major legal elements of informed consent that are inherent in the ethical imperative are information and consent.

Information

The information component of informed consent includes both disclosure and understanding of the essential information. Box 11.1 lists the information that must be included in an informed consent. People need access

---

BOX 11.1 Content of Informed Consent

- The nature of the health concern and prognosis if nothing is done
- Description of all treatment options, even those that the healthcare provider does not favor or cannot provide
- The benefits, risks, and consequences of the various treatment alternatives, including nonintervention

---

to sufficient information to help them understand their health concerns and make decisions regarding treatment. The information provided need not be in "textbook" detail, but it does need to offer enough explanation for the person to have a clear picture of the situation, what is being offered, and the alternatives (including nonintervention), as well as their risks, benefits, and consequences. Determining the adequacy of information disclosed in an informed consent is based on one or more standards: (1) the professional practice standard—the disclosure is consistent with the standards of the profession; (2) the reasonable person standard—the disclosure is what a reasonable person in similar circumstances would need to make an informed decision; and (3) the subjective standard—the disclosure is what the particular person wants or needs to know. The outcomes of the court cases noted earlier have led to more of an emphasis on the reasonable person standard, or patient point of view, regarding the information that must be included in informed consent. Informed consent implies that the person has received the information and understands what is provided. Verification of understanding can be accomplished through discussion in which patients have an opportunity to ask questions and are asked to describe their understanding of the nature of the intervention, alternatives, risks, and benefits.

Consent

Consent to something implies the freedom to accept or reject it. This means that consent to healthcare interventions must be voluntary, without coercion, force, or manipulation from healthcare providers, family, or others. Force entails making someone do something against her or his will. Coercion and manipulation may be overt or subtle and may include threats, rewards, deception, or inducing excessive fear. The voluntary nature of consent does not prohibit healthcare providers from making recommendations or attempting to persuade patients to accept their suggestions. However, we must be alert to situations in which persuasion takes on qualities of coercion or manipulation.

Special Considerations Regarding Informed Consent

Transcultural Considerations

As mentioned previously, understandings of autonomy, rights and duties of individuals, and approaches to decision making vary among cultures. Such cultural differences have an impact on understanding patient self-determination and approaches to obtaining informed consent. For example, in cultures where there is more emphasis on duty and responsibility to family and community than on the rights of the individual, it would be important to include the family in discussion and deliberation regarding consent. Another example is a belief in some cultures that even talking about the possibility of negative outcomes can increase the chance of their occurring. Members of such cultures may say they do not want to know about risks related to a treatment. In such situations, healthcare practitioners may face the dilemma of respecting autonomy and fulfilling the legal requirements of providing information necessary for an informed choice while avoiding potential harm to the patient's well-being by discussing risks (Lasser & Gottlieb, 2017). Assuring that both written and verbal information related to the process of obtaining informed consent is provided in a language understood by the patient/family is an essential transcultural consideration. Cultural competence, including linguistic competency (discussed in Chapter 18), is a key component of the nursing role related to obtaining informed consent.

Vulnerable Populations

Vulnerable populations include groups such as the elderly, prisoners, children, homeless persons, those with low literacy or mental/emotional challenges, and various high-risk groups. With vulnerable groups, nurses must be sensitive to the possibility of coercion. The very act of asking a patient to sign a form giving permission for a particular treatment that they may not fully understand may constitute a form of coercion. Poor comprehension of the informed consent process is associated with low literacy, lower educational levels, and a primary language different from that of the dominant culture. To increase comprehension among persons with these challenges, Heerman et al. (2015) suggest creating informed consent materials that use low-literacy health communication techniques, visual aids, and graphics focused on explaining key concepts, avoiding medical jargon, and having the healthcare provider seated with a relaxed and open body posture when talking with the patient/family.

Children and Adolescents

In most situations, parents are the key decision makers regarding consent for medical interventions for children younger than 18 years. There are three circumstances in which minors (primarily adolescents) can legally make healthcare decisions for themselves: (1) they are considered mature minors, (2) they are legally emancipated, and (3) their care involves specific diagnostic or care categories such as sexually transmitted infections or prenatal care. Including children in decision making occurs through the process of giving *assent* for the intervention. The American Academy of Pediatrics recommends that several elements be incorporated into assent with children (AAP, 2016; Katz & Webb, 2016). These elements include (1) helping patients achieve a developmentally appropriate awareness of the nature of their condition; (2) telling patients what they can expect with tests and treatments; (3) making clinical assessments of patient understanding of the situation and the factors influencing how the patient is responding (including whether there may be elements of coercion to accept testing or therapy); and (4) soliciting an expression of the patient's willingness to accept the proposed care. Readers are encouraged to review the full American Academy of Pediatrics Policy Statement: Informed Consent in Decision-Making in Pediatric Practice at https://publications.aap.org/pediatrics/article/138/2/e20161484/52512/Informed-Consent-in-Decision-Making-in-Pediatric?searchresult=1.

As is true for adults, healthcare decisions for children and adolescents are influenced by cultural, religious, and social factors that may at times conflict with medical recommendations or contribute to poor outcomes. It is important for nurses and other clinicians to respect culture and beliefs as they work with and support the autonomy of parents/families. However, healthcare providers also have an ethical and legal obligation to protect children from imminent or potential harm. When parental refusal of an intervention could mean harm to the child, the decision about what is best for the child may be determined by the legal system.

Nursing Role and Responsibilities: Informed Consent

Although the practice of documenting informed consent for a procedure usually ends with the signing of a consent form, the process is much more complex. It is the responsibility of the physician or other healthcare provider to explain a medical intervention, its risks, alternatives, and risks of nontreatment to the patient in language the patient can understand. The provider should also verify that the patient understands the information given and recognizes the implications that each option will have on his or her lifestyle. Although the provider may delegate the task of obtaining the patient's signature on the consent form to another member of the healthcare team, such as the nurse, the task of providing the necessary education cannot be delegated (Rock & Hoebeke, 2014). It is the nurse's responsibility as advocate for the patient to ensure that all criteria for autonomous decision making are met. If the nurse believes that the patient does not understand the implications of any part of the process, including nontreatment

and alternative options, or that the patient is unable to deliberate and to reason about the various choices, it is the responsibility of the nurse to intervene. Legally, the nurse must act if it becomes apparent that the patient is not informed. Actions may include notifying the provider and requesting further information for the patient or stopping the process until it is ensured that the decision can be made autonomously. Although the mechanics of the process usually require the nurse to obtain the patient's signature on a consent form, the primary concern of the nurse is to ensure that all criteria for autonomous decision making are met.

CASE PRESENTATION

Language and Informed Consent

Mohano is a 67-year-old deaf man who was admitted to the hospital with atrial fibrillation. The nurse notes that he is alert, apparently oriented, and able to follow simple directions that she acts out, although he does look apprehensive as she cares for him. Mohano's social history indicates that he was brought into the hospital by a community worker, who looks in on him because he is deaf and illiterate and has no family in the area. She indicated that he came to the area as a migrant worker a number of years ago, along with a brother who died the previous year. She also noted that two of his five siblings were also deaf, and they had developed a type of sign language that was understood only by family members. At the interdisciplinary care conference, the medical resident who is in charge of his case voices frustration because of the need to get the patient's permission to do a stress test and to talk to him about medications and risk for stroke. She suggests that they should just get the patient to make an X on the form so they can go ahead with the treatment protocol because it is in the patient's best interest to do so. The social worker suggests that they get an interpreter for the deaf to come in and try to talk to him through sign language, although she is not sure he will understand.

Think About It

Obtaining Informed Consent When There Is No Common Language

- What ethical dilemmas are evident in this case?
- What do you think about Mohano's decision-making capacity?
- Do you think it is possible to obtain an informed consent from Mohano? Support your position with discussion of elements of informed consent and decision-making capacity. Are there things clinicians can do to help Mohano understand his health situation?
- In a situation such as this, it is evident that the patient has a language, although it is not understood by the healthcare providers, and that he has been able to care for himself with some assistance. How would these factors enter into the determination of his decision-making capacity?
- How does the inability of the healthcare provider to communicate with a patient affect the determination of the patient's decision-making capacity?
- What are the implications of denying Mohano important services because of a lack of common language and subsequent inability to ensure informed consent?

Federal, state, and institution policies govern expectations regarding a properly executed informed consent (including who can legally obtain this consent), and nurses need to be familiar with these policies. Merely witnessing a patient's signature on a consent form that has previously been discussed with the patient by the provider is not considered obtaining informed consent (Petersen, 2010). Rather, witnessing a patient's signature

implies accountability on the part of the nurse to ensure that the patient is giving consent willingly, is competent in that moment to give consent, and that the patient's signature is authentic. An important part of the nursing role is to verify that the patient understands the procedure, determine whether there are any questions that need to be discussed with the provider, and be alert for any indication of coercion (Plawecki & Plawecki, 2009).

Nursing documentation of communication with the patient and with the provider regarding any questions, concerns, or teaching related to the informed consent is of utmost importance. Any special circumstances should also be documented, such as the patient's inability to read or write, or the use of an interpreter if the patient speaks a language that is different from the dominant language.

Advanced practice nurses (e.g., Nurse Practitioner, Doctor of Nursing Practice, and Nurse Midwife) are accountable for providing information and obtaining informed consent for interventions that they initiate under their scope of practice. The question of the right of nurses other than those in advance practice to inform a patient of the risks inherent in a certain procedure or alternative courses of action in other settings is not as clear. In 1977, in the course of initiating chemotherapy, Jolene Tuma, a nursing instructor, answered an elderly patient's questions about cancer treatment alternatives. The patient indicated that she did not want to question the physician because he was not open to considering other therapies. Tuma was also asked to describe the therapies to the patient's son, who was upset by this. Although the patient decided to continue chemotherapy, she died two weeks later. After the patient's death, the son told the physician of Tuma's action. The physician subsequently brought charges against Ms. Tuma for disrupting the physician–patient relationship. She was fired from her job and lost her nursing license as a result. Ms. Tuma pursued an appeal of the decision. In 1979 the Idaho Supreme Court ruled that she could not lose her license for "unprofessional behavior" because there was no statutory description of this offense. The court did not address, however, the nurse's right to inform the patient (*Tuma v. Board of Nursing of the State of Idaho*, 1979).

Unfortunately, this leaves the nurse in a sort of limbo with regard to ensuring informed consent. Although the nurse is legally required to act on behalf of the patient to guarantee true informed consent, there is no clear course of action when a nurse believes that the patient has not been informed or does not understand the information, and the provider is uncooperative in remedying the situation. Institutional and legal constraints may impede the nurse from following the ethically correct course of action. Nurses need to advocate for the development of clear institutional guidelines regarding professional responsibility related to obtaining informed consent.

ASK YOURSELF

What Is the Nurse's Responsibility Regarding Informed Consent?
- In the case described previously, do you feel that Jolene Tuma's actions were appropriate? Support your position. How would codes of nursing ethics inform your position?
- What ethical issues are apparent in situations such as this?
- How does the nurse–patient relationship factor into such a situation?

ADVANCE DIRECTIVES

Given the dilemmas that can arise regarding the use of life-sustaining interventions, an important nursing role is to encourage and assist people to make their wishes known concerning the use of such interventions. For those who are mentally alert and capable of making decisions, informed consent is needed before initiating any life-sustaining interventions. To ensure that our wishes regarding treatment are followed in the event that we have lost decision-making capacity, advance directives are needed. Advance directives are legal documents that indicate healthcare interventions to initiate or withhold, or that designate someone who will act as a surrogate in making such decisions in the event that we lose decision-making capacity (Fig. 11.1). Such directives can be considered a kind of informed consent for future interventions. Advance directives support people in making decisions on their own behalf and help ensure that patients have the kind of end-of-life care that they want. To help patients be as clear as possible about their choices, the various life-sustaining measures that may be considered in end-of-life care should be discussed openly and clearly. Patients should be encouraged to express verbally or in writing their wishes about life-sustaining measures such as tube feedings, respirators, extracorporeal membrane oxygenation machines, cardiopulmonary resuscitation, artificial sources of nutrition, and dialysis. Choices about cardiopulmonary resuscitation and do-not-resuscitate (DNR) orders that are routinely part of advance directives are discussed in Chapter 10. Consideration of interventions should include how long they might want to stay on an intervention if it is initiated and their condition continues to decline or is not improving. In addition to enabling

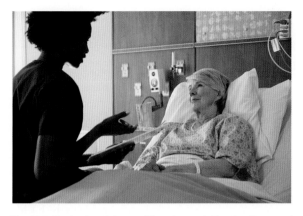

Fig. 11.1 Reviewing Advance Directives—A Nursing Responsibility. (©iStock.com/monkeybusinessimages.)

people to have choices in their dying process, the presence of clearly understood advance directives can alleviate stress on family and clinicians when dealing with end-of-life concerns.

The most important factor in decision making regarding end-of-life care is clear and open communication between the patient or the healthcare surrogate and healthcare providers. We need to do more than merely seek to know which potential life-sustaining technology a person does or does not want. We need to see and get to know the person who is making these decisions. Eliciting a clear statement of personal values is basic to this process. What does the person value in life? What constitutes quality of life for the person? What are his or her personal beliefs and concerns about dying? We must recognize the influence of cultural, societal, spiritual, and familial norms and perspectives on personal values. For example, in some cultures, speaking of death and dying is believed to bring bad luck. Family wishes may influence personal choices, and in some cultures, the patient may defer decisions about end-of-life care to the family. When discussing different interventions, we need to ensure that patients understand what the procedure is and what it involves. They also need to appreciate that the risks and benefits of life-sustaining interventions vary with age, health condition, and circumstances that prompt the consideration of the intervention. For example, the literature shows no evidence that tube feedings prolong life or improve the quality of life for patients with dementia or multisystem illness (ANA, 2017; Geppert et al.,

2010). We need to understand why the patient or family wants a particular intervention and what it is that they think it will do for them.

Advance directives include living wills and medical or durable powers of attorney for healthcare. Living wills are legal documents giving directions to healthcare providers related to withholding or withdrawing life support if certain conditions exist. Statutes regulating living wills vary from state to state, so nurses must be familiar with their own state laws. Living wills guide decisions by indicating a person's desires regarding life-sustaining interventions; however, they also raise issues of concern. Directives in living wills may be vague and can address only the interventions a person does not want. In some states, only persons who are terminally ill or whose death is imminent are allowed to make living wills. Particularly in emergency situations, there may be a concern that a document that had been developed when a person was in good health may not reflect the patient's current desires.

A durable power of attorney for healthcare (which may also be referred to as medical power of attorney, healthcare surrogate, or healthcare proxy) allows a competent person to designate another as a surrogate or proxy to act on her or his behalf in making healthcare decisions in the event of the loss of decision-making capacity. The designation must be in writing and must be signed and dated by the person making the designation and two witnesses other than the designated surrogate. A sample form is available on the West Virginia Center for End-of-Life Care at https://wvendoflife.org/media/1292/2022-new-mpoa-faq.pdf. The designating person may revoke the designation at any time by changing the person named as surrogate or by destroying the document. The authority of the surrogate does not become effective until it has been determined that the person has lost decision-making capacity. The authority of the surrogate is effective only for the duration of the loss of decision-making capacity. For example, in the case of a person who has a temporary loss of consciousness, the surrogate's authority to make decisions would end once the person regained consciousness and the ability to make decisions for himself or herself.

The presence of a living will or durable power of attorney and surrogate designation should be documented in a patient's health record. Nurses can seek opportunities to explore with patients whether they have such documents and to discuss the importance of such directives with patients and families. Discussion can begin with providing materials on advance directives to patients and families or by asking patients whether they have discussed end-of-life choices with their family or healthcare provider and by asking whether they have, or would like to develop, an advance directive. All states have advance directive laws, as well as definitions regarding who can serve as healthcare surrogate for a person who is incapacitated, although elements of these laws vary among states (Miller, 2017). Definitions of incapacitation and guidelines for determining incapacitation also vary among states. Copies of advance directive forms and instructions for each state and territory in the United States can be found on the *Hospice and Palliative Care Organization's Caringinfo* website at https://www.caringinfo.org/planning/advance-directives/by-state/. Similar information for Canada can be found through the Health Law Institute, Dalhousie University *End-of-life Law & Policy in Canada:* http://eol.law.dal.ca/?page_id=231. Readers are encouraged to review guidelines for advance directives for their own state, territory, or province.

It is well known that patients may indicate concerns to nurses that they have not discussed with their physicians. Issues related to advance directives may be one such concern. Thus, it is important that nurses develop skills and comfort in talking with patients about end-of-life wishes.

Decision-Making Capacity

Informed consent requires that the patient or healthcare surrogate have the ability to make a reasonable decision regarding healthcare concerns. As noted earlier, a surrogate or healthcare proxy is someone who makes medical decisions on the patient's behalf if the patient is incapable of doing so. Conscious adults are presumed to have decision-making capacity unless there is evidence to the contrary. Decision-making capacity is a medical determination relating only to the issue at hand, as people may have the ability to make decisions about some areas but not about others (Box 11.2). For example, a person may be able to make decisions about health but unable to make reasonable decisions about household matters such as finances. Persons may have decision-making capacity at some times and not others, and in each specific situation, there must be a determination that they have, or do not have, the capacity. The fact that a person

> ### BOX 11.2   Elements of Decision-Making Capacity
>
> The patient must:
> - Have the ability to understand all information
> - Have the ability to communicate understanding and choices
> - Have personal values and goals that guide the decision
> - Have the ability to reason and deliberate

makes a decision that seems unreasonable to the healthcare provider does not necessarily mean a lack of decision-making capacity; it may merely reflect a difference in values. If the decision seems unreasonable, however, it is wise to explore the patient's capacity regarding decision making, as well as beliefs and values that underlie the decision.

Elements of Decision-Making Capacity

When evaluating a patient or surrogate for decision-making capacity, several elements must be present. These are listed in Box 11.2. First, the patient must be able to understand all relevant information, including the nature of the healthcare problem; the prognosis; treatment options and recommendations; the risks, benefits, and consequences of each; and the risk of doing nothing. Second, the patient must be able to communicate this understanding and her or his choices. Third, the patient must possess a set of values and goals that enable evaluation regarding whether this healthcare decision will be of benefit in terms of personal goals. Fourth, the patient must have the ability to reason and to deliberate about available choices, which includes the ability to grasp notions such as risk and percentage, cause and effect, and chance and probability. Although it is not unreasonable to see some indecision, or even a change of mind, once a choice has been made, a great deal of vacillation between choices suggests the need to reevaluate decision-making capacity. Nurses are in a key position to observe patients and families for the presence of these elements of decision-making capacity. As patient advocates, nurses need to assess, document, and communicate to appropriate members of the healthcare team any concerns in this regard.

Physicians usually have the legal authority and responsibility to determine decision-making capacity.

In at least one state, however, an advanced practice nurse, a physician assistant, or a psychologist can also legally certify incapacity (West Virginia Healthcare Decisions Act, 2022). Determining incapacity is best done in consultation with family or others who have the patient's best interests in mind. There is a distinction between decision-making capacity and competence. Decisions about competence, which is the ability to make meaningful life decisions, require a legal action. Legally, persons are considered competent unless there is a ruling by a judge that they cannot make meaningful life decisions. Legal declarations of incompetence generally stay in effect for the remainder of the person's life and include a court-appointed guardian to be the surrogate decision maker for the person.

When a patient lacks decision-making capacity and does not have advance directives or a medical power of attorney, someone else must be identified as a healthcare surrogate to make decisions for the patient. In the case of children, the surrogate is usually a parent or legal guardian. With adults, the surrogate may be a spouse, parent, adult children, other relatives, or other person named as surrogate in the patient's advance directives. In situations where a patient has no advance directives or has not named a surrogate to make decisions in the event of incapacity, healthcare providers should work with family and others to identify a surrogate. The legal process for choosing a healthcare surrogate varies in different states and provinces, and you need to be familiar with the process where you live and work (see http://www.caringinfo.org/i4a/pages/index.cfm?pageid=3289 for the United States and http://eol.law.dal.ca/?page_id=231 for Canada). The person chosen as healthcare surrogate should be someone who knows the patient well, is willing to serve in this role, is calm in a crisis, and can make healthcare decisions that are in accordance with the patient's wishes, or that are consistent with the patient's best interests if these wishes are not known or cannot be reasonably discerned. The surrogate should demonstrate care and concern for and have regular contact with the patient. In addition, the surrogate should be willing to ask questions and advocate for the patient, be able to participate fully in the decision-making process, and be willing to engage in face-to-face contact and communication with caregivers and family. Close family members such as parents, adult children, adult siblings, and adult grandchildren are often considered first if the patient has not designated a healthcare surrogate. However, close friends or neighbors may at times be better qualified to make these decisions. The decisions made by the healthcare surrogate should reflect the patient's values, including the patient's cultural and spiritual perspective, to the extent that these are reasonably known.

Patient Self-Determination Act

The US Patient Self-Determination Act (PSDA), which went into effect in December 1991, is a federal law requiring institutions such as hospitals, nursing homes, health maintenance organizations, and home care agencies receiving Medicare or Medicaid funds to provide written information to adult patients regarding their rights to make healthcare decisions. Such decisions include the right to refuse treatments and the right to write advance directives for guiding decisions should they become incapacitated. Nurses have an ethical responsibility to educate and support patients in making informed decisions regarding self-determination (ANA, 2015, 2016a, 2016b; CNA, 2017, Part I.C; ICN, 2011; 2015; 2021). Nurses have a critical role in implementing the PSDA within all healthcare settings. This role includes ensuring that patients and families understand both the decisions they make and their consequences. Nurses need to ensure as much as possible that discussions utilize the patient's primary language and incorporate respect for the patient's cultural and spiritual perspectives. Nurses must also advocate for patients to ensure their wishes are followed by healthcare surrogates and the healthcare team.

In spite of the PSDA, only a small percentage of patients have advance directives, and many clinicians are not always aware of the wishes of seriously ill patients for whom they care (Miller, 2017). Paternalistic attitudes of some clinicians may result in their disregarding advance directives because of their belief that they know what is best for the patient in the current circumstances. Developing advance directives is part of the ongoing process of communication between patients or their healthcare surrogates and clinicians (ANA, 2016a; CNA, 2021. Part I.C; Levi & Green, 2010). Open discussion on end-of-life decisions should occur routinely within primary care settings, before the physical and emotional stress of serious illness or hospitalization.

CASE PRESENTATION

Terri Schiavo

The well-publicized case of Terri Schiavo illustrates a number of ethical issues regarding end-of-life care decisions made in the absence of advance directives. It is an example, as Quill (2005) notes, of medicine, ethics, law, and family working together poorly to meet the needs of a patient in a persistent vegetative state. Terri Schiavo had a cardiac arrest in 1990, reportedly triggered by severe hypokalemia related to an eating disorder, and was left paralyzed and severely brain damaged. For 15 years she was sustained by artificial nutrition and hydration via a feeding tube. Reports of her neurological exams indicated that she was in a persistent vegetative state, which includes some reflexive response to noise and light, basic gag response, and periods of alternating sleep and wakefulness, but without signs of cognition, emotion, or willful activity. In the absence of advance directives, her husband was made her legal guardian and healthcare surrogate. Reports indicate that the relationship between Ms. Schiavo's husband and her family (parents and siblings) had been strained since around 1993 and that they held vastly different opinions about what Ms. Schiavo would want and should have. Based on reports of medical experts and diagnostic tests, the state court of appeals ruled that there was clear and convincing evidence that supported the diagnosis of a persistent vegetative state. Stating that his wife would not want to be kept alive indefinitely in this condition (because of a reported statement she had made when she was cognizant that she would not want to be kept alive on machines), her husband requested that the feeding tube be discontinued. Ms. Schiavo's family, however, found other medical practitioners who believed that her condition could improve with therapies (for which there was no research evidence), and they would not accept the diagnosis of persistent vegetative state. Between 2001 and 2003, the courts authorized removing the feeding tube two different times, ruling that the evidence showed that she would not have chosen life-prolonging interventions given her condition. Because of legal action

initiated by her family, the tube was reinserted each time. In the midst of an ongoing legal battle (during which a guardian ad litem was appointed) and massive media attention, public debate, and political and religious rhetoric, her feeding tube was again removed on March 18, 2005. Multiple legal appeals to reinsert the tube were denied, and she died 13 days later.

Think About It

- What do you see as the ethical issues in this case?
- What is your opinion of the ethical nature of the various decisions that were made? What values, beliefs, and information have shaped your opinion?
- Based on your understanding of the case, if you were appointed guardian ad litem for Ms. Schiavo, what would you recommend regarding life-sustaining measures? Support your position with what you understand to be the facts in the case and the ethical reasoning that would guide your recommendation.
- How might have Ms. Schiavo's end-of-life care been different if she had completed advance directives?
- Quill (2005) notes that the media coverage, distortion by interest groups, and emotional overtones associated with this case show what can happen when someone becomes more of a precedent-setting symbol than a unique human being. How do you feel about public treatment and discussion of a situation such as this? How do you think you would have felt if she were your family member?
- How might you deal with a situation in which family members of a patient who is terminally ill (and unable to make decisions for himself or herself) or in a persistent vegetative state hold vastly different views of both the patient's condition and of what the patient would want regarding end-of-life care?
- How might the healthcare system, ethics, law, and the family work more effectively together to preserve the dignity and meet the needs of a patient in Ms. Schiavo's condition? What guidance would nursing codes of ethics provide for nurses situations like this?

Nursing Role and Responsibilities: Advance Directives

As noted above, nurses have an ethical responsibility to educate and support patients in making informed decisions regarding self-determination (ANA, 2015, 2016a, 2016b; CNA, 2017, Part I.C. I.D.9,10; ICN, 2015). This requires that nurses be knowledgeable about end-of-life care and about state, provincial, and national laws and

statutes that guide and govern advance directives and end-of-life care. Whatever the work setting, we as nurses have a key role and responsibility in ensuring that patients have an opportunity to discuss and complete advance directives. We also need to be aware of the policies and procedures regarding advance directives where we work. Completing our own advance directives helps us reflect on our own values, beliefs, and concerns associated with end-of-life issues. Through this process, we learn more about the specific forms and processes involved and ultimately have more empathy with patients going through this process. Information concerning advance directives is often provided to patients on admission to a facility by a clerical worker. Because there may be limited explanation of this information to patients or limited opportunity for questions, we need to explore patient and family understanding of the information received. We can use this as an opening to stress the importance of having such directives and to advocate for patients who may need assistance in developing advance directives. This is also a beginning opportunity for us to help patients explore personal values, their understanding of themselves in the context of their current situation, and significant cultural

or other issues that may influence decision making. As nurses, we need to be familiar with our patients' directives for care and ensure that care is consistent with the patient's wishes as expressed in the advance directives. Nursing's advocacy role in this regard includes informing other health team members of the presence and content of advance directives, alerting appropriate team members to changes in patient wishes or to evidence of changes in the patient's decision-making capacity, and intervening on behalf of the patient when wishes expressed in advance directives are not being followed. Nurses have an important role in increasing public awareness about advance directives through patient and community education, through research, and through education of nurses and other healthcare providers.

CASE PRESENTATION

The Absence of Advance Directives

Ninety-year-old Mr. Moshe did not have advance directives when he was admitted to the hospital with Alzheimer disease and renal failure. Although he was coherent at times and could converse with caregivers, the doctor determined that Mr. Moshe did not have decision-making capacity and named his daughter, Zelda, with whom Mr. Moshe had been residing, as his surrogate. The nursing staff questioned this choice because of their concerns about the quality of care Mr. Moshe had been receiving from Zelda and her husband, Josh. As Mr. Moshe's health began to deteriorate rapidly, the nurses inquired about his DNR status. Josh replied he wanted Mr. Moshe kept alive and that this was what Mr. Moshe wanted also. Zelda concurred with this. Although Zelda's four siblings called frequently inquiring about their father, Zelda would not inform them about Mr. Moshe's condition nor allow them access to him. Because of this conflict and their concerns regarding the motives for his DNR status, the nurses notified the physician about the family issues and requested an ethics committee consultation to determine the best interests of the patient. The nurses also noted that the physician had not signed the surrogate form as required by their state law, so legally there was no surrogate. The ethics committee representative convened a family meeting that included all five siblings, the physician, the primary nurse, and a member of the pastoral care team. After explaining that the purpose of the meeting was to discuss the type of care that would be in the best interests of their father, not to resolve family issues, the physician was asked to discuss Mr. Moshe's current health status and prognosis. All of the children were given the opportunity to ask questions of the physician and primary nurse. Then each family member was asked to voice what their father valued in life

and what they believed to be his wishes regarding end-of-life care. Even though some of the siblings had not spoken to each other for nearly 10 years, they each stated that their father had told them he would never want to be on life support. Zelda, who was asked to speak last, agreed, much to the dismay of her husband, that her father would not want to be placed on life support. The siblings also requested that they be allowed to visit their father and to call and check on him. When they were informed that there currently was no legal surrogate for their father, they all agreed to have Zelda continue in that role, provided that she allowed them access to him. They stated that even though they were upset with her, they believed she loved him and provided good care for him. To close the meeting, all family members were invited to go together to their father's bedside, where they shared prayer and family stories. Mr. Moshe died that night.

Think About It
Considering the Patient's Best Interests
- Because Mr. Moshe was coherent at times, do you think the physician should have asked him what he would want regarding life support?
- What do you think of the physician's choice of a surrogate for Mr. Moshe? What factors do you think he considered in appointing Zelda as surrogate? Are there factors you think he should have considered that he may not have?
- As the nurse caring for Mr. Moshe, what would be your concerns regarding his situation? How do you think you would have responded in this situation?
- How was nursing's advocacy role evident in this situation?
- How did the process of the family meeting address the communication that is needed for making end-of-life decisions?

ETHICAL CONSIDERATIONS RELATED TO LIFESTYLE AND HEALTH CHOICES

Although discussion of patient autonomy frequently focuses on issues of informed consent and end-of-life decisions, issues related to self-determination can arise in any area of nursing practice. In every area of practice, nurses must deal with the effects of lifestyle and health-related choices on patients' health and healing. Many people who come into our care are suffering from ill effects of such things as overeating; tobacco, drug, or alcohol use; sexual activity; or work-related stress. Our job is to deal with the present health concern while encouraging change toward healthier living. However, patients are often not willing to follow the treatment plan and make the changes needed for healthier living. Dealing with patients whose health problems are clearly related to lifestyle choices yet who are not willing to change their behaviors may present dilemmas for nurses. Although nurses may acknowledge that the autonomous person has the right to choose healthy or unhealthy behaviors, it may be difficult to be as caring toward those who are perceived to have brought problems on themselves.

This is another area where the principle of justice may temper the bounds of autonomy. In situations where resources are limited, questions arise regarding whether it is ethical to put resources into treatments for people whose health problems are brought on by unhealthy life choices. This is countered by the question of whether it is ethical to refuse treatment or provide a lesser level of care to someone because the healthcare provider does not agree with that person's lifestyle choices.

Choices Regarding Recommended Treatment

What are nurses to do when patients are well informed and apparently able to follow plans of care, yet do not? Certainly one hears of physicians who refuse to continue to care for patients who do not comply with instructions—smoking cessation, for example. In a climate of limited resources, this is a question worthy of contemplation. The ANA's *Code of Ethics for Nurses with Interpretive Statements* (2015) states that nurses in all professional relationships practice "with compassion and respect for the inherent dignity, worth, and unique attributes, and human rights [of] all individuals …

regardless of the factors contributing to the person's health status" (Provisions 1.1 and 1.3). Further, "nurses establish relationships of trust and provide nursing services according to need, setting aside bias or prejudice" (Provision 1.2). Similar directives are found in the CNA (2017) and ICN (2021) codes of ethics. Healthcare practices are an integral part of patients' backgrounds, cultures, customs, and beliefs. Therefore, it is clear that refusal to participate in a plan of care, regardless of the outcome, is the prerogative of the patient and must not affect the professional care given by the nurse. Nurses do, however, have an obligation to address unhealthy or risky life and health practices in a nonjudgmental way and to offer resources and opportunities to modify behaviors as part of a patient's plan of care.

Ultimately, choices about healthcare practices belong to patients. If allowed to choose, patients should not be labeled in a negative way for choices with which nurses do not agree. It is not appropriate for professionals who express the belief that all competent patients have the right to autonomous choice to then make value judgments about the choices made and subsequently label patients as noncompliant. In fact, it is worth pondering whether the term *noncompliant* even belongs in nursing vocabulary. The notion of compliance relates to a paternalistic view that healthcare providers know what is best for patients and that, providing patients follow these directions, they will get well. Nurses should speak more appropriately in terms of motivation to follow a mutually agreed-on plan of care that incorporates patient and family values and beliefs. We must remember that patients have a right to refuse interventions, and they have a right to seek therapies other than those offered by conventional Western medicine.

Complementary Therapies

Many people utilize therapies that may be termed *complementary, alternative,* or *integrative* with regard to Western allopathic medicine. As noted in Chapter 18, complementary therapies include acupuncture, herbal and nutritional interventions, energy healing modalities, biofeedback, relaxation techniques, massage, and spiritual healing processes. Most people tend to use such therapies along with conventional modalities, but some will choose to use them in lieu of what is offered by medical practitioners. Many people do not inform their medical practitioners that they are using these therapies.

CASE PRESENTATION

A Challenging Patient

Rochelle, a 36-year-old woman who is a known cocaine addict, presented to the emergency room (ER) with severe left leg pain and swelling. The triage nurse reviewed her chart and presenting problem, noting that she had been seen two days prior for chest pain and left leg pain. Assuming these complaints were evaluated then, the nurse sent her to the "fast track" area to be seen by the nurse practitioner (NP). The NP noted that her chart was flagged regarding her cocaine addiction and that the physician who had seen her at the previous visit ordered an electrocardiogram, complete blood count, electrolytes (which were normal), and a urine drug screen (which was positive for cocaine). She was then discharged with diagnoses of chest pain and illicit drug use. The NP's assessment revealed no shortness of breath, cough, or chest pain. Severe swelling and skin tightness of the left leg, with exquisite tenderness and positive Homan's sign, were suggestive of deep vein thrombosis. When the NP went to the ER physician saying that the patient needed to be evaluated by him, she was told to keep the patient over there and do the work-up because he had a patient with a similar problem in the ER.

When the ultrasound confirmed extensive deep vein thrombosis, the NP told the patient the situation and that she needed to be hospitalized. The patient immediately said that she could not stay because she had no one to watch her nine-year-old daughter, and she began to put on her shoes to leave. The NP told Rochelle that she could choose to leave but that the reason the NP wanted her to stay was that this was a very serious problem from which she could die. Rochelle's response was to start crying, saying that she thought she would go home anyway because she had nothing to live for since her husband had died, so she would go home to die. When the NP called Rochelle's primary physician to alert him to the situation, he responded that he would come in to see her only if Rochelle agreed to stay; otherwise, it would be a waste of his time. After considerable effort, the NP contacted Rochelle's mother, who reluctantly agreed to keep her granddaughter when the NP explained the situation, and Rochelle agreed to stay.

Think About It
Dealing With Patients Who Make Apparently Unhealthy Choices

- What issues of patient self-determination are evident in this case?
- How do you see lifestyle choices affecting Rochelle's care? What ethical issues must be considered here?
- Take an honest look at how you think you might react to Rochelle, knowing that she frequently shows up in the ER and is a cocaine addict.
- As the nurse in this situation, how would you deal with the patient's saying she could not stay? What do you think of the way the NP handled it?
- Evaluate ethical issues involved in the responses of the various healthcare providers in this case. Did the NP's response align with professional nursing ethical codes? Give examples.
- Interestingly, Rochelle was indigent, African American, and without health insurance, and the woman in the ER with similar complaints was middle class, White, and had health insurance. Discuss the implications of these factors in this case. What health disparities are evident in this situation?

Nurses need to be alert to several issues regarding patient self-determination when complementary therapies are considered. First, people have a right to use modalities other than conventional medicine to address their healthcare needs. Second, nurses and other healthcare practitioners need to develop at least a talking knowledge and, better yet, a working knowledge of such therapies to be better able to discuss their use with patients. Many therapies work as an adjunct to medical interventions, some may interact in unhealthy ways, and the efficacy of many modalities has not yet been studied scientifically. Third, nurses should create an atmosphere that encourages nonjudgmental discussion of all modalities being considered or employed, with a goal of using whatever is beneficial for the particular patient. Nurses need not be practitioners of other modalities to discuss them with patients any more than they need to be able to do surgery to discuss it. Transcultural considerations (discussed in Chapter 18) may influence a person's choice of treatment modalities. Fourth, complementary modalities should not be discounted merely because they are not understood within the Western medical framework; however, it is important to counsel patients to explore the validity of claims made about a particular therapy. Fifth, as research continues and expands in the area of complementary therapies, the question of whether informed consent will need to at least acknowledge these therapies as treatment options must be addressed. Sixth, nurses who are skilled in complementary therapies need to be clear about what is within their scope of practice according to their state's nurse practice act. The ethical stance with complementary therapies, as with other interventions, requires explaining the intervention and receiving permission from the patient or family before initiating the therapy. Because these therapies can affect conventional interventions, practitioners should apprise other health team members of their use and document both treatments and their effects. More information about research and other considerations regarding complementary therapies is available through the National Institutes of Health and the National Center for Complementary and Integrative Health (https://nccih.nih.gov/health).

Ethical Issues Related to Selected Health Concerns and Personal Choice

The value of patient self-determination is cited to support two decisions that have been the focus of much discussion in this country for many years: abortion and assisted dying. Both of these choices are surrounded by ethical, philosophical, and religious opinions and debates. Abortion in particular is an example of an issue in which legal answers have been sought for ethical dilemmas. The potential for transmission of HIV infections within the community and in healthcare settings raises controversial issues regarding testing and disclosure. The choice of individuals and of parents to not follow vaccination policies for themselves or their children gives rise to ethical issues related to public health and professional ethics. A number of ethical issues surround lifestyle choices that lead to addiction, particularly related to the opioid crisis. Following is a brief discussion of various perspectives related to these health and lifestyle choices and associated ethical issues. Readers are encouraged to further explore these issues as they relate to their own experience and professional practice.

Nurses need to be very clear about their own values regarding each of these issues and need to find a balance between personal values and professional obligations to patients and families. Through understanding their own beliefs about what is right and wrong, nurses can differentiate between tasks and roles that are consistent with their ethical stance and those that are not and make responsible practice decisions accordingly. Decisions regarding care are guided by professional ethical codes that include the directives to respect the rights of others and to not abandon patients, yet to practice within the integrity of one's own values and beliefs. If a nurse feels a strong ethical conflict in caring for a particular patient, it is appropriate to ask that the patient be assigned to another nurse. Aligning one's care with the Golden Rule of "do unto others as you would have them do unto you," even when there is disagreement with patient choices, is a good practice.

Abortion

The abortion debate sparks passionate, emotion-laden arguments in political, social, legal, religious, and moral arenas. Issues of self-determination arise regarding the mother's right to control her body and her life (right to choose) in contrast to the rights of the unborn fetus to a chance at life (right to life). Those in the right-to-life camp believe that abortion constitutes murder of an unborn person, suggesting that it is a legal as well as an ethical matter. This has raised questions about the role of government in dealing with this ethical concern. Those who support the right to choose maintain that autonomy and the right to privacy regarding healthcare decisions includes a woman's reproductive choices, implying that governmental regulation is an infringement on this autonomy and privacy.

Values in relation to life are fundamental considerations with regard to abortion. Such values include beliefs about when life begins, considerations regarding the quality of life for children who are unwanted, and concerns about the mother's life and health. Some believe that life starts at conception, whereas others hold that life begins only when a fetus is viable outside the womb. Discussions regarding viability continue to change as technology enables the survival of babies of lower and lower birth weights, resulting in saving some imperiled newborns of the same gestational age as some aborted fetuses.

Opponents of abortion hold the position that because a fetus possesses humanity, it must be accorded all human rights, including the right to life. Proponents of abortion argue that, based on autonomy, a woman has a right to her own body and that no woman should be forced to bear a child that she does not want. Because abortion is a situation in which two lives are involved, dilemmas arise regarding who has rights and whose rights take precedence. Those who support the right to abortion base their argument on the woman's autonomy and feel that the woman's rights override those of the fetus. Those who oppose abortion argue from the stance of the sanctity of life of the fetus, believing the rights of the fetus overshadow those of the pregnant woman. Depending on one's stance, there is concern that either the woman or the fetus becomes viewed as an object or a thing. From either perspective, the consideration of abortion presents a dilemma for those involved.

In spite of vehement public discourse and legal decisions, there is no agreement about the morality of abortion in our society. It is a complex issue with many facets to consider. Although debate generally focuses on areas related to the rights of the woman or the fetus, Mahowald (2000) suggests that it is also important to consider the morality of circumstances that provide fertile ground for abortion. She notes that immoral conditions that sometimes contribute to a woman's seeking abortion include poverty, lack of social and medical supports for pregnancy and parenthood, stereotypical views of sex roles and biological parenthood, and a eugenic mentality that welcomes only those babies that meet the parents' desired specifications. She stresses the need for society to direct more effort into rectifying these conditions.

A Broader Look at Reproductive Rights

Roberts (2000) raised ethical concerns about the need to include in reproductive rights discussion areas such as contraceptive choices, decisions about cesarean sections, and reproduction-assisting technologies. These concerns continue to be pertinent. Her discussion incudes how race and gender affect the ethics of policies and practices in these areas. One example is how the early birth control movement in the United States became tied to the **eugenics** movement. This movement advocated policies encouraging so-called "genetically superior" people to have children, while discouraging so-called "genetically inferior" people from having children—even through forced sterilization. She points to the historical example of the first public birth control clinics in the United States that were established in the South and directed toward poor Black women. Another example is a class-action lawsuit in Alabama that uncovered that hundreds of thousands of women in the United States, the majority of whom were Black, were being coercively sterilized through government welfare

programs that conditioned healthcare and benefits on sterilization. This lawsuit prompted the 1970s federal regulation requiring informed consent and a waiting period before sterilization.

Although one aspect of the abortion debate relates to compulsory motherhood, where women's value is linked to their ability to reproduce, contraceptive policies often devalue poor women and women of color as mothers, in that such policies are aimed at preventing these women from having children. Roberts (2000) cautions that various societal norms can lead to reproductive regulation of women and that we need to expand the meaning of reproductive freedom to include the right to have a child—the right to decide to be a mother. She notes that there are as many policies that have sought to deter women from having children as there are those that have sought to force women to have children.

Nurses need to consider the ethical implications of issues such as the dangers of eugenics in population control, deciding that some people are unfit to have children because of their biology or socioeconomic status and suggesting that reproduction is the cause of social problems. Another important ethical issue is the racial disparity in reproductive policies and practices. Technologies that help women have children are more available to White women, in contrast to policies and practices aimed at deterring women from having children that are being targeted toward poor women, particularly women of color. Such policies raise questions about who is valued in society and how we use reproductive technologies to encourage the birth of certain "valued" children versus those perceived to be of less value. Reproductive policies that flow from such attitudes affect group status and social structure as well as individuals. Dealing with issues regarding the ethics of reproduction requires that nurses address social determinants of health, social justice, and power relationships in the broader society.

Assisted Death

As noted in Chapter 10, technology has caused death to become an unnatural event in the lives of many people. Because of concern that healthcare providers will not adhere to personal wishes regarding end-of-life issues, fears about prolonged suffering resulting from prolongation of dying, and the lack of control that each of these engenders, many people consider the possibility of **assisted death**. Assisted death is an act in which the means of death, such as a lethal dose of medication, is provided by a health professional but is administered by the patient, family member, or friend. This is different from **euthanasia** in which someone other than the person administers a lethal dose with the intent of hastening death. With assisted death patients receive the means of ending their life from someone, such as a physician, but activate the process themselves. Public dissatisfaction with end-of-life care has prompted efforts to legalize these acts. Multiple views and controversies about assisted death fueled public debate surrounding these efforts. Several states, including Oregon, Washington, Vermont, Maine, New Jersey, Hawai'i, and California, have passed *Death with Dignity* legislation that enables patients to end their lives on their terms when pain and suffering become intolerable (Miller, 2017; https://deathwithdignity.org/2023). Justification offered by proponents of these acts includes respect for the person's autonomy in choosing to end her or his life if it is deemed intolerable due to conditions of a lingering terminal illness and compassion exhibited in relief of the patient's suffering. Opponents argue from a stance of the sanctity of life, saying that any such act violates the prohibition against killing human beings. They hold that suffering can almost always be relieved, and they voice concerns about potential abuses related to these acts, such as involuntary euthanasia to contain healthcare costs (ANA, 2019; Lo, 2013). Even in states in which assisted death is legal, the position of the ANA (2019) is that "nurses are ethically prohibited from administering medical aid in dying medications"; however, they may still be involved in the patient's care. Nurses need to be aware of personal values and beliefs related to assisted death and how their values may affect patient care. Taking care never to abandon a patient, nurses whose values conflict with assisted death have a right to decline to participate in a patient's care, providing they inform supervisors ahead of time that they conscientiously object to such care based on personal values so other arrangements for care of the patient are in place (ANA, 2015, 2019; CNA, 2017, Part I.C.12, I.G.7; ICN, 2021, Element 2.8).

It is particularly important to consider the reason for a patient's request for assisted death. When the patient indicates that life has become intolerable, we must determine why this is so. Often, inadequate pain management and depression are factors that enter into this perception, which, when treated appropriately, can change the patient's perspective. This may not always be the case, however, and nurses need to be able to support patients and families as they struggle with questions regarding whether natural death is always the best and most loving choice (ANA, 2019, 2016a; Baumrucker et al., 2009; ICN, 2012). Attending to the nature and cause of a person's suffering and providing comfort care throughout the dying process are important components of the nursing role that may influence choices regarding active voluntary euthanasia or assisted suicide.

HIV/AIDS

We know that HIV/AIDS continues to be a major worldwide health concern and that the virus is generally transmitted from an infected person through the exchange of body fluids such as blood, semen, vaginal secretions, or breast milk. Because HIV infections are most often associated with having unprotected sexual relations or sharing IV drug needles with someone who is infected with HIV, there is frequently a stigma surrounding HIV diagnosis. Nurses need to be aware of how this stigma may evoke judgmental attitudes toward persons with HIV/AIDS, and be alert to how these attitudes may affect the quality of care they receive. Nurses are guided by codes of nursing ethics to treat each person with dignity and respect and to provide compassionate care for patients regardless of their values or lifestyle.

Due to the risk of exposure to HIV in healthcare settings, primarily through accidental needle sticks, questions arise regarding issues of autonomy and confidentiality in relation to HIV testing and status. One issue relates to whether patients can be required to submit to HIV testing in situations of potential or actual percutaneous exposure of healthcare workers to their blood. To protect persons from potential discrimination, confidentiality of HIV testing and status is generally ensured by law. Information on HIV laws by state is available through the Centers for Disease Control and Prevention (CDC) at https://www.cdc.gov/hiv/policies/law/states/index.html.

Prior written informed consent to HIV testing that was previously the norm is generally no longer required (Bayer et al., 2017; CDC, 2021). CDC guidelines (CDC, 2015, 2021) recommend incorporating HIV screening into the general consent for medical care rather than requiring a separate written consent. These guidelines also recommend screening patients ages 15–65 in healthcare settings at least once after notifying that testing will be performed (unless the patient declines); testing people at high risk for HIV yearly; screening all people requesting sexually transmitted infection testing; and including HIV screening as part of routine prenatal screening (unless the patient declines). Because testing for HIV without the patient's consent violates the patient's autonomy and privacy, the CDC recommendations continue to emphasize voluntary testing. The recommendation to screen more routinely for HIV is based on the awareness that around 15 percent of the estimated 1.2 million people living with HIV in the United States do not know they are infected; thus, they unknowingly continue to spread the disease. These people could receive counseling and treatment, and their prognosis would be better with an earlier diagnosis.

Concerns about potential stigma and discrimination in work or home settings related to having a documented HIV test, regardless of its result, may lead patients to refuse a test even if they are sure it will be negative. Considerations of routine screening of all patients for HIV may reduce this stigma. To ensure confidentiality and to encourage patient agreement to testing in the event of exposure of a healthcare worker to a patient's blood, anonymous testing of the patient may be a consideration. Anonymous testing would necessitate paying for the test by a source other than the patient's insurer (such as an employee health fund), recording the results in a location other than the patient's medical record (such as a special occupational health file), and labeling the specimen with a code rather than the patient's name. In this way, the healthcare worker could know if he or she is at risk, while protecting the patient from potential stigma resulting from the test. Some of these concerns may be less of an issue with the advent of self-testing for HIV that provides results quickly at home or other private settings. The CDC provides information on self-tests at https://www.cdc.gov/hiv/basics/hiv-testing/hiv-self-tests.html.

Another issue that has become a public concern relates to potential exposure of patients to the blood of a seropositive healthcare worker. Questions arise whether HIV testing among healthcare workers, or at least those involved in certain invasive procedures, should be mandatory; whether seropositive healthcare workers should have restrictions on their practice; and whether the HIV status of healthcare workers should be made known to patients. Some argue that if it is mandatory for healthcare workers to be tested, then it should be mandatory for all patients as well. Principles of autonomy, confidentiality, and nonmaleficence become part of this discussion. Healthcare workers, as well as patients, have a right to autonomy and confidentiality regarding health matters, particularly where discrimination could result from disclosure. At the same time, nonmaleficence directs them to do no harm to patients, and the doctrine of informed consent requires advising patients of potential risks related to interventions being considered. Economic factors enter into the discussion as well. At the present time, presuming healthcare workers follow universal infection control precautions, the risk of a patient contracting HIV from a seropositive healthcare worker is low, in contrast to the cost of mandatory testing. Johnson (2022) notes that healthcare institutions may be within their rights to ask employees about HIV status. He also notes that under the *Americans with Disabilities Act* people with HIV cannot be discriminated against based on their HIV status as long as it does not interfere with their job performance.

Current issues related to HIV/AIDS may become less of a concern with the development of more effective approaches to prevention and advances in medical treatment of the disease such as antiretroviral therapy (ART). Some concerns with ART relate to cost and availability, raising ethical issues of health disparities and fair distribution. Ethical concerns surrounding these issues apply to other health problems of a similar nature. Nurses and other healthcare workers must be aware of any factors in their own health that might put their patients at risk (e.g., testing positive for hepatitis or for COVID-19) and take necessary precautions to protect patients from harm. It is also essential that nurses follow universal precautions aimed at protecting themselves and others from harm. If behaviors on the part of healthcare workers are observed that might put patients at risk, the imperatives of beneficence and nonmaleficence direct nurses to do what is necessary to protect the patient. Actions may include approaching the person involved, reporting the situation to appropriate persons within the agency, and working with groups to institute changes to prevent similar situations from occurring (ANA, 2015, Provision 3.5; CNA, 2017, Part I.F.8, I.G.6; ICN, 2021, Element 2.10).

Although all infectious diseases must be reported, including cases of HIV/AIDS, caregivers cannot disclose a person's HIV status without consent. The legal and ethical right to confidentiality regarding HIV/AIDS raises an ethical issue related to the protection of others when the infected individual continues behaviors that may expose others to the infection. In some circumstances, physicians are allowed limited disclosure without consent, such as to the patient's spouse. In such situations, the imperative of confidentiality must be weighed against the duty to warn others to protect them from potential harm.

Immunization Policy, Antivaccination Attitudes, and Vaccine Hesitancy

Outbreaks of communicable diseases in recent years have raised awareness of complex issues related to immunization policy, **antivaccination** attitudes, and **vaccine hesitancy**. (In this discussion the terms *vaccines* and *immunizations* are used interchangeably.) Self-determination is a key factor because a person must give informed consent for self (or a parent/guardian for a child) to receive an immunization. The principle of autonomy implies that one can also choose not to be immunized. People who refuse or limit immunizations for themselves or their children do so for a variety of reasons. These reasons include concern about the safety and effectiveness of vaccines, limited knowledge or misinformation about the vaccine, lack of understanding or concern about the risk related to vaccine-preventable disease, issues of accessibility and affordability of vaccines, and personal religious or philosophical beliefs (SAGE, 2014; WHO, 2015; Milliken & Uveges, 2022). Among people who are not immunized, Milliken and Uveges (2022) make a distinction between those who are antivaccination versus vaccine hesitant. They note that whereas those who are antivaccination tend to base their vaccine refusal on disinformation, conspiracy theories, personal liberty, or political choice, vaccine hesitancy is more often the result of insufficient and sometimes misinformation, lack of availability of vaccines and healthcare providers, language barriers, and a consequence of social determinants of healthcare such as structural racism. They also note that although antivaccination adherents are found in different socioeconomic, ethnic, and geographic groups, they most frequently come from well-educated, White, higher socioeconomic populations, while vaccine hesitancy is more frequent among people of color.

Refusal of immunizations for self or a child brings up issues related to public health policy versus personal choice (Hendrix et al., 2016; ANA, 2021). An important factor in the effectiveness of immunizations in preventing disease is **herd** or **community immunity**, which is a critical threshold of immunity within a community that helps prevent the spread of a communicable disease to those who cannot be immunized. When immunization rates within a community are low, there can be outbreaks of communicable diseases. For example, effective community immunity related to measles requires that 90–95 percent of the population be immunized against measles (Hendrix et al., 2016; ANA, 2021).

Since vaccines were first developed some people have refused to be vaccinated; however, the voice of "antivaxxers" garnered greater attention when COVID-19 vaccines became available. Although the percentage of the US population that has received at least one COVID vaccine is around 80 percent, the percentage of those considered to be fully vaccinated is only around 69 percent, and both vary by state. Those who remain unvaccinated jeopardize the health of others and have a significantly greater risk of becoming seriously ill with COVID-19 and being hospitalized and dying from complications of the illness. Milliken and Uveges (2022) discuss ethical challenges faced by nurses who must care for unvaccinated people who are critically ill with COVID-19. Caring for such patients through the pandemic has caused traumatic stress, moral distress, and burnout for many nurses who were pushed to the limit dealing with the challenges of patient care and many personal and professional hardships. Now that there are vaccines readily available some nurses may feel patients who choose not to be vaccinated are placing an unnecessary burden on them and the healthcare system. Because nurses may experience frustration, anger, and moral outrage toward these patients, ethical concerns arise related to nurse burnout and to nurses' obligations to respect the inherent dignity of each person and practice with compassion. Milliken and Uveges (2022) note that a nurse's ethical response in caring for unvaccinated patients includes being alert for personal attitudes that may impact the quality of care these patients receive and assuring that all patients receive safe, compassionate, respectful care. Because of a nurse's ethical responsibility to self, it is critical for nurses in such situations to seek appropriate outlets for reflecting on, expressing, and dealing with feelings of anger, frustration, and moral outrage.

CASE PRESENTATION

Ethical Concerns—Unvaccinated Patients Critically Ill With COVID-19

In a scenario described by Milliken and Uveges (2022), Simon, a nurse in an ICU that has a high census of patients critically ill with COVID-19, has heard disparaging comments from other staff during report and at the nurses' station about unvaccinated patients and their families. He has observed increased frustration and dismay among his colleagues toward COVID-19 patients who they feel "chose" not to be vaccinated. He understands that the anger and frustration can lead to burnout among nurses in an already shore-staffed unit. He is also concerned that care for these patients may suffer because of the sense of moral outrage some nurses feel toward these patients.

Think About It

- How do you think you would feel toward the current unvaccinated patients if you were a nurse who had been working on this unit throughout the COVID-19 pandemic?
- What potential ethical issues are evident in this scenario?
- What are nurses' ethical obligations toward patients who are unvaccinated or who make other choices that may frustrate and anger nurses and even place their health at risk?
- What do you think Simon should do about his concerns about the attitudes of his colleagues and the quality of patient care?

- Milliken and Uveges aptly note that the guidance and support that Simon needs in addressing his concerns is found in nursing's professional codes of ethics. Review the sections of the codes noted in the following examples that highlight nursing's ethical obligations in this scenario. Give examples of other sections of nursing codes of ethics pertinent to this situation.
- Nurses respect the dignity and worth of each person and provide safe, ethical, and compassionate care to all persons (ANA, 2015, Provision 1.1, 1.3, 2.1; CNA, 2017, Part I, A.2, D.1, 2, 4; ICN, 2021, Element 1.2, 1.8).
- Nurses take into account a patients' values and beliefs, respect their right to self-determination, and refrain from labeling or stigmatizing them (ANA, 2015, Provision 1.2,1.3, 1.4; CNA, 2017, Part I, D.3, F.3; ICN, 2021, Element 1.2, 2.9).
- Nurses promote an ethical environment and the safety of persons receiving care and, individually or collectively, express and report any concerns regarding unethical behavior to the appropriate persons (ANA, 2015, Provision 6.1, 6.2, 6.3; CNA, 2017, Part I.A.14, I.B.5, I.D.4; ICN, 2021, Element 2.11, 3.5).
- Nurses have a responsibility to preserve their integrity and promote their personal health and well-being (ANA, 2015, Provision 5.1, 5.2, 5.4; CNA, 2017, Part I.B.5, I.G.5, I.G.6; ICN, 2021, Element 2.2, 2.4).

Vaccine refusal for any reason brings up ethical issues related to health disparities, distributive justice, beneficence, and nonmaleficence. Recall that distributive justice relates to fair, equitable, and appropriate distribution in society, determined by justified norms that structure the terms of social cooperation, including policies that allot diverse benefits and burdens among members of the society. Immunization policies are considered justified norms that support a social contract to protect the health of the community by mandating that all individuals are immunized. According to distributive justice, for everyone to receive the benefits of being protected by immunizations, all those who are able should share the burden of receiving immunizations (recognizing that there are some situations in which immunization is contraindicated). Recall as well that beneficence requires one to act in ways that benefit another, and nonmaleficence requires one to act in such a manner as to avoid causing harm to another,

including risk of harm. All members of society have a social responsibility to consider how individual choices affect others. Those who choose not to be immunized are putting others (and themselves) at potential risk for harm. Questions arise related to whether children and others who are not immunized should be excluded from some activities or work settings so as not to put others at risk. There are some who raise the question of whether those who choose not to be immunized should be held ethically and legally responsible for costs related to a communicable disease outbreak (Hendrix et al., 2016; Moser et al., 2015).

Nurses have a professional and ethical obligation to promote and protect the health of individuals and the community. This responsibility includes providing evidence-based education to patients, parents, and others regarding risks and benefits of immunizations, including the importance of community immunity (Johnstone, 2016; ANA, 2021; Fig. 11.2). Although nurses have a

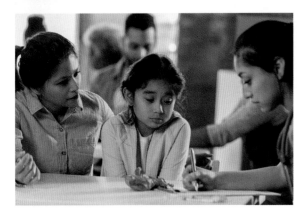

Fig. 11.2 The Nurse Discusses Benefits and Risks of Immunizations With Mother Before Consent Is Signed. (©iStock.com/asiseeit.)

right to their personal opinions related to immunizations, professional ethical responsibility and being part of the larger community direct that they support policies that benefit the public good even when counter to their own beliefs. To protect the public health, the ANA (2021) supports immunization for all against diseases preventable by vaccines (with exceptions solely for medical contraindications). In relation to the ongoing debate about whether immunizations should be mandated, the ANA (2021) and others (Giubilini et al., 2018; Ivanković, & Savić, 2021) argue that it a professional and ethical obligation for nurses and others to be vaccinated. Ethical grounding for this argument is found in the *Code for Nurses with Interpretive Statements* (ANA, 2015) particularly Provisions 1, 2, 5, and 7.

Substance Use Disorder, Pain Management, and the Opioid Epidemic

Substance use disorder is a complex health concern of which the opioid epidemic is only a part. This section highlights a few of the ethical considerations related to this issue that are particularly pertinent to nursing. An important consideration is whether substance use is a choice or a disease. Emerging evidence in neuroscience suggests that although taking drugs for the first time is voluntary, continued use alters the structure of the brain and causes impaired brain function (Hardee, 2018). This happens more quickly with some substances than with others, and there is no single factor that determines who will or will not become addicted. Drugs affect the brain by mimicking the natural chemical messengers of the

brain and by overstimulating its reward circuits (Hardee, 2018). Description of the complexity of brain changes that occur in addiction is beyond the scope of this book. What is important to understand is that once brain circuits are disrupted, the person loses control of the ability to "choose" not to take the drug. The circuits related to drug taking become so strong that it is hard for the person to counter this urge (Hardee, 2018). The disease of addiction includes social, genetic, and environmental factors that influence its development and symptoms. Along with the impaired brain circuitry noted earlier, behaviors such as craving, lack of control over drug use, compulsive use, and continued use despite harm are characteristic of the disease (Wakim, 2018).

Because of the opioid epidemic, issues of pain management and substance use disorder overlap. Appreciating that substance use disorder is a disease may enable nurses to be more sensitive to some of the issues related to care for patients, although there will still be challenges in dealing with patient behaviors. Nursing care is based on the "ethical obligation to provide respectful, individualized care to all patients experiencing pain regardless of the person's personal characteristics, values, or beliefs" (ANA, 2018, p. 2). Nurses need to be aware of personal biases and tendency to label and judge those with chronic or acute pain or with substance use disorder. Stigmatizing and blaming patients for their illness and using derogatory terms such as *junkie* or *frequent flyer* in the ED in reference to patients promotes attitudes that such patients do not want to get better, and this can affect the quality of nursing care provided. Remember that nurses are expected to practice with compassion and respect for the inherent dignity and worth for each person (ANA, 2015; CNA, 2017; ICN, 2021).

The ethical responsibility to ensure treatment for pain (acute, chronic, and end of life) and the suffering it causes may present challenges for nurses and contribute to moral distress (ANA, 2018). Nurses may encounter patients whose pain is ineffectively treated, yet they are not able to provide adequate pain relief due to inadequate treatment orders, the patient's condition, or doubting the patient's reports of pain by the healthcare provider. These circumstances may be associated with personal bias, lack of knowledge regarding effective pain control, or institutional policies and legal restrictions related to limiting use of controlled drugs. The goal of such policies may derive from the duty to prevent harm by assuring that the medications are used for legitimate pain control and are not diverted from the patient to others. These policies may also create hurdles for those who need these medications to control their pain or for whom nonnarcotic medications are legitimately medically contraindicated. Many institutions require that all patients receiving controlled drugs sign a contract that includes agreeing to such things as getting prescriptions from only one pharmacy, not giving medications to anyone else, understanding that lost or damaged medication will not be replaced, and submitting to periodic urine drug tests. Some patients may resist this practice because of feeling stigmatized and not receive the treatment they need. It is worth pondering whether principles of beneficence and nonmaleficence outweigh considerations of coercion when signing the contract is a condition of care.

Recognizing the tension that can occur between a nurse's duty to manage pain and the duty to avoid harm, the ANA's (2018) position statement *The Ethical Responsibility to Manage Pain and the Suffering It Causes* offers guidance and support to nurses. The basic elements of this statement are as follows: (1) nurses have an ethical responsibility to relieve pain and the suffering it causes; (2) nurses should provide individualized nursing interventions; (3) the nursing process should guide the nurse's actions to improve pain management; (4) multimodal and interprofessional approaches are necessary to achieve pain relief; (5) pain management modalities should be informed by evidence; (6) nurses must advocate for policies to ensure access to all effective modalities; and (7) nurse leadership is necessary for society to appropriately address the opioid epidemic (p. 1). Providing optimal care for patients requires that nurses reflect on their own biases related to the issue, advocate for policies that support effective pain control, and are knowledgeable about various approaches to effective pain management, including holistic and nonpharmacological interventions.

Dealing with and balancing the many aspects of caring for patients with health issues related to pain control and substance use can contribute to moral distress and burnout for nurses. As noted in Chapter 10, nurses need to be attentive to caring for themselves as they deal with challenging situations with patients. The ANA and the American Holistic Nurses Association (AHNA) both encourage nurses to incorporate evidence-based processes for nonpharmacological pain relief into patient care. Many of these modalities are self-care practices for nurses as well. A link to the AHNA tool kit Pain Relief Tools for Patients and Self Care can be found in the "Discussion Questions and Activities" section of this chapter. Nurses can use these processes for their own self-care, as well as to support pain control with patients. Readers are encouraged to explore these modalities and integrate them into both patient care and their own self-care practices.

ASK YOURSELF

Who Should Pay for Ill Effects of Unhealthy Lifestyles or Choices That Affect Public Health?

It is interesting that in the time of Hippocrates, physicians were taught that they should not treat persons whose bodies were overmastered by their disease because it was an inappropriate use of medical resources.

- How do you feel about this?
- Would this same stance be considered ethical today?
- To what extent do personal lifestyle choices impinge on the rights of others if significant healthcare resources are needed to pay for the ill effects of these choices?
- Is it just to expect society to pay for the healthcare services required for treating the effects of unhealthy behaviors or choices, such as refusing immunization, that can cause risk to others?
- How would you go about allocating healthcare resources in relation to unhealthy lifestyle choices?

■ SUMMARY

This chapter discusses considerations for nursing practice related to patient self-determination. The concept of self-determination derives from the principle of autonomy and denotes the right and freedom to make choices about issues that affect one's life. Principles of justice, beneficence, and nonmaleficence may temper the bounds of autonomy in some circumstances. The doctrine of informed consent is both a legal and ethical imperative for protecting a person's right to self-determination in healthcare decisions. Informed consent implies the right to accept or reject recommended treatment plans. As patient advocates, we need to be alert for situations in which patient autonomy may be limited or in which there is a lack of sufficient information for the patient or family to make informed decisions. Nurses have a particular responsibility for facilitating informed decision making regarding patient choices for end-of-life care. Nursing professional codes of ethics direct nurses to provide services with respect for the rights and dignity of the patient, regardless of a person's background or the nature of the health concern. If professional responsibilities expected of a nurse in a patient care situation are inconsistent with the nurse's ethical stance, integrity, and accountability, she or he should remove herself or himself from that situation after ensuring that there are others to assume care for the patient. A nurse's attention to the many-faceted issues surrounding patient self-determination may be the factor that ensures the patient's involvement in important healthcare decisions.

CHAPTER HIGHLIGHTS

- Self-determination derives from the principle of autonomy and implies having the freedom to make choices about issues affecting one's life, an ability to make decisions about personal goals, and an appreciation for self in relation to others.
- Autonomy may be threatened by factors such as paternalism; presumptions that a patient's values, knowledge level, and ways of dealing with issues are consistent with those of healthcare providers; and greater attention to technology than caring. In some situations, principles such as justice or nonmaleficence may temper the bounds of autonomy.
- Decisions about healthcare require attention to patient values, culture, and beliefs; effects of lifestyle and role; and others who are affected by a patient's choices; as well as evaluation of risks, benefits, and economic considerations.
- healthcare providers are not required to honor requests for interventions that are outside accepted standards of care or contrary to the practitioner's ethical views.
- Informed consent provides legal and ethical protection of a patient's right to personal autonomy regarding plans for healthcare, including the right to refuse interventions and to choose from available alternatives. Information necessary in an informed consent includes the nature of the concern and prognosis if nothing is done; description of treatment options; and benefits, risks, and consequences of treatment options or nonintervention.

- Decision-making capacity, which is a medical determination and essential for informed consent, includes evidence of the ability to understand information, to communicate understanding and choices, to evaluate decisions in relation to personal values and goals, and to reason and deliberate. Conscious adults are presumed to have decision-making capacity, unless there is evidence to the contrary.
- Nursing responsibility regarding informed consent includes verifying that the patient is aware of options and the implications of each and advocating for patients to ensure that criteria for autonomous decision making are met in situations where the healthcare provider has not attended to these criteria. Nurses in advanced practice must obtain informed consent for interventions that they initiate within their scope of practice.
- Advance directives, which include living wills and durable power of attorney for healthcare, provide instructions regarding healthcare interventions in the event that one loses decision-making capacity. The PSDA provides legal support for ensuring that patients are informed of their rights regarding healthcare decisions.
- In dealing with patient lifestyle choices, nurses must remember the instructions in nursing codes of ethics to provide services with respect for human dignity and to avoid value judgments related to differences in background, customs, attitudes, and beliefs.
- Nurses need to be aware of their own values and beliefs regarding patient lifestyle and healthcare choices and know how these affect their care with patients.
- Nurses must recognize the patient's right to use complementary therapies, become more knowledgeable about other modalities, and create an atmosphere encouraging of nonjudgmental discussion of such interventions.

DISCUSSION QUESTIONS AND ACTIVITIES

1. Discuss your understanding of patient self-determination, including its ethical and legal basis, and nursing practice considerations.
2. Describe dilemmas that nurses may face related to patient self-determination and suggest approaches for dealing with such dilemmas.

3. Explore how nurses in your institution perceive their role regarding informed consent. What dilemmas related to consent have they encountered, and how did they deal with these issues? Does the institution have a policy related to nursing responsibility with informed consent?

4. Analyze your own values regarding the patient lifestyle and health choices discussed in this chapter. How would you respond to a patient under your care who was affected by or deliberating such a choice?

5. Explore your state's statutes regarding advance directives, HIV testing and disclosure, euthanasia, assisted dying, abortion, immunization policies, and controlled drug policies. What are the implications of these regulations for nursing practice in your state? Advance directive forms for your state can be found at http://www.caringinfo.org/i4a/pages/index.cfm?pageid=.

6. What are your views on mandatory immunization, drug testing, and HIV testing for healthcare professionals? What about limiting the practice of seropositive healthcare workers or those who are inadequately immunized? Review current literature, nursing codes of ethics, and position statements to determine recommendations by professional organizations concerning these issues. ANA Immunize Website https://www.nursingworld.org/practice-policy/work-environment/health-safety/immunize/ provides research, education, tools, and other resources related to immunizations.

7. Determine how your institution meets the requirements of both the PSDA and Health Insurance Portability and Accountability Act. Discuss the adequacy of each process and nursing's involvement.

8. What is the process for obtaining support and guidance for dealing with ethical concerns and dilemmas in your institution? If there is an ethics committee, how are referrals made? Who is on the committee, and how are members chosen? Talk with a member of an ethics committee, and discuss how that person sees his or her role and the effectiveness of the committee. If possible, attend an ethics committee meeting. Review and discuss the ethics committee tools available online at http://www.wvnec.org/ethics-committee-tools/.

9. Create a hypothetical case situation in which there are ethical concerns that warrant referral to the ethics committee. With classmates, role-play the ethics committee discussion, decisions, and actions regarding the case. Use the tools at the website noted in Question 8 to guide this process. Explain why you take your position and how you feel about the outcome.

10. Choose one of the issues discussed in this chapter and explore the websites of the ANA, CNA, ICN, and the NCSBN regarding policies or position statements on the issue. Compare and contrast positions of the various organizations. Discuss your views about the issue and how they compare with the positions of the professional organizations.
ANA—http://www.nursingworld.org
ICN—http://www.icn.ch
NCSBN—https://www.ncsbn.org/index.htm

11. Review the *Pain Relief Tools for Patients and Self Care* available through the AHNA at https://www.ahna.org/Portals/66/Docs/Resources/Pain%20Tools/Pain%20Relief%20Tool%20Kit%20combined.pdf?ver=2017-12-19-161954-113. Integrate one or more of the processes described into your own self-care. With another student, role-play a nurse–patient interaction in which the patient is experiencing pain. Guide the "patient" through one of the nonpharmacological processes for pain relief. Take turns in being the nurse and the patient.

REFERENCES

American Academy of Pediatrics (AAP). (2016). Informed consent in decision-making in pediatric practice. *Pediatrics*, 138(2), 1–7. https://publications.aap.org/pediatrics/article/138/2/e20161484/52512/Informed-Consent-in-Decision-Making-in-Pediatric?searchresult=1.

American Nurses Association (ANA). (2015). *Code of ethics for nurses with interpretive statements*. http://nursingworld.org/DocumentVault/Ethics-1/Code-of-Ethics-for-Nurses.html

American Nurses Association (ANA). (2016a). *Position statement: Nurses' roles and responsibilities in providing care and support at the end of life*. https://www.nursingworld.org/~4af078/globalassets/docs/ana/ethics/endoflife-positionstatement.pdf

American Nurses Association. (2016b). *Position statement: The nurses' role in ethics and human rights: Protecting* and promoting individual worth, dignity, and human rights in practice settings. https://www.nursingworld.org/~4af078/globalassets/docs/ana/ethics/ethics-and-human-rights-protecting-and-promoting-final-formatted-20161130.pdf

American Nurses Association (ANA). (2017). *Position statement: Nutrition and hydration at the end of life.* https://www.nursingworld.org/~4af0ed/globalassets/docs/ana/ethics/ps_nutrition-and-hydration-at-the-end-of-life_2017june7.pdf

American Nurses Association (ANA). (2018). *Position statement: The ethical responsibility to manage pain and the suffering it causes.* https://www.nursingworld.org/~495e9b/globalassets/docs/ana/ethics/theethicalresponsibilityto-managepainandthesufferingitcauses2018.pdf

American Nurses Association (ANA). (2019). *Position statement: The nurse's role when a patient requests medical aid in dying.* https://www.nursingworld.org/~49e869/globalassets/practiceandpolicy/nursing-excellence/ana-position-statements/social-causes-and-health-care/the-nurses-role-when-a-patient-requests-medical-aid-in-dying-web-format.pdf

American Nurses Association (ANA). (2021). *Position statement: Immunizations.* https://www.nursingworld.org/~4afdf9/globalassets/docs/ana/practice/official-position-statements/immunizations-position-statement-nov-2021.pdf

Baumrucker, S. J., Sheldon, J. E., Stolick, M., Oertli, K. A., Morris, G. M., Harrington, D., & VandeKieft, G. (2009). Comfort care versus euthanasia. *American Journal of Hospice and Palliative Care, 26*(2), 119–128.

Bayer, R., Philbin, M., & Remien, R. H. (2017). The end of written informed consent for HIV testing: Not with a bang but a wimper. *American Journal of Public Health, 107*(8), 1259–1265.

F. Canterbury v. Spence, 1972 (464 F.2d 772 (d.c. 1972)).

Canadian Nurses Association (CNA). (2017). *Code of ethics for registered nurses.* https://cdn1.nscn.ca/sites/default/files/documents/resources/code-of-ethics-for-registered-nurses.pdf#:~:text=The%20Canadian%20Nurses%20Association%20%28CNA%29%20Code%20of%20Ethics,receiving%20care.%20The%20Codeis%20both%20aspirational%20and%20regulatory

Centers for Disease Control and Prevention (CDC). (2006). *CDC recommendations and reports: Revised recommendations for HIV testing of adults, adolescents, and pregnant women in health-care settings.* https://www.cdc.gov/mmwr/preview/mmwrhtml/rr5514a1.htm.

Centers for Disease Control and Prevention (CDC) (2021). Sexually transmitted infections treatment guidelines, 2021. *Morbidity and Mortality Weekly Report: Recommendations and Reports, 70*(4). https://www.cdc.gov/std/treatment-guidelines/STI-Guidelines-2021.pdf.

Centers for Disease Control and Prevention (CDC). (2015). HIV infection: Detection, counseling, and referral—2021 STI treatment guidelines. *Morbidity and Mortality Weekly Report: Recommendations and Reports, 64*(3). https://www.cdc.gov/mmwr/pdf/rr/rr6403.pdf.

Curtin, L. (1982). Autonomy, accountability, and nursing practice. *Topics in Clinical Nursing, 4*, 7–14.

Geppert, C. M., Andrews, M. R., & Druyan, M. E. (2010). Ethical issues in artificial nutrition and hydration: A review. *Journal of Parenteral and Enteral Nutrition, 34*(1), 79–88.

Giublini, A., Douglas, T., & Savulascu, J. (2018). The moral obligation to be vaccinated: Utilitarianism, contractualism, and collective easy rescue. *Medicine, Healthcare, and Philosophy, 21*, 547–560. https://doi.org/10.1007/s11019-018-9829-y.

Hardee, J. E. (2018). The neuroscience of addiction. In: *Presentation at West Virginia Network of Ethics Committees 31st Annual conference: Addiction across the lifespan: Ethically treating those affected by substance use disorder.* WV: Stonewall Jackson Conference Center, Roanoke, WV.

Hardwig, J. (2000). What about the family? In J. H. Howell & W. F. Sale (Eds.), *Life choices: A Hastings Center introduction to bioethics* (2nd ed., pp. 145–159). Georgetown University Press.

Heerman, W. J., White, R. O., & Barkin, S. L. (2015). Advancing informed consent for vulnerable populations. *Pediatrics, 135*(3), e562–e564.

Hendrix, K. S., Stunn, L. A., Zimet, G. D., & Meslin, E. M. (2016). Ethics and childhood vaccination policy in the United States. *American Journal of Public Health, 106*(2), 273–278.

International Council of Nurses (ICN) (2011). *Position statement: Nurses and human rights.* https://www.icn.ch/sites/default/files/inline-files/E10_Nurses_Human_Rights%281%29.pdf.

ICN. (2012). *Position statement: Nurse's role in providing care to dying patients and their families.* https://www.icn.ch/sites/default/files/inline-files/A12_Nurses_Role_Care_Dying_Patients.pdf

ICN. (2015). *Position statement: Informed patients.* https://www.icn.ch/sites/default/files/inline-files/E06_Informed_Patients.pdf.

ICN. (2021). *The ICN code of ethics for nurses.* https://www.icn.ch/system/files/2021-10/ICN_Code-of-Ethics_EN_Web_0.pdf

Ivanković, V., & Savić, L. (2021). Three harm-based arguments for a moral obligation to vaccinate. *Healthcare Analysis, 30*, 18–24. https://doi.org/10.1007/s10728-021-00437-x.

Jensen, L. A. (2015). *Moral development in a global world: Research from a cultural-developmental perspective.* Cambridge University Press.

Johnson, J. (2022). HIV confidentiality laws by state: What to know. *Medical News Today.* https://www.medicalnewstoday.com/articles/hiv-confidentiality-laws-by-state#law-implementation.

Johnstone, M. J. (2016). Ethics, evidence, and anti-vaccination debate. *Australian Nursing and Midwifery Journal, 24*(8), 27.

Katz, A. L., & Webb, S. A. (2016). Informed consent and decision-making in pediatrics: Technical report. *Pediatrics, 135*(3), e1–e16. http://pediatrics.aappublications.org/content/138/2/e20161485.

Lasser, J., & Gottlieb, M. C. (2017). Facilitating informed consent: A multicultural perspective. *Ethics and Behavior, 27*(2), 106–117.

Leclercq, W. K., Keulers, B. J., Scheltinga, M. R., Spauwen, P. H. M., & vander Wilt, G. J. (2010). A review of informed consent: Past, present, and future. A quest to help patients make better decisions. *World Journal of Surgery, 34,* 1046–1415.

Leever, M. G. (2011). Cultural competence: Reflections on patient autonomy and patient good. *Nursing Ethics, 18*(4), 560–570.

Levi, B. H., & Green, M. J. (2010). Too soon to give up: Re-examining the value of advance directives. *American Journal of Bioethics, 10*(4), 3–22.

Lo, B. (2013). *Resolving ethical dilemmas: A guide for clinicians* (5th ed.). Lippincott Williams & Wilkins.

Mahowald, M. B. (2000). Is there life after *Roe v. Wade*? In J. H. Howell & W. F. Sale (Eds.), *Life choices: A Hastings Center introduction to bioethics* (2nd ed., pp. 188–203). Georgetown University Press.

Miller, B. (2017). Nurses in the know: The history and future of advance directives. *Online Journal of Issues in Nursing, 22*(3). https://doi.org/10.3912/OJIN.Vol-22No03PPT57http://ojin.nursingworld.org/MainMenu-Categories/ANAMarketplace/ANAPeriodicals/OJIN/TableofContents/Vol-22-2017/No3-Sep-2017/Articles-Previous-Topics/History-and-Future-of-Advance-Directives.html.

Milliken, A., & Uveges, M. K. (2022). Nurses' ethical obligations toward unvaccinated individuals. *AACN Advanced Critical Care, 33*(2), 220–226. https://doi.org/10.4037/aacnacc2022491.

Moser, C. A., Reiss, D., & Schwartz, R. L. (2015). Funding the costs of disease outbreaks caused by non-vaccination. *Journal of Law, Medicine & Ethics, 43*(3), 633–647.

Petersen, C. (2010). Clinical issues: Responsibility for obtaining the surgical informed consent. *AORN Journal, 92*(5), 585–586.

Plawecki, L. H., & Plawecki, H. M. (2009). Simply stated: Obtaining informed consent can be a very complex task. *Journal of Gerontological Nursing, 35*(2), 3–4.

Quill, T. E. (2005). Terri Schiavo—A tragedy compounded. *New England Journal of Medicine, 352*(16), 1630–1633.

Roberts, D. (2000). *Race, gender, justice, and reproductive health policy.* Presentation at New Century, New Challenges: Intensive Bioethics Course XXVI. Kennedy Institute of Ethics, Georgetown University, Washington, DC.

Rock, M. J., & Hoebeke, R. (2014). Informed consent: Whose duty to inform. *Medsurg Nursing, 23*(3), 189–191.

Strategic Advisory Group of Expert (SAGE). (2014). *Report of the SAGE working group on vaccine hesitancy.* https://www.who.int/immunization/sage/meetings/2014/october/SAGE_working_group_revised_report_vaccine_hesitancy.pdf?ua=1.

Sakalys, J. A. (2010). Patient autonomy: Patient voices and perspectives in illness narratives. *International Journal for Human Caring, 14*(1), 15–20.

Salgo v. Leland Stanford, Jr. (1957). 317 P. 2d 170 (Cal. Dis. Ct. App; 1951).

Schloendorff v. The Society of New York Hospital. (1914). 211 NY125, 105 N.E. 92 (1914).

Slater v. Baker & Stapleton. (1767). High Court of Justice, King's Bench Division. *English Reports, Vol. 95,* 860–863.

Supreme Court of Minnesota (1905) Mohr v. Williams (104 N.W. 12 Supreme Court of Minnesota)

P. Truman v. Thomas, 1980 (611 P.2d 902 (Cal 1980)).

Tuma v. Board of Nursing of the State of Idaho. (1979). 593 P 2d 711 (1979).

Wakim, R. J. (2018). The opioid epidemic: Ethics & evidence. In: *Presentation at West Virginia Network of Ethics Committees 31st annual conference: Addiction across the lifespan: Ethically treating those affected by substance use disorder.* Stonewall Jackson Conference Center.

West Virginia Healthcare Decisions Act. (2022). *Article 30. West Virginia Healthcare Decisions Act: §16-30-8. Selection of a surrogate.* https://code.wvlegislature.gov/16-30-8/

Will, J. F. (2011). A brief historical and theoretical perspective on patient autonomy and medical decision making: Part II: The autonomy model. *Chest, 139*(6), 1491–1497.

World Health Organization (WHO). (2015). *Vaccine hesitancy: A growing challenge for immunization programs.* https://www.who.int/news/item/18-08-2015-vaccine-hesitancy-a-growing-challenge-for-immunization-programmes

12

Ethical Issues Related to Nursing Education, Research, and Scholarship

My experience tells me that people instinctively trust those whose personality is founded upon correct principles.

(Covey, 1992, p. 18)

OBJECTIVES

After completing this chapter, the reader should be able to:

1. Describe ethical issues related to education, research, and scholarship encountered by students and nurses in academic and clinical settings.
2. Discuss principles basic to academic honesty and the ethical treatment of research data.
3. Describe ethical principles and nursing standards undergirding the protection of human rights in research.
4. Explain why informed consent is mandated for research involving human subjects, and describe the elements required for this consent.

5. Discuss the nursing role regarding the protection of human rights in research.
6. Describe principles guiding a personal response to dilemmas regarding nursing scholarship.
7. Discuss elements of codes of nursing ethics that inform ethical accountability and responsibility in nursing education, research, and scholarship.

INTRODUCTION

Ethical issues related to academic pressures, research, and scholarship face students, teachers, researchers, and clinicians from the moment a person enters a nursing program and throughout that person's professional career. This chapter discusses principles that undergird ethical behavior in academic matters, in conducting research, in the treatment of data during the research process, and in reporting findings through presentations or publication. Respect for all persons, including ourselves, is basic to ethical behavior regarding scholarship. Personal values affect how we approach situations that present ethical dilemmas. It is essential that nurses be knowledgeable about principles and values guiding ethical conduct in academic settings and during all phases of the research process, particularly research involving human subjects.

ACADEMIC HONESTY

The ethical practice of nursing begins when a person enters a nursing educational program and is expected behavior in academic work, continuing education, and scholarly inquiry as well as in clinical practice. Integrity in upholding the principles of veracity and fidelity is expected of nurses in any setting and is at the core of academic honesty (ANA, 2015, Provisions 4.2, 5.4; CNA, 2017, Part I.A.1, IA.5, I.G.2; ICN, 2021, Element 1.8). Veracity refers to truth telling, which is an essential ingredient for trust among humans. True interaction and communication cannot occur where there is no trust. Recall from Chapter 3 that fidelity relates to faithfully keeping promises. In a manner of speaking, fidelity is the form that truth takes in an agreement between persons, such as nurse–patient, researcher–participant, or student–teacher. Integrity implies respect for self and others, and a personal commitment to principled behavior over time in our personal and professional lives. When integrity is present, there is no need to monitor a person's behavior; rather, there is an implicit trust that we represent ourselves in a truthful way. Honesty and integrity are key considerations in both academic and clinical situations. Personal values such as honesty serve as the basis for professional integrity.

Students at all levels face many stresses with regard to academic performance, and nursing students are no exception. Pressures may come from many areas, such as family expectations, personal goals of being accepted into graduate school or a particular job, needing a certain grade to receive tuition reimbursement, or self-expectations that say, "I always get good grades." When pressures become intense, values such as honesty and integrity may become challenged.

Academic institutions provide written policies that address issues of academic honesty. These issues include plagiarism, cheating, and forgery. **Plagiarism** is taking another's ideas or work and presenting them as our own. Sources of another's work include printed materials as well as materials found on the Internet such as portions of books, journal articles, or content from websites. Examples include submitting written, oral, or visual materials (such as a paper, a report, PowerPoint slides, a speech, or a thesis) that have been knowingly copied or obtained, in whole or in part, from another's work without appropriate acknowledgment. In addition to copying another's work and submitting it as one's own, summarizing or minimally paraphrasing another's work without giving appropriate credit is plagiarism. The Office of Research Integrity (ORI) of the US Department of Health and Human Services offers a free module on ethical writing that includes guidelines for avoiding plagiarism (Roig, 2015). The first eight guidelines of this module are outlined in Box 12.1. Students are encouraged to review these guidelines, found on the ORI website (http://ori.hhs.gov/avoiding-plagiarism-self-plagiarism-and-other-questionable-writing-practices-guide-ethical-writing).

Cheating refers to dishonesty and deception regarding examinations, projects, presentations, or papers. Examples include receiving help from or giving help to another student during an exam, allowing another to copy our work, doing work for another student that is

---

BOX 12.1 Acknowledging the Source of Our Ideas

- **Guideline 1:** An ethical writer always acknowledges the contributions of others to his or her work.
- **Guideline 2:** Any verbatim text taken from another source must be enclosed in quotation marks and be accompanied by a citation to indicate its origin.
- **Guideline 3:** When we summarize others' work, we use our own words to condense and convey others' contributions in a shorter version of the original.
- **Guideline 4:** When paraphrasing others' work, not only must we use our own words but we must also use our own syntactical structure.
- **Guideline 5:** Whether we are paraphrasing or summarizing, we must always identify the source of our information.
- **Guideline 6:** When paraphrasing and/or summarizing others' work, we must ensure that we are reproducing the exact meaning of the other author's ideas or facts and that we are doing so using our own words and sentence structure.
- **Guideline 7:** To be able to make the types of substantial modifications to the original text that result in a proper paraphrase, one must have a thorough command of the language and a good understanding of the ideas and terminology being used.
- **Guideline 8:** When in doubt as to whether a concept or fact is common knowledge, provide a citation.

(Excerpted from Roig, M. (2015). *Avoiding plagiarism, self-plagiarism, and other questionable writing practices: A guide to ethical writing.* U.S. Department of Health and Human Services. https://ori.hhs.gov/avoiding-plagiarism-self-plagiarism-and-other-questionable-writing-practices-guide-ethical-writing.)

---

to be submitted by that student, or unauthorized use of notes or other materials (including electronic devices) during an exam. The academic policy regarding the use of (and restrictions on) handheld electronic devices in both class and clinical settings may vary in different academic settings, and students are advised to be familiar with the policy at their school. **Forgery** includes fraud or intentional misrepresentation—for example, altering or causing a grade to be altered in an academic record or presenting false data on admission records or a resume.

Implicit in academic honesty is a trust that work submitted by a student, whether papers, projects, presentations, or exams, is indeed that of the student. When material from another source is included in a student's work, the student must appropriately reference the material to avoid plagiarism. Academic dishonesty engenders an atmosphere of mistrust, disrespect, and insecurity. The breach of trust and potential consequences within a student–teacher relationship that academic dishonesty creates are self-evident. Litigation is another potential consequence in severe situations. Because of the value of honesty, academic dishonesty may carry consequences as serious as the student being suspended, failed, or expelled for dishonest practices (Fig. 12.1).

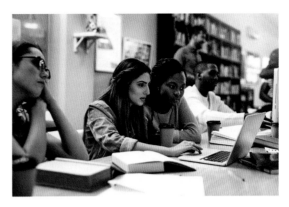

Fig. 12.1 Honesty and Integrity Are Key Considerations in Both Academic and Clinical Situations. (©iStock.com/PeopleImages.)

ASK YOURSELF

What Are Your Perspectives on Academic Honesty?

- One of your closest friends is in a different section of the same course, and his section meets two days after yours. You know he has been very stressed because of his mother's illness and the fact that he needs good grades to keep his scholarship. You have just taken the midterm exam, and he asks you to give him an idea of the topics covered so he can focus his studying. What would you do? How do you feel in this situation? What principles would guide your decisions?
- During an exam, you notice two students passing what appear to be notes between them. You also notice another student texting on her cell phone. You are fairly sure that the instructor has not seen these activities. How do you feel in response to these situations? What would you do, and why? What ethical principles and nursing values would guide your decision?
- You are struggling with an assignment that is due in just a few days. A classmate says she has a paper that her cousin did for this same course three years ago that she is using as a guide, changing the text so that it seems like her own writing. She offers to let you see her cousin's paper to do the same. What do you think about her plan? How would you respond? What would guide your decision?
- How would codes of ethics from the ANA (2015, Provision 5.3), or the CNA (2017, Part I. A.1), and the ICN (2021) Elements (1.2, 2.5, 3.5) guide your responses in each of these situations?

CASE PRESENTATION

Suspicions of Dishonesty

Case 1. Sabrina and Jude have been close friends and study partners throughout their nursing program. They discuss their readings and class notes and frequently choose the same topic when writing papers and share articles between them. After a recent submission of papers, the instructor called them in and noted that their papers were almost identical, including mistakes in grammar, and said that it appeared that one had copied the other's paper. They each denied copying from the other.

Case 2. During an exam in a nursing course, the instructor observed a student leaning over to ask a classmate for the answer to a question. The student denied this when confronted by the instructor. Since the exam was given electronically and the system was able to track and document the incident, the instructor was able to provide evidence of the attempt to cheat. The student was ultimately dismissed from the nursing program.

Think About It
Considering Consequences for Academic Dishonesty

- What ethical issues, principles, and nursing values are evident in these situations?
- What impact does academic dishonesty have on students and the nursing profession?
- How do you think these situations should be handled? What consequences would you consider?
- In light of the standards that guide nursing practice, what is your position on allowing a student who has violated academic honesty through plagiarism, cheating, or forgery to continue in a nursing program?
- What components of the codes of ethics of the ANA, or the CNA and the ICN would inform your response?

RESEARCH ISSUES AND ETHICS

Nurses must be accountable for the quality of care they deliver, and research is one way of documenting the efficacy of nursing practice. Both the art and science of nursing are expanded through research and scholarly inquiry and are necessary for advancing the profession of nursing. All nurses have a role in the ongoing development of the unique body of knowledge that undergirds the discipline of nursing and provides an organizing framework for nursing practice (ANA, 2015, Provision 7.1; CNA, 2017, Part A,1.10; ICN, 2021, Elements 3.2, 3.3, 3.6).

Participating in research can be exciting and encourage professional growth. It can also present some dilemmas for the nurse and nurse researcher in the academic and clinical realms. Seeking new knowledge and understanding is the expected motivation for conducting research. However, personal or institutional gains related to rewards such as grant funds, prestige, the need to succeed, or promoting a product can be other motivating factors that may challenge principled behavior with regard to research.

A nurse who works in clinical areas where research is being conducted must be aware of principles for the conduct of research, regardless of whether the nurse has an active role in the research project. Nursing Codes of Ethics speak to the relationship of trust between nurse and patient and respect for the inherent dignity and human rights of individuals that are the foundations of nursing practice. These principles apply to research as well. There must be a relationship of trust between the researcher and the research participant that requires the researcher to make the safety of the participant a priority (ANA, 2015, Provision 3.1, 3.2; CNA, 2017, Part I.A.11; ICN, 2021, Element 1). Nurses, whether they are the researcher or the nurse caring for the person clinically, have an ethical obligation to ensure the safety of participants in research. This means recognizing that persons have the right to choose whether or not to participate in research as a human subject, and ensuring that they have received sufficient information to make an informed decision and that they understand it is their right to decline to participate in or withdraw from the study at any time without fear of consequences (ANA, 2015, Provision 3.2; CNA, 2017, Part I.A.11; ICN, 2021, Element 2.9).

Ethical Issues in Research

Many research texts focus their discussions of ethical issues in research primarily on the protection of human rights. This emphasis is understandable because of violations that have occurred. The most cited violations of human rights in research are those that were perpetrated by the Nazis during World War II and that came to public awareness during the Nuremberg trials. International efforts to provide guidelines for the protection of human rights have been documented in the Nuremberg Code and the Declaration of Helsinki. The Nuremberg Code was developed as a set of principles for the ethical conduct of research against which the experiments in the Nazi concentration camps could be judged. The Declaration of Helsinki was issued by the World Medical Assembly in 1964 to guide clinical research and was revised in 1975 and 2008. Included in the Belmont Report, the principles set forth in these codes serve as the basis for policies developed by the United States National Commission for the Protection of Human Subjects of Biomedical and Behavioral Research (DHHS-OHRP, 1979). Readers are encouraged to review the Belmont Report that is available at https://www.hhs.gov/ohrp/regulations-and-policy/belmont-report/index.html. These regulations are part of the *Code of Federal Regulations* (CFR) (2018), which is also called the *Common Rule* because the various US departments involved in research on human subjects have a chapter in the CFR to guide that department's research. These regulations, which were updated in 2017, are available online at the *Electronic Code of Federal Regulations*. See the relevant website under "Discussion Questions and Activities."

In spite of these policies and guidelines, ethical lapses continue to occur in research with human subjects (Clark & Thompson, 2020; George, 2016; ORI, 2023; Ward-Smith, 2016). Ongoing concerns prompt questions about whether current regulations adequately protect the rights and welfare of research subjects. To oversee and enforce federal regulations pertaining to research with human subjects, the US Department of Health and Human Services formed an Office for Human Research Protection. Efforts to bolster protections for human research subjects focus on the education and training of clinical investigators and institutional review board (IRB) members; auditing records for evidence of compliance with informed consent; improved monitoring of clinical trials; managing conflicts of interest so that research subjects are appropriately informed; and imposing monetary penalties for violations of important research practices, such as informed consent (US Department of Health and Human Services, n.d.; https://ori.hhs.gov/index.php/about-ori).

Principles of beneficence, respect for persons, and justice underlie the ethical conduct of research (ANA, 2015; Childress et al., 2005; CNA, 2017; DHHS-OHRP, 1979; ICN, 2021). Recall from Chapter 3, the principle of beneficence implies the right to protection from harm and discomfort, including a balance between the benefits and risks of a study. The principle of respect for human dignity implies the rights to full disclosure and self-determination or autonomy. The principle of justice implies the rights of fair treatment and privacy, including anonymity and confidentiality. A brief discussion of each principle as it relates to research follows.

Beneficence

In research situations, the maxim that says "above all, do no harm" means that researchers need to design and conduct studies so as to protect the participants from physical, mental, emotional, spiritual, economic, and social harm. Discomfort can range from no anticipated effects to certainty of permanent damage and includes such things as fatigue, physical pain, anxiety, embarrassment, confronting meaning and purpose in life, threats to self-esteem or to values, lost earnings for time given to participate in research, and social stigma (Gray, Groves, & Sutherland, 2020). If discomfort is anticipated as part of the research protocol, the participant, after being given all relevant information, must be willing to experience the discomfort, and the risk for harm must be balanced with anticipated benefits. In general, a minimal risk is that which is no more than would be expected within the context of routine life activities. When risks are greater than minimal, the researcher's aim must be to minimize risks while maximizing the benefits to participants. Because our role as nurses impels us to protect those in our care from unnecessary physical or mental suffering, if the risks of the research outweigh the benefits, the study should be redesigned or discontinued. A well-publicized example of this occurred with the National Institutes of Health, Women's Health Initiative (WHI) study. When preliminary findings of the study indicated that long-term use of hormone replacement therapy (HRT) was associated with increased health risks among the participants, the HRT arm of the WHI study was discontinued.

Respect for Human Dignity

The right to self-determination acknowledges the autonomy of the potential participant in research. This means that persons have the right to choose whether they wish to participate in the research—participation is voluntary and free from coercion of any type. Coercion includes threat of harm or penalty for not participating in the research or offering excessive rewards for participation. The right of self-determination means that the person has the right to withdraw from participation in the study at any time without imposed consequences, such as denial of healthcare or benefits. Voluntary participation requires full disclosure. The potential participant must be fully informed of the nature of the study, the anticipated risks and benefits, time commitment, what is expected of the participant and the researcher, and the right to refuse to participate. This is addressed through the process of informed consent, which is discussed later.

Justice

The principle of justice includes the rights to privacy and to fair treatment. The nature of research is to gather information about that which is being studied. When persons are the focus of study, the right to privacy is a critical issue. Attentiveness to privacy means the participant determines when, where, and what kind of information is shared, with an assurance that information, attitudes, behaviors, records, opinions, and the like that are observed or collected will be treated with respect, kept secure, and kept in strict confidence. Privacy is maintained through anonymity, confidentiality, and informed consent (ANA, 2015, Provision 3; CNA, 2017, Parts I.A.10,11; ICN, 2021, Elements 1.2, 1.4, 1.5). Because the concept of privacy may vary in different cultures, the kinds of information participants feel comfortable allowing to be shared may also vary (Calloway, 2009; Wu et al., 2015). Anonymity exists when even the researcher cannot link information with a particular participant. Confidentiality refers to the researcher's assurance to participants that the information provided will not be made public or available to anyone other than those involved in the research process without the participant's consent. Confidentiality is maintained by using codes rather than personal identification on data collection forms and restricting access to raw data to those on the research team who need to use the data.

The right to fair treatment is related to the right to self-determination. Equitable treatment of participants in the selection process, during the study, and after the completion of the study is the foundation of this right. Factors to consider in fair treatment include the following:

- Selecting participants based on the research needs, not on the convenience or compromised position of a group of people
- Equitably distributing the risks and benefits of the research among participants, regardless of age, gender, socioeconomic status, race, or ethnic background
- Honoring any agreements made or benefits promised
- Treating participants with respect, providing access to research personnel or other professionals as needed
- Treating persons who decline to participate or withdraw from the study without prejudice
- Debriefing as needed to clarify issues or when information had been withheld before the study

Informed Consent

As noted previously, voluntary participation in a research study requires full disclosure. Informing potential participants of the research purpose, expected commitment, risks and benefits, any invasion of privacy, and ways that anonymity and confidentiality will be addressed are included in the process of informed consent. The researcher must ensure that the person who is agreeing to participate in the study understands the information included in the consent and has a chance to receive clarifications and additional information when needed. It is important to ensure that individuals from vulnerable populations do not feel compelled to participate to receive a stipend or treatment (Gehlert & Mozersky, 2018; Fig. 12.2). Printed consent forms should be written in the common language without jargon and be accurately translated into the participant's primary language. Because literacy level affects how people understand both written and verbal instructions and documents, researchers need to assess and document the literacy level of the person signing the informed consent and verify their understanding of the content. Additionally, the person agreeing to participate in the research must be mentally and emotionally competent to make the decision (Bios, 2018).

CASE PRESENTATION

Protecting Patients Who Are Research Subjects

Annissa, a nurse in a primary care clinic, talked with her coworker, Bill, about his nonnursing graduate program. Bill said he plans to study the emotional attitudes of patients using a standardized instrument for his required research project. When Annissa asked about recruiting participants, he said he will have all his patients complete the instrument when he sees them for routine visits over the next few weeks. In response to Annissa's questions about the possibility of patients not wanting to participate, Bill said that he will just tell them it is for a student project, and he is sure they will fill out the form to help him out and keep on his good side. Annissa recalled from her research course that proposals for research involving human subjects must be approved by an IRB to assure the protection of the rights of participants. She asked which IRB reviewed his proposal, and Bill replied that his school does not have an IRB, so only his advisor had to give approval.

Think About It
What Principles Guide Ethical Conduct of Clinical Research?

- What principles and nursing values are involved in this situation?
- What dilemmas may arise with Bill's research project? What do you think about his plan for recruiting participants?
- What are Annissa's ethical responsibilities in this situation? How might codes of ethics from the ANA (2015, Provision 3.1, 3.2), or the CNA (2017, Part I.A.4.11), and the ICN (2021, Elements 1.2, 1.8, 2.7) guide Annissa in choosing a course of action in this situation?
- What is the responsibility of the primary care agency related to research conducted within the agency?

Munhall (2012) suggests that the process of informed consent provides a way of including the person as a collaborator in the research rather than as a mere "subject." We must, however, guard against the element of coercion. When the nurse who cares for the patient is on the research team and is the one obtaining the informed consent, determining whether the patient is giving consent to the "nurse" or to the "researcher" can be somewhat tricky. The nurse researcher must determine

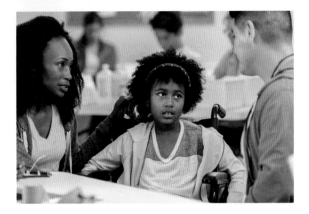

Fig. 12.2 Nurses Are Attentive to Protection of Human Rights With Vulnerable Populations—Ensuring the Parent Has Given Consent and the Child Has Given Assent to Participate in the Research Study. (©iStock.com/asiseeit.)

whether the patient truly feels the freedom to refuse to participate in the study.

The Department of Health and Human Services, Office for Human Research Protection (DHHS-OHRP, 2022) lists basic elements that need to be included in informed consent:

- A statement that the study involves research, an explanation of the purpose of the research and the expected duration of the subject's participation, a description of the procedures to be followed, and identification of any procedures that are experimental.
- A description of any reasonably foreseeable risks or discomforts to the participant.
- A description of any benefits to the participant or to others that may reasonably be expected from the research.
- A disclosure of appropriate alternative procedures or courses of treatment, if any, that might be advantageous to the subject.
- A statement describing the extent, if any, to which confidentiality of records identifying the subject will be maintained.
- For research involving more than minimal risk, an explanation as to whether there will be any compensation and an explanation as to whether medical treatments are available if injury occurs and, if so, what they consist of or where further information may be obtained.
- An explanation of whom to contact for answers to pertinent questions about the research and research

subjects' rights and whom to contact in the event of a research-related injury to the subject.
- A statement that participation is voluntary, that refusal to participate will involve no penalty or loss of benefits to which the subject is otherwise entitled, and that the subject may discontinue participation at any time without penalty or loss of benefits to which the subject is otherwise entitled.

Nurses who are assisting with research or who work on units where research is being conducted must be familiar with these elements of informed consent. If consent forms do not contain these elements, nurses should bring this to the attention of the investigators or the institution's ethics committee. Nurses also need to be familiar with the Health Insurance Portability and Accountability Act (HIPAA) policies and guidelines of the institutions in which they work. HIPAA requires institutions to establish procedures for handling individually identifiable patient health information (PHI) for all areas of patient contact. The goal of these procedures is to protect privacy and ensure confidentiality regarding PHI. HIPAA regulations may add more privacy protection for patients regarding their participation in a research study and researcher access to PHI necessary for a research study. The written, signed authorization from research participants to use PHI for research purposes must include the purpose for which the PHI will be used, what PHI will be disclosed, who will have access to the PHI, and the right of the participant to review the PHI that is recorded for research (DHHS-NIH, 2003; https://www.hhs.gov/hipaa/for-professionals/privacy/index.html).

Special Considerations: Vulnerable Populations

Nurses must be especially attentive to protection of human rights in research with vulnerable populations. These populations include persons with physical, mental, or emotional disabilities or challenges; children or elderly persons; those who are dying, sedated, or unconscious; persons who are institutionalized or incarcerated; pregnant women; fetuses; and immigrants. Because people in these populations are often vulnerable to deception and coercion and may have decreased ability to give informed consent, advocates or guardians who have the person's best interests in mind may need to be involved in decisions regarding their participation in research. In both research and clinical care, the less able the person is to give informed consent, the more important it is for nurses to advocate for the person, ensuring that rights are protected. Guidelines for research involving children age 7–18 provide one example of special considerations regarding consent. In addition to the consent by the parents or guardians, researchers seek the assent of the child to participate in a research study. The principle of respect for persons acknowledges that persons, to the degree that they are capable, have the right to choose what will or will not happen to them. In accordance with this principle, US federal guidelines direct researchers to inform children of any intended research activity, even if the parents or guardians have already agreed to the child's participation in a research study. Oulton and colleagues (2016) suggest approaching assent as a way to gain the child's trust and to engage the child in the research process throughout the study. They present a model that suggests the need to address several components for assent to be meaningful. These components are *child-related factors* such as literacy level, language spoken, health status, maturity, and knowledge of health condition; *family dynamic* such as level of agreement within the family and cultural values; *study design* and *complexity* such as what is required, risks and benefits, and research burden; and *researcher and organizational* factors such as culture, tools, and experience. In general, the process of obtaining the child's *assent* includes describing, in language appropriate for the age and competence of the child, the purpose of the research and providing an explanation of the risks and benefits associated with the child's participation in the research. Younger children are asked to assent orally to participate in the proposed research, whereas older children may be asked to sign an assent form or the parent's permission form indicating their willingness to participate in the study. Assent needs to be documented in the research protocol. Nurses who work with these populations need to be especially aware of their roles as advocates, particularly when research is proposed or being conducted in their clinical settings.

Characteristics of Ethical Research

Ethical considerations related to research must be addressed at each stage of the process, beginning with the research proposal and continuing through the dissemination of findings. When nurses are working in agencies or institutions where research is being conducted, whether or not they are directly involved in the

---

CASE PRESENTATION

Nurses, Research, and Informed Consent

Juan, a registered nurse, works in a small rural hospital clinic that has a strong commitment to the underserved population in its area. The hospital has been struggling financially because of the large number of indigent patients and the recent federal cutback of funding for health services. There has been talk of possibly eliminating some positions because of the financial crisis. In a recent staff meeting, he learned that a pharmaceutical company has negotiated an agreement with the physicians at the clinic to use a new medication with their hypertensive patients and to gather data about the side effects of this medication. A sizable financial reimbursement for the hospital is part of the agreement. As the registered nurse (RN), Juan will be responsible for checking patients' blood pressures and completing the side effect surveys. Juan asks about informed consent and is told that the pharmaceutical company said it is not needed because this medication has been through clinical trials already. Juan does not feel comfortable about participating in the project but recognizes that the money is needed by the hospital and, in fact, may make the difference in avoiding the elimination of staff positions.

Think About It
Decisions About Participating in Research
- What ethical issues do you identify in this case situation?
- What ethical principles are being violated or potentially violated?
- What ethical dilemmas do you think Juan is experiencing?
- What do you think Juan should do, and why? How might codes of ethics from the ANA (2015, Provisions 3.2, 3.4, 3.5), or the CNA (2017, Parts I.A.11, I.C.3,5), and the ICN (2021, Element 2.7, 2.8, 2.10) guide Juan's ethical decision making?
- How might potential consequences affect the decision-making process?

---

research, they must be aware of standards for ethical research to guard against violations of these standards. Characteristics of ethical research discussed by Wilson (1999) are still applicable. These include:

Cooperation—submitting proposals to and following recommendations of those authorized to review the research for protection of human rights—generally IRBs

Nobility—working actively to ensure the protection of participants from harm, deceit, coercion, and invasions of privacy, even when this may inconvenience the study

Integrity and truthfulness—honestly describing the research process, including the purpose, procedures, methods, risks, discomforts, benefits, and findings

Impeccability—ensuring anonymity and confidentiality of data and using discretion with information learned about people

Illumination—publishing and presenting research findings to enhance nursing's body of scientific knowledge

Scientific objectivity—reporting all data, both supportive and unsupportive of hypotheses, and not engaging in misconduct, fraud, or acts of bad faith

Equitability—noting contributions of others in publications and presentations

Forthrightness—disclosing funding sources and sponsorship in publication and presentation of research findings

Courage—being willing to request public clarification of apparent distortions of research findings made by others

Nurses who participate in conducting research may at times experience role conflict. A nurse is held to standards of professional practice that delineate the nurse's concern as safeguarding the health and well-being of the patient. A researcher is focused on the processes and outcomes of a study in which patients may be used as sources of data. Nurse researchers need to incorporate humanistic values in decisions regarding research participants. When questions arise regarding potential harm to a patient involved in a research study, the advocacy role of the nurse and the therapeutic imperative take precedence over the integrity of the research protocol (Gray & Groves, 2020; Munhall, 2012). Ignorance of ethical and legal guidelines related to research is no excuse for a nurse failing to be a patient advocate in research situations. Although research is necessary for the development of scientific and therapeutic knowledge, a balance between principles guiding scientific inquiry and those guiding nursing practice must be maintained.

When nurses are employed, particularly in institutions that are research focused, they need to clarify what is expected of them with regard to research. Nurses should know before accepting a position whether they will be required to gather data or administer treatments

> ## ASK YOURSELF
>
> **What Takes Precedence—Research or Nursing Care?**
> Questions that Fowler (1988, p. 354) posed over 30 years ago continue to be worth pondering:
> - Is the good of the patient ever subservient to the acquisition of nursing knowledge?
> - Does the therapeutic imperative of clinical care and the good of the patient always preempt the mandate to enlarge the nursing profession's body of knowledge?
> - At what point must a nurse stop a specific nursing research project?
> - When must a nurse intervene to halt a specific medical research project?
> - Are there conditions under which a nurse should not include a specific subject in a study, even though consent has been secured?

as part of research protocols and whether such treatments may have potential risks to patients. Nurses in such settings need to know whether their positions will be jeopardized if they refuse to participate as part of a research team. When participation in research is expected as part of a nurse's job, the nurse must know the protocol, whether it has been approved by the IRB, and whom to consult with any concerns about the research process and its effect on patients.

Ethical Treatment of Data

Scholarship issues regarding data include how the data are handled during the collection and analysis process and how the data are reported. Ethical treatment of data implies integrity of research protocols and honesty in reporting findings. The honesty and integrity of the researcher are of utmost importance in the ethical treatment of data. Taking care to ensure that only those who are involved in the research process have access to the data and to maintain confidentiality was mentioned previously. A critical ethical obligation of qualitative nursing researchers is to present and describe the experiences of others as authentically and faithfully as possible, even when it is contrary to our own aims (Munhall, 2012). Reporting findings as accurately as possible is an ethical obligation as well in quantitative research.

Nurses involved in research are accountable to professional standards for reporting findings. Principles that guide academic honesty apply as well to nurse researchers in reporting outcomes of studies. It is dishonest to exaggerate results, withhold negative findings, or adjust the facts of a study to maximize or minimize particular outcomes or hypotheses. When information or ideas from someone else are included in a report without appropriate referencing, this is plagiarism. Scientific misconduct continues to be a concern within the scientific community. Articles have been published in professional journals reporting studies that were never conducted, findings that were fabricated, or findings that were intentionally distorted by researchers (Clark & Thompson, 2020; George, 2016; Horner & Minifie, 2011; Karcz & Papadakos, 2011; ORI, 2023; Ward-Smith, 2016). Although these reports have related more to biomedical studies than to nursing research, such reports present problems to disciplines whose clinical practice may be changed based on research findings. They also serve as reminders to nurses to be vigilant regarding ethical reporting of research findings.

CASE PRESENTATION

Ethical Issues in Handling Research Data

A classmate and good friend is in the process of doing a research project required for graduation. You know she is frustrated because the surveys she sent out are not being returned, and the project needs to be completed soon if she is to graduate on time. She also needs to do well on this project to graduate with honors. To have a large enough sample, she tells you that she is going to fill in several forms herself and asks if you will do some for her too, noting that several other friends have already completed forms. She says that, after all, the object of the assignment is to see if one can collect and analyze the data. You are also aware that the best studies will be published in the student nursing newsletter.

Think About It
Honesty in Nursing Research
- What is your reaction to her plan and request?
- Discuss the ethical issues involved in this scenario.
- Describe the appropriate ethical stance in this situation. What factors would support you in taking this stance or prevent you from taking this stance? List particular components of nursing codes of ethics that would guide your response.
- What would you do with this information, and what principles would guide your actions?

ASK YOURSELF

Consequences of Reporting Fraudulent Research
Pause and think about the havoc rendered by the publication of fraudulent research.
- How might this affect how others view the integrity of the profession?
- How might this affect a reader's response to other research published in the same journal?
- How would this affect your ability as a nurse to determine whether you should adjust your practice based on reported research?
- Imagine that you have just read the report of a research project for which you gathered data and discovered that the process described was quite a bit different from what you had done, making the results take on a different meaning. How would you react? What would you do?

SUMMARY

Nurses are expected to exhibit principled behavior in all situations. This chapter has focused on principles related to education and scholarship issues facing nurses. Decisions related to academic honesty face nursing students before they ever encounter a patient. Personal values and nursing codes of ethics inform professional behavior. Choices made in the academic arena concerning actions such as plagiarism, cheating, or forgery may foreshadow values used to guide future professional decisions. Nurses must be familiar with principles guiding ethical practices in research and reporting of research findings. These principles guide nursing decisions about research protocols, participation, and advocacy for patients related to research issues. Ethical conduct in education, research, and scholarship is essential to the integrity of both the professional and the profession.

CHAPTER HIGHLIGHTS

- Principles of veracity and integrity are core to academic honesty and to ethical treatment of research data.
- Nursing research and researchers must adhere to nursing standards regarding the ethical conduct of research that affirm a participant's right to freedom

from intrinsic risk of injury, right to privacy, and right to anonymity.

- Protection of human rights, a prime focus of research ethics, is based on principles of beneficence, respect for human dignity, and justice. These principles imply protection from physical, emotional, spiritual, economic, and social harm; voluntary participation in research; and assurance of privacy and equitable treatment of all research participants.
- Informed consent for research studies, which helps ensure that a participant's rights are protected, must include the elements contained in the Code of Federal Regulations (2018).
- When there is a question of potential harm to a patient involved in a research study, the nurse's advocacy role and the therapeutic imperative take precedence over the integrity of the research protocol. Nurses need to be especially attentive to the protection of the rights of vulnerable groups in clinical and research settings.
- When considering employment, nurses should clarify expectations regarding potential participation in research.
- Nursing codes of ethics offer guidelines for ethical conduct and action for students and for nurses involved in doing research.

DISCUSSION QUESTIONS AND ACTIVITIES

1. Review your school's policy regarding academic honesty, and discuss ethical principles that are violated in cases of academic dishonesty. Explore issues and policies related to academic honesty at the following websites:
   https://ori.hhs.gov/avoiding-plagiarism-self-pla-giarism-and-other-questionable-writing-prac-tices-guide-ethical-writing
2. Describe factors that persons reviewing cases of academic dishonesty should consider.
3. How did protection of human rights come to be required for research involving human subjects? Explore the following websites for information about the Belmont Report and the Declaration of Helsinki:
   Belmont Report—
   http://www.hhs.gov/ohrp/humansubjects/guid-ance/belmont.html
   Declaration of Helsinki—World Medical Association

https://www.wma.net/policies-post/wma-decla-ration-of-helsinki-ethical-principles-for-medi-cal-research-involving-human-subjects/

4. What guidance do nursing standards and codes of ethics offer nurses who are participating in or conducting research? What principles underlie the ethical conduct of research? Discuss nursing roles and responsibilities related to these codes of ethics, principles, and standards.
5. Interview a nurse researcher regarding how human rights are protected in the study. Have all the required elements been included in the informed consent?
6. Give examples of situations in which the nursing role of patient advocate and the role of researcher might be in conflict. Which role takes precedence and why?
7. Discuss the potential effects of fraud and deceit in medical or nursing research on patient care. Review cases found on the ORI website, and discuss the implications of research misconduct in these cases: https://ori.hhs.gov/content/case_summary
8. Compare and contrast what the ANA (www.ana.org), the CNA (https://www.cna-aiic.ca/en/home), and the ICN (www.icn.ch) say about human rights in research and in nursing practice. Start with reviewing their position statements.
9. Explore one or more of the following websites and report back to the class what you discovered about informed consent and protection of human rights in research:
   Regulations and Ethical Guidelines—
   http://www.hhs.gov/ohrp/humansubjects/guid-ance/belmont.html
   Office of Human Research Protection—
   https://www.hhs.gov/ohrp/regulations-and-policy/informed-consent-posting/index.html
   CFR—Section on informed consent
   https://www.ecfr.gov/search?search%5Bdate%5D=current&search%5Bquery%5D=in-formed+consent&view=standard
   US Department of Education—
   http://www2.ed.gov/about/offices/list/ocfo/humansub.html
   Alliance for Human Research Protection—
   http://www.ahrp.org
   HIPAA regulations—
   https://privacyruleandresearch.nih.gov/pdf/HIPAA_Booklet_4-14-2003.pdf https://www.hhs.gov/

hipaa/for-professionals/special-topics/research/index.html

10. Review the code of ethics from the ANA (2015), the CNA (2017), or the ICN (2021), whichever is most appropriate for your situation, and discuss how pertinent statements in the codes relate to each of the issues discussed in this chapter.

UNCITED REFERENCES

Office of Research Integrity (ORI) (2023).

REFERENCES

ANA. (2015). *Code of ethics for nurses with interpretive statements.* http://nursingworld.org/DocumentVault/Ethics-1/Code-of-Ethics-for-Nurses.html

Bios, M. (2018). Capacity, vulnerability and informed consent for research. *Journal of Law, Medicine & Ethics, 46,* 72–78.

Calloway, S. J. (2009). The effect of culture on beliefs related to autonomy and informed consent. *Journal of Cultural Diversity, 16*(2), 68–70.

CNA. (2017). *Code of ethics for registered nurses.* https://cdn1.nscn.ca/sites/default/files/documents/resources/code-of-ethics-for-registered-nurses.pdf#:~:text=The%20Canadian%20Nurses%20Association%20%28CNA%29%20Code%20of%20Ethics,receiving%20care.%20The%20Code%20is%20both%20aspirational%20and%20regulatory

Childress, J., Meslin, E., & Shapiro, H. (Eds.). (2005). *Belmont revisited: Ethical principles for research with human subjects.* Georgetown University Press.

Clark, A. M., & Thompson, D. R. (2020). How to minimize research misconduct? Priorities for academics in nursing. *Journal of Advanced Nursing, 76*(3), 751–753. https://doi.org/10.1111/jan.14273. Epub 2019 Dec 13. PMID: 31777081.

Code of Federal Regulations. (2018). *Protection of Human Subjects. Title 45, Part 46.* https://www.ecfr.gov/current/title-45/subtitle-A/subchapter-A/part-46

Covey, S. R. (1992). *Principle-centered leadership.* Fireside.

Fowler, M. D. M. (1988). Ethical issues in nursing research: A call for an international code of ethics for nursing. *Western Journal of Nursing Research, 10,* 352–355.

Gehlert, S., & Mozersky, J. (2018). Seeing beyond the margins: Challenges to informed inclusion of vulnerable populations in research. *Journal of Law, Medicine & Ethics, 46,* 30–43.

George, S. L. (2016). Research misconduct and data fraud in clinical trials: Prevalence and causal factors. *International Journal of Clinical Oncology, 21,* 15–21.

Gray, J. R., & Groves, S. K. (2020). *Burns and Grove's' the practice of nursing research* (9th ed.). Elsevier.

Horner, J., & Minifie, F. D. (2011). Research ethics III: Publication. practices and authorship, conflicts of interest, and research misconduct. *Journal of Speech, Language & Hearing Research, 54*(1), 346–362.

ICN. (2021). *The ICN code of ethics for nurses.* https://www.icn.ch/system/files/2021-10/ICN_Code-of-Ethics_EN_Web_0.pdf

Karcz, M., & Papadakos, P. J. (2011). Consequences of fraud and deceit in medical research. *Canadian Journal of Respiratory Therapy, 47*(1), 18–27.

Munhall, P. L. (2012). *Nursing research: A qualitative perspective* (5th ed.). Jones & Bartlett Learning.

Office of Research Integrity (ORI). (2023). *Research misconduct: Case summaries.* Rockville, MD: Office of Research Integrity. https://ori.hhs.gov/case_summary.

Oulton, K., Gibson, F., Sell, D., Williams, A., Pratt, L., & Wray, J. (2016). Assent for children's participation in research: Why it matter and making it meaningful. *Child Care, Health, and Development, 42*(4), 588–597.

Roig, M. (2015). *Avoiding plagiarism, self-plagiarism and other questionable writing practices: A guide to ethical writing.* https://ori.hhs.gov/avoiding-plagiarism-self-plagiarism-and-other-questionable-writing-practices-guide-ethical-writing

US Department of Health and Human Services. (n.d.). *Office for Human Research Protections (OHRP).* https://www.hhs.gov/ohrp/index.html

US Department of Health and Human Services—National Institutes of Health (DHHS-NIH) (2003). *Protecting personal health information in research: Understanding the HIPAA privacy rule.* Author. (NIH Publication Number 03-5388). https://privacyruleandresearch.nih.gov/pdf/HIPAA_Booklet_4-14-2003.pdf

US Department of Health and Human Services—Office of Human Research Protection (DHHS-OHRP). (1979). *The Belmont report: Ethical principles and guidelines for the protection of human subjects of research.* https://www.hhs.gov/ohrp/regulations-and-policy/belmont-report/index.html

US Department of Health and Human Services—Office of Human Research Protection (DHHS-OHRP). (2022). *Informed consent.* https://www.hhs.gov/ohrp/regulations-and-policy/guidance/checklists/index.html

Ward-Smith, P. (2016). Evidence based nursing: When evidence is fraudulent. Urological. *Nursing, 36*(2), 98–99.

Wilson, H. S. (1999). *Introducing research in nursing* (2nd ed.). Addison-Wesley.

Wu, E., Wang, T., Lin, T., Chen, X., Guan, Z., Cao, C., & Lok, A. S. (2015). A comparative study of patients' attitudes toward clinical research in the United States and urban and rural China. *Clinical and Translational Science Journal, 8*(2), 123–131.

Nursing Ethics, Global Health Care Challenges, and Social Justice

Part IV recognizes each person as part of an interrelated global population affected by many interacting forces. With a focus on ethical nursing practice, this part addresses issues that require global consciousness on the part of nurses. This section explores considerations related to ethical and professional responsibility and accountability of nurses, individually and as a profession, in ever-changing local, national, and global health care settings. These chapters focus on nursing's ethical imperative to address planetary health and social justice and to provide holistic health care to diverse populations in both routine and challenging situations. In addition, these chapters encourage nurses to be responsible professionals and citizens in acknowledging and participating in advocacy, decision making, and shaping health policy related to issues that influence health care delivery and outcomes worldwide.

13

Nursing Ethics in a Diverse Global Society

What we remember, we can change; what we forget, we always are.

(Tafoya, 1996)

OBJECTIVES

After completing this chapter, the reader should be able to:

1. Discuss the relationship between Earth health and human health.
2. Describe the role and ethical responsibility of nursing in addressing local, national, and global environmental issues.
3. Discuss health and ethical issues related to local, national, and global issues such as climate change, disaster, displaced persons, immigrants, war and violence, epidemics and pandemics, toxic chemicals, and other pollutants.
4. Describe the impact on vulnerable populations of global humanitarian and health crises.
5. Discuss the nursing role, responsibility, and ethical stance in addressing local, national, and global

healthcare needs of people and communities affected by these global issues.
6. Describe the challenges of accessibility and financing facing healthcare delivery systems around the globe.
7. Identify how traditional healing systems can be resources for health care worldwide.
8. Briefly describe factors affecting healthcare delivery for rural and urban aggregates.
9. Discuss the practical application of nursing codes of ethics for nurses in caring for and advocating for people affected by selected global health concern.

INTRODUCTION

Many global concerns have a significant impact on the health and well-being of people and the planet. Ethical and other issues associated with these concerns call for both personal and professional responses from nurses at local, national, and international levels. Examples of these issues include Earth health, natural and other disasters, migrants and displaced persons, famine and malnutrition, violence against children, human trafficking, use of torture, war and violence, genocide, unexploded bombs and land mines, pollution, global warming, epidemics and pandemics, drug-resistant organisms, bioterrorism, and access to and financing of health care (both Western and traditional systems). Nurses need

to be aware of both overt and covert human rights violations that are at the heart of, or result from, many of these global concerns. Discussion of the nursing role, responsibility, and ethical considerations for several of these concerns is included in this chapter. Students are encouraged to explore and discuss appropriate nursing roles and responses related to other global health issues not discussed here.

EARTH ETHICS AND HEALTH

Discussions of ethics, especially healthcare ethics, generally refer to principles and practices related to human experiences, values, and ways of being in the world. Rarely is there any consideration of ethical treatment of the more-than-human world—indeed, the Earth as a whole—the health of which is so intricately connected to human health. The more-than-human world includes all beings and elements of Earth that are not human beings. Our sense of relationship with the natural world is based on our worldview or cosmology. The Western scientific perspective flows from a worldview that holds that there is a radical distinction between humans as subjects and the natural world as object (Ausubel, 2004, 2012; Berry, 2009; Foster et al., 2020; Swimme & Tucker, 2011; Uhl, 2004). This sense of human experience being separate from and in opposition to nature has engendered and permitted a destructive attitude toward Earth and has supported the belief that all species and resources of the Earth have been put here primarily for human use. One significant assumption of the Western worldview (which is now spreading globally) is that the more we try to control and "fix" nature, the more we are doing what is right and good. This idea is based on a view that began emerging in the 17th century of Earth and all its inhabitants (including the human body) as a complex machine with ordered, predictable laws. This shift from an organic understanding of reality where everything is alive to a mechanistic view of reality engendered the belief that humans have a right to do anything they want with nature. Such an attitude results in little sense of ethical responsibility toward the more-than-human world. On the contrary, it has allowed us to turn a blind eye to our complicity in the exploitation of the planet. After several hundred years of demoting the natural world to a collection of material objects available for exploitation, we are now realizing that the complete disregard for the realities of ecological systems and the limited capacity of the natural world to sustain such exploitation and destruction are contributing to the ill health of humans and to the planet itself.

When we destroy the source of our life and sustenance, our health (physical, mental, emotional, and spiritual) suffers. Indigenous peoples continue to teach what many people in the West are only now beginning to remember: that all things are connected and that we belong to a whole universe, not just to a city, culture, or nation. They remind us that, as part of the interconnected web of life, what we do to the Earth, we do to ourselves. Indigenous peoples, mystics of many traditions, and contemporary scholars understand the world to be a seamless garment in which there is no separation between humans and nature, the sacred and the secular.

They also recognize that we cannot have healthy minds or communities without healthy land and environment (Ausubel, 2012; Myers & Frumkin, 2020; Foster et al., 2020; Luck, 2022; Nelson, 2004). Understanding that we are all one single, sacred, Earth community, we recognize the interdependence and unity of all in the natural world and appreciate that all species have an intrinsic right to exist. As we move beyond a human-centered focus, we begin to relate to the Earth community as having core value in itself and incorporate Earth ethics into our nursing ethics. When we understand that, as humans, we are only one part of the interconnected Earth community, we recognize that our ethical principles must address the integrity and health of the entire community of life, and we understand the moral imperative to apply principles of respect, beneficence, nonmaleficence, and justice to our treatment of the whole Earth community. This in no way diminishes human rights; rather, it augments human well-being by fostering the rights of humans to live within healthy ecosystems and receive the life-supporting benefits of the diversity, community, and beauty of the natural world.

Earth health is a critical global issue because, as noted, we cannot be healthy if the Earth is not healthy. The manipulation of nature through scientific and technological exploration has brought many benefits to human health, life, and general well-being. These benefits, however, have come with a high price—a disruption of the life systems of Earth, violence toward and degradation of much of the natural world, and disruption of both the human and bioregional communities. These disruptions have led to poisoning of the air we breathe, the water we drink, and the soil and seas that provide us food. Examples of health problems or potential problems related to disruptions of the natural balance in nature include asthma; birth defects; deformed frogs; trees dying from acid rain; toxins in air, water, soil, and human tissues (including breast milk); drug-resistant organisms; and malnutrition. Recognizing that some healthcare practices and products (during manufacture, use, or disposal) can harm both humans and the environment, nurses are taking a leadership role in issues of environmental health (ANA, 2015, Provision 9.4; Canadian Nurses Association (CNA), 2017b; ICN, 2018a; Foster et al., 2020; McDermott-Levy, 2023; Luck, 2022).

Environmentally responsible health care requires awareness and action at many levels. One level involves seeking to move beyond the symptoms of an illness to address the source of the health concern. This may need to be done on an individual, community, or global level. The impact of smoking and secondhand smoke on asthma and pregnancy outcomes is one example of linking an environmental pollutant to a health concern and taking action to decrease the pollutant. Many health problems are related to toxic chemicals and other pollutants in the environment. These pollutants come from many sources, such as industrial production, everyday use in homes, health care and other institutions, manufacturing, agribusiness, waste disposal, and military actions. We take these chemicals into our bodies through the food we eat, the water we drink, the air we breathe, and our skin. It is alarming to realize the impact of these toxins on human health (CNA, 2017b; Crinnion, 2010; Li, 2017; McDermott-Levy et al., 2023; Myers & Frumkin, 2020). Addressing the source of these toxins requires action at the personal level, such as responsible use and recycling of plastic; at the professional or local level, such as reducing the use of and providing for the responsible disposition of disposable plastic equipment in the hospital; and at the global level, such as working for legislation that mandates industry to provide a process for recycling components of disposable products that they manufacture in a way that does not create more pollution.

Nurses are positioned to be proactive in addressing the impact of the healthcare system on the health of the environment. This includes considerations such as attention to the health impact of chemicals found in products used in healthcare institutions; how the institution disposes of toxic and other waste; the proper disposal of unused or outdated medications; the impact of antibiotics, hormones, and chemotherapy that get into water and soil through human waste; and unnecessary water and electric consumption. Nurses can take leadership roles in instituting recycling programs by helping develop institutional policies aimed at using energy-efficient, recycled, and environmentally friendly products wherever possible. The **precautionary principle** provides a useful guide for ethically addressing the potential risk or harm to human health or the environment of new products, processes, interventions, or technologies. This principle states "when an activity raises threats of harm to human health or the environment, precautionary measures should be taken even if some cause and effect relationships are not fully established scientifically" (Raffensperger, 2004, p. 44). The precautionary approach affirms that when there is reasonable suspicion of harm and scientific uncertainty regarding cause and effect, people have a duty to act to prevent harm. With this approach, the developer or proponent of a product must provide sufficient information about and reasonable assurances of its safety before it can be marketed. (Currently, the burden of proof of the harmfulness of a product lies with the public or government, generally after the product is already in use.) The precautionary approach suggests action steps that include setting goals; examining all reasonable alternatives for achieving the goal and choosing the least harmful way; monitoring results; heeding early warnings; making midcourse corrections as needed; and ensuring that all decisions include the affected parties and be open, informed, and democratic (Chaudry, 2008; Foster et al., 2020; Myers & Raffensperger, 2006; Pinto-Bazurco, 2020). The ultimate goal of the precautionary approach is to determine how little harm is possible with a new product or development.

The Earth Charter and Nursing

The Earth Charter (https://earthcharter.org) can provide guidance to nurses and others for promoting ethically responsible relationships with Earth and the global community. This charter is a people's treaty resulting from a decade-long, worldwide, cross-cultural conversation about shared vision and goals for global interdependence and shared responsibility for the well-being of the human family and the larger living world. As a declaration of fundamental principles for building a just, peaceful, and sustainable global society, the Earth Charter recognizes that issues of human rights, environmental protection, equitable human development, and a culture of peace are interdependent and indivisible. The charter provides a framework and ethical vision for addressing these issues (Box 13.1).

Climate Change

Climate change is a global concern that has significant health implications. In its position paper, *Nurses, Climate Change and Health*, the International Council of Nurses (ICN, 2018a) notes that "climate change presents the single largest threat to global development." The ICN, CNA, and ANA all call on nurses to take leadership roles in mitigating climate change, supporting individuals and communities around the world in adapting to the impact of these changes, and developing healthcare

BOX 13.1 Principles of the Earth Charter: A Summary

Respect and care for the community of life, which includes:
- Respecting Earth and life in all its diversity
- Caring for the community of life with understanding, compassion, and love
- Building democratic societies that are just, participatory, sustainable, and peaceful
- Securing Earth's bounty and beauty for present and future generations

Ecological integrity, which includes:
- Protecting and restoring the integrity of Earth's ecological systems with special concern for biological diversity and the natural processes that sustain life
- Preventing harm as the best method of environmental protection and, when knowledge is limited, applying a precautionary approach
- Adopting patterns of production, consumption, and reproduction that safeguard Earth's regenerative capacities, human rights, and community well-being
- Advancing the study of ecological sustainability and promoting open exchange and wide application of the knowledge acquired

Social and economic justice, which includes:
- Eradicating poverty as an ethical, social, and environmental imperative
- Ensuring that economic activities and institutions at all levels promote human development in an equitable and sustainable manner
- Affirming gender equality and equity as prerequisites to sustainable development and ensuring universal access to education, health care, and economic opportunity
- Upholding the right of all, without discrimination, to a natural and social environment supportive of human dignity, bodily health, and spiritual well-being, with special attention to the rights of indigenous peoples and minorities

Democracy, nonviolence, and peace, which includes:
- Strengthening democratic institutions at all levels and providing transparency and accountability in governance, inclusive participation in decision making, and access to justice
- Integrating into formal education and lifelong learning the knowledge, values, and skills needed for a sustainable way of life
- Treating all living beings with respect and consideration
- Promoting a culture of tolerance, nonviolence, and peace

From Earth Charter International. (2023). Earth Charter. http://earthcharter.org.

ASK YOURSELF

What Is an Ethic of Care for the Earth?
- What does your culture teach about your relationship with Earth and the more-than-human part of a global community of life?
- How do you see principles of respect, beneficence, nonmaleficence, and justice reflected in the Earth Charter?
- What can you do, personally and professionally, to promote environmentally conscious practices in your local area and healthcare setting?
- What do you see as the role of nursing in developing and promoting an ethic of care for the Earth? What guidance for this is provided in nursing codes of ethics and position statements?

systems to deal with health issues related to climate change (ICN, 2018a; CNA, 2017b; ANA, 2008, 2022). Excerpts from the ICN position statement are found in Box 13.2. Nurses need to be alert to the many social and environmental determinants of health that are affected by climate change, including sufficient food, clean water and air, and secure shelter (AHNE, 2023; ANA, 2015, Provision 9.3, 9.5; Anderko & Chalupka, 2023; CNA, 2017a, Part II; CNA, 2017b; ICN, 2021, Element 4.5; Li, 2017; Rossati, 2017; WHO, 2018a).

Climate change affects health in direct ways such as the impact of severe drought, storms, floods, tornados, and other natural disasters. Examples include deaths and injuries from the disaster; lack of food, shelter, water, and access to health care; spread of infectious diseases; and mental health issues such as depression and posttraumatic stress disorder. Health is also affected in indirect ways such as long-term loss of clean air, water, biodiversity, and productivity of agricultural land; changes in the geographic range of vectors for infectious diseases; loss of land needed for housing and agriculture; and civil conflict (Fig. 13.1).

Examples of the health effects of climate change include food and water insecurity (which may lead to conflict over limited resources), malnutrition, increases in infectious diseases (leading to epidemics and pandemics), pollution (causing an increase in respiratory

BOX 13.2   Excerpts from ICN: Nurses, Climate Change, and Health

As the global voice of nursing, ICN:

- Strongly believes that nurses have a shared responsibility to sustain and protect the natural environment from depletion, pollution, degradation, and destruction.
- Recognizes that building climate change resilience must include efforts to improve and sustain the social and environmental determinants of health through sustainable development.

ICN encourages national nurses' associations to:

- Work to enable nursing leadership and nurses to support healthcare organizations to contribute to climate change mitigation through the implementation of environmental policies and sustainable practices.
- Engage in national and multisectoral measures to mitigate the impact of climate change on the population with a focus on vulnerable groups and those more exposed to disease and injury.
- Be involved in developing national action plans and policies for mitigation, adaptation, and resilience strategies, as well as contribute to environmental health and justice policymaking.
- Raise awareness of the health implications of climate change and how to assess and address climate change

risks to health by developing policy documents on the subject.

- Support the introduction of incentives for nurses to incorporate environmentally responsible health practices into their interventions.

The ICN calls on individual nurses to:

- Advocate for policies that promote the reduction of healthcare waste and ensure correct waste management.
- Actively engage in environmental health committees and policymaking that focus on the safety and protection of health workers and the management and regulation of the healthcare environment.
- Empower individuals, families, and communities to make healthy lifestyle choices and change their own practices (i.e., active transportation, use green energy, and dietary changes) to decrease the contribution to greenhouse gases.
- Work with communities to build resilience to the impacts of climate change in a way that is driven by the local context and needs and that goes beyond reactivity but seeks to address underlying vulnerabilities.

(From International Council of Nurses. (2018). *Position statement.* https://www.icn.ch/sites/default/files/inline-files/PS_E_Nurses_climate%20change_health_0.pdf)

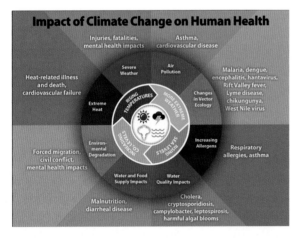

Fig. 13.1 Impact of Climate Change on Human Health. (From Centers for Disease Control and Prevention. (2014). *Climate effects on health.* https://www.cdc.gov/climateandhealth/effects/.)

and other health issues), chronic stress, civil and domestic violence, poor pregnancy outcomes, and impaired childhood development (Table 13.1). Globally, vulnerable populations such as older adults, women and children, and the poor (particularly in developing countries) are more affected by and susceptible to the health impacts of climate change (WHO, 2018a). For example, Zalon (2019) notes that common physiological changes of aging, such as changes in sweating and ability to regulate body temperature, decreased cardiac reserve and respiratory muscle strength, decreased immune response, and decreased mobility, make the elderly more vulnerable to the effects of climate change. Limited social support, poverty, multiple health concerns, and polypharmacy exacerbate their vulnerability. She reflects that healthcare systems are not prepared to address the impact of climate change particularly on the elderly. She urges nurses to assist older patients in preparing for, managing, and adapting to the impact on their health of adverse environmental events. Nurses need to be knowledgeable about global and local health concerns related to climate change and advocate for policies, regulations, and practices designed to support individuals and communities in addressing these concerns. Resources that will assist readers in beginning to explore this area more fully are included at the end of this chapter.

TABLE 13.1 **Climate Change and Human Health**	
Environmental Occurrence	**Health Impact**
Acute natural disasters such as hurricanes, floods, heat waves, forest fires, and tornados	Deaths and traumatic injuries Mental illness: acute stress and posttraumatic stress disorder Infections and other health issues related to air, water, and soil pollution Inadequate shelter, displaced persons Interruptions in food and water supply Medication and healthcare access issues
Long-term drought Compromised agricultural production due to alterations to and shrinking of arable land Damaged crops Food insecurity Water insecurity	Malnutrition, undernutrition, famine Impaired childhood development Lack of drinkable water and water for hygiene Lack of water for agriculture and manufacturing Violence and civil conflicts Exacerbation of chronic diseases Exacerbation of stress-related illnesses
Heat waves	Complications for those with chronic health conditions Increases in rates of heat stress, heat stroke, and exhaustion Increased risk of death in vulnerable groups, particularly the elderly
Air pollution	Increases in acute respiratory symptoms Exacerbation of chronic respiratory conditions Increases in emergency room visits for respiratory issues (especially for the elderly)
Change in habitats and geographic ranges of insects and pathogens that cause disease and that damage food crops	Increases in infections related to water-borne diseases and vector-borne diseases Increases in communicable disease epidemics Malnutrition and famine

DISASTERS: NURSING RESPONSE AND ETHICAL CONSIDERATIONS

Nurses throughout the world play an important role in providing emergency care and in meeting the ongoing humanitarian needs of people affected by disasters. Disasters are generally described as sudden events of massive proportion that result in large numbers of victims, displacement of people, material damage, disruption to society, or a combination of these (ANA, 2017; ICN, 2019; Leider et al., 2017). Disastrous situations around the world, which may be linked to sudden events and require long-term as well as immediate interventions, include drought, famine, epidemics, and pandemics (such as Ebola, Zika, COVID-19, or HIV/AIDS). Disasters may be termed *natural* (such as hurricanes, earthquakes, or tsunamis), *technological* (such as major chemical leaks or nuclear plant malfunction), or *accidental* (such as a train derailing or a ship capsizing). The proportion of the disaster may be due to a combination of these factors. For example, the 2011 Japan tsunami and Haiti earthquake, the 2017 hurricanes Harvey and Maria, and the 2023 earthquake in Turkey and Syria were natural disasters, whereas the nuclear power plant failure brought on by the tsunami in Japan was a technological disaster. Another example is human alteration of the land through activities such as massive logging and deforestation that contribute to the severity of some flood-related disasters. Scientists see a link between the increase in the number and severity of natural disasters over recent years and climate change, which is occurring in great part through human activity (Mcdermott-Levy, 2023; Myers & Frumkin, 2020; Rockström & Gaffney, 2021; WHO, 2018a).

Emergency and continuous health care are essential parts of any disaster response. Disasters, from the health professional's view, are situations in which there is an often sudden, unforeseen imbalance between the needs of people whose health and well-being are threatened and the resources and capacity of the healthcare system to meet these needs (Leider et al., 2017; World Medical Association, 2017). Many health-related problems arise in a disaster. Disasters require prompt action, yet responders must often deal with inadequate supplies and resources as well as the need to get to victims who are in places that may present health risks, be dangerous, or be difficult to reach. The World Medical Association offers guides for ethical practice for physicians in a disaster situation, which are summarized in the following discussion. These apply to nurses as well (ANA, 2017; CNA, 2017b, Part I.A.9, I.F.6; ICN, 2019). See also the American Nurses Association (ANA) disaster preparedness webpage (https://www.nursingworld.org/practice-policy/work-environment/health-safety/disaster-preparedness/).

In the emergency phase, prioritizing treatment and management, or triage, is the first ethical consideration. Triage must be done quickly and by an experienced person (often a nurse) who is aware of available resources. Based on medical needs and intervention capabilities, victims are separated into groups of those who can be saved and those whose condition exceeds the available therapeutic resources. Victims who have a chance of being saved are separated into groups of those whose lives are in immediate danger and require urgent attention, those who are not in immediate danger and who need urgent but not immediate attention, those needing only minor treatment, and those with primarily psychological trauma. Because of the nature of trauma, regular reassessment of victims in each group must be done.

Perhaps the most difficult ethical consideration of triage is the sense of abandoning a person whose injuries or care needs are beyond the available resources. In the aftermath of hurricanes Katrina and Rita and the Haiti earthquake, a number of nurses reported having to make very difficult decisions about which patients would receive lifesaving treatment when electricity, medications, and other needed supplies and equipment were not available. Issues faced by those providing emergency care in disasters such as the earthquake in Haiti, the tsunami in Japan, Hurricane Maria in Puerto Rico, and the earthquake in Turkey-Syria include difficulty reaching victims; lack of basic necessities such as food, water, shelter, and sanitation; large numbers of victims and very limited resources such as medical supplies; language and cultural barriers; and limited transportation. The ethical stance in these situations is to save the greatest number of persons who have a chance of recovery,

restrict morbidity to a minimum, and do as much as possible to show compassion and respect for those who are dying. Those involved in responding to disasters are often faced with moral dilemmas. For example, conflicts arise between principles such as duty to care for patients and justice in use and distribution of scarce resources. In international disaster situations especially, dealing with large numbers of patients who need the same limited resources is often a source of moral distress, posttraumatic stress disorder, and burnout (Leider et al., 2017; Sloand et al., 2012).

Ethical care of victims in disasters requires nurses to provide impartial assistance to every victim without waiting to be asked, incorporating emotional as well as technical care. Nurses need to obtain a person's consent and address cultural differences as often as possible. Triage decisions should be based on a person's emergency status and not on nonmedical criteria such as socioeconomic status, ethnicity, or political position. Nurses need to do their best to respect cultural customs, religious practices, and other traditions, especially those associated with dying, mourning, and emotional and psychological response and needs. Other considerations are to ensure confidentiality as much as possible, particularly when dealing with media and other third parties, and to be objective and respectful of the emotional and political climate associated with the disaster.

The lack of preparedness to deal with the rapid spread of COVID-19 and the resulting global pandemic created crisis situations in many hospitals and healthcare settings worldwide. Unlike emergency disaster situations in which crisis care may be needed for a few weeks, the crisis care required during the COVID-19 pandemic began in 2020 and persisted for months during the initial phase of the pandemic and subsequent peaks related to new variants of the virus. Issues related to caring for large numbers of critically ill patients with COVID-19 who needed the same limited supplies and medical equipment, along with insufficient personal protective equipment for nurses and other care providers went on for months. Issues like these and the persisting need for working in a crisis mode led to moral distress, posttraumatic stress disorder, and burnout among nurses and other healthcare providers.

The challenge of adhering to professional standards of care when faced with often overwhelming need that far exceeds resources in disaster situations prompted the development of *Guidance for Establishing Crisis Standards of Care for Use in Disaster Situations* (IOM, 2009, 2012). This document defines crisis standards of care (CSC) as a "substantial change in usual healthcare operations and the level of care it is possible to deliver, which is made necessary by a pervasive (e.g., pandemic influenza) or catastrophic (e.g., earthquake and hurricane) disaster" (p. 18). Hick and colleagues (2021) note that CSC "occur when the degree of resource shortage requires decisions that place a patient or provider at risk of a poor outcome" (p. 1). Implicit in these standards is the expectation that nurses and other professionals provide the optimal level of health care possible given the circumstances. These guidelines were developed to assist policymakers (primarily in the United States) at local, state, tribal, and national levels in developing uniform policies and protocols for planning a response that can be applied in any disaster situation. The IOM (2009, 2012) identified five key elements that should be included in CSC protocols:

- A strong ethical grounding
- Integrated and ongoing community and provider engagement, education, and communication
- Assurances regarding legal authority and environment
- Clear indicators, triggers, and lines of responsibility
- Evidence-based clinical processes and operations

The overarching ethical goal of CSC is fairness to all affected parties that include equity of triage decisions and allocation of resources (IOM, 2009, 2012; Hick et al., 2021). Other ethical considerations include duty to care, duty to steward resources, transparency, consistency, proportionality, and accountability, all of which are congruent with directives in codes of nursing ethics. The CSC guidelines also include legal protections for healthcare providers and institutions. Leider and colleagues (2017) note that CSCs have been implemented in response to global disasters more than in the United States. According to Hick and colleagues (2021), during COVID-19 in the United States, CSC healthcare plans were utilized inconsistently. Some jurisdictions declared CSC at state or county levels, others made no formal declaration authorizing CSC, and some states even ignored CSC plans they had in place. Hick and colleagues (2021) note the need to utilize what has been learned from the issues and dilemmas that arose during COVID-19 to update and revise CSC guidelines to ensure consistency in providing the best care possible when faced with similar crisis situations in the future. In light of the ever-increasing local and global need for nurses to

respond in disaster situations, students are encouraged to explore the IOM guidelines at https://www.nursing-world.org/~4ad845/globalassets/docs/ana/stds-of-care-letter-report-2.pdf.

Nurses are key healthcare providers in disaster situations and are generally very willing to respond in times of crisis. However, there may be situations in which responding jeopardizes the health or safety of the nurse or the nurse's family. The ANA *Issue Brief: Who Will Be There?* (2017) raises the question of whether nurses have an ethical obligation and contractual duty to respond in every disaster situation. The brief notes that two different provisions in the *ANA Code of Ethics with Interpretive Statements* (2015) may present a conflict of obligations for the nurse. Provision 2 of the code states that the "nurse's primary commitment is to the patient," and Provision 5 states, "the nurse owes the same duties to self as to others, including the responsibility to promote health and safety." This document highlights several important considerations for nurses relative to choosing between duties based on moral grounds regarding responding to disasters (Box 13.3). Implicit in nurses' duty to uphold the standards of their profession is the "commitment to help care for and protect their patients while protecting their own right to self-preservation and self-care" (ANA, 2017, p. 2). Similarly, the ICN (2019) writes "disaster risk reduction, response and recovery planning must include strategies to support the resilience of nurses. This involves ensuring nurses' personal safety and physical and psychological health and wellbeing in the short and long term" (p. 2). Ethical codes and position statements of ANA (2015), CNA (2017a), and ICN (2021) encourage nurses to be proactive in addressing issues related to the conflict between a nurse's duty to care versus duty to self through active involvement in shaping policy and protocols at institutional and governmental levels.

Many nurses choose to volunteer locally, nationally, and internationally in times of disaster, both as individuals and as part of organized medical rescue teams. Two position statements of the ANA offer guidelines related to work release during a disaster for both nurses and their employers. Links to these position statements are noted in Table 13.2. Another support for nurses who provide services in a disaster in a state in which they are not licensed is the Uniform Emergency Volunteer Health Practitioners Act, initially developed in 2006 by the Uniform Law Commission. States that adopt this model legislation recognize, in a declared disaster, licensure of

CASE PRESENTATION

Challenges of Providing Health Care in Disaster Situations

After the 2010 earthquake in Haiti, many nurses volunteered to assist in humanitarian and health relief efforts. They provided care in emergency trauma, inpatient, and primary care settings on land and on hospital ships. The following are examples of some of the situations they encountered taken from Sloand and colleagues' (2012) study of experiences of nurse volunteers who cared for children after this disaster. Consider the ethical issues nurses faced in each of these situations.

General Issues

- The overwhelming need and impossibility of seeing everyone needing care
- Limited overall supplies, medications, and equipment and lack of proper pediatric resources such as smaller size equipment and ability to provide medication in appropriate pediatric doses
- Shortage of clean water to reconstitute medications
- Children with devastating injuries who had been separated from family or whose parents were dead
- A lack of reliable rehabilitation for those with severe injuries
- Insufficient numbers of healthcare practitioners particularly with pediatric expertise
- A chaotic and crime-rampant environment that jeopardized the safety and well-being of many survivors

Particular Case Situations

- A girl exhibited signs of sexual and physical abuse; however, the nurse had difficulty reporting this due to a lack of infrastructure in Haiti at the time to handle these types of abuse cases.

- A child had an acute exacerbation of asthma, and there was no medicine other than steroids. The nurse had to choose whether to send the only inhaler they had home with the child.
- A six-month-old baby required suctioning to survive and no pediatric suctioning equipment was available.
- A child had continuous seizures and, after deliberating whether to intubate the child, the team decided it was not a viable option because there was no pediatric nurse in the intensive care unit (ICU) to care for the patient on the ventilator.
- The only nurse on a night shift in a neonatal ICU had six babies who needed to be fed every three hours.

Think About It
Applying Crisis Standards of Care

- What is your initial reaction to each of the situations described?
- Did the care the nurses provided meet the expected standards of nursing care and follow ethical codes? How would CSCs apply to these situations?
- How do you think you would have responded in these situations? What would have made them most challenging for you?
- What ethical conflicts did these nurse volunteers have to deal with?
- What guidance is offered to those providing health care in disasters by professional codes of ethics, position statements, and other guidelines?
- How might the experiences of these volunteer nurses contribute to moral distress?
- What parallels can you see between the ethical dilemmas in these situations and what nurses faced during the COVID-19 pandemic?

BOX 13.3   Choosing Between Duties Based on Moral Grounds

Pondering the following questions may be helpful when considering a nurse's moral duty to respond in a disaster:
- How much high-quality care can the nurse provide to others and still take care of oneself?
- Does the response situation feel physically safe?
- Is there potential danger to the nurse in providing patient care?
- Is there adequate support for meeting the nurse's own family needs?

- Is there any concern about professional ethical and legal protection for the nurse during the response situation?
- Are there legal obligations for the nurse to respond?
- Is what the nurse is being asked to do within the parameters of the nurse's professional license, knowledge, and clinical expertise?
- What line will the nurse not cross when it comes to maintaining professional integrity?

TABLE 13.2 Resources: Disaster and Climate Change: Advocacy and Preparedness	
American Nurses Association—Disaster preparedness	https://www.nursingworld.org/practice-policy/work-environment/health-safety/disaster-preparedness/
Work release during disaster—Employer guidelines	https://www.nursingworld.org/practice-policy/nursing-excellence/official-position-statements/id/work-release-during-a-disaster-guidelines-for-employers/
Work release during disaster—Employee responsibilities	https://www.nursingworld.org/practice-policy/nursing-excellence/official-position-statements/id/RN-rights-and-responsibilities-related-to-work-release-during-a-disaster/
Advocacy	https://nursingworld.org/practice-policy/advocacy/
International Committee of the Red Cross—Disaster preparedness	https://media.ifrc.org/ifrc/what-we-do/disaster-and-crisis-management/disaster-preparedness/
US Department of Homeland Security— Make a plan	https://www.ready.gov/make-a-plan
American Association of Diabetes— Emergency preparedness	https://diabeteseducator.org/living-with-diabetes/disaster-preparedness
American Red Cross—Disaster preparedness for seniors by seniors	https://www.redcross.org/content/dam/redcross/atg/PDF_s/Preparedness___Disaster_Recovery/Disaster_Preparedness/Disaster_Preparedness_for_Srs-English.revised_7-09.pdf
Centers for Disease Control and Prevention—Emergency preparedness for older adults	https://www.cdc.gov/aging/publications/features/older-adult-emergency.html
Alliance of Nurses for Healthy Environments—Environmental advocacy	https://envirn.org
Health Care Without Harm—Environmental advocacy	https://noharm.org/
World Health Organization—Climate change and health	https://www.who.int/news-room/fact-sheets/detail/climate-change-and-health
United Nations—Climate change toolkit	https://unfccc.int/news/new-toolkit-to-boost-capacity-building
Environmental Protection Agency—Climate change and extreme heat: What you can do to prepare	https://epa.gov/sites/production/files/2016-10/documents/extreme-heat-guidebook.pdf
ReliefWeb—Humanitarian inclusion standards for older people and people with disabilities	https://reliefweb.int/report/world/humanitarian-inclusion-standards-older-people-and-people-disabilities
US Department of Health and Human Services—Primary protection: Enhancing health care resilience for a changing climate	https://toolkit.climate.gov/sites/default/files/SCRHCFI%20Best%20Practices%20Report%20final2%202014%20Web.pdf
National Oceanic and Atmospheric Administration—US climate resilience	https://toolkit.climate.gov

healthcare practitioners from another state if the practitioner is registered with a public or private registration system. At the time of this writing, 19 states and the District of Columbia have enacted this legislation. The list of states can be found on their website (https://www.facs.org/advocacy/state/uevhpa). The Nurse Licensure Compact (NLC) is a process for enabling nurses to more easily work in states other than where they have their primary nursing license that is not limited to disaster situations. The NLC is an agreement among states to honor each other's nursing license by enabling nurses to apply for a multistate nursing license in addition to their local state license. For information about the NLC visit https://www.nursecompact.com/.

Nurses need to be aware of emergency response plans where they work, be familiar with disaster preparedness efforts in their communities, and know what their expected roles might be. Nurses need to be aware as well of healthcare issues and be prepared to intervene with health needs beyond the emergency response to a disaster. Principles of humanitarian action basic to this care include meeting critical human needs and restoring personal dignity. Critical human needs that may become serious problems during and after a disaster include nutrition (availability, quality, and special needs of children); economic security; environmental health (water, sewage, air quality, and vector control); communicable disease control; emotional and mental health (including attention to rape and other forms of violence); basic health care (both preventive and curative); and family and social support. Disaster preparedness is becoming a very important set of skills for nurses worldwide. Students are encouraged to explore the resources related to disaster preparedness at the websites noted in Table 13.2.

DISPLACED PERSONS, MIGRANTS, REFUGEES, AND VICTIMS OF ARMED CONFLICT

In the past decades, disasters, wars, political instability, and armed conflict have forced growing numbers of people worldwide to become refugees or displaced persons. This is a global humanitarian disaster of immense proportions (Box 13.4). As noted in Box 13.5, refugees are persons who have fled their countries and who cannot or do not want to return due to well-founded fears of death or persecution because of their religion, race, political opinion, nationality, or membership in a

---

BOX 13.4   Consider the Numbers: Displaced Persons Worldwide (UNHCR, 2023b; United Nations Children's Fund [UNICEF], 2023)

100 million—the record number of people in the world forcibly displaced due to persecution, conflict, and human rights violations at the end of May 2022. This number included:

- **27.1 million** refugees (the highest number ever seen).
- **53.2 million** IDPs.
- **4.6 million** asylum seekers.
- This represents nearly **1.2 percent** of people globally.

36.5 million children (nearly **1 in every 70** children worldwide) live outside their country of birth. This number includes (as of the end of 2021):

- **12.5 million** child refugees and **1.2 million** asylum seekers.
- **22.8 million** displaced within their own country due to violence and conflict.
- Nearly **30 percent** of children living outside their country of birth are refugees—children comprise **40 percent** of all refugees.

(Data from USA for UNHCR, 2023b. *Refugee statistics.* https://www.unrefugees.org/refugeefacts/statistics/; United Nations Children's Fund (UNICEF). (2023). *Child displacement.* https://data.unicef.org/topic/child-migration-and-displacement/displacement/.)

BOX 13.5   Key Terms in Migration and Displacement

Migrants are individuals who are moving or have moved across an international border or within a state away from their habitual place of residence, regardless of (1) the person's legal status, (2) whether the movement is voluntary or involuntary, (3) what the causes for the movement are, or (4) what the length of the stay is. (Refugees may be considered a subset of the migrant population.)

Refugees are, in accordance with the 1951 Convention Relating to the Status of Refugees (and its 1967 Protocol), individuals who, due to a well-founded fear of being persecuted for reasons of race, religion, nationality, or membership of a particular social group or political opinion are outside the country of their nationality and are unable or, due to such fear, unwilling to avail themselves of the protection of that country; or who, not having a nationality and being outside the country of their former habitual residence as a result of such events, is unable or, due to such fear, is unwilling to return to it. For statistical purposes, since 2007 the refugee population has also included people in refugee-like situations facing the same protection concerns as refugees but whose refugee status has not been formally ascertained.

Internally displaced persons (IDPs) are individuals or groups of people who have been forced or obliged to flee or to leave their homes or places of habitual residence, in particular as a result of, or to avoid the effects of, armed conflict, situations of generalized violence, violations of human rights, or natural or human-made disasters and who have not crossed an internationally recognized state border. For statistical purposes, since 2007 the population of IDPs has also included people in an IDP-like situation.

(From United Nations Children's Fund (UNICEF). (2016). *Uprooted* (p. 14). https://www.unicef.org/media/50011/file/%20Uprooted_growing_crisis_for_refugee_and_migrant_children.pdf.)

particular social or ethnic group. Internally displaced persons (IDPs) are those who, because of war, persecution, or other threats, have been forced to leave their homes but who have not crossed an internationally recognized border (USA for UNHCR, 2023a). The 53.2 million IDPs in the world are legally under the protection of their own government and are not protected by international law or eligible to receive many types of aid (USA for UNHCR, 2023b). Asylum seekers are those who, when fleeing their own country, seek sanctuary in another country with hopes of receiving material support and legal protection. Victims of major disasters and those in areas of famine or severe economic upheaval can become displaced persons either temporarily or long term. Victims of human trafficking (discussed in Chapter 16) are a less visible group of displaced persons.

Displaced persons, migrants, and refugees are highly vulnerable populations. They often have serious health and social problems related to social determinants of health, deprivation (including basic human rights), detention, physical hardship, stress, poor nutrition, sexual violence, social exclusion, and generally poor health status (ICN, 2018b). Displacement often separates family members and cuts people off from community support, employment, educational opportunities, and cultural ties. Refugee settlements are frequently overcrowded and may lack sufficient resources, including food and sanitation, to meet basic necessities and healthcare needs. The majority of displaced persons around the world are women and children. The conditions in refugee settlements engender emotional cruelty and gender-specific violence such as rape, sexual abuse and harassment, spousal battering, and forced prostitution, and may also give rise to political unrest, particularly when internment in these camps becomes long term.

The impact of displacement and violence on children is a particular concern worldwide. The trauma and uncertainty of displacement and resettlement in temporary or long-term situations create a unique form of toxic stress. In addition, displaced children, especially those who travel on their own or become separated from their families, are at high risk for numerous health concerns, including violence, abuse, exploitation, and trafficking (UNICEF, 2016). Violence against children comes in many forms. Among displaced children, it may occur as state action (during migration enforcement or detention), abusive attitudes and xenophobic attacks from the general public, through child labor practices, through bullying and abuse in schools, or

related to domestic violence within families (which can be worsened by prolonged and extreme stress related to displacement) (UNICEF, 2016). The World Health Organization (WHO, 2022) describes six main types of violence that children may experience at some point in their lives (Box 13.6). The WHO notes that the health impact of this violence includes severe injuries and death; impaired cognitive and physical development; negative coping skills; unintended pregnancies and sexually transmitted infections; and behaviors that contribute to an increased risk for health concerns, such as substance abuse, smoking, depression, and suicide. Although violence is most often described in physical terms, its impacts extend far beyond the physical dangers, including long-standing psychological, emotional, and social effects on the child's health and well-being.

Although international humanitarian law provides for the protection of civilians in times of war, large humanitarian aid groups such as the International Committee of the Red Cross and United Nations organizations must have the permission of those in power to work in a country. IDPs are often victims of repressive governments. Because humanitarian aid is generally unavailable to them, they may be left without basic necessities to suffer and die because the ruling government persecutes the group in various ways, provides no assistance, and denies permission for outside aid. The ongoing situations and resulting genocide in Xiaxing, China (against the Uyghurs), Sudan (against the Darfuris), and Myanmar (against the Rohingya) are examples of such treatment of IDPs.

Nursing involvement with refugees and displaced persons can occur at levels of emergency needs, care and maintenance of health, and seeking ongoing solutions to the plight of refugees and to meeting their healthcare needs (Fig. 13.2). The ICN (2018b) suggests a number of action areas for nursing involvement with issues of displaced persons. These include raising public awareness and lobbying governments regarding the situation, identifying nursing and health needs of displaced persons and mobilizing resources to address these needs, assisting with emergency and resettlement programs, planning for provision and evaluation of health services for displaced persons, implementing educational programs for nursing personnel, and assisting nurse refugees. Recognizing that we live in a global community, principles of beneficence, justice, and respect for human dignity compel nurses to advocate for those who are suffering both close to home and globally.

BOX 13.6   Types of Violence Against Children

Most violence against children involves at least one of six main types of interpersonal violence that tend to occur at different stages in a child's development.

- Maltreatment (including violent punishment) involves physical; sexual and psychological/emotional violence; and neglect of infants, children, and adolescents by parents, caregivers, and other authority figures, most often in the home but also in settings such as schools and orphanages.
- Bullying (including cyberbullying) is unwanted aggressive behavior by another child or group of children who are neither siblings nor in a romantic relationship with the victim. It involves repeated physical, psychological, or social harm and often takes place in schools and other settings where children gather, as well as online.
- Youth violence is concentrated among children and young adults aged 10–29 years, occurs most often in community settings between acquaintances and strangers, includes bullying and physical assault with or without weapons (such as guns and knives), and may involve gang violence.

- Intimate partner violence (or domestic violence) involves physical, sexual, and emotional violence by an intimate partner or ex-partner. Although males can also be victims, intimate partner violence disproportionately affects females. It commonly occurs against girls within child marriages and early/forced marriages. Among romantically involved but unmarried adolescents, it is sometimes called "dating violence."
- Sexual violence includes nonconsensual completed or attempted sexual contact and acts of a sexual nature not involving contact (such as voyeurism or sexual harassment), acts of sexual trafficking committed against someone who is unable to consent or refuse, and online exploitation.
- Emotional or psychological violence includes restricting a child's movements, denigration, ridicule, threats and intimidation, discrimination, rejection, and other nonphysical forms of hostile treatment.

When directed against girls or boys because of their biological sex or gender identity, any of these types of violence can also constitute gender-based violence.

(From World Health Organization (WHO). (2022). *Fact sheet: Violence against children.* https://www.who.int/news-room/fact-sheets/detail/violence-against-children.)

ASK YOURSELF

Nursing Response to the Plight of Displaced Persons

Baroness Cox of Queensbury (Interview, 2003), former coeditor of the *International Journal of Nursing Studies*, is actively involved in international humanitarian work. She calls for nurses to address the ethical, legal, and professional implications of the plight of displaced persons worldwide by posing the following questions:

- If nursing is concerned for all humanity, why are we silent when vast numbers of people are left to suffer and die unaided?
- Should nursing not be raising the issue of denial of access to those suffering under repressive regimes?
- Where is the nursing profession's voice urging governments to press repressive regimes to allow humanitarian and human rights organizations access to groups in need in their countries?

- How can nurses use professional conferences, journals, and media to try to find professional, legal, and ethical solutions to these problems?
- If nurses, who have a professional mandate to advocate for those who are suffering, remain silent, who else will speak (p. 445)?

How would you respond to Baroness Cox? How would principles of beneficence, justice, and respect for human dignity guide your response?

How do her suggestions compare with the recommendations of the ICN and directives found in nursing codes of ethics?

What action steps are needed individually and as a profession to address these issues?

It should be self-evident that nursing care for refugees and immigrants, both locally and internationally, must be grounded in nursing's professional codes of ethics. Recognizing that people in these populations often experience stigma and discrimination within society at large and within healthcare settings, nurses "must recognize the potential impact of unconscious bias and practices contributing to discrimination, and actively seek opportunities to promote inclusion of all people in the provision of quality health care while eradicating disparities"

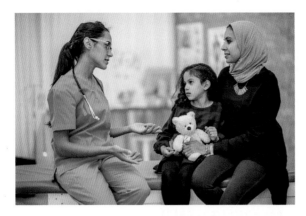

Fig. 13.2 Nurses Provide and Advocate for Just Care for All Patients. (©iStock.com/FatCamera.)

(ANA, 2018, p. 1). Similar directives are found in ethical codes and position statements of the CNA (2009, 2017a) and the ICN (2018b, 2021). This requires self-awareness regarding personal biases, as well as seeking ways to address discriminatory attitudes and practices toward immigrants within the work setting. One form of discrimination faced by immigrants is limited access to health care for a variety of reasons. Immigrants in the United States (even those with legal status) often do not have health insurance due to low-paying jobs and exclusion from or limited access to publicly funded health insurance programs (Parmet et al., 2017). Patients who cannot pay for health care generally do not seek timely evaluation and treatment for health concerns. This often leads to higher use of emergency departments (which are required to evaluate and treat all patients who arrive, including undocumented immigrants). Lack of interpretive services, a subtle form of discrimination, may also deter immigrants from seeking care in a timely manner. In addition to being unethical, there is a broader impact of discrimination on healthcare services. As Parmet and colleagues (2017) remind us, "discrimination against immigrants with respect to health undermines efficient and effective health policy … when we deny immigrants access to health insurance, we cause them to delay treatment, shifting costs to U.S. safety net providers" (p. 58). Parmet and colleagues note that most immigrants in the United States are either citizens or have legal status; only a small percentage (about 3.5 percent) are undocumented. Caring for patients who are undocumented immigrants may present ethical challenges for some nurses. Noting that caring for undocumented patients

is a daily concern for many clinicians and healthcare organizations, Sorrell (2017) calls on us to reflect on the ethics of advocacy for undocumented individuals who become our patients. What is our ethical responsibility to a patient who, for example, is an undocumented immigrant ready for discharge from the hospital for posttraumatic injuries and who needs rehabilitation or other services, yet has no family or financial resources for these services? She notes that principles of autonomy may be violated if a patient is discharged without giving consent. She also notes the potential conflict healthcare providers and institutions may face between ethical principles of doing good and avoiding harm for the patient and ensuring principles of justice related to how healthcare delivery is authorized and paid for. She calls on nurses and other healthcare providers to "advocate for the development and implementation of equitable and sustainable healthcare policies that can help to ensure just care for this vulnerable population." Ultimately, whatever a person's status as migrant or refugee, nurses are directed by professional codes of ethics to respect the intrinsic worth, dignity, and unique attributes of all persons, and advocate for the human rights of all individuals. Nursing's advocacy role is exemplified in the joint statement by the ANA and the American Academy of Nursing (ANA, 2019) calling on the US Congress "to take swift action to address the needs of migrant, refugee, and asylum-seeking children and families impacted by the Administration's separation policy at the border" (p. 1). This statement highlights the human rights issue related to the health impact of the separation on both children and parents. It calls particular attention to the effects of toxic stress created by the separation on immediate and long-term physical, mental, and emotional health, especially of the children.

Opinions about the presence, status, and rights of immigrants in the United States and elsewhere (both legal and undocumented) have engendered contentious political and social debate. Nurses are entitled to hold personal political views about social issues. However, regardless of personal and political beliefs, nurses, by virtue of their professional license, have an implicit right and duty to uphold ethical norms in providing care that respects the dignity, worth, rights, and unique aspects of each person (ANA, 2015, 2018; CNA, 2017a; ICN, 2018b, 2021).

When the incivility toward immigrant groups that have increased in recent years manifests in healthcare settings, it can jeopardize patient care. Nurses who witness such incivility and racism in comments and behavior may feel caught between the ethical obligation of advocating for their patients and fear related to possible repercussions from peers, supervisors, or others if they speak out (Fitzgerald et al., 2017). Incivility in the workplace, whether it is directed toward patients or other staff, creates an unhealthy environment that affects patient care and can contribute to moral distress and burnout. Fitzgerald and colleagues (2017) reflect that nurses who witness unjust and unethical acts and remain silent indirectly perpetuate and contribute to the injustice and become *guilty bystanders*. They remind us that nurses have an ethical duty to promote justice and safe patient care. A first step may be indicating disagreement with the incivility by addressing the comment or behavior directly. Nurses who feel uncomfortable in doing this can choose not to participate in harassing or derogatory comments by removing themselves from the situation. Noting that nurses are not responsible

for changing the prejudiced attitudes of others, these authors reiterate that the ethical duty to make appropriate persons aware of prejudicial and uncivil attitudes and behavior is similar to the duty to alert those in leadership to a substance-impaired nurse. The focus in both situations is the prevention of potential harm to patients and coworkers. Nurses need to be aware of how to access resources and follow protocols in this process. It is wise for nurses to engage in self-reflection and to seek support from others regarding ways of addressing the concern.

WAR AND VIOLENCE

We live in a troubled world, perhaps made more so by the ease of global travel and instant electronic communication. Conflict, violence in many forms, and war touch our lives in many ways, either directly if we live in an area experiencing the violence or indirectly through the media or the presence of family or friends in

---

CASE PRESENTATION

Discriminatory Attitudes and Immigrant Health Care

Sabrina works at a hospital that serves a multiracial and multiethnic population, many of whom are immigrants. She is caring for Mrs. H., a middle-age Middle Eastern woman who was just admitted with severe pneumonia. Several family members are in the room with her. A nursing colleague, Louella, comments to Sabrina, "this is another ignorant foreigner who let things go too long" and tells her "to be careful because there may be terrorists in the room." Louella also adds that they should all be arrested and sent back to where they came from. Sabrina feels offended by Louella's comment but hesitates to say anything because Louella is good friends with the charge nurse, and she is concerned about repercussions. When Sabrina talks to Mrs. H., she discovers that the family came as refugees from Syria several years prior. Mrs. H. has legal immigration status and has been working in a day care center. Because she has no health insurance, she tries to take care of health issues at home as best she can.

Think About It
The Impact of Ethnic Bias on Patient Care and Work Environments
- What ethical issues are evident in this situation?

- How do you feel about Louella's comments, especially in light of what you know about Mrs. H.'s background? Would you feel differently if she did not have legal immigration status?
- What would nursing codes of ethics and position statements on human rights, discrimination, and health of migrants say about Louella's comments? Give specific examples.
- How would you feel if you were Sabrina? What do you think about her decision to not respond to Louella? How do you think you would have responded if you were Sabrina?
- Would you consider Sabrina a "guilty bystander"? What else could Sabrina do to address the ethical issues in the situation?
- How do attitudes and comments like those of Louella affect patient care? How do they affect the work environment? How do they affect healthcare-seeking behavior of immigrants?
- What healthcare disparities are evident in this case situation? What impact do these disparities have on the overall public health?

violence-torn areas. We cannot escape the impact of war and violence on our lives, nor can we escape the need, as nurses, for an appropriate ethical response to these realities. Inherent in national and international codes of nursing is respect for the life and dignity of people and adherence to principles of beneficence, nonmaleficence, and justice. In the face of modern warfare and increasing acts of violence worldwide (including genocide, torture, and terrorism), we need to ask ourselves what the ethical stance of nursing needs to be.

As you are aware, the principle of beneficence directs nurses to do good and prevent or remove harm. This includes defending and protecting another's rights, seeking ways to keep people out of harm's way, and intervening to assist if the person is in danger. Nonmaleficence directs nurses to do no harm, which includes the directives not to inflict suffering or to kill another. Justice refers to fair and equitable treatment of individuals, regardless of their backgrounds. As discussed in Chapter 15, fair, equitable, and appropriate distribution of resources in society is termed *distributive justice*. Applying these ethical principles to issues of war and violence raises many ethical considerations which are discussed only briefly here. Students are urged to pursue further reflection and discussion about these critical global issues.

Applying the principles noted earlier impels nurses to understand the effects of war and violence to know what and where the needs are and how to intervene. One tragic effect of modern warfare is that civilian casualties, especially women and children, are frequently more extensive than those of the soldiers (ICN, 2012a). Even after a war is over, unexploded land mines and bombs left in the region continue to create casualties. The devastating effects of war and violence affect individuals and society and include physical, emotional, spiritual, and social components. Soldiers and civilians alike suffer physical injuries that require multiple surgeries and long-term rehabilitation and may result in their dealing with chronic pain. Personal, family, and societal resources are often stretched to provide even minimal care for these people who are casualties of war. Physical and emotional trauma sustained in war is compounded by poverty; destruction of societal infrastructure, such as roads, sanitation, and communication; spread of infectious diseases, sometimes in epidemic proportions; and strain on or destruction of resources necessary to meet basic healthcare needs. Traumas that have become common in armed conflict around the world, such as

rape, torture, and maiming, and the stress of displacement and having to rely on charity for basic needs contribute to the increase of both physical and mental health concerns such as hypertension and posttraumatic stress disorder. Fear, depression, insomnia, flashbacks, and nightmares are part of the often lifelong psychological fallout of war and violence. An example of this is a man who survived imprisonment in a concentration camp during the Nazi Holocaust and moved to a small town in the United States after World War II. He became a successful businessman and was well respected in the community. He owned a nice house in a friendly and safe neighborhood but rarely lived there because he felt insecure there. He lived instead (until his death at age 82) in a small apartment, with several locks on the door, above a store in the downtown area because of fear that someone would come for him in the night.

Environmental degradation resulting from war and armed conflict includes soil and water pollution; destruction of crops, trees, other vegetation, and animal habitats; and general ecological disturbances. This affects the ability of the land to support the needs of the people for even the basic requirements of food and water. A country's resources are strained and possibly depleted by warfare, limiting its ability to provide for the basic needs of its people. The lack of care and the physical and emotional traumas sustained during the war can cause the impact of war to affect a person's health throughout life. The cost of war includes not just the resources needed for the military action but also the impact on the lives and health of individuals and communities and the resources needed for cleaning up, rebuilding, and repairing the various levels of devastation caused by the war.

Nurses have an ethical responsibility to work to prevent war and conflict and the consequences of devastation that they cause. The response to war and violence must move beyond local and national considerations and embrace a global consciousness. This response requires taking leadership roles at the national and international levels "advocating the prevention of conflict, developing and teaching nonviolent ways to resolve conflict, being aware of international issues of professional concern, learning how to exercise the profession's political voice, and making politicians and governments aware of the devastation and misery caused by aggression and its drain on national and international economic, ecological, humanitarian, and emotional resources" (Tschudin &

Schmitz, 2003, p. 358). The nursing imperative to address social justice and health disparities that are consequences of war and violence is grounded in codes of nursing ethics (ANA, 2015, Provision 8,9; CNA, 2017a, Part II; ICN, 2021, Element 1.7, 1.8, 3.7).

Understanding that world peace is a prerequisite for developing, fostering, and maintaining health, the ICN (2012b) affirms the ethical responsibility of nurses to eliminate threats to life and health caused by weapons of war and conflict. The ICN calls on national nurses' associations to work toward the elimination of these weapons and land mines and to work to prevent the consequences of all types of weapons. Action steps that the ICN poses for nurses individually and collectively include educating the profession and the public about the social, economic, and environmental consequences of weapons that cause large-scale devastation; collaborating with human rights and health groups, disaster prevention agencies, the media, and other groups in lobbying manufacturers and governments against the production, distribution, and use of these weapons; developing strategies for taking action to reduce the threat of these weapons; and actively participating in disaster preparedness and response planning.

Along with working to prevent and avert war and armed conflict, nurses are called on to deal with issues related to the immediate experience of war and violence. This includes working to alleviate the suffering of and providing equitable care for injured persons on all sides of the conflict. It is important as well to ensure, to the best of our ability, that human rights and dignity are maintained for all in our care and to ensure that our practice is aligned with the ethical standards of the profession. In areas of armed conflict, nurses may be called on to care for civilian as well as military casualties, provide basic health care for displaced persons, and work with both private and governmental agencies in procuring and providing basic necessities for those in need. Considerations discussed in the previous section on disasters apply as well in situations of war and armed violence. In times of war, nurses and other healthcare professionals may be asked or directed to participate in the treatment of or practices related to patients or other persons that they consider ethically questionable. In such circumstances, the ethical stance for nurses is to provide care that is aligned with directives in nursing professional codes of ethics and to seek support and guidance from professional organizations and others as necessary. Professional codes mandate that nurses provide ethical and equitable care with respect for human dignity for all victims of war, including civilians, military, and even prisoners of war.

ASK YOURSELF

What Is My Personal Response to War and Armed Conflict?

Morally justify your responses to the following questions using ethical principles.
- Have I personally or professionally spoken out against the global devastation caused by war and armed conflict?
- How many people must be injured, killed, or displaced and where must the violence occur for me to find my voice and take action?
- Are war and its multilevel costs ever justified?
- Who is most affected by war and armed conflict and its aftermath?
- Who should pay for the cost of war?

(Adapted from Silva and Ludwick (2003).)

HEALTHCARE ACCESS AND FINANCING

Addressing global health issues at their source requires an awareness of the interconnectedness of the whole Earth community. The challenge to provide health care for people worldwide requires increasing effort, creativity, and global consciousness. Many variables play a part in this challenge, not the least of which is the health of the Earth itself. In addition to issues discussed previously, other critical factors include economics, culture, politics, national crises, and global travel. The problems are further compounded by limited appreciation of what it means to live in a global community, national versus private health insurance, methods of health promotion contrasted with curative methods of treating illness, tenuous relationships between conventional medicine and traditional healing systems, and ignoring the health of the environment in healthcare policies and practices. These factors all affect the functioning of health systems and the care they provide around the world (Ausubel, 2012; Berry, 2009; Holtz, 2017; Myers & Frumkin, 2020).

The fundamental principles and model on which the healthcare delivery system is based and the way it is financed define the parameters within which nurses and other healthcare personnel function. Issues of healthcare delivery and the effectiveness of the healthcare delivery system are concerns worldwide. In the United States and most of the Western world, delivery of health care is much like a runaway train of high technology with its proliferation of markets for new medications and expensive treatments. Further, this system is challenged to provide for an ever-increasing global population with decreasing resources, both natural and monetary. Basic to this global concern is the state of the health of the planet itself and the ever-increasing cost of health care and the issue of its sustainability. Developed and developing countries recognize that the current and future healthcare systems in the Western model have at their foundation expensive technologies and medication, many of which have to be imported from other regions of the globe. Traditional healing systems that have supported the health and healing of many people around the globe for centuries are often discounted.

Healthcare systems must address global changes and challenges if they are to survive in the 21st century. Important questions arise about how best to meet the healthcare needs of people worldwide.

ASK YOURSELF

What Is Nursing's Role in Addressing the Health Needs of People Worldwide?

Reflect on the following questions and consider the appropriate nursing role and response in addressing the issues implicit in the questions.

- Can countries address the needs of their people without relying on expensive medications and treatments?
- Can local existing systems of health care be utilized to provide basic health services to rural and urban poor communities?
- In both developing and developed countries, can traditional methods and systems of health care be utilized to promote health and prevent disease, working collaboratively with the conventional system?
- Has modern Western healthcare practice been lax in preserving and utilizing traditional healing methods along with Western medical interventions, and at what cost?
- What ethical principles need to be considered when addressing issues of cost limits, access, rationing, justice, need and medical necessity, and quality of care?
- How can nurses take on a leadership role in addressing the issues implicit in these questions? Give examples from codes of nursing ethics that guide nursing role and response.

GLOBAL NEEDS AND FINITE RESOURCES

Healthcare resources are limited worldwide. Making choices regarding who receives these resources is difficult at all levels of care and these decisions can have far reaching consequences. Although ethical principles direct us to distribute healthcare resources justly and equitably, there are powerful local and global social, political, and economic forces that create disparities in the availability of and access to health care worldwide (Holtz, 2017). The political controversy over making the COVID-19 vaccines available in an equitable way to people in developing countries is an example of disparities that can affect individuals, local communities, and the global community. Lack of access to the vaccine left huge populations unprotected leading to the development of new variants and further endangering the global population.

In developing countries, access to Western-model health care may be very limited for much of the population because of limited governmental resources for health care, insufficient healthcare workers, distance from facilities, and limited ability to pay. Basic healthcare services that we take for granted in the West, such as immunizations, antibiotics and other medications, and common surgical and other treatments, are unavailable or too expensive. Healthcare needs may be addressed by traditional healing practices, local outreach workers who do their best with limited resources, periodic visits from healthcare teams from the government or abroad, or not at all. As noted earlier, difficulty accessing health care is often compounded by political unrest; economic instability; impact of Earth changes; and social, cultural, and other factors that contribute to a large gap between the rich and the poor. Ultimately, a large portion of the global population suffers from poor health.

Access to health care in industrialized nations is addressed at least in part through various forms of private or public health insurance. Most industrialized nations (with the United States and South Africa as notable exceptions) have some form of universal health coverage that covers basic healthcare needs. However, all of these programs are not equal, and most function less smoothly than one would hope. These systems vary with regard to the amount of government and private involvement in healthcare delivery and contributions for health insurance. Some countries have a combination of several methods. Germany, France, and Japan, for example, mandate benefits coverage, the cost of which is shared by employers, employees, and government tax revenues. These healthcare delivery systems share three traits with the system in the United States: medical care is offered through private physicians and through private and public hospitals, patients may choose their providers, and most people in these countries have health insurance coverage through their place of employment. Health insurance is offered to the citizens of these countries through multiple third-party insurance agencies. Similar problems to those in the United States exist, such as high costs and increased spending on technology. However, every citizen has some type of healthcare coverage. In an attempt to hold down rising healthcare spending, all have instituted direct controls on the price of health care. Canada and Great Britain have developed national healthcare systems that provide health care for their citizens. The government-run plans provide cradle-to-grave services that are financed through taxes. These plans enable patients to receive healthcare services and to choose their own hospitals and physicians. The British plan employs physicians and operates its own hospitals. In the Canadian healthcare system, plans are developed by each province based on federal guidelines. It is funded by a single-payer system through both federal and provincial taxes. No system is perfect, and there are both champions and critics of the various approaches to financing health care worldwide. The important thing is that nurses recognize the role that economics plays in access to health care around the world (Box 13.7).

In the United States, the burden of dealing with issues of healthcare access, limited resources, justice, rationing, and quality involves many players, including insurance companies, governmental agencies, managed care organizations, individual clinicians, and patients. A workgroup convened by the American College of Physicians and the Harvard Pilgrim Health Care Ethics

Program developed a statement of ethics of managed care (Povar et al., 2004). The interdisciplinary group consisted of patients, nurses, physicians, social workers, medical ethicists, and managed care representatives. The four principles set forth in this statement are still pertinent and are summarized as follows:

1. Relationships are critical in the delivery of health services. They should be characterized by respect, truthfulness, consistency, fairness, and compassion. This implies truthfulness and openness among patients, clinicians, and health plan purchasers; maintaining accurate and honest records; supporting the importance, intimacy, and ethical obligations of the patient–clinician relationship; and honesty on the part of patients regarding their health conditions and needs.

2. Health plan purchasers, clinicians, and the public share responsibility for the appropriate stewardship for healthcare resources. This implies including all parties in public dialog to shape policies on access to and quality of care and on resource allocation decisions, recognizing that a clinician's duty is to promote the good of patients, practice effective and efficient care, use resources responsibly, and advocate as vigorously for vulnerable and disadvantaged patients as for any other patient. Included in this principle is the understanding that all involved parties (patients, clinicians, and insurers) are in discussion about what healthcare needs can reasonably be met with available resources, that all parties understand and honor the rules and coverage of their contracts, and that all commit to effective, quality health care with consistency and fairness.

3. All parties should foster an ethical environment for the delivery of effective and efficient quality health care. Implicit in this principle is the understanding that agreements between clinicians, health plans, and healthcare organizations are congruent with professional ethical standards and that all parties share the ethical obligation to protect the confidentiality of patient health information.

4. Patients should be well informed about care and treatment options and all financial and benefit issues that affect the provision of care. This implies that patients receive sufficient and appropriate information to support informed consent for or refusal of treatment, that clinicians disclose any potential conflict of interest to patients, and that purchasers and health plans inform patients of any arrangements that may influence care.

BOX 13.7   Information About National Healthcare Systems Worldwide

Students are encouraged to visit this website to compare and contrast what is offered by healthcare systems in various countries. Click on the country and then click on *healthcare system*.

http://www.allianzworldwidecare.com/national-health care-systems.

These principles do not solve the socioeconomic and political problems contributing to the rising cost and limited resources faced by the healthcare system. Although nurses need to work to address these issues individually and as a profession, they must continue to deal with the ethical and moral dilemmas associated with these difficult issues in the changing healthcare environment. The purpose of these principles is to provide some guidance for ethical practice in a healthcare system where resources do not always meet the need, regardless of the setting.

ASK YOURSELF

Access to Health Care: Rights and Responsibilities

Much of the discussion regarding the healthcare delivery systems of countries around the world is a commentary on access to what is termed *modern medical care*.

- How does access to health care affect an individual's participation in the healthcare system?
- What is our individual responsibility in the big picture of these vast healthcare systems?
- Do you consider health care a basic right? If it is a right, what are our individual responsibilities in ensuring this right for all citizens?
- What ethical issues arise when access to care is limited for some people and available to others? What directives to codes of nursing ethics give regarding nursing's role in addressing health disparities?

TRADITIONAL SYSTEMS OF HEALING AND HEALTH CARE

Many cultures throughout the world have traditional forms of health care that view humanity as connected to the wider dimensions of the Earth and nature. In developing countries, these traditional healing systems provide comprehensive approaches to the prevention of illness and promotion of health that are grounded in models different from Western medical care. The WHO refers to these systems as holistic—that is, viewing a person in totality within a vast ecological spectrum and emphasizing the notion that illness or disease occurs as a result of an imbalance between the person and his or her ecological systems (WHO, 2013, 2019).

An important component of traditional systems of health care is their basis in models that consider mental, spiritual, physical, and ecological factors in assessing health and well-being. A basic concept of all traditional healthcare systems is that of balance between mind and body; function and need; and individual, community, and environment. Illness or disease is thought to be a breakdown in the balance in one or more of these areas. Treatments are designed to restore health and balance between the individual and his or her internal and external environments. Although these models of traditional healthcare systems have been considered primitive and unsophisticated by modern practitioners, increasing numbers of developing countries are showing a new interest in program development toward revitalizing these traditional systems. Recognizing the value and importance of traditional systems, the WHO (2013, 2019) encourages nations to develop policies that build the knowledge base for these systems; strengthen the quality assurance, safety, and effectiveness of the systems; and incorporate these systems into healthcare coverage and delivery services, including self-health care. Commitment to holistic care of patients positions nurses to take leadership roles in promoting the policies put forth by the WHO to ensure that traditional healing systems that support the health of populations around the world remain available. Respect for various healing traditions and healers is a component of culturally congruent nursing care.

ASK YOURSELF

What Do You Know About Traditional Healing?

Traditional methods of healing and health care have kept populations healthy and functioning for thousands of years. Many countries are trying to reinstate these practices to promote health and reduce the cost of healthcare and healthcare delivery.

- How do you think traditional and modern healing systems should relate to each other?
- What traditional methods of health care are available in your community or nearby area?
- With what traditional healing practices are you familiar? Have you or persons you know utilized these practices?
- What guidance to codes of nursing ethics give regarding nursing's response to traditional healing and healers?

CHALLENGES FOR RURAL AND URBAN AGGREGATES

Problems in the delivery of health care to populations around the world occur not only because of expensive technology or lack of money to pay for insurance but also because of geographic barriers. Rural populations in the United States and globally often have to do without services because of a lack of healthcare providers and facilities within a reasonable distance from their homes. Healthcare for persons in these populations may require time off of work for travel and waiting in crowded waiting rooms. Many rural areas lack healthcare personnel, and emergency care is often nonexistent. In one mid-Atlantic state in the United States, all counties boast of access to a 911 emergency number, but for some, the switchboard and emergency medical technician vehicle are three counties away, and travel is over narrow mountain roads. Patients often delay treatment or do not become involved with prevention or health education plans because they require so much effort to accomplish. In addition, many rural citizens tend to be older persons for whom travel and finances are a great consideration in healthcare services.

The urban poor face similar access problems, not because care is geographically distant, but because access requires trips to places they cannot afford or free clinics, where lines are long and workers are few. Individuals are often required to take time from work, like their rural counterparts, to see a provider. Medications for both urban and rural poor may be unaffordable. Large immigrant populations often live in overcrowded situations in the urban setting. In addition to financial constraints, there may be language and cultural barriers and lack of knowledge about how to access the system.

SUMMARY

Global consciousness is needed to address 21st-century healthcare needs and issues. Nurses must be aware of and prepared to address the global concerns that have a significant impact on the health and well-being of people and the planet. Nursing care and response to these concerns need to be grounded in codes of nursing ethics. Nurses need to apply principles of beneficence, nonmaleficence, and justice to their relationship with Earth, as well as to humans. Recognizing that human health depends on the health of Earth, nurses must engage in

and promote environmentally responsible health care locally and internationally. Examples of issues that need to be addressed include natural and other disasters, displaced persons, migrants, famine and malnutrition, violence against children, human trafficking, use of torture, war and violence, genocide, unexploded bombs and land mines, pollution, global warming, epidemics and drug-resistant organisms, bioterrorism, and access to and financing of health care. Although some countries ensure access to basic healthcare services for their citizens, many individuals throughout the world have limited or no access to basic health care. There is a renewed interest in traditional healing systems of various cultures to provide needed healthcare services. Nursing professional codes of ethics direct nurses to work individually and collectively to address the impact of these issues on local, national, and global health.

CHAPTER HIGHLIGHTS

- Earth health and human health are intricately interconnected, and nurses need to include ethical considerations of our relationship with Earth into nursing practice.
- Twenty-first-century healthcare needs and issues require global consciousness.
- Emergency and continuous health care are essential parts of any disaster response. Disasters, from the health professional's view, are situations in which there is an often sudden, unforeseen imbalance between the needs of people whose health and well-being are threatened and the resources and capacity of the healthcare system to meet these needs. Disasters require prompt action, yet responders must often deal with inadequate supplies and resources, as well as the need to get to victims who are in places that may present health risks, be dangerous, or be difficult to reach. Nurses play an important role in providing emergency care and in meeting the ongoing humanitarian needs of people affected by disaster.
- The number of displaced persons worldwide has created a humanitarian crisis of immense proportions. Displaced persons, migrants, and refugees are highly vulnerable populations. They often have serious health and social problems related to deprivation (including basic human rights), detention, physical hardship, stress, poor nutrition, sexual violence, social exclusion, and generally poor health

status. The impact of displacement and violence on children is a particular concern worldwide. Nursing involvement with refugees and displaced persons can occur at levels of emergency needs, care and maintenance of health, and seeking ongoing solutions to the plight of refugees and to meeting their health care. Difficult decisions emerge with issues of access, cost, and justice.

- Nurses have an ethical responsibility to work to prevent war and conflict and the consequences of devastation that they cause. The response to war and violence must move beyond local and national considerations and embrace a global consciousness. This response requires taking leadership roles at the national and international levels.

- Addressing global health issues at their source requires an awareness of the interconnectedness of the whole Earth community. The challenge to provide health care for people worldwide requires increasing effort, creativity, and global consciousness. Some nations provide basic healthcare services for their citizens, whereas people in many areas suffer from limited access to or availability of such services. Problems of access to and payment for healthcare services are of special concern among rural populations and the urban poor. People in both developing and industrialized countries are exploring ways to incorporate traditional healing practices into the broader healthcare systems in an effort to utilize the benefits of both systems in meeting the healthcare needs of society.

- Nurses are guided by professional codes of nursing ethics to work individually and collectively both to meet the needs of those affected by global issues such as war, violence, disaster, famine, epidemics, and displaced persons and to prevent the devastation these issues cause.

DISCUSSION QUESTIONS AND ACTIVITIES

1. Read the Earth Charter at https://earthcharter.org/ and compare the principles it sets forth with those found in nursing codes and position statements, such as those found at:
   https://www.nursingworld.org/practice-policy/nursing-excellence/ethics/
   https://www.nursingworld.org/practice-policy/nursing-excellence/official-position-statements/

   https://www.cna-aiic.ca/en/nursing/regulated-nursing-in-canada/nursing-ethics
   https://www.cna-aiic.ca/en/policy-advocacy/policy-support-tools/position-statements
   https://www.icn.ch/system/files/2021-10/ICN_Code-of-Ethics_EN_Web_0.pdf
   https://www.icn.ch/nursing-policy/position-statements
   How can the Earth Charter help us integrate Earth ethics into nursing practice?

2. Explore the websites listed in Box 13.5. Compare and contrast information and policies related to climate change and disaster preparedness and advocacy. Discuss with classmates.

3. Investigate disaster preparedness plans and policies in your town or city and healthcare agency.

4. Work with classmates to create a mock disaster scenario in which you must provide care to large numbers of disaster victims with limited resources. Discuss ethical issues related to decisions that are made for the various patients who need both urgent and ongoing care.

5. Explore the humanitarian and health impact of the global refugee crisis. Discuss with classmates your personal reaction and how you feel nursing should respond to this global concern. These websites are a place to start:
   https://www.unrefugees.org/refugee-facts/what-is-a-refugee/
   https://www.unrefugees.org/refugee-facts/statistics/
   https://www.unicef.org/reports/uprooted-growing-crisis-refugee-and-migrant-children
   https://www.who.int/news-room/fact-sheets/detail/violence-against-children

6. Discuss with classmates how the nursing codes of ethics and pertinent position statements guide nursing care of and response to immigrants and refugees.

7. Discuss global issues related to healthcare delivery. Which of these issues would have the greatest impact on your nursing practice and why? Share with classmates how these issues might affect your nursing practice.

8. Describe the impact of healthcare access and financing on patient care and health outcomes. Identify potential ethical dilemmas related to current systems of delivery or financing. Have you known people who delayed seeking health care because of financial or other access issues? Discuss with classmates.

9. Explore the WHO's Traditional Medicine Strategy 2014-2023 at https://www.who.int/publications/i/item/9789241506096 and WHO *Global report on traditional and complementary medicine 2019* at https://apps.who.int/iris/handle/10665/312342. License: CC BY-NC-SA 3.0 IGO. What do you think about the WHO's recommendations regarding incorporating traditional healing systems into healthcare coverage and delivery services?

REFERENCES

Alliance of Nurses for Healthy Environments (AHNE). (2023). *Climate change, health, and nursing.* https://envirn.org/climate-change-health-and-nursing/.

American Nurses Association (ANA). (2008). *American Nurses Association 2008 House of Delegates Resolution: Global climate change.* https://www.nursingworld.org/~4afb0e/globalassets/practiceandpolicy/work-environment/health--safety/global-climate-change-final.pdf.

ANA. (2015). *Code of ethics for nurses with interpretive statements.* http://nursingworld.org/DocumentVault/Ethics-1/Code-of-Ethics-for-Nurses.html.

ANA. (2017). *Who will be there? Ethics, the law, and a nurse's duty to respond in disaster (Issue brief).* https://www.nursingworld.org/~4ad845/globalassets/docs/ana/who-will-be-there_disaster-preparedness_2017.pdf.

ANA. (2018). *The nurse's role in addressing discrimination: Protecting and promoting inclusive strategies in practice settings, policy, and advocacy. (Position statement).* https://www.nursingworld.org/~4ab207/globalassets/practice-andpolicy/nursing-excellence/ana-position-statements/social-causes-and-health-care/the-nurses-role-in-addressing-discrimination.pdf.

American Nurses Association. (2019). *ANA and AAN joint statement on family separation policy (Position statement).* https://www.nursingworld.org/practice-policy/nursing-excellence/official-position-statements/id/family-separation-policy/.

ANA.(2022). *News release: ANA acts on climate change and key nursing issues.* https://www.nursingworld.org/news/news-releases/2022-news-releases/ana-acts-on-climate-change-and-other-key-health-care-issues/.

Anderko, L., & Chalupka, S. (2023). Climate change. In, R. McDermott-Levy, K. P.Jackman-Murphy, J. Leffler, & A. G. Cantu (Eds.), Environmental health in nursing (3rd ed.) (pp. 265-284). Alliance of Nurses for Healthy Environments. https://www.enviRN.org.

Ausubel, K. (Ed.), (2004). *Ecological medicine: Healing the earth, healing ourselves.* San Francisco, CA: Sierra Club Books.

Ausubel, K. (2012). *Dreaming the future: Reimagining civilization in the age of nature.* White River Junction, VT: Chelsea Green Publishing.

Berry, T. (2009). *The sacred universe: Earth, spirituality, and religion in the 21st century. Mary Evelyn Tucker.* New York: Columbia University Press.

CNA. (2009). *Global health and equity: position statement.* https://hl-prod-ca-oc-download.s3-ca-central-1.amazonaws.com/CNA/2f975e7e-4a40-45ca-863c-5ebf0a138d5e/UploadedImages/documents/PS106_Global_Health_Equity_Aug_2009_e.pdf.

CNA. (2017a). *Code of ethics for registered nurses.* https://cdn1.nscn.ca/sites/default/files/documents/resources/code-of-ethics-for-registered-nurses.pdf#:~:text=The%20Canadian%20Nurses%20Association%20%28CNA%29%20Code%20of%20Ethics,receiving%20care.%20The%20Codeis%20both%20aspirational%20and%20regulatory.

Canadian Nurses Association (CNA). (2017b). *Climate change and health: Position statement.* Retrieved from https://hl-prod-ca-oc-download.s3-ca-central-1.amazonaws.com/CNA/2f975e7e-4a40-45ca-863c-5ebf0a138d5e/UploadedImages/documents/Climate_change_and_health_position_statement.pdf.

Chaudry, R. V. (2008). The precautionary principle, public health, and public health nursing. *Public Health Nursing, 25*(3), 261–268.

Crinnion, W. J. (2010). The CDC Fourth National Report of Human Exposure to Environmental Chemicals: What it tells us about our toxic burden and how it assists environmental medicine physicians. *Alternative Medicine Review, 15*(2), 101–108.

Fitzgerald, E. M., Myers, J. G., & Clark, P. (2017). Nurses need not be guilty bystanders: Caring for vulnerable immigrant populations. *The Online Journal of Issues in Nursing, 22*(1), 8.

Foster, A., Cole, J., Petrikova, I., Farlow, A., & Frumkin, H. (2020). Planetary health ethics In S. Myers & H. Frumkin (Eds.), *Planetary health: Protecting nature to protect ourselves* (pp. 453–473). Island Press.

Hicks, J. L., Hanfing, D., Wynia, M. K., & Toner, E. (2021). *Discussion paper: Crisis standards of care and COVID-19: What did we learn? How do we ensure equity? What should we do?* National Academy of Medicine. https://www.ncbi.nlm.nih.gov/pmc/articles/PMC8486425/pdf/nampsp-2021-202108e.pdf.

Holtz, C. (2017). *Global health care: Issues and policies* (3rd ed.). Burlington, MA: Jones & Bartlett Learning.

Institute of Medicine (IOM). (2009). *Guidance for establishing crisis: Standards of care for use in disaster situations: A letter report.* National Academies Press. https://www.ncbi.nlm.nih.gov/books/NBK219958/.

Institute of Medicine (IOM). (2012). *Crisis standards of care: A systems framework for catastrophic disaster response.* National Academies Press.

ICN. (2021). *The ICN code of ethics for nurses.* https://www.icn.ch/system/files/2021-10/ICN_Code-of-Ethics_EN_Web_0.pdf.

ICN. (2012a). *Armed conflict: Nursing's perspective (Position paper).* https://www.icn.ch/sites/default/files/inline-files/E01_Armed_Conflict.pdf.

ICN. (2012b). *Towards elimination of weapons of war and conflict (Position statement).* https://www.icn.ch/sites/default/files/inline-files/E14_Elimination_Weapons_War_Conflict.pdf.

ICN. (2018a). *Nurses, climate change, and health (Position paper).* https://www.icn.ch/sites/default/files/inline-files/PS_E_Nurses_climate%20change_health_0.pdf.

ICN. (2018b). *Health of migrants, refugees and displaced persons (Position paper).* https://www.icn.ch/sites/default/files/inline-files/PS_A_Health_migrants_refugees_displaced%20persons.pdf.

ICN. (2019). *Position statement: Nurses and disaster risk reduction, response and recovery.* https://www.icn.ch/sites/default/files/inline-files/PS_E_Nurses_and_disaster_risk_reduction_response_and_recovery.pdf.

Interview. (2003). Baroness Cox of Queensbury. *Nursing Ethics, 10*(4), 441–445.

Leider, J. P., DeBruin, D., Reynolds, N., Koch, A., & Seaberg, J. (2017). Ethical guidance for disaster response, specifically around crisis standards of care: A systematic review. *American Journal of Public Health: Law & Ethics, 107*(9), e1–e9.

Li, A. M. L. (2017). Ecological determinants of health: Food and environment on human health. *Environmental Science and Pollution Research, 24,* 9002–9015. https://doi.org/10.1007/s11356-015-5707-9.

Luck, S. (2022). Environmental health In M. A. Blaszko Helming, D. A. Shields, K. M. Avino, & W. E. Rosa (Eds.), *Dossey & Keegan's holistic nursing: A handbook for practice* (8th ed., pp. 427–442). Jones & Bartlett Learning.

McDermott-Levy, R., Jackman-Murphy, K. P., Leffers, J., & Cantu, A. G. (Eds.), (2023). Environmental Health in Nursing (3rd ed). *Alliance of Nurses for Healthy Environments.* https://www.enviRN.org.

Myers, N. J., & Raffensperger, C. (2006). *Precautionary tools for reshaping environmental policy.* MIT Press.

Myers, S., & Frumkin, H. (2020). *Planetary health: Protecting nature to protect ourselves.* Island Press.

Nelson, M. (2004). Stopping the war on Mother Earth In K. Ausubel (Ed.), *Ecological medicine: Healing the Earth, healing ourselves* (pp. 228–230). San Francisco, CA: Sierra Club Books.

Parmet, W. E., Sainsbury-Wong, L., & Prabhu, M. (2017). Immigration and health: Law, policy, and ethics. *The Journal of Law, Medicine & Ethics, 45*(1), 55–59.

Pinto-Bazurco, J. F. (2020). *The precautionary principle.* International Institute for Sustainable Development (IISD). https://www.iisd.org/articles/deep-dive/precautionary-principle.

Povar, G. J., Blumen, H., Daniel, J., Daub, S., Evans, L., Holm, R. P., & Campbell, J. D. (2004). Ethics in practice: Managed care and the changing health care environment. *Annals of Internal Medicine, 141*(2), 131–137.

Raffensperger, C. (2004). The precautionary principle In K. Ausubel (Ed.), *Ecological medicine: Healing the earth, healing ourselves* (pp. 41–52). Sierra Club Books.

Rockström, J., & Gaffney, O. (2021). *Breaking boundaries: The science of our planet.* DK – Penguin Random House.

Rossati, A. (2017). Global warming and its health impact. *International Journal of Occupational and Environmental Medicine, 8,* 7–20.

Silva, M. C., & Ludwick, R. (2003). Ethics and terrorism: September 11, 2001 and its aftermath. *Online Journal of Issues in Nursing, 8*(1) https://ojin.nursingworld.org/table-of-contents/volume-8-2003/number-1-january-2003/ethics-and-terrorism/.

Sloand, E., Ho, G., Klimmek, R., Pho, A., & Kub, J. (2012). Nursing children after a disaster: A qualitative study of nurse volunteers and children after the Haiti earthquake. *Journal for Specialists in Pediatric Nursing, 17,* 242–253.

Sorrell, J. M. (2017). Ethics of advocacy for undocumented patients. *The Online Journal of Issues in Nursing., 22*(3)

Swimme, B., & Tucker, M. E. (2011). *Journey of the universe.* New Haven, CT: Yale University Press.

Tafoya, T. (1996, May). Embracing the shadow: Mending the sacred hoop. In: *Paper presented at the South Texas AIDS Training (STAT) for mental health providers: The human, transcultural, and spiritual dimensions of HIV/AIDS.* San Antonio, TX.

Tschudin, V., & Schmitz, C. (2003). The impact of conflict and war on international nursing and ethics. *Nursing Ethics, 10*(4), 354–366.

Uhl, C. (2004). *Developing ecological consciousness: Path to a sustainable world.* Lanham, MD: Rowman & Littlefield.

United Nations Children's Fund (UNICEF). (2016). *Uprooted: The growing crisis for refugee and migrant children.* https://www.unicef.org/media/50011/file/%20Uprooted_growing_crisis_for_refugee_and_migrant_children.pdf.

United Nations Children's Fund (UNICEF). (2023). *Child displacement.* https://data.unicef.org/topic/child-migration-and-displacement/displacement/.

USA for UNHCR. (2023a). *What is a refugee?* https://www.unrefugees.org/refugee-facts/what-is-a-refugee/.

USA for UNHCR. (2023b). *Refugee statistics.* https://www.unrefugees.org/refugee-facts/statistics/.

World Health Organization (WHO). (2013). *WHO's traditional medicine strategy 2014-2023.* https://www.who.int/publications/i/item/9789241506096.

World Health Organization (WHO). (2018a). *Fact sheet: Climate change and health.* Available fromhttps://www.who.int/news-room/fact-sheets/detail/climate-change-and-health.

World Health Organization (WHO). (2019). *WHO global report on traditional and complementary medicine 2019.* https://apps.who.int/iris/handle/10665/312342 License: CC BY-NC-SA 3.0 IGO.

World Health Organization (WHO). (2022). *Fact sheet: Violence against children.* https://www.who.int/news-room/fact-sheets/detail/violence-against-children.

World Medical Association. (2017). *WMA statement on medical ethics in the event of disasters.* https://www.wma.net/policies-post/wma-statement-on-medical-ethics-in-the-event-of-disasters/.

Zalon, M. L. (2019). Preparing older citizens for global climate change: Collaborate and advocate to meet patient needs and implement policy change. *American Nurse Today, 14*(2), 5–9.

14

Nursing Ethics and Health Policy Issues

Every community is established for the sake of some good (for everyone performs every action for the sake of what he takes to be good).

(Aristotle, 350 B.C.E./1998)

OBJECTIVES

After completing this chapter, the reader should be able to:

1. Describe the various processes by which health policies are established.
2. Distinguish between the terms *political* and *partisan*.
3. Give examples of specific political issues related to health care.
4. Describe the health policy process.
5. Discuss the role of ethics in policymaking.
6. Discuss how personal values affect one's perspective on contemporary political issues.
7. Explain the role of nurses in the policymaking process.
8. Describe various methods of influencing public policy.

INTRODUCTION

As you read the past few chapters, you learned that nursing ethics extends broadly—far beyond the person-to-person, nurse–patient realms. Because nurses are the largest group of healthcare workers and because they have intimate knowledge about healthcare delivery, they have a responsibility to be involved in promoting the health of individuals, communities, and the global population. Codes of nursing ethics call on nurses to be involved in a number of specific issues within and outside the workplace including the following: patients' right to privacy, workplace safety, professional competency, human rights, health disparities, resource allocation, disasters, pandemics, and the natural environment (ANA, 2015; CNA, 2017; ICN, 2021). To solve problems surrounding these issues, professional codes of nursing ethics compel nurses to become involved in health policy at the institutional and civic levels. The American Nurses Association (ANA) challenges nurses to participate in nursing health policy development as advocates or as elected or appointed representatives through local, regional, state, national, or global initiatives (ANA, 2015). Laws and policies that address the interests of the health of individuals and the legal practice of licensed nurses all require the involvement of nurses. Therefore, it is incumbent upon nurses to become knowledgeable and active in the health policy arena.

Nurses involved in policy development must be informed by personal values, ethical principles, and codes of professional nursing ethics. Nurses must critically examine the source of their own values, especially as they become involved in emotionally laden political issues. They must clearly understand the principles of ethics. For example, the principle of justice should guide policies that establish how goods and services are distributed, such as those that regulate Medicare and Medicaid policies; and the principle of beneficence should guide policies regarding licensure of professionals. Nurses must also look to the professional codes of nursing ethics for guidance. Nurses in the United States should rely specifically on the ANA *Code of Ethics for Nurses with*

Interpretive Statements (2015) and be familiar with the *ICN Code of Ethics for Nurses* (2021). Nurses in Canada should rely on the *Code of Ethics for Registered Nurses* (2017).

In the current divisive political climate, some people view health policy as a political process, strongly influenced by ideology and party politics. Others view the health policymaking process as a thoughtful one, by which decisions are made based on data and the rational analysis of needs, outcomes, and costs. In reality, the health policy process is a combination of both informed rational judgments and ideological partisan politics. The process requires nurses with self-awareness, scientific knowledge, motivation, and communication skills to tackle health policy issues. This chapter features examples of selected political issues that relate to health policy, describes the health policy process, and outlines specific methods that nurses can employ to influence policy.

POLITICAL ISSUES

The term *political* relates to the complex process of policymaking within the government. Government is an essential element of society, and politics is inherent in government. Political policies are those that are created, affected, or regulated by decisions within either the executive, judicial, or legislative branches of government. Any issue can become political, depending on the existence of legitimate need or the interest or whims of society at large, special-interest groups, individuals, or government. Political parties are organized groups with distinct ideologies that seek to control government. When political parties take opposing positions on an issue, the different opinions and subsequent decisions are said to be **partisan**. For example, during the COVID-19 worldwide pandemic, liberals were much more likely to favor policies that required social distancing, immunizations, and the use of masks in public; whereas conservatives were more likely to favor personal freedom to choose which recommendations to follow. Though individuals may genuinely and independently agree with the position of a particular political party because it is congruent with their core values, partisanship is often seen in a negative light—that is, consisting of blind, prejudiced, and unreasoning allegiance to the ideals of one political party. When one political party takes over the executive or legislative branch of government, partisan issues

become hotly debated and laws are passed. The executive branch sets priorities and may propose, sign, or veto legislation. Laws that are passed in the legislative branch of government become the regulatory responsibility of administrative government agencies. Constitutional challenges to laws are referred to the judicial branch, so that any given law may eventually involve all branches of government. Fig. 14.1 depicts the three branches of the US government.

The **executive branch of government** in the United States is led by the president at the national level and governors at the state level. The executive branch has many functions, some of which impact health policy. Activities of this branch of government that are most likely to influence health policy include the following: setting healthcare priorities based on ideals of the political party of the president or governor; proposing healthcare bills to legislative bodies; writing executive orders; and appointing people to leadership positions such as Secretary of the Department of Health and Human and Human Services. At the national level, the president submits nominations to fill openings on the Supreme Court. These functions of the executive branch can have enormous influence on the health of people. Following are some recent examples of executive actions that have impacted health: President Obama proposed the legislation that resulted in the *Affordable Care Act*; President Trump nominated three justices to the Supreme Court; state governors' signed executive orders during the peak of the COVID-19 pandemic; and President Biden set a priority to reduce the cost of prescription drugs (The Council of State Governments, 2022; The White House, 2022, n.d.; United States Senate, n.d.). So, the executive branch of government can have a tremendous impact on the health care of citizens.

The **judicial branch of government** influences healthcare professions and healthcare delivery through the common law system. The Supreme Court selects certain cases to hear on appeal and can either affirm or overturn lower courts' decisions. It also has the power to declare an action of the executive or legislative branch in breach of the US Constitution. The Supreme Court is the ultimate arbiter, and all decisions are final—unless the same issue, via another case, returns to the Court. As noted in Chapter 8, judicial precedents take on the force of the law. Consider, for example, the profound effects on the American healthcare system of the landmark Supreme Court decision in *Roe v. Wade* (1973) and the 2022 Supreme Court turnaround in the 2022

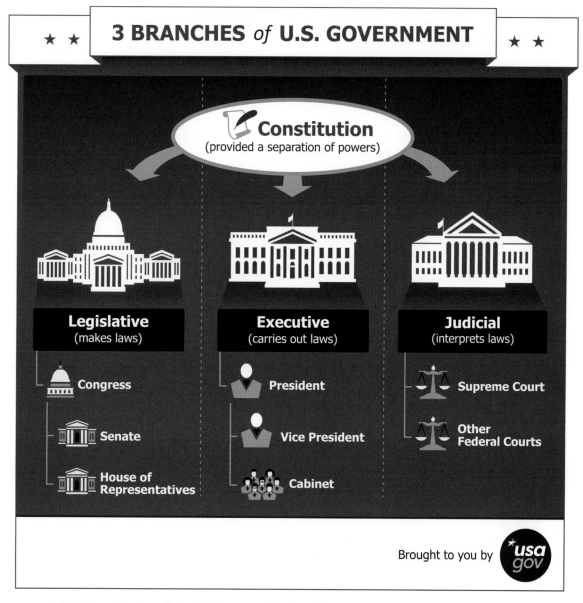

Fig. 14.1 Three Branches of the US Government. Reprinted from the government website https://www.usa.gov/branches-of-government.

Dobbs v. Jackson Women's Health Organization decision that overturned *Roe v. Wade*. Although the country's founding leaders envisioned the Supreme Court as nonpartisan, over time partisan politics has played a tremendous role in judicial appointments. Supreme Court appointments are particularly important to political parties because of the potential to apply party ideology through the unusual power granted the Supreme Court in the United States, the small number of justices, the durability of Supreme Court decisions, the court's relative freedom from special-interest groups, and the fact that Supreme Court justices are appointed for their lifetimes. Supreme Court decisions can have far-reaching and long-lasting effects.

ASK YOURSELF

Abortion—A Moral and Political Issue

Abortion, a moral issue, raises questions about basic beliefs regarding life and death, the sanctity of life, the beginning of life, and women's rights to make decisions about their own bodies. Over time, abortion has become a political issue. Examples of this change include legal arguments over women's choice versus the right to life; congressional discussions regarding public funding of abortions, including debate related to the level of coverage; which abortion procedures are legal; and the definition of acceptable circumstances surrounding conception and abortion. For the last half-century, the two major American political parties have been polarized on the issue, creating a fiercely partisan debate. One party supports the freedom of a woman to make her own decision, whereas the opposing party advocates for the fetus's right to life. As a result, abortion continues to be a hot-button partisan issue.

- What is your personal moral stand on abortion?
- How did you develop this stand?
- Does your political party affiliation affect your opinion about abortion?
- Would you support a particular party based solely on this one issue?
- What is the government's role related to moral issues? Explain your position.
- How would your opinion influence your ability to give quality patient care in the event you were assigned to care for a patient who requested an abortion?

ASK YOURSELF

Is the Supreme Court Partisan?

Supreme Court justices are appointed by the president of the United States, with the advice and consent of the Senate. The Senate Judiciary Committee holds a series of hearings, during which the appointee is questioned on judicial and legal matters. The committee makes a recommendation on the suitability of the appointee; the entire Senate then votes to confirm or reject the president's appointment. Search the Internet for contentious Supreme Court nomination hearings and scan the reports.

- Did the Senate Judiciary Committee members question the court nominees about issues with moral/ethical implications?
- Did the Senate Judiciary Committee members question the nominees about their positions on specific partisan issues such as abortion?
- Why do political parties want to appoint judges with known partisan leanings to the Supreme Court?
- What role does the Supreme Court have in shaping the country's health policy?

Nurses are most familiar with political issues in the **legislative branch** of government. Legislative issues are the ones decided through the passage of federal or state laws. Within the legislative arena, nurses can influence the outcome of various political issues. Examples of well-publicized legislative issues with healthcare implications include Medicare and Medicaid revisions; health insurance reform, such as the Affordable Care Act (Obamacare); and policies related to public health such as mandatory immunization. Nurses who advocate in the legislative arena should rely on the scientific body of nursing knowledge to support policies that will improve the health and welfare of all people.

Nurses function in a variety of roles. They are citizens, knowledgeable consumers of health care, professionals whose practice is regulated by government, and advocates for patients. Responsible political involvement is an important function of each of these roles. Because nurses are individuals with a variety of backgrounds, experiences, beliefs, and values, their opinions about political issues are diverse. This diversity, when coupled with sensitivity to moral and ethical implications, scientific knowledge, and experience working with patient populations, provides a foundation for productive and fair policy discussions.

Political issues of particular interest to nurses fall into four categories as follows: moral values, professional regulation, the health of individuals in society, and distributive justice. Nurses' opinions on these issues are based on personal experience, ethical orientation, religion, cultural bias, and a number of other factors. Naturally, there is a healthy diversity of opinion among nurses on most issues—particularly those involving moral values. Box 14.1 shows examples of selected political issues of interest to many nurses.

As discussed in Chapters 6 and 8, the **administrative branch of government**, sometimes known as the fourth branch of government, is involved in the operation of

---

BOX 14.1   Selected Examples of Health-Related Policy Issues

Issues Involving Moral Values
Healthcare Issues
- Medicare and Medicaid funding
- Pandemic preparedness
- Privacy of electronic health records
- Opioid abuse
- Undocumented immigrant health care

Beginning-of-Life Issues
- Use of fetal stem cells
- Contraception and sterilization
- Genetic testing
- Abortion

End-of-Life Issues
- Home care at the end of life
- Active and passive euthanasia
- Physician-assisted suicide
- Patient self-determination

Issues Involving Professional Regulation
Nursing Education
- Faculty shortage

- Funding for nursing education
- Access to technological innovations

Workplace Issues
- Workplace violence
- Equitable compensation
- Safe staffing
- Discrimination in the workplace

Advanced Practice Issues
- Full scope of practice
- Use of titles and credentials in all settings

Issues Involving the Health of Individuals in Society
Environmental Health
- Clean energy
- Clean water
- Global warming

Public Health
- Emerging pandemic diseases
- Bioterrorism
- Immunization and population health
- Gun control

---

government agencies. State boards of nursing and medicine, for example, are administrative agencies charged with regulating the activity of physicians and nurses. Rules and regulations promulgated by professional boards can have a profound effect on healthcare delivery. Because positions on these boards are often granted through political appointment, decisions are occasionally viewed as partisan. Examples of current nursing issues influenced by the administrative branch include scope and boundaries of practice, nursing education for entry into practice, and multistate licensure.

HEALTH POLICY

Because health plays a critical role in the physical, psychological, and economic condition of individuals, it affects society in general. Therefore, the central purpose of health policy is to improve the overall health of the population. Health policy is far reaching; it influences the behavior and decisions of people in relation to their environment and living conditions; it affects lifestyle and personal behavior; and it affects availability, accessibility, and quality of healthcare services. Health-related

issues receive considerable attention in the policy-making forum. Public policy for health care is often expressed through public health efforts. Public health comprises what the organized society does to assure, as far as is reasonably possible, the necessary conditions for its members to remain healthy (Gostin & Wiley, 2015).

Different people define health in different ways. The culture's prevailing definition of health affects the investment society is willing to make in specific healthcare programs. For example, if society defines health narrowly in terms of the absence of illness, policymakers might choose to fund programs that focus on the treatment of illness but neglect programs that support health-promoting behaviors. In contrast, a society that defines health positively, in terms of wellness, would place more emphasis on funding programs to prevent illness or maximize health potential.

Health policies are formal and authoritative decisions focusing on health. Health policies are made in the legislative, executive, or judicial branches of government and are intended to direct or influence the actions, behaviors, or decisions of others. Examples of the different forms health policy can take include legislation, rules, and regulations guiding the implementation of legislation, rules and regulations established to operate the government and its various programs, and judicial decisions related to health. Statutes or laws are pieces of legislation that have been enacted by legislative bodies and approved by the executive branch of government. Rules or regulations are policies that are established to guide the implementation of laws and programs. Judicial decisions are authoritative court decisions that direct or influence the actions, behaviors, or decisions of others. In addition to these different types of policies, there are two broad categories of health policies: allocative and regulatory.

Allocative policies determine what programs are funded—that is, where the resources are allocated. This is the area in which we see distributive justice in practice. Allocative policies are essentially economic in nature. In most countries, these policies are geared toward guaranteeing access to goods and services for the disadvantaged. Allocative policies are based on fundamental beliefs about which groups or classes of individuals or organizations should receive the benefits. Policymakers realize that there is a distribution of both benefits and burdens: some people will receive benefits while others will bear the expense. In a democratic system, these decisions should be based on public opinion. Some of the most well-known examples of allocative health policies in the United States are those of that regulate Medicare, Medicaid, workers' compensation, Veterans Health Administration, Children's Health Insurance Program, and Indian Health Service. The major nursing associations actively promote various allocative policies. For example, the Canadian Nurses Association (CNA) actively pursues legislation focused on human resources in the workforce; the International Council of Nurses (ICN) pursues international policies on health services for migrants, refugees, and displaced persons; and the ANA promotes equitable third-party reimbursement for advanced practice registered nurses.

Regulatory policies are those designed to achieve society's objectives to deliver better economic and social outcomes and enhance the life of individuals and groups using regulations and laws. Regulatory policies establish rules for healthcare delivery. They standardize and control groups of people by monitoring and enforcing penalties when policies are violated. The most basic and familiar regulatory health policies are the ones requiring nurses and physicians to be licensed to work. Many

nurses today do not realize the impact regulatory policies have on nursing practice. For example, in the late 1980, the American Medical Association (AMA) proposed a new category of healthcare professional that would be subordinate to physicians and would be prepared to assume many of the same functions as registered nurses. These new healthcare workers were to be called *registered care technicians* (Chernomas & Chernomas, 1989). The ANA and other state and national nursing organizations joined forces in their lobbying efforts against the proposal. Calling the establishment of this new group a major step backwards, nursing was successful, and AMA abandoned their plans (Dermody, 1990). Had the AMA succeeded, organized healthcare and professional nursing would look entirely different today. In addition to the type of administrative duties described above, all legislation goes through a second major step after being passed by legislatures and signed into law. Newly passed laws are distributed to appropriate regulatory bodies, which develop rules and regulations that explicitly describe how the laws will be implemented. Clearly, the health policy process is complex.

The Health Policy Process

The process of health policy includes three distinct phases. These phases are consecutive but can be repeated. The first phase is that of policy formulation. This phase includes such actions as agenda setting and the subsequent development of legislation. The second phase is that of policy implementation. This phase follows the enactment of legislation and includes taking actions and making additional decisions necessary to implement legislation, such as rule making and policy operation. The final stage is policy modification. The purpose of this stage is to improve or perfect legislation previously enacted. This might entail only minor adjustments made in the implementation phase, or it may involve major changes or the elimination of particular statutes (Longest, 2015).

Policy Formulation

The first phase of policymaking is policy formulation. Policy formulation can occur outside of government or within the government at the executive, administrative, or legislative levels. An example of policy formulation outside the government is the initial development of the nurse practitioner role in which state nurses' associations in the 1960s through the 1980s initiated legislation to create this new professional category. The policy formulation phase is divided into two distinct, sequentially related sets of activities: setting the agenda and developing the legislation (Longest, 2015). At any point in time, there is a complex mix of three variables: health-related problems, possible solutions and alternatives, and diverse political interests. As agenda setting progresses, the emerging issues can proceed to the development of legislation.

Problems. Real or perceived problems are the impetus for the policy formulation phase of policymaking. Problems may become evident in a number of ways. For example, the initial nurse practitioner legislation addressed the problem of a shortage of primary care providers in rural areas. Sometimes problems occur as the result of variables related to previous policy (Longest, 2015). For example, it is often predicted that the future shortfall in Social Security could be related to policies that failed to consider future inequities between promised benefits and escalating costs. Other problems may gain attention as they reach unacceptable levels. An increase in the number of children with vaccine-preventable communicable illness is an example of this type of problem. Other problems emerge because of some specific event that forces public attention. A dramatic

example of this type of problem was the sudden need for healthcare services and resources during the early days of the COVID-19 pandemic. However, the mere existence of problems is not always sufficient to ensure policy formulation. There must also be feasible solutions to the problems and the political will to enact legislation.

Solutions. Someone must come up with an idea to solve a problem before legislation is initiated. The process of offering solutions to problems involves generating ideas for solving the problems, refining the ideas, and selecting from among the options (Longest, 2015). Nursing's Agenda for Health Care Reform (ANA, 1991) is an important example of the profession's early attempt to participate in the formulation of specific solutions to problems of healthcare access.

Even if nurses identify a serious problem and offer feasible solutions, they may not be able to influence legislation. Legislation can only progress through the process with the sponsorship of influential policymakers who believe in the issue and invest time and energy. Potential sponsors are sensitive to the political will of their party, constituents, and colleagues. Factors that influence political will include public attitudes, concerns, and opinions surrounding an issue; the preferences and

ASK YOURSELF

Healthcare Reform Initiatives

Healthcare access has been a critical social issue since the 1980s and has become one of the most divisive political issues of the past four decades. On September 22, 1993, President Bill Clinton introduced the American Health Security Act. Following months of high-level negotiation and planning, this reform package included many of the ideas presented in at least 11 separate proposals made within the preceding five years. Administration officials thought the public and many special-interest groups were demanding a radical reform of the healthcare system. Leah Curtin (1996), a nursing leader and ethicist, predicted in May 1991 that there would be a universal access system within three to eight years. Yet Clinton's proposal, along with all of its predecessors, failed. Universal access did not become a reality. In 2010 President Barack Obama signed into law the *Patient Protection and Affordable Care Act*, a law that phased in reforms of some aspects of private and public insurance programs by prohibiting the exclusion of preexisting conditions and expanding insurance access to millions of Americans (Patient Protection

and Affordable Care Act, 2010). This law had an extremely polarizing effect on the political parties, with many political leaders praising the law as landmark legislation and others vowing to repeal it. Rollback of many Affordable Care Act elements began in earnest with the change of power in the US legislative branch and a new president after the 2016 general election.

- A great deal of time and energy was invested in the policy formulation phase of healthcare reform. How effective do you believe leaders were in this phase of each bill?
- What was the problem being addressed? How clear was the problem?
- How do you think the influence of special-interest groups affected the evolving outcomes of healthcare reform? Explain your thinking.
- At what point in the policymaking process do you think the proposals succeeded or failed?

relative ability to influence political decisions; the positions of key political leaders on the issue; the influence of outside special-interest groups; and the other competing items on the policy agenda. Creating a political thrust forceful enough to cause policymakers to formulate and implement new policy is often the most difficult problem (Longest, 2015). Nurses are a significant percentage of the voting population. They are in a good position to collectively influence political decisions and enhance the political will essential to formulate health policy.

Policy Implementation

Policy implementation immediately follows the enactment of legislation. Because legislation seldom contains explicit language on how it is to be implemented, details are left to the process of rule making. For example, the various states' boards of nursing are responsible for developing legislative rules to specifically guide nursing practice. Generally, these organizations accept input from affected groups during the rule-making process. Interest groups routinely seek to influence rule making because they are so often the targets of rules established to implement health policies. Lobbying is one of the major means by which interest groups attempt to influence policymakers. Lobbying is especially intense when various interest groups disagree on the formulation of a particular policy.

Policy Modification

Policy modification occurs when outcomes, perceptions, and consequences of existing policies indicate that the original problems still exist or that new problems have arisen from unforeseen circumstances or from the policy itself. The policy modification phase is intended to spiral backward, with feedback, into the agenda-setting and legislation development stages of the formulation phase—potentially creating new legislation—and spiral forward into the rule-making and policy operation stages of the implementation phase, stimulating changes in rules or operations. Many programs are routinely amended, some of them repeatedly, over a period of many years. These modifications may reflect, among other things, the development of new technologies, changing economic conditions, and public demand (Longest, 2015). Rollbacks of elements of the Affordable Care Act in 2017 and 2018 are examples of the policy modification process affected by partisan politics. Fig. 14.2 depicts the iterative nature of the policy process.

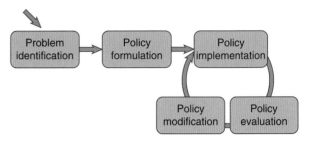

Fig. 14.2 The Policy Process Cycle.

Ethics in Policymaking

Policymaking is an inherently ethical endeavor because it affects people's lives, their relationships, and the distributive justice process. The outcomes and consequences of most health policies affect large groups of people. There are two equally important functions of ethics in public policymaking. In the policy formulation phase, ethics can guide the original development of new policies. Ethics is also useful in the policy modification phase as a means to examine the immediate and far-reaching effects of policies that are already implemented. There is, however, some practical difficulty in adhering strictly to specific ethical principles during the policymaking process. Policy formulation and criticism involve more complex data and forms of reasoning than ethical principles can handle. Disagreements about public policy can turn on differences in basic beliefs and interpretations, as well as uncertainties. Ethical principles provide the moral background for policy decisions, but participants must consider complex empirical data and specialized disciplinary knowledge, such as that of nursing and medicine (Beauchamp & Childress, 2019). Thus, health policy is so complex that it prohibits the strict and exclusive use of specific rules or principles in guiding policy formulation; rather, ethical considerations must be accompanied by the rational use of empirical data.

Research Data in Policymaking

When nurses want to influence health policy, they must furnish officials with important and reliable information. If policymakers have reliable facts and research findings, they can identify problems, make comparisons, confirm trends, and establish policy based on evidence. Because time is a precious commodity, officials are more interested in research findings than unsubstantiated

ASK YOURSELF

Ethics and Politics of Tobacco Sales

The sale and distribution of tobacco products, including cigarettes and cigars, smokeless tobacco, and E-cigarettes, have been a highly publicized political issue for many years. The tobacco industry is increasingly affected by legislative and judicial decisions regarding the health effects of tobacco.

- What are the ethical issues of which the policymakers should be aware?
- What are some ethical arguments in favor of regulating the production and sale of tobacco products?
- What are some ethical arguments in favor of allowing the industry to operate on the free market, unrestricted?
- There are judicial precedents that assign at least some responsibility for the health problems of smokers to the tobacco companies. Is this a legal, ethical, or political issue, or some combination of these?
- What factors determine whether nurses should be interested in this issue?

opinion. When preparing to discuss policy with officials, nurses should carefully review objective data, pertinent research findings, and a few particularly attention-getting personal stories. Cost savings often get attention when other facts elicit little response.

The federal government recognizes the importance of healthcare research in the development of policy. Established by Congress as part of the 1989 Omnibus Budget Reconciliation Act, the Agency for Healthcare Research and Quality (AHRQ) was created to improve the quality, safety, efficiency, and effectiveness of health care for all Americans. The agency supports and disseminates health services research to improve the quality of health care and promote evidence-based decision making. The AHRQ is a bridge between clinicians, consumers, policymakers, payers, and other health officials.

NURSING, POLICY, AND POLITICS

Not since the days of Lavinia Lloyd Dock (1858–1956) have nurses been so actively involved with health policy. Through the perspective of knowledge, experience, and intimacy with the healthcare needs of people, nurses are in the unique position to bring insight and balance to the policymaking process. Moreover, professional codes of ethics identify the goals and values of the profession and explicitly call for nurses to be involved in policy formulation. For example, the *ICN Code of Ethics for Nurses* calls for nurses to initiate and support action to meet the health and social needs of all people by leading or contributing to sound health policy development (ICN, 2021, Elements 1.6 and 4.3), and the CNA calls for all nurses to address broad societal issues (CNA, 2020, Part II). The ANA Code of Ethics for Nurses (2015) calls for individual nurses' participation in the roles of advocates or elected or appointed officials for health policy initiatives at the local, regional, state, national, or global levels (ANA, 2015, Provision 7.3). ANA also calls for the organized profession to actively engage in the political process, especially in regard to legislative and regulatory issues that most affect public health and the profession of nursing (ANA, 2015, Provision 9.4). In addition, the American Association of Colleges of Nursing (n.d.), National League of Nursing (n.d.), National Council of State Boards of Nursing, American Association of Nurse Practitioners (n.d.), and specialty nursing organizations are all active in advocacy and encourage nurses to participate in the policy arena.

The formulation of health policy requires strong nursing leadership and an understanding of the crucial role of local and national policymaking. Nurse leaders must develop the ability to think, teach, research, and communicate. They must be aware of the short- and long-term impact that policies have on health and on clinical practice. They must conduct research on health policy issues and find strategic ways to influence state and national policy agendas. They must step beyond the familiar practice setting. Recognizing health problems as policy issues is the first step toward policy formulation.

Nursing's Political Strengths

Nursing enters the political arena with notable strengths. Nurses have the strength of numbers because they comprise the largest group of healthcare providers (American Association of Colleges of Nursing, 2022). Acting together, nurses are a formidable political force. Nurses have traditionally been perceived favorably by the public. Research has repeatedly shown that the public views nurses with respect, trust, and admiration. They view nurses as being honest and having ethical integrity. In fact, throughout the early 21st century, the

Gallup poll has placed nurses on top as the profession the public views as the most ethical and honest—except for 2001, when firefighters earned that distinction (Brenan, 2023). High levels of public trust give nursing a strong voice in health policy, and once nurses become involved, they usually continue to be active. Through involvement, nurses become familiar with political leaders and health policy processes. They retain interest in policy issues and become more politically sophisticated as time passes.

Nursing's Political Weaknesses

The profession also has a few political weaknesses. First, being relatively new to the political arena, many nurses are not astute or comfortable in policymaking or lobbyist roles. Second, there has historically been a lack of ideological and political unity within the profession, which may stem from a wide diversity of educational preparation and titles. Third, though nurses comprise the largest number of professionals, they have fewer funds specifically earmarked for intense lobbying than many other special-interest or high-income groups.

Policy Goals for Nursing

How do nurses become aware of the issues that are important and require energy and focus? Each nurse is responsible to reflect on health-related problems and potential solutions. In addition, one of the major functions of professional organizations is to provide leadership and assistance to members in political and other matters. Congruent with nursing codes of ethics, each of the major nursing associations provides specific issues and strategies for nurses interested in policymaking. Each organization clearly highlights its legislative and policy agendas on its website. Organizations such as the ANA, the CNA, and the ICN share the goals of maintaining control of nursing practice, making a positive impact on healthcare policy, advocating on behalf of the vulnerable, and instituting workplace reforms.

NURSING ADVOCACY IN THE POLICY PROCESS

Political advocacy includes activities by individuals or groups that aim to influence policy decisions. Sometimes nurses are privileged to be legitimate members of governmental or institutional policymaking bodies. More often, the nurse's role in policy formulation, implementation,

---

ASK YOURSELF

Nurses Take Positions on Political Issues

The ANA has been a powerful lobbying force for many years. Issues of interest to members of the organization are freely accessible through the ANA's advocacy website (n.d.) at https://www.nursingworld.org/practice-policy/advocacy/. The ANA has been active in advocating policy for many issues, including the following: opioid abuse, telehealth, pandemic preparedness, child and elder care, civil rights, collective bargaining, domestic violence, family and medical leave, gun control, homelessness, malpractice/liability reform, migrant and seasonal farm worker health issues, pay equity, rural health care, and sexual harassment. These are but a few of the issues the ANA has been involved in over the years.

- Why do you think the professional organization of nursing in the United States is concerned with issues such as homelessness and gun control?
- What impact do you think the profession could make if each nurse became familiar with all of the issues and advocated for them to policymakers?
- Identify any issues within your state that affect the health of your patients or your practice.
- How could you begin the process of health policy formulation for this issue?

---

and modification is that of advocate. Advocacy involves promoting solutions to an issue that is affected by the decisions of policymakers. Political advocates have a powerful voice in determining the policymaking process, from agenda setting to policy modification. They cultivate relationships and employ the art of persuasion as they attempt to influence officials toward their point of view. Advocacy is essential to the proper functioning of the government and is specifically protected by the First Amendment of the Constitution, ensuring that Congress will not pass laws that abridge the rights of the people to peaceably petition the government (*U.S Const. Amend. I-X*). Political advocacy provides a forum in which to resolve conflicts among diverse and competing points of view. It also provides information, analysis, and opinion to policymakers, which promotes informed and balanced decision making.

To be effective in the political domain, nurses need to become politically astute. They must be aware of trends in the political climate, must be able to access powerful political leaders, and must learn how to play the game.

Knowing the power players in the political arena is one of the most important steps in the advocacy process.

In seeking help to promote a particular legislative agenda, nurses want to begin by enlisting policymakers who have the following characteristics: (1) legitimate power, (2) an interest in the problem, (3) an affinity for nursing or for healthcare issues in general, (4) time and energy to invest in the process, (5) the respect of colleagues, and (6) committee or other positions appropriate to the particular legislation. Finding an official with these characteristics will greatly improve the probability of success. Nurses who are new to political advocacy can waste valuable time and energy trying to influence officials who are uninterested, have conflicting loyalties, are powerless, or are not respected by their colleagues. Nurses and nursing students who are new to political advocacy should contact the health policy or legislative committee of their state nurses' associations. Nursing leaders with lobbying experience can identify the most appropriate policymakers, give novices focused information about current issues, and involve them in organized activities.

Types of Advocacy

Once nurses have identified the appropriate policy-making officials and are familiar with the issues and the legislative and regulatory process, strategies must be initiated. There are two basic types of political advocacy: **lobbying** through direct communication (Fig. 14.3)

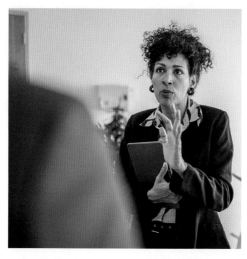

Fig. 14.3 Lobbying Can Occur in Formal or Informal Settings. (©iStock.com/AzmanL.)

and indirect **grassroots campaigning**. Grassroots campaigning is geared toward influencing public opinion, which in turn will influence policymakers. Grassroots campaigning includes many types of activities intended to generate a response from the wider public. Following are grassroots campaigning strategies:

1. Garner support within professional nursing organizations
2. Initiate and distribute messages via e-mail, social media, or postal mail
3. Gather signatures on petitions
4. Write opinion pieces and letters to the editor for newspapers
5. Contribute to professional newsletters
6. Partner with other grassroots organizations such as the American Association of Retired People
7. Contribute to web-based bulletins and online discussions
8. Organize public events such as marches
9. Initiate large-scale advertising campaigns
10. Participate in social media campaigns
11. Disseminate the results of opinion polls

Direct communication through lobbying is often more effective than grassroots campaigning. Lobbying is the art of persuasion—attempting to convince a legislator, a government official, the head of an agency, or a state official to comply with a request—whether it is convincing them to support a position on an issue or to follow a particular course of action. Many nurses who are involved in influencing policy are volunteer lobbyists who are exempt from registering or reporting their lobbying efforts. The following are seven methods of volunteer lobbying:

1. Participate in or testify at legislative committee meetings or hearings
2. Conduct prearranged formal face-to-face meetings with policymakers
3. Reach out personally on social media platforms
4. Meet with policymakers by telephone or video call
5. Approach a policymaker at a social event, such as an organized legislative reception
6. E-mail a policymaker
7. Write a personal letter to a policymaker

Skillful volunteer lobbyists are skilled communicators who understand that some strategies work better than others. The next sections discuss tips with effective techniques for personal visits and letter writing.

Personal Visits

A personal visit is usually a more powerful lobbying tool than messages sent via letters, e-mail, or social media. Whenever possible, nurses should seize the opportunity to meet face-to-face with policymakers. Following are a few suggestions for personal visits with policymaking officials:

- Be prepared. Develop your plan of action and know what you intend to say.
- Be on time for your appointment and be patient if the official is late.
- Be courteous and greet the official with a firm handshake, introduce yourself, and present your business card if you have one.
- Identify the subject of the meeting and present your facts in an orderly, succinct, calm, and direct fashion.
- Support your position with concise personal experiences and anecdotes; use valid research and statistics when appropriate.
- Keep your presentation simple. Avoid technical language and professional jargon. Your goal is to inform and influence, not to impress.
- Close the meeting strongly and effectively, asking for the official's support.
- Leave a short fact sheet summarizing the issue and your position. Include the names and telephone numbers of contact people.
- Send a message within a few days thanking the official for the meeting, restating your position, and including any information requested during the meeting.

Written Communication

Handwritten, personal, mass letter, e-mail, and social media messages can be powerful grassroots lobbying techniques. Certain techniques have been found to be more effective. Here are some practical tips for written communication:

- Write the letter, e-mail, or social media message in your own words, using your own thoughts and logic, and drawing pertinent inferences. Though more effective than no letters at all, form letters are much less likely to be read by officials than personal correspondence.
- Identify yourself as a nurse and state your reason for writing in the first paragraph, including the title and number of the legislation in which you are interested.
- Be specific and include key information and examples supporting your position.

- Be explicit. Tell the official exactly what you want. If you are writing to ask for cosponsorship or a vote for or against a bill, say so.
- Be brief but informative.
- Include only one topic.
- Never threaten or use hostility. This immediately destroys your chances of developing a cooperative relationship.
- Offer your assistance as a resource.
- Promptly thank the official for favorable votes.

Political Campaigns

One very effective key to successful advocacy is for nurses to become involved by either supporting candidates or running for elective office themselves. To begin, nurses can become involved in campaigns and elections. This can be done in any number of ways. Involvement may take the form of campaigning door-to-door, stuffing envelopes, or publicly endorsing candidates. Actively supporting candidates for public office helps forge relationships with officials and helps elect candidates who will sympathize with issues important to nurses. Involvement in a political party can also be helpful in developing a campaign platform sensitive to issues of interest to nurses. Relationships that nurses form with public officials during campaigns can also lead to nurses' candidacies and election or appointment to important policymaking positions. Political involvement can occur individually or through district and state nurses' associations. Professional organizations provide a vehicle for meeting candidates, forming relationships, and offering candidates forums. Forums remind a candidate that nurses are an organized group interested in politics and public policy and acquaint nurses with the candidate's position on important issues.

▌ SUMMARY

Many policy issues are important to nurses. Most issues for which nurses are actively concerned relate to health policy: Issues of a moral nature, issues related to professional regulation, issues related to public health, and issues related to distributive justice. Fulfilling the role of advocate, nurses are challenged to become politically active: to know and become involved with important issues, to learn the political process, to form relationships with public officials, and to become astute in methods of influencing health policy.

ASK YOURSELF

Be Careful of Your Wording

Nurses must choose the right words when lobbying. One nurse relates a story of her first experience testifying before a state legislative committee. Feeling that her presentation was well prepared and would be effective, the nurse decided at the last minute to substitute the words *nurse voters* for the word *nurses*. There were many people giving testimony that day. After the completion of the testimony phase, the legislators were given an opportunity to make comments or ask questions. There were no questions. Every comment was directed toward the nurse, who was surprised to learn that the legislators perceived the term *nurse voters* as a veiled threat. They did not hear the substance of the presentation, but rather perceived an unintended and unspoken threat, "If you do not support our position, we will vote you out of office." By giving this impression, the nurse ruined a productive relationship with these legislators. The legislation that the nurses were supporting failed.

- Why do you think the nurse changed the wording of her presentation in the first place?
- What words would you have used?
- Describe similar circumstances in which you were speaking and the reaction of the listeners was based on their inferences from your choice of words rather than their intended meaning.
- How can nurses avoid mistakes of this sort?

CHAPTER HIGHLIGHTS

- The term *political* relates to the policymaking process within the government.
- Political issues are those that are created, affected, or regulated by any of the government branches.
- Political parties are organized groups with distinct ideologies that seek to control government.
- Partisan issues are those issues for which the political parties have distinct ideology.
- Health policies influence the actions, decisions, and behaviors of people in the domain of health.
- Society's definition of health reflects the extent to which society is willing to move toward maximizing the health of citizens.
- Allocative or distributive health policies are designed to provide benefits to certain groups.

- Regulatory policies are designed to influence others through directive techniques.
- The process of health policy includes three phases: policy formulation, policy implementation, and policy modification.
- There are two important functions of ethics in public policymaking: guiding the original development of policy and criticizing previously implemented policy.
- Nurses can affect health policy through various political means.

DISCUSSION QUESTIONS AND ACTIVITIES

1. Explore the advocacy websites of three nursing organizations, paying close attention to health policy issues and strategies.
2. Review the *Federal Issues* page of the ANA website at https://www.nursingworld.org/practice-policy/advocacy/federal/. How do the listed issues fit with the ANA code of nursing ethics?
3. Visit the Kaiser Family Foundation website at https://www.kff.org/. Which of the issues highlighted on the website are health policy issues? Discuss how nurses could affect the policymakers on these issues.
4. Discuss five issues listed in Box 14.1 in class. How do classmates' positions compare to those of the major political parties? Are individual students' opinions politically consistent from issue to issue?
5. Discuss the following question in class: What purpose do political parties serve?
6. Compile a list of political issues related to allocation (distributive justice). Examine the ANA or CNA code of nursing ethics and discuss how the codes of ethics guide nurses who wish to advocate for a particular policy.
7. Discuss strategies for influencing health policy in the administrative and judicial domains.
8. Compile a list of at least three political issues related to health that have been decided in the court system. How have the judicial decisions affected healthcare delivery?
9. Compile a list of political issues related to moral values. Discuss the role of the professional organization in guiding members' actions related to these moral issues.

10. Discuss popular definitions of health and determine how each definition, if adopted by the government, would affect healthcare delivery.

11. Read the online article, *Lavinia Dock (1858–1856): Picketing, Parading, and Protesting* found at https://www.ncbi.nlm.nih.gov/pmc/articles/PMC4318304/ (Garofalo & Fee, 2016). Discuss with classmates how Lavinia Dock's activism relates to nursing today.

REFERENCES

American Association of Colleges of Nursing. (2022). *Nursing fact sheet*. https://www.aacnnursing.org/news-Information/fact-sheets/nursing-fact-sheet#:~:text=Nursing%20is%20the%20nation%27s%20largest,84.1%25%20are%20employed%20in%20nursing.&text=The%20federal%20government%20projects%20that,each%20year%20from%202021%2D2031.

American Association of Colleges of Nursing. (n.d.). *Policy & advocacy*. https://www.aacnnursing.org/Policy-Advocacy

ANA. (1991). *Nursing's agenda for health care reform*. Nursebooks.org.

ANA. (2015). *Code of ethics for nurses with interpretive statements*. Nursebooks.org. http://nursingworld.org/DocumentVault/Ethics-1/Code-of-Ethics-for-Nurses.html

ANA. (n.d.). *Advocacy*. https://www.nursingworld.org/practice-policy/advocacy/

Aristotle. (1998). *Politics (C. D. C. Reeve, Trans.)*. Hackett (Original work published 350 BCE).

Beauchamp, T. L., & Childress, J. (2019). *Principles of biomedical ethics* (8th ed.). Oxford University Press.

Brenan, M. (2023). *Nurses retain top ethics rating in U.S., but below 2020 high*. https://news.gallup.com/poll/467804/nurses-retain-top-ethics-rating-below-2020-high.aspx

Chernomas, R., & Chernomas, W. (1989). Escalation of the nurse-physician conflict: Registered care technologists and the economic crisis. *International Journal of Health Services, 19*(4), 635–650. https://doi.org/10.2190/2bmp-c0kq-614g-d9fg.

CNA. (2017). *Code of ethics for registered nurses*. https://cdn1.nscn.ca/sites/default/files/documents/resources/code-of-ethics-for-registered-nurses.pdf#:~:text=The%20Canadian%20Nurses%20Association%20%28CNA%29%20Code%20of%20Ethics,receiving%20care.%20The%20Code%20is%20both%20aspirational%20and%20regulatory.

CNA. (2020). *CNAs key messages on anti-Black racism in nursing and health*. https://hl-prod-ca-oc-download.s3-ca-central-1.amazonaws.com/CNA/2f975e7e-4a40-45ca-863c-5ebf0a138d5e/UploadedImages/documents/Anti-Racism-key-messages_e.pdf

Curtin, L. (1996). *Nursing into the 21st century: Health care reform, restructuring, practice, leadership*. Springhouse.

Dermody, B. (1990). KNA director reminisces about the registered care technician project. *Kentucky Nurse, 38*(6), 9.

Dobbs v. Jackson Women's Health Organization (U.S. Supreme Court 2022). https://supreme.justia.com/cases/federal/us/597/19-1392/

Garofalo, M. E., & Fee, E. (2016). Lavinia Dock (1858-1856): Picketing, parading, and protesting. *American Journal of Public Health, 105*(2), 276–277. https://www.ncbi.nlm.nih.gov/pmc/articles/PMC4318304/.

Gostin, L. O., & Wiley, L. F. (2015). *Public health ethics and law*. The Hastings Center Bioethics Briefings. https://www.thehastingscenter.org/briefingbook/public-health/

ICN. (2021). *The ICN code of ethics for nurses*. https://www.icn.ch/system/files/2021-10/ICN_Code-of-Ethics_EN_Web_0.pdf

Longest, B. B. (2015). *Health policymaking in the United States* (6th ed.). Health Administration Press.

National Association of Nurse Practitioners. (n.d.). *AANP advocacy: Championing the NP role and amplifying the NP voice*. https://www.aanp.org/advocacy

National League for Nursing. (n.d.). *NLN homepage*. https://www.nln.org/home

Patient Protection and Affordable Care Act, Pub. L. No. H.R. 3590 (2010). https://www.congress.gov/111/plaws/publ148/PLAW-111publ148.pdf

Roe v Wade, 410 (U.S. 1973).

The Council of State Governments. (2022). *COVID-19 resources for state leaders*. https://web.csg.org/covid19/2022-state-executive-orders/

The White House. (2022). Executive order on lowering prescription drug costs for Americans. Retrieved from https://www.whitehouse.gov/briefing-room/presidential-actions/2022/10/14/executive-order-on-lowering-prescription-drug-costs-for-americans/

The White House. (n.d.). *Health care that works for Americans*. https://obamawhitehouse.archives.gov/healthreform/healthcare-overview

U.S Const. *Amend. I-X*.

United States Senate. (n.d.). *Supreme court nominations (1789-present)*. https://www.senate.gov/legislative/nominations/SupremeCourtNominations1789present.htm

15

Ethical Implications of Healthcare Economics

Our faith in freedom does not rest on the foreseeable results in particular circumstances but on the belief that it will, on balance, release more forces for the good than for the bad.
(Hayek, 1960)

OBJECTIVES

After completing this chapter, the reader should be able to:

1. Describe the role of economics in health care.
2. Explain the concept of distributive justice.
3. Discuss utilitarian, libertarian, communitarian, and egalitarian theories of distributive justice.
4. Discuss basic questions related to the distribution of healthcare resources.
5. Describe recent trends in healthcare economics and the relationship of economic trends to the delivery of health care.
6. Examine nurses' codes of professional ethics for guidance in relation to healthcare economics issues.

INTRODUCTION

Nursing, other healthcare professions, and the overall healthcare delivery system exist to deliver health care to society. Over the past several decades, dynamic forces have worked together to create a complex system that has sometimes been called the best in the world. From advances in knowledge and technology to changes in healthcare financing, the system has experienced rapid and drastic changes. It is not unusual today to hear the term *crisis* used to describe the state of the current healthcare system. This crisis relates to problems with cost, quality, and access to healthcare services. Current debates about social justice are fueled by inequalities in access to health care and health insurance, combined with dramatic increases in the costs of care. Thoughtful, systematic consideration of ethics is necessary to the process of devising solutions to the current problems. This chapter discusses aspects of healthcare economics, distributive justice, and emerging trends.

OVERVIEW OF TODAY'S HEALTHCARE ECONOMICS

One of the main assumptions in traditional economics is that we should judge the institutions of a society by the preferences of the people affected by those institutions. There are different ways to judge the total preference of society. One method claims that one arrangement is better than another only if it satisfies the preferences of some people and does not frustrate the preferences of any others. Another method suggests that one arrangement is better than another only if it is preferred by people allowed to make a collective choice. Because institutions should be judged by the people they affect, the institution of health care should be judged by the people it serves. Discussion and debate about the current state of healthcare economics are integral to the process of evaluating and improving the present system.

Today's problems in the healthcare system have a long history, with many intervening factors. Before the 1940s, most health care was paid for by individuals. During World War II, the US War Labor Board froze wages. To attract workers in a scarce wartime labor force, industries initiated generous health insurance benefits. Health insurance benefits for some included "first dollar" 100 percent payment for health care in which individuals ended up paying nothing for health care. There was no incentive for physicians, hospitals, or individuals to limit costs because insurance paid for the best of everything. This system of third-party reimbursement, coupled with an increasing number of malpractice lawsuits, produced a healthcare system with progressively higher standards that required almost unlimited, high-tech care for a large segment of the population, regardless of cost. This led to a skewed model that focused heavily on expensive technology and personal autonomy and ignored the basic principles of social responsibility and distributive justice. This system still exists, though not to the degree of the last century. Managed care programs, expensive insurance premiums, increased copays, and increased deductibles have affected individuals and the healthcare system alike. Even so, there is a peculiar relationship between the patients and physicians who make the spending decisions and the third-party payers who must actually pay for those decisions. Moreover, there are staggering contrasts within this system. In an age when millions of dollars are spent on futile care, a portion of the population still has no access to healthcare services.

Before the advent of managed care, most health care was fee-for-service in which ethics was predominately driven by codes of ethical behavior and patients' rights statements, with a strong focus on the principle of autonomy. The fee-for-service model focuses on the individual patient, protects physician autonomy, promotes treatment that offers potential benefit or prolonged life, and assumes unlimited resources. Much of health care continues to be financed in this way. Analysts have recognized that there are ethical problems associated with this model, including the simultaneous extremes of overutilization by those who can pay and healthcare rationing for those who can't.

Although most people agree that modern health care in America is highly sophisticated and technologically advanced, they also recognize that there are many deficiencies in the system. First, healthcare services and resources have been inaccessible to a segment of the population. Second, healthcare costs are accelerating at

ASK YOURSELF

Paying for Futile Care

One hears stories about elderly patients with terminal illness—and even "no code" status—who remain in intensive care settings for extended periods, often because family members insist that everything should be done for their loved ones.

- Is the expenditure of expensive healthcare resources appropriate for these types of situations? Explain your position.
- Who should bear the financial burden for long-term, futile care?
- What ethical principles conflict in situations of this sort?

an unsustainable annual rate, consuming a huge portion of the gross domestic product. Third, the high cost of health care threatens the competitiveness and profitability of business and industry. Fourth, the benefits to the individual and corporate providers within the system are often pursued at the expense (and sometimes harm) of persons who need health care. Serious problems in the current system are related to the fundamental priorities that focus on a form of autonomy that gives more weight to individual interests than to the needs of society as a whole, profit as the primary motive for providing healthcare services, and the unquestioned use of expensive technology. The well-being of people subjected to a healthcare system driven by these values is threatened by the kinds of services offered, the way they are provided, and the underlying priorities that determine both. Nurses should be involved in challenging the values that drive the system and making ethical improvements that will promote health and well-being of people.

DISTRIBUTIVE JUSTICE

One of the primary purposes of government is to formulate and enforce policies that deal with the distribution of scarce resources. As mentioned in Chapter 3, the relevant application of the ethical principle of justice within the healthcare system focuses on the fair distribution of goods and services. This application is called distributive justice. Beauchamp and Childress (2019) define distributive justice as the fair, equitable, and appropriate distribution of diverse benefits and burdens such as property, resources, taxation, privileges, and opportunities. Because there is a scarcity of resources and competition for resources and services, it is impossible for all people to have everything they might want or need. It follows that giving to some will deny receipt to others who might otherwise have received these things. The "others" may be those in the same hospital, living in the same community, in other communities, or even those who are not yet born. For example, if Social Security becomes bankrupt through budget cuts or excessive expenditures in the present, others who would have received benefits in the future (even if they are not yet born) will be denied these benefits.

Three areas of health care are relevant to questions of distributive justice: What percentage of society's resources is it reasonable to spend on health care? Which population groups should be the recipients of healthcare resources? Recognizing that healthcare resources are limited, which aspects of health care should receive the most resources? These are important questions that are both practical and ethical in nature.

Entitlement

In deciding questions of distributive justice, we must ask, "Who is entitled to these services?" (Fig. 15.1). As with all of ethics, there is no universally accepted answer. Distribution of limited resources is the function of various levels of governing bodies. In attempting to distribute limited resources fairly, leaders will seek systematic means of deciding. Historically, these questions have been answered by material rules such as the following: to each person an equal share, to each person according to need, to each person according to merit, to each person according to social contribution, to each person according to their rights, to each person according to the effort, to each person according to ability to

pay, or to each person according to the greatest good to the greatest number. Von Platz (2020) offers examples of how decisions are made based on some of these principles as follows: each child in a group would receive an equal size piece of pie (distribute equally); the sick would receive medicine (distribute to those in need); people arriving at a restaurant would be seated as they arrive (distributed on a first-come, first-served basis); students would receive appropriate grades for their work (grades distributed according to merit); and a person freely chooses with whom to dance (distributed according to the principle of liberty). But these examples ignore the context. Of course, someone who is sick should receive medicine, but what happens if everyone is sick and there is only so much medicine? This kind of large-scale decision is usually the realm of public policy. Most societies will utilize several of these principles in establishing public policies. We find many of these principles in effect in the United States where, for example, welfare payments and many healthcare programs are distributed on the basis of need; jobs and promotions in

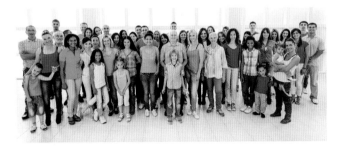

Fig. 15.1 Who Deserves Access to Health Care? (©iStock.com/skynesher.)

many sectors are awarded on the basis of demonstrated achievement and merit; comparably high incomes of some are awarded on the basis of superior effort, merit, or potential social contribution; and the opportunity for public education is distributed equally to all citizens (Beauchamp & Childress, 2019).

Right to Health Care

In examining who should receive care, we ask questions about the basic right to health care. Is health care a right or a privilege? This question is debated fiercely in the media, in professional and political arenas, and around the dinner table. Is society responsible for providing health care for all citizens and, if so, to what degree? Should each person be eligible for minimum basic health care, or should everyone be allowed to have everything there is to offer, from organ transplants to tummy tucks? Would the public benefit from a strict free-market system that would provide healthcare services only to those who can pay, or should the government be responsible for the healthcare needs of all citizens? If health care is a right and healthcare resources are scarce, which resources are allocated to which group of people? These and other questions fuel the debate about the right to health care.

Discussion of health care as a right is not new. In 1948 the General Assembly of the United Nations adopted the Universal Declaration of Human Rights, which declares that medical care is a necessary social service. Article 25 of the document states that "Everyone has the right to a standard of living adequate for the health and well-being of himself and of his family, including food, clothing, housing and medical care and necessary social services, and the right to security in the event of unemployment, sickness, disability, widowhood, old age or other lack of livelihood in circumstances beyond his control" (United Nations, 1948/2015, p. 52; Box 15.1). Thirty-five years later, the President's Commission for the Study of Ethical Problems in Medicine and Biomedical and Behavioral Research (1983) concurred that society has a moral obligation to ensure that everyone has access to adequate care without being subject to excessive burdens. The commission made a clear distinction between society and government, recognizing that a collective or societal obligation does not imply that government should be the primary institution involved in making health care available, but rather that government should participate with the private sector.

> ### BOX 15.1   The Universal Declaration of Human Rights
>
> Everyone has the right to a standard of living adequate for the health and well-being of himself and of his family, including food, clothing, housing and medical care and necessary social services, and the right to security in the event of unemployment, sickness, disability, widowhood, old age or other lack of livelihood in circumstances beyond his control.

From "The Universal Declaration of Human Rights," Copyright 2015 United Nations. Reprinted with the permission of the United Nations.

> ### BOX 15.2   US Constitution
>
> We the People of the United States, in Order to form a more perfect Union, establish Justice, insure domestic Tranquility, provide for the common defence, promote the general Welfare, and secure the Blessings of Liberty to ourselves and our Posterity, do ordain and establish this Constitution for the United States of America.
> (US Const. Amend. I-X)

The issue of health care as a right has some basis in constitutional law. Some argue that the "general welfare" clause in the Preamble of the US Constitution implies the protection of basic needs, including a right to the protection of health (Box 15.2). The President's Commission for the Study of Ethical Problems in Medicine and Biomedical and Behavioral Research (1983) reported that neither the Supreme Court nor any appellate court has found a constitutional right to health care, but many federal and state statutes have been interpreted to provide statutory rights in the form of entitlements to some vulnerable groups. Consequently, vulnerable groups have benefited from many legal decisions.

The concept of health care as a right is not universally accepted. There are those who believe that health care is a privilege. This position implies that health care can be enjoyed by some but would be beyond the common advantage of all citizens. The entrepreneurial model of libertarianism declares that health care is not a right, but rather a commodity that must be purchased on the open market like any other service. This model compares the healthcare professional's right to conduct a practice and charge fees to other business's right to do the same. This model provides health care only to those who can pay or those who are given health care as a gift. Some believe that a free-market system of healthcare delivery would force pricing competition and result in lower healthcare costs. This in turn would cause healthcare services to become more accessible to a larger portion of the population. Except for the fact that professionals can choose to provide services free of charge, this model makes little allowance for children and the very poor (Beauchamp & Childress, 2019).

How Much and to Whom?

If we accept that health care is a right or that society has an ethical obligation to provide healthcare services to vulnerable populations, then we must examine the question of how much health care should be provided and to whom. There are two broad views about the right to access to health care—some believe all people should have equal access health care, whereas others believe the right extends only to a basic level of health care. Consider the following case.

CASE PRESENTATION

Should Public Funds Pay for Extraordinary Procedures?

A middle-aged indigent woman with insulin-dependent diabetes mellitus demanded that Medicaid pay for a pancreas transplant. This patient was reported to be unco-operative in her previous diabetic regimen and disliked giving herself insulin injections. Even though Medicaid in that state had a fiscal policy that denied payment for this surgery to all program recipients, the state supreme court ruled that this woman had a right to the surgery because other people with insurance or adequate funds had access to the surgery. The decision was based on the principle of nondiscrimination.

Think About It
Decisions About Entitlements
- Do you think the patient had a "right" to this surgery? Why or why not?
- Should society (through taxes) pay for the surgery, even though the patient was known to be nonpartici-pative in her previous regimen? Why or why not?
- Should the government make arbitrary decisions permitting or prohibiting certain therapies?
- Do you think there were others who might have received benefits but were denied because of the extraordinary expense for this patient?
- What are the ethical implications of the court decision?
- What are the ethical arguments for and against the court decision?

Fair Distribution

The court's decision to require public payment for the pancreas transplant in the previous case study raises questions about the distribution of healthcare services. There are simply not enough resources to pay for all services for all people. Think about your household budget. If you have only $300 to spend on Christmas gifts for your three children and you also need to purchase groceries for the week and antibiotics for yourself, it would be foolish to spend $200 on a gift for one child. By doing that, you would ensure that your children would not be treated fairly, that you probably would not be eating very well for the next week, and that you would not feel well anyway because you could not afford your prescription medication. The same principle applies to healthcare dollars. The limited public budget must be divided among many interests. To maintain a functioning infrastructure, the government must ensure that public schools, highways, police, border security, national defense, Social Security, and other services in the public domain have a proportionate share of the total budget. Policymakers are charged with the difficult task of making equitable and rational decisions about the distribution of resources. Decisions must balance health care spending with other programs and must carefully avoid both extravagant excess spending and frugality that threatens the health of citizens.

Distribution of Resources

Limited healthcare dollars must be spent wisely. Several different criteria have been proposed to make distributive justice decisions. One method involves making judgments about the cost in relation to the predicted benefit. For example, we could question the practice of allowing patients in the last stages of terminal illness to monopolize limited and expensive intensive care beds, thus utilizing the most expensive kind of health care for the least benefit. Some propose that the best way to avoid making arbitrary decisions in these kinds of situations is to set mandatory guidelines. For example, some suggest that expensive therapies, such as dialysis or organ transplant, be reserved only for those below a certain age. A second method involves making judgments about the usefulness of given therapies. Some suggest that less costly therapies, such as immunizations, that are nearly guaranteed to help a large number of people should have priority over expensive therapies that benefit only a few people.

CASE PRESENTATION

COVID-19: A Crisis on Every Front

Although officials had been warned of the risk of emerging pandemics, to most people COVID-19 struck suddenly and without warning. Individuals, healthcare providers, hospitals, and the government were not ready to respond to a deadly and quickly spreading infectious disease affecting the global population. During the first year of the pandemic, there were shortages in critical supplies. Hospitals were overrun with sick and dying COVID-19 patients. Within a short time, nurses, physicians, and other healthcare staff were contracting the disease, while others were suffering from overwork and burnout. Patients with other critical illnesses either stayed home or waited for hours for emergency care—occasionally dying on the spot. There was a shortage of critical care beds, ventilators, masks, gloves, protective gowns, extracorporeal membrane oxygenation (ECMO) machines, and morgue space. Once diagnostic tests became available, there were shortages of swabs and reagent solution. Vaccines were developed, approved, and produced more quickly than ever before in history, but millions needed vaccine at once and it could not be produced and distributed quickly enough. When vaccines were finally available, there were scarce providers to administer them to the long lines of people who waited for hours—often without food or toilet facilities. Once treatments for COVID-19 were identified or developed, there were shortages of 29 of 40 critical medications (Paquin & Sanders, 2022). Some countries experienced a shortage of oxygen and India even reported a shortage of wood needed for funeral pyres (Colarossi, 2021). Individuals, hospitals, clinics, private medical offices, and government agencies scrambled to grab whatever was available. To make the crisis worse, the opinions of people around the world became ferociously divided and health policy became a daily public drama.

Think About It

- Many elderly COVID-19 patients occupied critical care beds during the early pandemic, sometimes for weeks, while other, younger patients, waited for the precious commodity. What ethical principle or guideline in the ANA, CNA, or ICN code of nursing ethics would assist in making decisions about distribution of critical care beds?

- In the United States, the first round of vaccines was distributed to nursing home residents and healthcare workers in most states. What rule of distributive justice supports this policy decision?

- One man, who chose not to be vaccinated contracted the disease, was hospitalized and quickly needed an ECMO machine. His daughter contacted 169 different hospitals before she found a machine available 1200 miles away. The man was transported by air and placed on the ECMO machine (Yan, 2021). The upper limit cost of ECMO and hospitalization can be as much as $500,000 (Lansink-Hartgring et al., 2021). Even the Hastings Center questioned vaccination status in decision making about triage and treatment of COVID-19 patients (Chuan et al., 2021). How does this case and the debate about vaccination status fit into your thoughts about distributive justice?

- When resources were scarce, some countries contemplated giving lower priority to COVID-19 patients who had chosen to be unvaccinated. What factors would you have taken into consideration when making decisions about distributing care between vaccinated and unvaccinated patients who had contracted the disease.

- What policies could the government put in place to prevent distributive justice crises such as the one described in this case presentation?

Theories of Justice

Distributive justice is based on morals and ethical principles. Several theories have been proposed to determine how resources and services should be distributed. Utilitarian, libertarian, communitarian, and egalitarian theories are examples of popular theories of justice. Because of society's fragmented beliefs about social justice, no single theory can be expected to bring coherence to the situation. Many countries seek the best possible health care for all citizens, while at the same time instituting cost containment programs. The US healthcare system promotes the ideal of equal access to health care while maintaining some aspects of free-market competition. The goals of superior, accessible, and affordable health care are very difficult to reach simultaneously. Pursuing one goal may cripple another (Beauchamp & Childress, 2019). Recognizing that no single theory will satisfy society by fulfilling all principles, we suggest that several theories of justice must be employed to satisfy competing social goals.

Utilitarian Theories

Generally based on the rule that it is good to maximize the "greatest good for the greatest number," utilitarian theories favor social programs that protect public health and distribute basic health care in a manner that maximizes the overall benefit. For example, with some exemptions and some recent current controversy, all states require children to be vaccinated when they enter public schools. Immunization is inexpensive and effective. Consider the case of polio, a disabling, potentially fatal, and uncurable infectious disease. In the 1940s polio outbreaks in the United States caused disabling disease to more than 35,000 people each year, with a death rate of 5 to 10 percent. The disease was especially prevalent among young children. Travel was sometimes restricted, quarantines were imposed, and thousands were crippled. Polio vaccines were developed and in the mid-1950s a widespread vaccination campaign began. Both children and adults were vaccinated. Most schools required polio vaccine, and by 1994 polio was declared eradicated from the Americas (The College of Physicians of Philadelphia, 2022). So, even if parents don't agree with immunizations, most states require them for the benefit of society as a whole. This is based on the belief that the outcome of these programs maximizes utility. Although utilitarian theories are the basis of many social programs, there are problems in their application. For example, because utilitarianism places aggregate social good before individual rights, social utility might be maximized by denying access to advanced health care for some of society's sickest and most vulnerable populations (Beauchamp & Childress, 2019).

Libertarian Theories

Libertarian theories propose that the just society protects the rights of property and liberty of each person, allowing citizens to improve their circumstances by their own effort. Libertarian theories support a private citizen's or group's right to own and manage a healthcare business. Libertarian theory does not classify health care as a right, but rather as a commodity that operates on the material principle of ability to pay. Strict libertarians view taxation as an unjust redistribution of private property but do not oppose other methods of distribution if they are freely chosen. Market strategies and managed competition are proposals in the United States that are influenced by libertarianism (Beauchamp & Childress, 2019).

CASE PRESENTATION

Rise in the Cost of Insulin

At the age of 24, Alec Smith was diagnosed with type 1 (insulin-dependent) diabetes. At that time, the cost of insulin and other supplies was $250 per month. When he was 26 years old, he was no longer eligible for his mother's health insurance. The insurance policy available to Alec had a $440 monthly premium and $7600 deductible. He couldn't afford insurance, so he decided to try to pay for his insulin out of pocket until he could save enough money to pay the insurance premiums and deductible. When Alec went to the pharmacy, he found that the cost of his insulin had risen to $1300 for a month's supply. Alec left the pharmacy without his insulin. He planned to make his remaining insulin last until he received his next paycheck. Alec was found dead of ketoacidosis, caused by lack of insulin, four days before payday (Rajkumar, 2020).

Think About It
Distributive Justice From the Personal Perspective

- How did you feel when you read the case presentation about Alec?
- How does Alec's situation fit into discussions of distributive justice?
- Do you know anyone who has needed to ration or forgo expensive medication?
- How would your thoughts about this situation differ if you were a legislator versus Alec's nurse?
- How does Alec's case apply to Libertarian theories of distributive justice?

Communitarian Theories

Communitarian theories place the community, rather than the individual, the state, the nation, or any other entity, at the center of the value system. Less fully developed than utilitarianism or libertarianism, communitarianism emphasizes the value of public good and maintains that values are rooted in communal practices. Communitarians believe that human life will be better if collective and public values guide people's lives. They have a commitment to facilities and practices designed to help members of the community develop their common lives and hence their personal lives (Honderich, 2005). Modern communitarian writers disagree on the application of these theories to healthcare access. Some propose a federation of interlinking community health programs that are democratically administered by citizen-members. In this model, each individual program would determine which benefits to provide, which care is most important, and whether expensive services will be included or excluded. Another communitarian theory holds that community tradition includes commitments of equal access to health care and suggests that as long as communal funds are spent, services must be equally available (Beauchamp & Childress, 2019).

Egalitarian Theories

Egalitarian theories are related to the concept of equality, in which people who are similarly situated should be treated similarly, though much depends on what kinds of similarity count as relevant and what constitutes similar treatment (Honderich, 2005). Promoting ideals of equal distribution of social benefits and burdens, egalitarian theories recognize the social obligation to eliminate or reduce barriers that prevent fair equality of opportunity. Egalitarian theories are cautiously formulated to avoid requiring equal sharing of all possible social benefits. A leading proponent of egalitarianism, John Rawls, suggested that in making decisions of justice, one should examine the situation behind a veil of ignorance. In Rawls's hypothetical situation, "no one knows his place in society, his class position or social status, nor does anyone know his fortune in the distribution of natural assets and abilities, his intelligence, strength, and the like" (Rawls, 1971, p. 567). This veil of ignorance ensures that no one will make decisions based on personal bias against the other person's characteristics. Supporters of Rawls's theory recognize a positive social obligation to eliminate or reduce barriers that prevent fair equality of opportunity and suggest that health policy formulated according to egalitarian principles would guarantee a safety net below which citizens would not be allowed to fall (Beauchamp & Childress, 2019).

ASK YOURSELF

Making Fair Decisions

- Which theory of distribution appeals to you as the most fair and equitable? Why?
- Do you think the theory you chose would be fair to all people in all circumstances?
- How could you combine two or more theories to make a system that is fair and equitable?

RECENT TRENDS AND HEALTH ECONOMIC ISSUES

Questions of ethics and distributive justice began to be discussed well before the 21st century. Claims that the United States was experiencing a crisis in healthcare economics have escalated in the last 50 years. Skyrocketing expenditures and a general tightening of healthcare dollars have resulted in fiscal scarcity. Both government and business have responded by attempting to gain control over expenditures. This economizing assumed a variety of forms, including managed care systems, prospective payment, Medicare and Medicaid cutbacks, and utilization review. Partially sacrificing a focus on the welfare of patients, healthcare corporations devised ways to cut costs, improve profits, increase efficiency, and branch out into more profitable ventures such as landscaping, catering, and laundry services.

Government was the prime mover of cost containment during the early 1980s. Because they had experienced virtually no incentives for cost controls up to that point, hospitals were unprepared in the 1980s when the government instituted the payment system for Medicare based on diagnosis-related groups (DRGs). DRGs totally restructured Medicare payment to hospitals. Whereas Medicare had paid hospitals based on their charges, the new DRG system paid hospitals a set amount for a specific diagnosis, regardless of the length of stay. This shift represented the first major change in the way hospitals were paid for Medicare patients because it placed the responsibility for efficiency and cost savings on hospitals and physicians. For example, before DRGs, many patients with low back pain were admitted to the hospital for up to two weeks for pelvic traction—a treatment with little scientific justification. This practice disappeared with DRGs.

Other cost-saving practices were established. Certificate-of-need programs at the state level were created to stop the building or purchasing of unnecessary and expensive technologies and capital construction. The Social Security Act provided for professional standards review organizations (PSROs) to promote effective, efficient, and economic delivery of healthcare services by assessing services to ensure that (1) the services are medically necessary, (2) services are provided in the most appropriate and economic facility, and (3) the quality of services meets professional standards (U.S. Social Security Administration, 2003). Similar to PSROs, peer review organizations (PROs) were established in 1982 to maintain and lower hospital admission rates, reduce lengths of stay, and ensure against inadequate treatment (Tax Equity and Fiscal Responsibility Act of 1982). PSROs and PROs require physicians to develop more efficient practice standards. By the early 1990s the healthcare system was in a state of disequilibrium. Large hospital corporations were finding ways to cut costs by eliminating support services, reducing waste, and eliminating nursing staff positions. Many small rural hospitals closed because of the financial strain. Inherent problems were unsolved. Care remained excellent for some, but inaccessible to many.

Economic influences also arose from outside the healthcare system. Two of the major outside influences were increased malpractice litigation and employment-negotiated health insurance plans. Malpractice litigation resulting in huge awards, and the subsequent birth of defensive medicine added to the expense of the system. As a result, a higher standard of medical care was established. Whereas the standard of medical care had traditionally been established at the community level, scientific invention; medical technology; specialization; Medicare and Medicaid; and regional heart, cancer, and stroke centers required nationalized, very high standards of care for physicians. This resulted in the routine practice of ordering batteries of (often unnecessary) diagnostic tests to meet new, stricter standards. Fearing malpractice lawsuits, physicians lost a measure of the autonomy that would previously have allowed them to choose only the diagnostic tests they thought were appropriate.

Employment-negotiated insurance plans fueled the practice of overspending and added to these pressures. Negotiated as part of employment contracts, many health insurance plans featured full coverage of healthcare costs with no deductible. As a result, a large percentage of patients did not pay directly for any healthcare services; thus, the cost of the doctor or hospital was rendered irrelevant (Califano, 1986). Everyone expected the most and the best. Because patients did not pay for healthcare services directly, they were much more likely to use more of them, even services that were marginally helpful or duplicated services they already had. Hospitals and physicians were more than happy to participate. Some physicians took advantage of the system by focusing on services that maximized their income. Hospitals purchased the latest and best medical equipment and encouraged physicians to order expensive tests. For hospitals and doctors alike, maximizing services resulted in increased income. This trend contributed to even higher standards of care that required very aggressive diagnosis and treatment, resulted in greater costs, and opened the door for more malpractice litigation. Increased healthcare delivery and costs produced an unsustainable spiral.

Healthcare Reform

The President's Commission on the Health Needs of the Nation (1953) concluded that access to health care is a basic human right, and the President's Commission for the Study of Ethical Problems in Medicine and Biomedical and Behavioral Research (1983) concluded that "society has an ethical obligation to ensure equitable access to health care for all. This obligation rests on the special importance of health care: its role in relieving suffering, preventing premature death, restoring functioning, increasing opportunity, providing information about an individual's condition, and giving evidence of mutual empathy and compassion. Furthermore, although life-style and the environment can affect health status, differences in the need for health care are for the most part undeserved and not within an individual's control" (p. 4). Even considering the 1983 President's Commission Report, the US federal government continued to face polarizing political controversy over various attempts to implement comprehensive healthcare legislation. Recognizing problems in the healthcare delivery system and sensing a groundswell of public support, the Clinton administration devised a healthcare reform proposal. Unveiled in the fall of 1993, this proposal called for universal access to health care through managed competition. It also described a system of financing that would be accomplished primarily through mandated coverage at places of employment, with employers required to pay a large percentage of the premiums. Subsidies were planned for small businesses, and the federal government assumed the employer responsibility for persons who were not covered by employer-based plans. After months of highly publicized debate, the Clinton health care reform proposal was defeated. Managed care was the only piece that emerged unscathed from Clinton's healthcare reform proposal. Existing as a small part of the US healthcare system for several decades, managed care gained prominence as a preferred method of delivery and financing of healthcare services.

CASE PRESENTATION

Cultivating Business

Lakeview is a small town of 25,000 people. The town has two competing community hospitals: Memorial Hospital and General Hospital. Memorial Hospital has owned a magnetic resonance imaging (MRI) machine for several years. This MRI machine served the needs of the people of Lakeview, and the charges were reasonable. For instance, whereas the cost of an MRI of the knee ranged from $800 to $4800 around the United States, Memorial Hospital charged $1000. Physicians wanted to be able to order MRIs for their patients, so they chose to send them to Memorial Hospital. Physicians are the customers of hospitals—hospitals carefully cultivate relationships with physicians because physicians bring along their patients. The General Hospital board of directors became aware that the Memorial MRI machine was drawing physicians and patients away from General Hospital. So, they procured a loan for $400,000 to purchase a new state-of-the-art MRI machine with more sophisticated capabilities than the older machine at Memorial Hospital. Physicians were pleased with the new machine and began sending their patients to General Hospital. But the cost of the machine was so high that General Hospital set the price of an MRI of the knee at $3000—three times higher than Memorial Hospital. As time passed, fewer patients had MRIs at Memorial Hospital, so to cover their expenses, Memorial Hospital had to raise the price of an MRI of the knee to $2000. General Hospital enjoyed the influx of patients and money, but the hospital continued to experience budget restraints. Knowing that their MRI machine was a great money maker, they increased the price of an MRI of the knee to $4000. Fifty miles away, Willow Garden Hospital was performing knee MRIs for $890. As is the usual custom in the United States, patients did not know the cost of the procedure in advance.

Jody is a 25-year-old college student who maintains a part-time, minimum-wage job at a small florist shop. She has no savings, and her parents, who are middle-class wage earners, took out a loan to pay for her college education. Her parents also pay $1000 monthly premiums for their health insurance policy that has an $8000 deductible. On a weekend trip, Jody slipped and injured her right knee and was unable to walk. The physician at the local urgent care center referred her to an orthopedist, who ordered an MRI at General Hospital. Jody had to borrow $500 to pay the two physicians. She has no funds to cover her $8000 deductible. If she knew about the price difference, she could go to Willow Garden Hospital.

Think About It

Are High Costs Ethical? Fair? Necessary?

- What are the ethical implications of wildly different hospital charges?
- What are the ethical implications of exorbitant costs for common procedures or medications?
- Should a patient be able to know the cost of a test at the different facilities?
- Should physicians consider cost when ordering tests?
- Are there any actions a nurse could take in this type of situation?
- Imagine that you are a lawmaker. What types of legislation might you devise to correct the situation?
- Imagine you are a hospital administrator at General Hospital in charge of ensuring the financial success of the facility. How should you react when approached by a local television news producer who asks for a list of charges of common procedures and tests?
- As this book goes to press, the US Congress and the Administration are continuing to advance efforts to require hospitals to comply with the Transparency in Coverage: Requirements for Public Disclosure (2020) and make their prices publicly available. How can nurses support the government in their efforts to make costs transparent?

There continued to be a global crisis of healthcare access in the early 21st century. Millions of people in the United States and billions of people worldwide continued to have limited access to healthcare services, often because of a lack of health insurance coverage. The uninsured population in the United States grew rapidly. In 1982 there were an estimated 32 million uninsured citizens. By 2010 the number of uninsured had swelled to 46.5 million, which constituted 17.8 percent of the population (Tolbert et al., 2022).

To solve the problem of inaccessible health care for uninsured indigent people, piecemeal and incremental efforts by disparate public and private groups moved toward relieving the problem of healthcare access. A network of free clinics was established to serve the indigent in all 50 states. In 2023 there were more than 1400 free and charitable clinics that served the uninsured and underinsured patients, donating billions of dollars in healthcare services (National Association of Free & Charitable Clinics, 2023). Registered nurses and nurse practitioners provide much of the care delivered in the nation's free clinics.

President Barack Obama sponsored a new plan for health reform in the United States. The bill passed both houses of Congress, and on March 23, 2010, President Obama signed the *Patient Protection and Affordable Care Act* (ACA) into law. The law reformed some aspects of public and private health insurance, increased coverage for preexisting conditions, and expanded access to insurance for more than 30 million Americans. Although the ACA addressed many problems that had plagued healthcare system in the United States, passage of the law was not the end of the story. Health care reform continued to be a controversial partisan issue. During his presidential campaign, Donald Trump promised to repeal the ACA. On his first day in office, he issued an executive order intended to reverse implementation of the law. Although the ACA remained largely intact during the Trump's administration, several features were eliminated. For example, the individual mandate that required all uninsured to purchase insurance was repealed. Subsequently, millions of people suddenly dropped their insurance, which resulted in healthcare facilities bearing the financial burden of uninsured care and higher cost premiums for those who maintained insurance coverage (Gusmano et al., 2021). Even with the high number of people dropping out of the program when the individual mandate was lifted, the ACA proved to be successful. The number of uninsured in the United States dropped from a high of 46.5 million in 2010 to 27.5 million in 2021 (Tolbert et al., 2022).

Aside from the ACA, government and private organizations have initiated numerous strategies to improve health care while reducing costs. Nurses should maintain a broad, nonpartisan appreciation for the importance of cost-effective strategies and must participate in ensuring their success. Following are some strategies that have been put in place to reduce healthcare spending while improving health:

- **Wellness incentives**. Some third-party payers initiated incentives to improve wellness and prevent illness. Health insurance and corporate websites describe wellness incentives that include wellness visits, wellness-center membership, tobacco cessation services, medication adherence programs, and weight reduction activities. Incentives to participate in these programs can take many forms, including vouchers, gift cards, discounts on health insurance premiums, free biometric screening, bonuses, raffles for all-expense paid trips, free Weight Watchers membership, flex benefit credits, and reimbursement for fitness club memberships.

- **Choosing Wisely**. Choosing Wisely is an educational campaign that asks healthcare providers to reduce or eliminate unnecessary health care. Providers are encouraged to avoid unnecessary tests, treatments, and procedures to those that are supported by research evidence, are free from harm, are truly necessary, and do not duplicate other tests or procedures already done. Choosing Wisely focuses on inappropriate medication use, unnecessary laboratory tests, unwarranted maternity care interventions, unwarranted diagnostic procedures, inappropriate nonpalliative services at the end of life, unwarranted procedures, unnecessary consultations, preventable emergency department visits and hospitalizations, and potentially harmful preventive services with no health benefits (American Board of Internal Medicine, 2019).

- **Complex care management**. Super-utilizers are patients who bounce from emergency department to emergency department and from hospital to hospital seeking care. These people may have complex physical, behavioral, or social needs. But their healthcare utilization turns out to be astronomically costly, chaotic, and ineffective. Studies have found that super-utilizers consume an amazing disproportion of healthcare expenditures. Medicare and Medicaid programs, hospitals, and communities are focused on finding more efficient and effective ways to identify and engage with these high-cost individuals. Targeted, intense case management of super-utilizers leads to reductions in unnecessary and inappropriate emergency and hospital use and fosters connections with less costly community-based resources (Weiner et al., 2017). Complex case management has shown great promise. One study demonstrated that complex case management resulted in decreased total medical expenditures, fewer inpatient hospital days, and fewer specialist visits (Powers et al., 2020).

- **Patient-centered medical homes**. Many patients move from provider to provider and from specialist to specialist with no coordination of care. This leads to fragmented expensive care with the potential for both duplication of services and gaps in care. The patient-centered medical home focuses on patient-centered, coordinated, accessible, continuous, and comprehensive primary care with a focus on quality and safety. With this model, a patient chooses or is assigned to a primary care provider who coordinates care across all health systems. When care is coordinated at the primary care level, high-cost services such as emergency room visits, unnecessary specialist appointments, and hospitalizations are reduced (AHRQ, 2021).

- **Accountable care organizations (ACOs)**. ACOs consist of groups of doctors, nurse practitioners, hospitals, and other healthcare providers who voluntarily agree to share responsibility for the healthcare delivery and outcomes of a defined population. The goal of ACOs is to make sure patients get the right care at the right time, avoid duplication of services, and prevent medical errors (Center for Medicare and Medicaid Services, 2022). Quality goals such as weight loss or control of blood sugar are defined and measured. When an ACO achieves its goals, it shares in the cost savings. ACOs are good for patients because they force providers to be accountable for improved patient outcomes and are good for providers because they offer monetary incentives. ACOs save Medicare hundreds of millions of dollars each year (Kaiser Health News, 2020).

- **Home- and community-based services** (HCBS). HCBS address the needs of people who have functional limitations and those who need assistance with everyday activities such as dressing or bathing. HCBS can prevent the elderly from entering nursing homes or other types of institutional settings. Proponents suggest that it is more effective and less costly than other types of care. A variety of healthcare services can be provided including skilled nursing care; occupational, speech, and physical therapy; dietary management by a registered dietician, and pharmacy services. HCBS can also include durable medical equipment, case management, personal care, and hospice care (Centers for Medicare & Medicaid Services, 2022b).

- **Antifraud strategies**. Healthcare fraud and abuse cost the public billions of dollars annually. The Center for Medicare and Medicaid Services (CMS) has an antifraud campaign that includes penalties to punish those who commit fraud, improved screening and enrollment requirements for providers, and better coordination of fraud prevention efforts. Examples of fraud include billing for services at a higher level of complexity than actually provided, billing for services or supplies that were not furnished, ordering medically unnecessary items or services for patients, and billing for missed appointments. New technology to rapidly identify fraudulent billing patterns is coupled with tough new rules and penalties for those who commit fraud. Healthcare providers found guilty of fraud can experience civil and monetary penalties; criminal proceedings and incarceration; exclusion from participating in all federal healthcare programs in the future; and loss of professional licensure (Center for Medicare & Medicaid Services, 2021).

- **Managed care**. Managed care reduces the cost of health care through the elimination of redundant facilities and services. Managed care integrates healthcare delivery and financing and attempts to control costs by modifying the behavior of providers and patients. Managed care moves away from a system based on patient and provider autonomy. Managed care organizations create policies that dictate aspects of healthcare delivery such as provider networks, medication formularies, utilization management, and financial incentives that influence how and where a patient receives their medical care. There are four basic types of managed care organizations: health maintenance organizations (HMOs), preferred provider organizations (PPOs), point-of-service (POS) plans, and exclusive provider organizations (EPO). HMOs are the most restrictive type of managed care, requiring members to select a primary care physician. HMOs typically require a referral before a patient sees a specialist or other physician. HMOs usually only pay for care within the provider network. PPOs usually allow members to receive care out of their network, but the member must pay more if they use a non-network provider. POS plans have features that are similar to both HMOs and PPOs. Like HMOs, POS plans usually require members to have primary care physicians. Like PPOs, POS plans allow members to go out of network for care. They must pay more for an out-of-network provider than they would for a network provider. Premiums for

PPO and POS plans are usually higher than those for HMO plans. EPO allow patients to choose their in-network providers but are not required to establish a primary care provider and receive referrals. Out-of-network expenses are not covered by EPOs. Each of these four types of managed care organizations has been shown to save money and improve outcomes (Heaton & Tadi, 2022).

- **Inflation Reduction Act** of 2022 (IRA). The IRA includes several health provisions to reduce healthcare costs. One of the most important provisions lowers prescription drug costs for Medicare recipients. Until 2022 Medicare was prohibited from negotiating prescription drug prices with manufacturers, which led to soaring prices, far above other countries. The IRA permits Medicare to negotiate prescription drug prices, which will enable Medicare to offer enhanced coverage to seniors. Specific provisions in the IRA that lower costs will be rolled in over three years and include the following: (1) a cap of $35 per month on insulin costs with no deductible for insulin; (2) elimination of cost-sharing during the catastrophic phase of healthcare coverage; (3) a yearly cap for prescription medication at $2000 per year; and (4) the ability to budget prescription medication costs over 12 months (Centers for Medicare & Medicaid Services, 2022a). Although changes mandated by the IRA focus on seniors, policy discussions continue.

SUMMARY

Because health care is a scarce resource, citizens rely on social institutions to make fair and equitable distributive justice decisions. There is little consensus on basic ethical questions such as: Who should receive healthcare resources? Is there a right to basic health care? How much should be spent on particular healthcare services? What percentage of the society's overall resources should be invested in health care? Utilitarianism, libertarianism, communitarianism, and egalitarianism are theories that attempt to describe fair means of distributing resources. Recent focus on problems related to the economic aspects of the healthcare delivery system of the United States has prompted debate on practical issues of distributive justice. A number of strategies have emerged from the struggle to reform the healthcare system. While moving from a traditional system that valued patient and provider autonomy to a system that values

the economic delivery of health care to broader populations, close attention must be paid to ethical standards in health care. Nurses have a responsibility to participate in formulating and supporting economic policies in health care that meets the goals outlined in codes of nursing ethics.

CHAPTER HIGHLIGHTS

- The traditional healthcare system in the United States is fee-for-service.
- Within a fee-for-service system, there is a strong focus on the principle of autonomy.
- Justice relates to fair, equitable, and appropriate treatment in light of what is due or owed to persons and recognizes that giving to some will deny receipt to others who might otherwise have received these things.
- Distributive justice is the fair, equitable, and appropriate distribution of benefits and burdens. Theories of distributive justice seek to render diverse principles coherent.
- Utilitarian theories are based on the rule that it is good to maximize the greatest good for the greatest number.
- Libertarian theories propose that the just society protects the rights of property and liberty of each person, allowing citizens to improve their circumstances by their own effort.
- Communitarian theories place the community—rather than the individual, the state, the nation, or any other entity—at the center of the value system.
- Egalitarian theories are related to the concept of equality in which people who are similarly situated should be treated similarly.
- Scarcity of healthcare resources has led to a rethinking of the structure of healthcare economics.
- Healthcare reform has introduced several strategies to improve healthcare access and quality while controlling costs.

DISCUSSION QUESTIONS AND ACTIVITIES

1. Read the Summary of Conclusions of the 1983 President's Commission for the Study of Ethical Problems in Medicine and Biomedical and Behavioral Research on the following website:

https://repository.library.georgetown.edu/bitstream/handle/10822/559375/securing_access.pdf?sequence=1&isAllowed=y. Discuss ways that the federal government has attempted to respond to the report.

2. Read Article 25 of the United Nations 1948 *Declaration of Human Rights* at http://www.un.org/en/universal-declaration-human-rights/. List current private national and international efforts toward ensuring this right.

3. Visit America's Health Insurance Plans online at http://www.ahip.org/ to find out current perspective on various economic and policy issues.

4. Discuss current problems in healthcare economics with classmates. Is there a consensus regarding root causes, the right to health care, or the role of the government as a payer for healthcare services?

5. Conduct an Internet search for a lay definition of the free-market system of economics. How do various economic aspects of the US healthcare system differ from basic free-market systems?

6. Discuss the influence of utilitarian theory on the economics of the current healthcare system.

7. Why do patient and provider autonomy affect healthcare delivery and financing?

8. Define *distributive justice*. In class, discuss the material rules of distributive justice. Which material rule do you think is fair and equitable? Which material rule is most popular among classmates?

9. Discuss healthcare ethics as they relate to strategies listed in this chapter that help reduce healthcare costs.

10. Discuss your opinion about healthcare reform efforts with classmates. Do opinions of your classmates seem to be based on a rational assessment of healthcare financing and quality, or are they based on partisan beliefs?

11. Explore the Healthcare Bluebook website for wide variations in the price of various procedures. The site can be found at https://www.healthcarebluebook.com/ui/consumerfront.

REFERENCES

AHRQ. (2021). *Defining the PCMH*. https://pcmh.ahrq.gov/page/defining-pcmh

American Board of Internal Medicine. (2019). *Choosing wisely*. https://abimfoundation.org/what-we-do/choosing-wisely

ANA. (2015). *Code of ethics for nurses with interpretive statements*. Nursebooks.org. http://nursingworld.org/DocumentVault/Ethics-1/Code-of-Ethics-for-Nurses.html.

Beauchamp, T. L., & Childress, J. (2019). *Principles of biomedical ethics* (8th ed.). Oxford University Press.

Califano, J. A., Jr. (1986). *America's health care revolution: Who lives? Who dies? Who pays?*. Oxford Univesity Press.

Center for Medicare & Medicaid Services. (2021). *Medicare fraud & abuse: Prevent, detect, report*. https://www.cms.gov/Outreach-and-Education/Medicare-Learning-Network-MLN/MLNProducts/Downloads/Fraud-Abuse-MLN4649244.pdf

Center for Medicare and Medicaid Services. (2022). *Accountable care organizations (ACOs)*. https://www.cms.gov/medicare/medicare-fee-for-service-payment/aco

Centers for Medicare & Medicaid Services. (2022a). *Fact Sheet: The inflation reduction act lowers health care costs for millions of Americans*. https://www.cms.gov/newsroom/fact-sheets/inflation-reduction-act-lowers-health-care-costs-millions-americans

Centers for Medicare & Medicaid Services. (2022b). *Home- and community-based services*. https://www.cms.gov/outreach-and-education/american-indian-alaska-native/aian/ltss-ta-center/info/hcbs

Chuan, V. T., Lower, A. E., Ferdinand, A. O., Liang, T. H., & Wynia, M. (2021). Should covid vaccination status be used to make triage decisions? *Hastings Bioethics Forum*. https://www.thehastingscenter.org/should-covid-vaccination-status-be-used-to-make-triage-decisions/.

CNA. (2017). *Code of ethics for registered nurses*. https://cdn1.nscn.ca/sites/default/files/documents/resources/code-of-ethics-for-registered-nurses.pdf#:~:text=The%20Canadian%20Nurses%20Association%20%28CNA%29%20Code%20of%20Ethics,receiving%20care.%20The%20Codeis%20both%20aspirational%20and%20regulatory.

Colarossi, N. (2021). India reports shortage of wood needed for funeral pyres as COVID deaths surpass 234K. *Newsweek*. https://www.newsweek.com/india-reports-shortage-wood-needed-funeral-pyres-covid-deaths-surpass-234k-1589571.

Gusmano, M. K., Sparer, M. S., & Brown, L. D. (2021). Trump v. the ACA. *Health Economics, Policy, and Law, 16*(3), 251–255. https://pubmed.ncbi.nlm.nih.gov/33138884/.

Hayek, F. A. (1960). The case for freedom: *The constitution of liberty*. University of Chicago Press. https://fee.org/articles/the-case-for-freedom/.

Heaton, J., & Tadi, P. (2022). *Managed care organization*. National Library of Medicine. https://www.ncbi.nlm.nih.gov/books/NBK557797/.

Honderich, T. (2005). *The Oxford companion to philosophy* (2nd ed.). Oxford University Press.

ICN. (2021). *The ICN code of ethics for nurses.* https://www.icn.ch/system/files/2021-10/ICN_Code-of-Ethics_EN_Web_0.pdf

Inflation Reduction Act of 2022 (2022). https://www.congress.gov/bill/117th-congress/house-bill/5376/text.

Transparency in coverage: Requirements for public disclosure, 45 C.F.R. § 147.212 (2020). https://www.federalregister.gov/documents/2020/11/12/2020-24591/transparency-in-coverage.

Kaiser Health News. (2020). *Medicare's ACO program, which offers doctors, hospitals rewards for better care, saved $749M last year.* https://khn.org/morning-breakout/medicares-aco-program-which-offers-doctors-hospitals-rewards-for-better-care-saved-740m-last-year/.

Lansink-Hartgring, A. O., van Minnen, O., Vermeulen, K. M., & van den Bergh, W. M. (2021). Hospital costs of extracorporeal membrane oxygenation in adults: A systematic review. *PharmacoEconomics, 5*(4), 613–623. https://doi.org/10.1007/s41669-021-00272-9.

National Association of Free & Charitable Clinics. (2023). *Building a health America, one person at a time.* https://nafcclinics.org/#:~:text=The%20National%20Association%20of%20Free,Charitable%20Pharmacies%20that%20serve%20them.

Paquin, T., & Sanders, D. (2022). To protect the medical supply chain, 'made in America' will be the key. *STAT.* https://www.statnews.com/2022/12/14/made-in-america-protect-medical-supply-chain/#:~:text=In%20the%20first%20year%20of,of%20essential%20medicines%20quickly%20arose.

Powers, B. W., Modarai, F., SPalakodeti, S., Sharma, M., Mehta, N., Jain, S. H., & Garg, V. (2020). Impact of complex care management on spending and utilization for high-need, high-cost Medicaid patients. *American Journal of Managed Care, 26*(2), 57–63.

President's Commission for the Study of Ethical Problems in Medicine and Biomedical and Behavioral Research. (1983). *Securing access to health care: A report on the ethical implications of differences in the availability of health services.* https://repository.library.georgetown.edu/bitstream/handle/10822/559375/securing_access.pdf?sequence=1&isAllowed=y

President's Commission on the Health Needs of the Nation. (1953). *The contribution of health education in meeting the health needs of the nation.* U.S.S.O. Documents. https://catalog.hathitrust.org/Record/001558303

Rajkumar, S. V. (2020). The high cost of insulin in the United States: An urgent call to action. *Mayo Clinic Proceedings, 95*(1), 22–28. https://doi.org/10.1016/j.mayocp.2019.11.013.

Rawls, J. (1971). A theory of justice In J. Feinberg (Ed.), *Reason and responsibility: Some readings in basic problems of philosophy* (pp. 567–572). Wadsworth.

Tax Equity and Fiscal Responsibility Act of 1982, 97th Congress (1982). https://www.congress.gov/bill/97th-congress/house-bill/4961.

The College of Physicians of Philadelphia. (2022). *Polio.* https://historyofvaccines.org/history/polio/overview.

Tolbert, J., Drake, P., & Damico, A. (2022). *Key facts about the uninsured population.* Kaiser Family Foundation. https://www.kff.org/uninsured/issue-brief/key-facts-about-the-uninsured-population/.

U.S. Const. Amend. I-X.

U.S. Social Security Administration. (2003). *Program operations manual systems.* https://secure.ssa.gov/poms.nsf/lnx/0600208080.

United Nations. (1948/2015). *Universal declaration of human rights.* http://www.un.org/en/udhrbook/pdf/udhr_booklet_en_web.pdf.

von Platz, J. (2020). *Theories of distributive justice: Who gets what and why.* Routledge. https://doi.org/10.4324/9780429318788.

Weiner, J. M., Romaire, M., Thach, N., Collins, A., Kim, K., Pan, H., Chiri, G., Sommers, A., Haber, S., Musumeci, M., & Paradise, J. (2017). *Strategies to reduce Medicaid spending: Findings from a literature review.* Medicaid. https://www.kff.org/report-section/strategies-to-reduce-medicaid-spending-findings-from-a-literature-review-issue-brief/.

Yan, H. (2021). After 169 hospitals, a dad finally got the Covid-19 care he needed – And changed dozens of skeptics's minds. *CNN Health.* https://www.cnn.com/2021/09/19/health/florida-man-inspires-covid-vaccinations/index.html.

16

Nursing Ethics, Social Issues, and Health Disparities

What we are doing is just a drop in the ocean, but if that drop was not in the ocean ... the ocean would be less because of that missing drop.

(Mother Teresa)

OBJECTIVES

After completing this chapter, the reader should be able to:

1. Explain how the social determinates of health are fundamental causes of health disparities, particularly among disadvantaged and vulnerable groups.
2. Discuss the scope of health disparities that result from poverty, food insecurity, homelessness, sexual violence, human trafficking, an increasing elderly population, and racism and ethnic inequities.
3. Discuss the practical application of nursing codes of ethics for nurses caring and advocating for people affected by social disparities.
4. Apply the concept of justice to vulnerable populations, elaborating on the implications for society and the healthcare system.
5. Discuss the application of beneficence and nonmaleficence to vulnerable groups in light of today's healthcare system.
6. Identify considerations related to promoting autonomy for healthcare decision making among vulnerable populations.

INTRODUCTION

Health can be significantly determined by social factors. The World Health Organization (WHO) defines social determinants of health as "the non-medical factors that influence health outcomes. They are the conditions in which people are born, grow, work, live, and age, and the wider set of forces and systems shaping the conditions of daily life" (WHO, 2023b). The social determinants of health can be the fundamental cause of health disparities, particularly among disadvantaged and vulnerable groups. Nurses come face to face with the consequences of social disparities every day. Codes of nursing ethics specifically refer to nurses' responsibility in relation to the social determinants of health. For example, the ICN states "nurses recognize the significance of the social determinates of health. They contribute to, and advocate for, policies and programmes that address them" (2021, p. 18). The CNA states that nurses are responsible for "Recognizing the significance of social determinants of health and advocating for policies and programs that address them...." (CNA, 2017, p. 18). The ANA (2015) is more specific stating "Structural, social, and institutional inequalities and disparities exacerbate the incidence and burden of illness, trauma, suffering, and premature death" (p. 32). Further, ANA proposes that nurses "educate the public; facilitate informed choice; identify conditions and circumstances that contribute to illness, injury, and disease; foster healthy life styles; and participate in institutional and legislative efforts to protect and promote health. Nurses collaborate to address barriers to health—poverty, homelessness, unsafe living conditions, abuse and violence, and lack of access...." (ANA, 2015, p. 32). Therefore, codes of nursing ethics specify nurses' responsibilities to address social determinants of health at the bedside, in the community, and in the larger society.

The WHO established five categories of the social determinants of health, each of which includes a broad spectrum of specific issues. The five categories are economic stability; education access and quality; healthcare access and quality; neighborhood and built environment; and social and community context. Every day, nurses come face to face with patients suffering from problems related to the social issues within these categories. These issues may create conflicts in values and ethical dilemmas that must be addressed to determine appropriate healthcare interventions. A number of the specific problems in each category are of special concern to healthcare providers, and many have been introduced in the "Ask Yourself and Think About It" exercises throughout this book. This chapter focuses on seven selected examples of social determinates of health that fall into the two broad WHO health disparities categories of economic stability and social and community context. Issues discussed in this chapter include poverty, food insecurity, homelessness, sexual violence, human trafficking, an expanding elderly population, and racial and ethnic inequities. Each of these social issues is reviewed in this chapter, along with reminders to readers of the dominant guiding ethical principles that can inform nursing care.

POVERTY

Poverty is a global problem. The United Nations (UN) defines poverty as a daily income of less than $1.90 per day. The UN estimates that worldwide poverty, which had been declining slowly in recent years, increased in 2020 due to the pandemic, global conflict, and climate change (United Nations Department of Economic and Social Affairs, 2023). Likewise, based on the raw data and federally established thresholds, the number of impoverished in the United States increased substantially in 2020 and slightly more during 2021 (Creamer et al., 2022; Office of Disease Prevention and Health Promotion, 2020). Poverty is more likely in communities with a higher percentage of individuals in certain racial and ethnic groups and in rural areas (Office of Disease Prevention and Health Promotion, 2020). In the United States, children, women, the disabled, those with lower education levels, noncitizens, and those who live in the south are more likely to suffer from poverty (Creamer et al., 2022). Children have the highest rate of poverty of any age group and, unfortunately, those who grow up in poverty are more likely to experience poverty as adults, thus perpetuating generational cycles of poverty (Office of Disease Prevention and Health Promotion, 2020).

Healthcare access is influenced more and more by the self-perpetuating loop of poverty which leads to illness and illness which leads to unemployment, which further increases poverty and the likelihood of illness. Access to health care is also influenced by limitations in employer-sponsored health insurance, unemployment, lack of access to available programs, and the high cost of health insurance. This remains a problem, even under the Affordable Care Act. In 2021 the total number of uninsured people in the United States was 27.5 million (Tolbert et al., 2022). Due to shifts in governmental budget priorities and changes in federal and state guidelines, a publicly financed healthcare system for medically indigent adults has become available to fewer people in recent years. Low-income individuals and families are more likely to be uninsured, and young adults, people of color, men, and noncitizens are at a higher risk for being uninsured (Cohen et al., 2022; Kaiser Family Foundation, 2022). Among people of color, Hispanics are the most likely to be uninsured, followed by non-Hispanic Blacks. Contrary to popular belief, the vast majority of uninsured people live in households with at least one employed person. Uninsured rates among the non-elderly indigent in the United States vary wildly, ranging from 4.7 percent in Massachusetts to 33 percent in Texas (Kaiser Family Foundation, 2021). Contrary to this data, many people in the United States believe the myth that all people below the poverty level have access to government-sponsored healthcare coverage. This is far from the truth.

Publicly funded healthcare programs such as Medicare, Medicaid, the Medicaid Children's Health Insurance Program, Veteran's Health Administration, and the Indian Health Service are all **categorical health insurance programs**. This means that publicly funded health insurance programs are restricted to certain categories of people (the elderly, children, veterans, and so forth). Poverty alone does not establish eligibility for these programs. Individuals who do not fit within well-prescribed categories, even though their income is below the poverty level, must do without health care altogether or search for privately administered healthcare delivery systems, such as free clinics, that provide care at no cost. Without healthcare coverage, the poor often postpone needed health care or cope with public clinics that are often impersonal and degrading. For this reason, many people living below the poverty level do not participate in basic preventive care programs and end up at healthcare facilities in desperate circumstances when catastrophic illness or injury occurs.

Poverty and widening income inequality increase health disparities. Poverty is known to have a negative impact on both the health of individuals and the utilization of healthcare services (Berman et al., 2018; Francis et al., 2018; Weeks, 2018). Poorer people are sicker than people with adequate financial resources. Poverty results in shorter life expectancy, higher infant mortality rate, and higher death rates for the leading causes of death, which in 2021 included heart disease, cancer, COVID-19, unintentional injuries, stroke, chronic lower respiratory diseases, Alzheimer's disease, diabetes, chronic liver disease, and kidney disease (America Academy of Family Physicians, 2021; Xu et al., 2022). Individuals living in poverty also have a higher incidence of obesity, smoking, substance use, chronic stress, disability, and violent injury.

Poverty is detrimental to the health of all individuals living with inadequate resources, and it also produces a next generation of citizens with more health problems than usual. Children living in poverty have a higher incidence of conditions associated with neglect, trauma, poor nutrition, drugs, burns, mental illness, HIV infection, poor social-emotional development, inadequate exercise, and diseases from environmental factors such as parasites, vermin, and lead exposure (Berman et al., 2018; Child Trends Data Bank, 2023; Cree et al., 2018; Kyunghee & Liangliang, 2022; Maguire-Jack & Sattler, 2023). Children in poverty are more likely to grow up with chronic illnesses that require extensive healthcare resources. Overall, poverty and health are inextricably enmeshed.

Nurses must be mindful of possible poverty-related issues. Patients who are impoverished will likely have problems with return visits due to travel expenses. They may not be able to pay for prescribed medication, therapeutic diets, recommended follow-up treatments, or further diagnostic testing. Because poverty is closely associated with educational level, nurses should be alert for illiteracy. Illiterate patients are often embarrassed and hesitant to tell their nurses that they cannot read

instructions for discharge care, follow-up appointments, or prescription medications. Nursing assessments should also include questions related to basic human needs such as food, shelter, and safety. For instance, an uninsured indigent patient should never be discharged with a prescription for an exorbitantly expensive medication and no reasonable plan for filling the prescription. Identifying issues of poverty enables nurses to advocate for patients by connecting them with sources of assistance such as free clinics and charity organizations or advocating for them when their physicians or nurse practitioners order costly medications or follow-up care. Expensive tests, treatments, and medications often have less costly alternatives and providers may be happy to substitute these rather than allow their patients to forgo treatment.

FOOD INSECURITY

Food insecurity and hunger are closely linked to poverty. **Food insecurity** refers to an economic and social condition in which a household has limited or uncertain access to adequate food. Food insecurity is most often sporadic, occurring only a few months or weeks each year. **Hunger** refers to a physiological response in an individual that may result from food insecurity. Hunger related to food insecurity is prolonged and involuntary and causes discomfort, illness, weakness, or pain and exceeds the usual uneasy sensation (USDA, 2022). Food insecurity and hunger are closely related but do not always occur together. According to the US Department of Agriculture, in 2021 about 34 million people, including five million children, lived in households that experienced food insecurity. Rates of food insecurity are higher in households with children, particularly those living in poverty; and within Black- and Hispanic-led households, single-parent households, and households of persons living alone (USDA, 2022). In ongoing research focused on seniors, Ziliak and Gunderson (2022) found that certain groups had significantly higher rates of food insecurity than others. Older individuals more likely to have food insecurity are those who are poor, Black and/or Hispanic, single, rural, unemployed, disabled, female, nonveteran, or disabled.

Hunger and poor nutrition related to food insecurity are public health issues that have a significant effect on health and health outcomes across the life span. In *children*, lack of sufficient healthy food intake is associated with health issues such as higher risk for birth defects; overall diminished physical and cognitive health; anemia; greater incidence of cognitive, educational, and developmental delays; higher hospitalization rates; school absenteeism; poor general health (including conditions such as asthma, depression, and behavioral problems); poor oral health; and greater risk of being exposed to violence in their homes (Francis et al., 2018; Gundersin & Ziliak, 2015; Murthy, 2016; Pai & Bahadur, 2020). For *nonsenior adults*, decreased nutrient intake related to food insecurity is associated with health issues such as overall poor-to-fair health, hypertension, hyperlipidemia, depression and mental health concerns, higher rates of hospitalization, and poor oral health (Gundersin & Ziliak, 2015; Phipps et al., 2016). In *older adults*, food insecurity is associated with health issues such as poor nutrient intake, overall poor-to-fair health, limitations in activities of daily living, anxiety, depression, higher rates of hospitalization and visits to the emergency department, lower cognitive functioning, and oral health concerns (Gundersin & Ziliak, 2015; Phipps et al., 2016; Portela-Parra & Leung, 2019; Steiner et al., 2018).

Because of the prevalence of food insecurity and its impact on health outcomes, nurses need to watch for issues related to food insecurity with patients in all clinical settings. Consider, for example, that patients who do not take medication as directed or follow a prescribed diet may be in the difficult situation of having to choose whether to use their limited funds to buy food or pay for needed medication, rent, or utilities. Faced with the higher cost of nutritious food, they may choose to purchase food of lower nutritional quality because it stretches further and fills the stomach. Nursing assessments should include questions related to food security such as "Do you always have enough money to buy food for your family? Do you ever worry about running out of food? Have you gone hungry because you did not have enough money to buy food or because you did not have enough food for everyone in your family?" Identifying issues of food insecurity enables nurses to advocate for patients by connecting them with sources of food assistance in their local areas such as food pantries, local church and service organizations, and US Department of Agriculture programs like the Supplemental Nutrition Assistance Program and the Special Supplemental Nutrition Program for Women, Infants, and Children.

HOMELESSNESS

The modern era of homelessness was caused by major forces in society that include inner-city gentrification; deinstitutionalization of the mentally ill; increasing unemployment rates; the emergence of infectious diseases such as HIV/AIDS and COVID-19; cuts to federal assistance programs; the decriminalization of public drunkenness; and a shortage of affordable housing (National Academies of Sciences Engineering and Medicine et al., 2018). Reflecting an upward trend in homelessness since 2016, estimates suggest that approximately 580,000 men, women, and children are homeless in the United States. Every night, more than 300,000 stay in sheltered locations such as emergency shelters or transitional housing, while nearly a quarter of a million are unsheltered, living on sidewalks or in locations such as subway cars, abandoned buildings, vehicles, and other places not suitable for human habitation (U.S. Department of Housing and Urban Development, 2022; University of Nevada, n.d.). Half of all homeless people reside in the nation's 10 largest cities (U.S. Department of Housing and Urban Development, 2022).

The homeless population is diverse. While the proportion of homeless veterans, families with children, and unaccompanied youth declined in recent years, numbers rose significantly for people with disabilities, those in unsheltered settings, single individuals, and the "chronically homeless." In addition, those who identify as Black, African American, African, Hispanic, and Indigenous are overrepresented in the homeless population. The homeless are not all mentally ill or substance abusers. The new homeless are often families, single women with children, veterans, and the elderly (Fig. 16.1). Approximately 28 percent of the homeless population are families with children, more than 30,000 are unaccompanied youth (mostly between the ages of 18 and 24), 60 percent are men or boys, and about 33,000 are veterans, an 11 percent decrease from previous years (Child Trends, 2023; U.S. Department of Housing and Urban Development, 2022).

Health problems of homeless individuals include those resulting from limited access to care, those coincident with homelessness, and those associated with the psychosocial burden of homelessness. Health problems resulting from limited access to care include exacerbated or advanced chronic conditions such as hypertension, diabetes, HIV/AIDS, and decreased cognitive

CASE PRESENTATION

Socioeconomic Influences on Health

Martha D. is a 69-year-old African-American woman who lives in a substandard, cold-water, third-floor, walk-up apartment in a housing project with a high crime rate. She draws a small Social Security check that does not cover living expenses. Her income is supplemented by food stamps, housing assistance, and working as a nanny for three small children for 20 hours a week. Ms. D. earns minimum wage for her job as a nanny and accepts cash for her work to avoid any interference with her Social Security check. She uses public transportation to go to and from her job, spending $5.50 for bus fare each day.

Ms. D. helps her 47-year-old alcoholic single daughter with two teenage children, especially when the daughter is experiencing a drinking binge. The children frequently stay with Ms. D. and rely on her for food, shelter, and love. Ms. D.'s husband is an alcoholic and has not been home for two years; however, he does occasionally call from a homeless shelter or treatment facility. Neither Ms. D's daughter nor husband contributes to household expenses, but Ms. D. is very devoted to her family, especially her two grandchildren.

Martha D. is 58" tall and weighs 285 pounds. She has hypertension, with her blood pressure ranging from 200/90 to 250/110 mm Hg. She is on medication for her blood pressure, and the physician has linked her with a county home health nurse to encourage a diet and simple exercise regimen for her obesity and hypertension. Ms. D. is beginning to show signs of type 2 diabetes and has been encouraged to lose weight and adhere to a diabetic diet. In addition, Ms. D. has some small ulcerations on her left ankle.

The home health nurse visits Ms. D. and instructs her in the care of her ulcers, advising her to keep her left foot elevated as much as possible. The nurse spends considerable time explaining a 1200-calorie diabetic diet with moderate sodium restriction to Ms. D. and talks with Ms. D. about the need to begin walking as soon as the ulcers on her foot heal. Ms. D. tells the nurse she used to attend a weight control group and understands low-fat and diabetic diets. However, she says coming home to a nice pot of beans, fried chicken, and biscuits is her only daily pleasure. "I've lived 69 years on this diet, don't wish to change, and have nothing to lose if I remain on it the rest of my life." She also points out that it is not safe to walk in her neighborhood, so she stays inside. In addition, she indicates that she is too tired to exercise after working all day.

Think About It
Who Decides What Is Best for a Patient?

- Consider Ms. D.'s decision to ignore recommendations regarding diet, exercise, and, perhaps, care of her ankle ulcerations in relation to autonomy, beneficence, and nonmaleficence. What factors might affect her decision? How might her decisions be associated with poverty and food insecurity?
- Because the principle of beneficence requires actively doing good for Ms. D., who decides what is good? Discuss sections of nursing codes of ethics that inform your response.
- Discuss the implications of justice and health care for Ms. D.
- How would you approach Ms. D. about her health issues? Are there resources in your community that might assist a patient such as Ms. D.?

function, that would likely have responded to early and thorough intervention; lack of early intervention for infectious diseases such as wound infections and sexually transmitted infections; lack of access to hygienic conditions such as bathing, which would help to keep wounds and bandages clean; and lack of access to mental health care, including substance abuse treatment (Public Health Ontario, 2019). Health problems coincident with homelessness include illnesses resulting from living in close quarters with others and having inadequate nutrition, warmth, hygiene, safety, privacy, and other basic needs. Common health problems coincident with homelessness include environmental exposure

problems, foot problems, hepatitis, tuberculosis, skin problems, and injuries. Homeless people in Denver, for example, are susceptible to frostbite from environmental exposure to subfreezing temperatures and asphyxia caused by fume exhaust from fires in makeshift shelters or tents, while the homeless in Phoenix suffer from heat exhaustion and dehydration (Colorado Coalition for the Homeless, 2022; Davis-Young, 2022). Health problems associated with the psychosocial burden of homelessness are primarily mental illnesses, suicide, assault, and substance abuse. Although estimates vary substantially, a systematic review of eight international research studies showed up to a 72 percent prevalence of at least

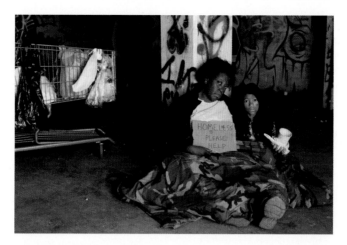

Fig. 16.1 The "New Homeless" Are Often Single Women With Children. Caring for People Experiencing Poverty, Homelessness, Food Insecurity, and Racial/Ethnic Inequities May Present Ethical Challenges for Nurses. (©iStock.com/AvailableLight.)

one mental disorder diagnosis among the homeless (Gutwinski et al., 2021). Mental health diagnoses common among the homeless include alcohol-related disorders, drug use disorders, schizophrenia, anxiety, suicide, major depression, cognitive disorders, bipolar disorders, psychosis, and personality disorders (Gutwinski et al., 2021; Hossain et al., 2020). Most mental health problems among the homeless are treatable.

The death rate among the homeless is high. A study conducted in cooperation with the University of Washington found that deaths among the homeless in the United States rose 77 percent between 2016 and 2020 (McCormick, 2022). The US government does not collect information on the cause of death of homeless people and many death certificates do not include housing status, so information is difficult to collect and deaths among unhoused individuals are often underestimated (Soriano et al., 2022). Local and philanthropic groups often fill in the gaps. Denver in 2022, for example, reported that 50 percent of homeless deaths were caused by drug overdoses, far exceeding chronic illness (Colorado Coalition for the Homeless, 2022; McCormick, 2022). In Marin County, California, homeless adults were found to be 50 percent more likely to die from any cause than an average adult with a 22-year difference between the median age at death among homeless people and all other county residents. Similar to Denver, the Marin homeless causes of death were drug overdose, cancer, and diseases of the circulatory system (Soriano et al., 2022).

Nurses may choose to work with homeless patients in street clinics, free clinics, or other charity facilities, or they may come across unhoused patients within established healthcare settings such as emergency departments or inpatient units. Whatever the setting, nurses must avoid stereotyping and honor nursing codes of ethics that require them to respect the "inherent dignity, worth, unique attributes, and human rights" of each individual (ANA, 2015). As the healthcare workers most likely to spend time with the patient, nurses must conduct careful and nonjudgmental assessment, addressing health problems common among the homeless and asking questions to elicit pertinent information. For example, one study found that homeless individuals had unmet health needs for vision treatment, dental care, sleep issues, pain, and sexual-reproductive problems (Semborski et al., 2022). Nurses should be alert for common problems among the homeless, even if they are not included in the presenting chief complaint. A homeless patient seen at an emergency department for frostbite, for example, might also have untreated diabetes, head-lice, tuberculosis, or syphilis. Nursing assessments should also include questions related to basic human needs such as food, shelter, and safety. The nurse must be aware that unhoused people are unlikely to be able to pay for prescribed medication, therapeutic diets, recommended follow-up treatments, or further diagnostic testing, and they are just as unlikely to have access to transportation for subsequent appointments. Identifying issues of homelessness enables nurses to actively advocate for patients by connecting them with sources of assistance such as soup kitchens, clothing closets, free clinics, domestic violence centers, homeless shelters, and other available social services.

CASE PRESENTATION

No Home to Go To

Ms. Brown, a 34-year-old White woman, comes into the emergency room to secure treatment for a head injury, plus minor bruises and abrasions that she reportedly received during an assault that happened about 20 hours ago. Ms. Brown is accompanied by her boyfriend, Roy. She indicates they were sleeping in a protected entrance to an elevator in the city parking garage when two young men began beating and kicking them. The two men took Ms. Brown's purse, a sack of food she and Roy had accumulated, and Roy's wallet, which contained $5.00. Ms. Brown indicates she has been homeless for over a year. She occasionally stays in city shelters but spends most of her time roaming the city and walking to secure meals at the various programs that feed the poor. She is tall and thin, with a variety of skin lesions. She came to the hospital due to dizziness that prevented her from walking to the church where she could eat. She and Roy occasionally work odd jobs, but they use the bulk of their income to support Roy's drug habit. She is trying to get Roy to quit using.

The physician has the nurse clean Ms. Brown's scalp and apply a dressing to the traumatic lesion. A contusion is expected, and the physician suggests that Ms. Brown rest for a few days and go to the neurological clinic if the dizziness worsens. The nurse reminds the physician that Ms. Brown has no place to rest and cannot get to the clinic without access to public transportation. The physician realizes this but indicates it is beyond her control.

Think About It
When Resources Are Lacking
- Apply the concepts of justice, nonmaleficence, and beneficence to Ms. Brown's care.
- What factors may have contributed to Ms. Brown's homelessness? Does society have any responsibility for Ms. Brown? If so, what? Are there resources in your community that could assist Ms. Brown?
- Can thorough treatment be denied if a client has no resources? If not, who pays for the treatment? What directives do nursing codes of ethics provide for nurses caring for Ms. Brown?

SEXUAL VIOLENCE

Sexual violence is pervasive in the United States and throughout the world. Sexual violence includes intimate partner (or domestic) violence, rape, stalking, unwanted sexual contact, and noncontact unwanted sexual experiences. Sexual violence is perpetrated against women and men, adults and children, in all socioeconomic, racial, ethnic, LGBTQ+, and religious groups (CDC, 2022; Futures Without Violence, 2023a; WHO, 2011, 2021). Intimate partner violence is the most common but least reported crime in the United States with homicide the most extreme consequence. Although low reporting of sexual violence makes it difficult to have an accurate number, it is estimated that the number of battered women in the US ranges from 2 to 12 million per year. The CDC (2022) describes four main types of intimate partner violence: sexual violence, stalking, physical violence, and psychological aggression. Women comprise the vast majority of victims of intimate partner violence, although a small percentage of men also report intimate partner violence. Twenty-five percent of women in the US report being physically or sexually abused by a partner at some point in their lives, one in five is sexually assaulted in college, and between 1 and 28 percent of pregnant women worldwide are victims of domestic violence (Futures Without Violence, 2023a; Leemis et al., 2022; WHO, 2011, 2021).

Intimate partner violence flows from a historical position of sexism. Eisler (1987) described how select tenets of Judaism, Christianity, and Islam support patriarchy, the inferiority of women, and women as the property of men. In the United States, it was legal until 1899 for a husband to beat his wife to maintain his authority (Barner & Carney, 2011). Remnants of these beliefs are still threaded through society, affecting the way families socialize their children and the way communities tolerate gender inequity. Women have long been defined in American society by their roles as mothers and caretakers, with an implied dependence on men. Although these role definitions are changing, daily events in society continue to perpetuate gender inequity. As long as gender inequity exists, domestic violence will remain a social problem affecting health and healthcare delivery.

The vast majority of abused women eventually leave their abusive partners. However, leaving is a process that takes time, energy, and resources. Many abused women will leave and return to their abusive partners several times before permanently terminating the relationship. Factors contributing to this include the inability to find housing or suitable jobs; the fear, loneliness, or poverty that results from being out on their own; concern for children who are experiencing relocation and other difficulties; relentless pressure from family and friends to try harder to make the relationship work; and poor support from the criminal justice system (Barner & Carney, 2011; Futures Without Violence, 2023a; National Coalition Against Domestic Violence, 2023). For some women, it is easier to return to a familiar, though unpleasant, situation than to start over and deal with numerous unknowns.

All persons living in violent relationships will experience poorer health. Women living in abusive situations may experience acute traumatic injuries and chronic physical and emotional problems (Fig. 16.2). They are especially vulnerable to battery during pregnancy and are at a higher risk than nonbattered women for poor pregnancy outcomes (Leemis et al., 2022; WHO, 2011). Victims of intimate partner violence may sustain acute injuries to the head, face, breasts, abdomen, genitalia, or reproductive system. Nonacute health conditions that may be associated with intimate partner violence include chronic headaches, palpitations, chronic pelvic pain, urinary frequency or urgency, irritable bowel syndrome, sexual dysfunction, sexually transmitted infections, abdominal symptoms, and recurrent vaginal infections. Psychosocial conditions associated with intimate partner violence may include sleep and appetite disturbances, anxiety, depression, posttraumatic stress disorder, isolation, alcohol and drug use, confusion, memory loss, homelessness, and suicide (ACOG

Committee on Health Care for Underserved Women, 2022).

The healthcare system may add insult to abused women's injuries. Women may feel humiliated by and blamed for the abuse by a healthcare system that minimizes the abuse, makes insufficient referrals, and fails to acknowledge abuse as the culprit (Barner & Carney, 2011). Women who leave healthcare settings without having the domestic violence addressed often remain isolated and uninformed about their options. However, women who have domestic violence issues addressed by a healthcare provider may be more likely to use an intervention and subsequently exit the abusive relationship (McCloskey et al., 2006).

The public has become more aware of and vocal about **unwanted sexual contact** and **noncontact unwanted sexual experiences** (Box.16.1). This was sparked by the Me Too Movement that began in October 2017 with the aim of bringing more public awareness to the prevalence of sexual harassment (which was discussed in Chapter 9) and sexual assault (U.N. Women, 2020). The increased public awareness has provided encouragement for many to speak up about their experience of being a survivor of sexual violence and seek help for issues related to this trauma. However, there are many survivors who, due to fear, shame, or other reasons, keep this trauma hidden, continue to suffer, and do not receive appropriate care. Because of this, nurses need to be alert to patient signs and symptoms that may indicate a current or past history of sexual violence. These signs include making excuses for injuries or bruises; having a partner present who speaks for the partner and does not want to leave the patient alone; constantly checking

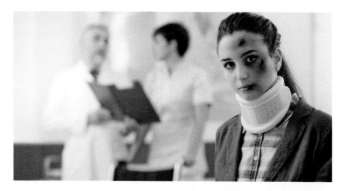

Fig. 16.2 Nurses Need to be Alert to Patient Signs and Symptoms That May Indicate Current or Past History of Sexual Violence, and Make an Effort to Address This With Patients. (©iStock.com/:demaerre.)

BOX 16.1   Description of Unwanted Sexual Contact and Noncontact Unwanted Sexual Experiences

- **Contact sexual violence** is a combined measure that includes rape, being made to penetrate someone else (males only), sexual coercion, and/or unwanted sexual contact.
  - **Rape** is any completed or attempted unwanted vaginal (for women), oral, or anal penetration through the use of physical force (such as being pinned or held down, or by the use of violence) or threats to physically harm and includes times when the victim was too drunk, high, drugged, or passed out from alcohol or drugs and unable to consent. Rape is separated into three types: (1) completed forced penetration, (2) attempted forced penetration, and (3) completed alcohol- or drug-facilitated penetration. Among women, rape includes vaginal, oral, or anal penetration by a male using his penis.
  - **Being made to penetrate someone else** (asked of males only) includes times when a victim was made to, or an attempt was made to make them, sexually penetrate someone without the victim's consent because the victim was physically forced (such as being pinned or held down, or by the use of violence) or threatened with physical harm, or when the victim was too drunk, high, drugged, or

passed out from alcohol and drugs and unable to consent.
  - **Sexual coercion** is unwanted sexual penetration that occurs after a person is pressured in a nonphysical way.
  - **Unwanted sexual contact** is unwanted sexual experiences involving touch but not sexual penetration, such as being kissed in a sexual way or having sexual body parts fondled, groped, or grabbed.
- **Physical violence** includes many behaviors from being slapped, pushed, or shoved to severe acts that include being hit with a fist or something hard, kicked, hurt by having hair pulled, slammed against something, beaten, burned on purpose, attempted to be hurt by choking or suffocating, and having a knife or gun used on them.
- **Stalking** involves a perpetrator's use of a pattern of harassing or threatening tactics that are both unwanted and cause fear or safety concerns.
- **Psychological aggression** includes expressive aggression (insulting, humiliating, or making fun of a partner in front of others) and coercive control and entrapment, which includes behaviors that are intended to monitor, control, or threaten an intimate partner.

(Excerpted from Leemis, R. W., Friar, N., Khatiwada, S., Chen, M. S., Kresnow, M., Smith, S. G., Caslin, S., & Basile, K. C. (2022). *The national intimate partner and sexual violence survey: 2016/2017 Report on intimate partner violence.* https://www.cdc.gov/violenceprevention/pdf/nisvs/NISVSReportonIPV_2022.pdf.)

---

in with the partner; being worried about pleasing the partner; being constantly put down by the partner in public; being isolated; and frequently seeking care for the conditions noted earlier. Providing a safe space in which patients can talk about experiences of sexual violence includes arranging to speak with patients privately, offering a nonjudgmental attitude, intentional listening, and a caring presence. Knowledge of how to connect patients with local and national resources for victims is important (Box 16.2). Links to several other national organizations for victims of sexual violence are found in the "Discussion Questions and Activities" section of this chapter. Remember that patients who seek to do what is good and just for themselves and perhaps their children often face dilemmas related to revealing their experiences of sexual violence that may include threats of harm and losing friends, family, and home. Although nurses may feel frustrated and discouraged,

BOX 16.2   Domestic Violence, Elder Abuse, and Human Trafficking Hotlines

- Human Trafficking
  - Department of Health and Human Services Human Trafficking Hotline at 888-373-7888
  - To report suspected human trafficking to federal law enforcement: 866-347-2423
- Domestic Violence
  - National Domestic Violence Hotline at 800-799-7233, or
  - Text START to 88788 (help available in numerous languages)
- Elder Abuse
  - Eldercare Locator at 800-677-1116 (open Monday through Friday, 9 a.m. to 8 p.m. Eastern Time; specially trained operators refer you to a local agency that can help; see https://eldercare.acl.gov/Public/About/Index.aspx; if urgent, call 911).

CASE PRESENTATION

Suspicions of Abuse

Maria P. is a 25-year-old woman who made an initial visit to the clinic for prenatal care when she was 18 weeks pregnant. She has returned for a second prenatal visit at 22 weeks of gestation. Maria has a four-year-old son and a two-year-old daughter. Her record indicates she had several bruises, lacerations, and a black eye during her last pregnancy that she attributed to clumsiness. Her two-year-old weighed 4 pounds, 8 ounces at birth and was 17 inches long.

As part of routine prenatal care for the most recent pregnancy, Maria was tested for HIV antibodies. The test was positive, and the physician and nurse conveyed this information to Maria during her second prenatal visit. Maria, of course, was quite upset. She admits that her spouse has been physically abusing her for some time and that both have used intravenous drugs in the past. She has had no sexual partners other than her spouse, though she has suspected that he has been with other women.

The nurse encourages Maria to tell her spouse that she is HIV positive so that he can be tested for HIV. She also encourages the use of condoms during sexual intercourse to help avoid transmission to her spouse should he not be infected. Maria insists that her husband refuses to use condoms, as they interfere with his pleasure. In addition, she says he would kill her if he knew she was HIV positive.

The nurse encourages Maria to go to a shelter for abused women and links her to both a counselor and a social worker to help her devise a safety plan. However, Maria ultimately decides to go home because she cannot abandon her children, and she does not want them in a shelter. She knows she cannot make it on her own, as she has neither income nor job skills. She requests that the clinic not interfere and that the clinic workers allow her to decide if, when, and how she will notify her spouse about her HIV status.

Think About It
When Patient Choices Place Them at Risk for Harm
- Consider the principle of autonomy when determining the appropriate decision in this situation. Remember that confidentiality is an inherent part of autonomy.
- Who is the patient in this situation? Maria? Her husband? The community? What is the nurse's responsibility to Maria? Does the nurse have a responsibility to her husband? To the community? How would you approach this situation?
- What would be the ethical implications if Maria's husband is notified by the clinic of her HIV status and he does significant harm to Maria? Would liability become an issue?
- If Maria's husband discovers he is HIV positive in the future, blames Maria, and discovers the clinic has known she was HIV positive for some time, what ethical concerns would arise? Is there any liability? Explain.

it is important to continue to support victims of sexual violence as they take even small steps toward leaving violent situations and healing the trauma.

HUMAN TRAFFICKING

Human trafficking, also known as modern-day slavery, is another form of violence that is often unrecognized. The United Nations Office on Drugs and Crime defines human trafficking as "the recruitment, transportation, transfer, harboring or receipt of people through force, fraud or deception for exploitation" (United Nations Office on Drugs and Crime, n.d.). Consistent with the UN definition, the complex US. definition of human trafficking is found within the *Victims of Trafficking and Violence Protection Act of 2000*. Victims of trafficking may be exploited for forced labor, their organs,

and sexual services. In the United States, victims are forced to engage in sex for money or to work in legal or illicit industries. In addition to sex work, they may be compelled to work in hospitality, agriculture, janitorial services, construction, landscaping, restaurants, factories, massage parlors, retail services, fairs and carnivals, peddling and begging, drug smuggling and distribution, religious institutions, child care, and domestic work (U.S. Department of State, nd). The full extent of this global issue is hard to determine due to the covert nature of trafficking. However, it is estimated that there are over 50 million victims of modern slavery worldwide, including nearly 28 million in forced labor, 22 million in forced marriage, 5 million in forced sexual exploitation, and 3.3 million children (Futures Without Violence, 2023b; International Labour Organization, 2022).

Traffickers are at the heart of this phenomenon. Their aim is to profit from the exploitation of the trafficked victims. Traffickers can be strangers, acquaintances, or even family members. They prey on the vulnerable for profit using violence, blackmail, emotional manipulation, removal of official documents (passports), fake employment agencies, and empty promises of education or job opportunities (U.S. Department of State, n.d.; United Nations Office on Drugs and Crime, n.d.).

Who are the victims of human trafficking? Victims can be of any age, race, ethnicity, sex, gender identity, nationality, immigration status, cultural background, religion, socioeconomic class, or education level. Young women and children trafficked for sexual exploitation are the largest group of those who are trafficked (Fig. 16.3). Children vulnerable to human trafficking include those in the child welfare and juvenile justice systems and foster care; runaway and homeless youth; unaccompanied, undocumented immigrants; children with substance use issues; racial or ethnic minorities; migrant laborers; foreign national domestic workers in diplomatic households; persons with limited English proficiency; persons with disabilities; LGBTQ+ individuals; and victims of intimate partner violence (U.S. Department of State, n.d.). According to the estimates noted earlier, one in four of those trafficked are children. Women and girls account for 99 percent of human trafficking in the commercial sex industry and 58 percent of those in other sectors (Futures Without Violence, 2023b; International Labour Organization, 2022). Trafficking victims have many faces, ranging from the poor in developing countries to the adolescent girl next door.

Nurses may encounter victims of human trafficking when they are brought to healthcare facilities with acute physical, emotional, or sexual health concerns. Their overall health may be poor. They often present in ways similar to victims of domestic violence, in that they seldom self-identify, have often been subjected to threats, intimidation, and physical and sexual violence; and are often accompanied by a person who is controlling, speaks for them, and does not leave the room. A more complete list of indicators of human trafficking is listed in Box 16.3. Victims of human trafficking may appear fearful and depressed, not have control of personal identification documents, not know their own address, have inconsistencies in their presenting story, may not know their legal rights, may not trust the police, and may not speak English (US Department of Homeland Security, 2022). Nursing responsibility related to victims of trafficking includes recognizing signs and providing appropriate interventions and support, as well as working toward the prevention of this form of violence. Trafficking survivors will likely need mental health services as well as general health care. They often need assistance identifying legal and benefits options, particularly if they have been trafficked into the country illegally (Futures Without Violence, 2023b). Human trafficking is illegal, and suspected cases should be reported (Box 16.2). Students are encouraged to explore the online resources related to human trafficking listed at the end of this chapter and to complete the free human trafficking awareness training available at http://www.dhs.gov/xlibrary/training/dhs_awareness_training_fy12/launchPage.htm.

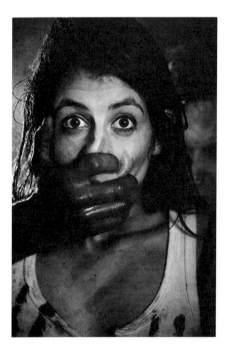

Fig. 16.3 Young Women and Children Are the Largest Group of Those Who Are Trafficked Primarily for Sexual Exploitation. Nurses need to be alert for and report suspected human trafficking. (©iStock.com/filadendron.)

EXPANDING ELDERLY POPULATION

An expanding elderly population presents another major social issue (Fig. 16.4). People are living longer. Factors such as healthier diets, vaccines, advances in

BOX 16.3 Indicators of Human Trafficking

Recognizing key indicators of human trafficking is the first step in identifying victims and can help save a life. Not all indicators listed here are present in every human trafficking situation, and the presence or absence of any of the indicators is not necessarily proof of human trafficking. Here are some common indicators to help recognize human trafficking:

- Does the person appear disconnected from family, friends, community organizations, or houses of worship?
- Has a child stopped attending school?
- Has the person had a sudden or dramatic change in behavior?
- Is a juvenile engaged in commercial sex acts?
- Is the person disoriented or confused, or showing signs of mental or physical abuse?
- Does the person have bruises in various stages of healing?
- Is the person fearful, timid, or submissive?
- Does the person show signs of having been denied food, water, sleep, or medical care?
- Is the person often in the company of someone to whom he or she defers? Or someone who seems to be in control of the situation (e.g., where they go or who they talk to)?
- Does the person appear to be coached on what to say?
- Is the person living in unsuitable conditions?
- Does the person lack personal possessions and appear not to have a stable living situation?
- Does the person have freedom of movement? Can the person freely leave where they live? Are there unreasonable security measures?

(From US Department of Homeland Security. (2022). *Indicators of human trafficking.* https://www.dhs.gov/blue-campaign/indicators-human-trafficking)

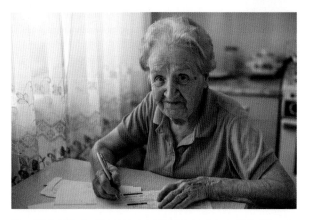

Fig. 16.4 Elderly Persons on Limited Incomes May Have to Choose Between Buying Medications or Paying for Food and Utilities. (©iStock.com/DimaBerkut.)

Although people are living longer, many face health challenges related to worsening chronic diseases such as cardiovascular disease, hypertension, and pulmonary disease; cognitive decline; behavioral health issues such as depression (with the risk of self-harm and suicide), anxiety, dementia, and substance abuse; social isolation; and falls. Aging adults may experience sensory changes such as hearing loss, decreased visual acuity, and vestibular function changes which lead to dizziness. The aging adult will likely lose muscle mass and have declining strength, which may also lead to falls. They may have osteoarthritis with back, neck, and other joint pain, which will further impede mobility. Their immune systems decline and decrease their capacity to fight infection. They likely have a combination of multiple chronic conditions and may gradually add more and more medications until they experience what is known as "polypharmacy" (Barron, 2017; Nickel et al., 2021). They may suffer from geriatric syndromes such as frailty, urinary incontinence, falls, delirium, functional decline, and pressure ulcers (WHO, 2022). Today's elderly are also known to be more susceptible to drug and alcohol abuse than previous generations (Nickel et al., 2021).

With the rise in the elderly population, the incidence of ageist stereotyping, prejudice against elders, and elder abuse is increasing. The WHO (2023a) defines elder abuse as "an intentional act, or failure to act, by a caregiver or another person in a relationship involving an expectation of trust that causes harm

healthcare knowledge, and improvements in the environment have contributed to greater longevity. The WHO predicts that the elderly population age 60 and over will increase from 1 billion in 2020 to 1.4 billion in 2030 and will more than double by 2050 (WHO, 2022). In the United States, older adults are expected to outnumber children by 2034, and by 2060 nearly a quarter of Americans will be 65 years or older. The number of people 85-plus is expected to triple, and the country will have 500,000 people over 100 years (U.S. Census Bureau, 2019).

to an adult 60 years and older." Elder abuse is often a hidden problem that is significantly underreported, however an estimated 10 percent of people 60 years and above have experienced some form of abuse in the United States, with some estimates ranging as high as five million elders abused each year. Rates in institutional settings are even higher (National Council on Aging, 2021; WHO, 2023a). Elder abuse includes physical abuse, sexual abuse, emotional abuse, confinement, passive neglect, and financial exploitation (National Council on Aging, 2021). See Box 16.4 for signs of elder abuse and neglect. Social isolation and mental impairment such as dementia make the elderly particularly vulnerable (National Council on Aging, 2021). Those who commit abuse within the community are most often adult children or spouses of the victims (National Council on Aging, 2021). Elders who have been abused have a 300 percent higher risk of death as compared to those who have not been mistreated (National Council on Aging, 2021).

Access to appropriate health care for this population is affected by socioeconomic, geographic, racial, ethnic, cultural, and other factors. For example, in the United States, those in higher socioeconomic groups have better health and access to health care than those in lower socioeconomic groups (Du & Xu, 2016; Fleary et al., 2016). Many elderly, especially from minority populations, live on limited incomes close to or below the poverty level and may have financial, transportation, and other concerns that cause delays in seeking health care (Administration for Community Living, 2021; Du & Xu, 2016). Healthcare insurance is less of a problem for the elderly population than those with social problems discussed previously. Older adults have a variety of insurance types including private insurance Medicare and Medicare Advantage, and other programs such as military coverage. Altogether, less than one percent of older adults in the United States are uninsured (National Center for Health Statistics, 2021).

Many elderly are socially isolated and susceptible to economic hardship. Some must work for pay in order to survive. Chronic illnesses, pain (especially from arthritic processes), frailties, cognitive problems, disabilities, and other health problems contribute significantly to the social isolation, financial burden, and general discomfort that may accompany aging. It is often presumed that the frail elderly will be cared for at home by family and friends. In reality, family members may be unable to provide needed support due to geographical distance from the frail elderly family member or personal responsibilities. Caring for the elderly, particularly those with dementia, can lead to emotional, relational, and financial strain for the caregivers. The caregivers often have to help with the finances of the elderly because their fixed incomes cannot cover the basic cost of living as well as healthcare expenses. Reliance on friends and family for health care of the frail elderly is especially problematic for the elderly without the necessary social or financial resources.

Nurses must approach the elderly with respect, recognizing their inherent dignity. When communicating with elderly patients, nurses should be aware of possible sensory deficits, particularly vision and hearing which can affect exchange of information. Nursing assessments should include questions focused on common problems of aging as well as those related to basic needs such as food, shelter, and safety. When elder abuse is suspected, nurses have the ethical and legal obligation to report their suspicions to the authorities (Box 16.2). As with other social problems, identifying issues of concern enables nurses to advocate for patients by connecting them with sources of assistance such as Social Security, Medicare, Medicaid, the Veterans Health Administration, and elder abuse resources.

Aging, Poverty, and Illness

Mr. Chang is a 65-year-old widower who is diabetic with chronic kidney disease. He is supposed to receive dialysis three times a week but frequently misses his appointments due to not having transportation or not feeling well. His only hope for a cure is a kidney transplant, which Mr. Chang really wants. Mr. Chang is very frail with many health problems. He lives alone in a small garage apartment. The landlord is threatening to evict Mr. Chang because he is behind on his rent payments. Mr. Chang lives on a small pension and Medicare. His prescription costs are excessive, and his Medicare Part D prescription plan requires large copayments on the brand-name medications needed for his care.

A home health nurse used to transport Mr. Chang to dialysis occasionally, as Mr. Chang lives outside the township limits and is unable to access public transportation services. The clinic, which does not believe Mr. Chang is a candidate for a transplant, has revised its policies regarding home visits due to changes in reimbursement mechanisms. The home health nurse can no longer visit Mr. Chang unless there is a reimbursable need such as a dressing change, and for liability reasons, she can no longer transport Mr. Chang to dialysis.

Think About It
What Health Care Should Society Provide for Its Citizens?

- Medicare pays for the medical care for patients with end-stage kidney disease who are on dialysis, regardless of age. Do you believe it should be society's responsibility to pay Mr. Chang's healthcare costs?
- There is often an undercurrent of political discussion regarding cuts to entitlement programs such as Medicare. Consider the principle of justice and ask yourself, if there comes a time when health care must be dramatically rationed, who should decide what services to eliminate?
- Do you think there should be a level of care that society should provide to all citizens, with private financing providing all care beyond the set level? Explain.
- What is fair for Mr. Chang? How would you approach this dilemma regarding Mr. Chang's care?

RACISM AND ETHNIC INEQUITIES

Unfair racial and ethnic disparities are a persistent challenge to healthcare status and healthcare delivery in the United States. The term *race* generally refers to biological traits related to a person's genetic heritage that allow classifications of human beings on the basis of characteristics such as skin color, facial features, and hair type and color. *Ethnicity*, on the other hand, refers to a shared cultural background such as nationality, language, practices, and beliefs. Although people within a racial group ascribe to many different cultural beliefs and practices, it is often race that stereotypes a group of people or engenders ethnocentric beliefs and moral conflicts in values. Racism and ethnic discrimination are ethical issues that violate the principle of respect for persons and contribute to human rights abuses.

Racial and ethnic minorities continue to experience disparities in health status and health care (Caraballo et al., 2022; Hill et al., 2023; James et al., 2017; LeCook et al., 2017; Ng et al., 2014). According to public health indicators, African Americans, Hispanics, Native Americans, Alaska Natives, Native Hawaiian, and other Pacific Islanders have the worst health status of all American groups. They fare worse than White people across the social determinants of health and most measures of health, itself. They have poorer cancer survival rates and higher incidences of obesity, asthma, heart disease, stroke, hypertension, diabetes, maternal mortality, and other problems. In addition, the life expectancy of non-Hispanic Black Americans is four years lower than White Americans and Black children have a 500 percent higher death rate from asthma as compared with White children. The COVID pandemic is a stark of example of the disproportionate impact among racial and ethnic minority populations (CDC, 2021; Government Accountability Office, 2021; Harvard School of Public Health, 2016; Lopez et al., 2021). In addition, African-Americans and Hispanics have the lowest levels of health insurance and the most inappropriate use of expensive emergency rooms. People in these groups have high rates of risk behaviors for disease. Although socioeconomic conditions contribute to these health conditions, it is easy to discern how racial and ethnic inequities influence health and healthcare options.

Problems of access to care and inequity of treatment for racial and ethnic minorities are frequently cited as evidence of racial bias within the healthcare system. In addition, traditional solutions to health problems, such as health education and health promotion programs, are often not designed for minority groups. More importantly, minority groups tend to demonstrate poorer health outcomes in some areas, revealing inadequate health care—for example, mortality from cancer is disproportionately high among people from racial and other ethnic minorities (Singh & Jemal, 2017). As you recall from Chapter 9, racism and discrimination of any kind are ethical issues that nurses need to be alert for and address in their care with patients, assuring that all patients are treated equitably and with respect.

THE INTERFACE AND OVERLAP OF SOCIAL ISSUES

As you read this chapter, you surely noticed the significant interface of poverty, food insecurity, homelessness, sexual violence, human trafficking, an expanding elderly population, and racism. Like falling dominos, each problem affects the next. Poverty can lead to food insecurity and homelessness. Sexual violence occurs more often in homeless and lower-income families. Sexual trafficking often leads to sexual violence. The elderly population is often poor and food insecure. Significant health disparities occur more often in these groups than other social groups. Racial and ethnic factors seem to be a thread that runs through all these issues. African-Americans, Native Americans, and Hispanics are overrepresented among the homeless. Women experiencing intimate partner violence more frequently and often deal with homelessness and poverty as they try to improve their situations. Poverty and homelessness are linked to a high abuse rate, and there is a link between violence and poverty. Elderly people are often made homeless as they face mounting health care and living costs on a fixed income. They may be subjected to abuse or neglect when being cared for by family or in institutions. Persons experiencing poverty, homelessness, aging, sexual violence, and racial or ethnic inequities are vulnerable to poor health and inadequate healthcare delivery. Often, these vulnerable groups are the least powerful and vocal persons in society, yet they are the groups most affected by ethical decisions regarding health care.

These social conditions represent examples of classism, sexism, ageism, and racism. Each indicates generations-long prejudice or discrimination against a particular class, gender, or racial group. The implication is that one group of people is held to standards espoused by another group. Statistical data on these social conditions, and the health of persons experiencing these social situations, explain why a feeling of helplessness may emerge when social situations are so intrinsically intertwined with health. Yet treating a person's symptoms without attending to the root causes of the problem may be viewed as inadequate health care.

NURSING ETHICS APPLIED TO SOCIAL DISPARITIES AND HEALTH CARE

Ethical problems involving classism, sexism, ageism, and racism are imbedded in society and difficult to resolve. Nurses live within family and community structures and are susceptible to common perceptions and beliefs, some which might be antithetical to the caring profession. Nurses must overcome biases and strive to administer care equitably, among all population groups. That is why, as professionals, nurses must look to professional standards for guidance. Nursing codes of ethics outline nurses' responsibility to all persons and direct nurses to be especially mindful of those with social disadvantages. Nurses should also look to common principles of bioethics that are essential to understanding and combatting healthcare disparities of vulnerable groups. Although the principles of justice, nonmaleficence, beneficence, and autonomy have been discussed in other chapters, a brief example of each principle as it relates to social issues is provided here.

Respect for Persons

Recall in Chapter 3 that we discussed respect for persons as a pillar of all other ethical principles. Respect for persons directs nurses to consider all other people as worthy of high regard, since genuine regard and respect for others is the moving force behind the caring professions. Respect for persons is reflected in nurses' caring behaviors. In Chapter 6 we discussed the history of caring in the nursing profession, acknowledging that care is the root of ethics. We discussed two distinctly different aspects of care: "caring about" and "taking care of" (Reich, 2003). Nursing codes of ethics guide nurses to practice both types of caring. Many contend that "caring about" goes to the heart of nursing. Caring is mindful and reflective, delivered with conscious intentionality (Watson, 2002) and compassionate concern. A nurse who cares about a patient is authentically committed to alleviating vulnerabilities, centering attention and concern on the person, preserving dignity and humanity, and supporting every facet of wellbeing (Smith, 1999). The second type of care, "taking care of," encompasses competence in the technical aspects of delivering care. This type of care focuses more on knowledge of the scientific aspects of health care and on skillful practice. Our examination of the social determinates of health in this chapter includes discussion about both aspects of caring—caring about patients with social disadvantages and caring for them with knowledge and expertise—both of which reflect nursing ethics in action. Working with people who are poor, homeless, victims of sexual violence, victims of human trafficking, aged, or of a different racial or ethnic background challenges nurses to explore their personal values to ensure that negative bias does not interfere with health care. One of the key strategies in beginning to respect and care about persons experiencing social disadvantages is to avoid blaming the victims.

Victim blaming is a real phenomenon that can affect attitudes and interactions (Center for Relationship Abuse Awareness, 2019; Côté et al., 2022; Felson & Palmore, 2018). Victim blaming suggests that people burdened by social conditions or victims of violence are accountable for their own situations and are responsible for needed solutions. Victim blaming is often evident in language such as "she was asking for it," "he should have quit smoking," or "they're not willing to work; they just want to live off the state." When there is evidence of personal or system-wide victim blaming, the ethical stance is to treat each person with dignity and fairness while working to change attitudes toward the victim. To respect others by allowing them to make choices and decisions, when they are capable of doing so, requires an attitude of caring with a focus on advocacy. This implies facilitating patient empowerment, acknowledging their values, guarding their rights, and promoting social justice in health care. Educating nurses and other healthcare providers to be aware of situations of victim blaming and enhancing the advocate role may improve care within a healthcare agency.

Socially Disadvantaged Groups and Codes of Nursing Ethics

Throughout this book, we have referenced codes of nursing ethics and asked you to think about cases and issues that command attention in relation to professional codes of ethics. In an examination of nine Western countries, and those of the European Union and the International Council of Nurses, there are several strikingly similar themes that are especially important when caring for people from socially disadvantaged groups. These themes include the following:

1. The nurse should respect the inherent worth, dignity, and rights of every person.
2. The nurse's primary responsibility is to the person seeking care.
3. The nurse has a duty to do good and avoid harm.
4. The nurse is responsible for the ethics of his or her own practice and must carry out daily actions with integrity.
5. The nurse must deliver care that is safe, compassionate, competent, and ethical.
6. The nurse must protect an individual when health is endangered by another person.
7. The nurse promotes justice.
8. The nurse is concerned with broader societal issues that affect health.

These broad themes, common to all Western codes of nursing ethics, set the standard for nursing care.

Principles of Ethics

Nurses should consider all principles of ethics in all professional situations. However, four principles are especially pertinent to the discussion in this chapter—the principles of justice, beneficence, nonmaleficence, and respect for autonomy.

Justice

Justice involves the duty to treat all people fairly without regard to age, socioeconomic status, race, or gender. This implies a fair distribution of the benefits and burdens among members of a society, with equal treatment to all or to those most in need. This could mean extending necessary treatment to those in need, even though they may not have the requisite means to pay for the treatment. For example, a frail elderly gentleman, beloved by his family, might receive an expensive but desired procedure based on justice, even though there is only a moderate chance that the extensive surgery will prolong life or improve the quality of life.

Nonmaleficence

Nonmaleficence is the duty to prevent or avoid doing harm, whether intentional or unintentional. This could

Who Should Receive Limited Healthcare Resources?

In this day of declining healthcare resources, should those with the greatest need or those who have contributed more to society receive expensive restorative procedures? Or should these procedures be available to all? Support your position.

The Impact of Social Conditions on Vulnerable Groups

Consider how social conditions affect other vulnerable groups, such as children, people who are mentally or physically disabled or challenged, undocumented immigrants, and people who are institutionalized or incarcerated.

- What factors make these populations vulnerable?
- What issues related to these populations give you concern as a nurse?
- What ethical concerns are related to the needs and care of people in these groups?
- How would you apply the principles of justice, nonmaleficence, beneficence, and autonomy to healthcare concerns with people in each of these groups?

mean refusing to discharge an abused woman to her home if there is a possibility of further injury or refusing to discharge a very ill homeless person to an under-bridge encampment. It might also entail ensuring a safe, hygienic environment before hospital release of a newborn infant and mother suffering from poverty or homelessness.

Beneficence

Beneficence is the duty to actively do good for patients. This requires us to act in ways that benefit others with attention to the psychological, social, and spiritual dimensions of disease or injury as well as the physical problems. This principle directs the nurse to try to ensure that the homeless lady—with leg ulcers and diabetes, who walks all day in poor shoes to secure free meals and safe sleeping quarters—will receive treatment for the leg ulcers that includes adequate diet and rest, elevation of the legs, and proper hygiene. Treatment would have to go beyond the usual prescriptions for drugs and address the social conditions contributing to the physical problems.

Respect for Autonomy

Respect for autonomy recognizes the patient's right to self-determination without outside control. Little (2000) reminds us that people must develop a sense of autonomy. She suggests that autonomy involves a set of skills that people possess to greater or lesser degrees. These skills often require someone to help us cultivate them, a context that sustains them, and help in exercising them when we are in a vulnerable position. One of these skills is the capacity to think through different options and imagine possibilities. Our social context, however, can get in the way of seeing our options. For example, respect for autonomy would direct us to work with the victim of sexual violence to develop a stronger sense of

herself and to help her see various options and available support. We also recognize that limitations on autonomy that occur within an abusive relationship affect a person's ability to act autonomously. Thus, respect for autonomy would direct us to honor her choice to return home—even if her safety is a concern—while continuing to offer support as she struggles with difficult decisions.

SUMMARY

This chapter focused on health disparities and the social determinants of health that present ethical problems in health care. Ethical problems related to health care for vulnerable populations confront nurses who work with those experiencing the social conditions of poverty, food insecurity, homelessness, sexual violence, human trafficking, unhealthy aging, racism, and ethnic inequities. Because values affect professional behavior, nurses must analyze personally held values as well as those of the healthcare agency where they are employed for appropriate consideration of justice, beneficence, nonmaleficence, and autonomy. Nurses who work with vulnerable groups need to utilize these principles in ethical decision making. Awareness of social issues that shape the health and healthcare management of their patients enables nurses to be alert for any conflicts in values and ethical dilemmas that may arise and be better prepared to provide needed support, appropriate interventions, and advocacy for those in their care.

CHAPTER HIGHLIGHTS

- The social determinates of health are fundamental causes of health disparities, particularly among disadvantaged and vulnerable groups.
- The scope of health disparities that result from poverty, food insecurity, homelessness, sexual violence, human trafficking, an expanding elderly population, and racism and ethnic inequities is immense.
- Limited choices and inappropriate treatment options often interfere with the best health care for vulnerable populations.
- Applying the concept of justice to vulnerable populations can change the way society and the healthcare systems provide health care. Addressing the social conditions of the individual with an illness or disease is basic to health care.
- Nonmaleficence and beneficence may clash with autonomy when providing care for vulnerable populations.
- Advocacy and caring require letting go of the power relationships that often dominate healthcare delivery.
- Codes of nursing ethics specify nurses' responsibilities to address social determinants of health at the bedside, in the community, and the larger society.

DISCUSSION QUESTIONS AND ACTIVITIES

1. Visit a homeless shelter or shelter for abused women. Interview staff or residents about their health and ability to access health care.
2. Spend a few afternoons volunteering in a soup kitchen or food pantry. Talk with people who come in for free meals about their health problems and ability to secure health care.
3. Spend some time with a home health nurse or a Meals-on-Wheels volunteer who contacts the elderly who live at home alone. Explore the individual's perceptions of quality of life, health dilemmas, and needs.
4. Work with classmates to develop a "health fair" for the homeless, discussing the value of typical activities and materials made available at traditional fairs, while designing a more relevant approach.
5. How many examples of toys, advertisements, acting roles, literature, childrearing practices, and the like can you identify that continue to perpetuate the woman's role as one of caregiver or sexual object? Discuss how the examples contribute to gender inequity for women.
6. Investigate racial and ethnic disparities in health at these or other websites:
   - https://www.gao.gov/assets/gao-21-105354.pdf
   - https://www.kff.org/racial-equity-and-health-policy/report/key-data-on-health-and-health-care-by-race-and-ethnicity/
   - https://www.cdc.gov/minorityhealth/index.html
   - https://minorityhealth.hhs.gov/
7. Explore information on the issues addressed in this chapter at several of the following websites and report to the class on issues, incidence, prevention, and ethical considerations related to these issues.

Sexual Violence
- Futures Without Violence—https://www.futureswithoutviolence.org/
- Office on Women's Health—https://www.womenshealth.gov/relationships-and-safety
- CDC Intimate Partner Violence—https://www.cdc.gov/violenceprevention/intimatepartnerviolence/resources.html
- National Coalition Against Domestic Violence—https://ncadv.org/learn-more
- WHO, violence against women—https://www.who.int/news-room/fact-sheets/detail/violence-against-women

Human Trafficking
- United Nations Office on Drugs and Crime—http://www.unodc.org/unodc/en/human-trafficking/
- US Department of State Human Trafficking Report—https://www.state.gov/united-states-advisory-council-on-human-trafficking-annual-report-2022/
- Futures Without Violence—https://www.futureswithoutviolence.org/human-trafficking-a-hidden-problem/
- Polaris Project—https://polarisproject.org/human-trafficking
- Department of Homeland Security Blue Campaign—https://www.dhs.gov/blue-campaign/what-human-trafficking
- Human trafficking awareness training—https://www.dhs.gov/xlibrary/training/dhs_awareness_training_fy12/launchPage.htm

Poverty and Food Insecurity

- Child Trends Data Bank—https://www.childtrends.org/research-topic/poverty-and-inequality and https://childtrends.org/publications/community-driven-approaches-to-addressing-food-insecurity
- Kaiser Family Foundation—https://www.kff.org/other/state-indicator/nonelderly-up-to-100-fpl/?currentTimeframe=0&sortModel=%7B%22colId%22:%22Location%22,%22sort%22:%22asc%22%7D
- Food Action Research Center—https://frac.org/
- Feeding America—https://www.feedingamerica.org/hunger-in-america/food-insecurity
- US Department of Agriculture—Household food security in the United States—https://www.ers.usda.gov/amber-waves/2022/february/food-insecurity-for-households-with-children-rose-in-2020-disrupting-decade-long-decline/

Homelessness

- National Coalition for the Homeless—http://www.nationalhomeless.org/
- National Alliance to End Homelessness—https://endhomelessness.org/homelessness-in-america/
- US Department of Housing and Urban Development Annual Homelessness Assessment Report—https://www.huduser.gov/portal/sites/default/files/pdf/2022-AHAR-Part-1.pdf

Aging Population

- WHO—https://www.who.int/news-room/fact-sheets/detail/ageing-and-health#:~:text=By%202050%2C%20the%20world%27s%20population,2050%20to%20reach%20426%20million
- National Council on Aging—https://www.ncoa.org/healthy-aging/
- National Institute on Aging—https://www.nia.nih.gov/health/elder-abuse
- Administration for Community Living—https://acl.gov/sites/default/files/Profile%20of%20OA/2021%20Profile%20of%20OA/2021ProfileOlderAmericans_508.pdf

REFERENCES

ACOG Committee on Health Care for Underserved Women. (2022). *Intimate partner violence.* https://www.acog.org/clinical/clinical-guidance/committee-opinion/articles/2012/02/intimate-partner-violence#:~:text=Consequences%20of%20Intimate%20Partner%20Violence,-Some%20women%20subjected&text=This%20stress%20can%20lead%20to,ongoing%20or%20past%20violence%2010.

Administration for Community Living. (2021). *2021 Profile of older Americans.* https://acl.gov/sites/default/files/Profile%20of%20OA/2021%20Profile%20of%20OA/2021ProfileOlderAmericans_508.pdf.

America Academy of Family Physicians. (2021). *Poverty and health: The family medicine perspective (position paper).* https://www.aafp.org/about/policies/all/poverty-health.html.

ANA. (2015). *Code of ethics for nurses with interpretive statements. Nursebooks.* http://nursingworld.org/DocumentVault/Ethics-1/Code-of-Ethics-for-Nurses.html.

Barner, J. R., & Carney, M. M. (2011). Interventions for intimate partner violence: A historical review. *Journal of Family Violence, 26*, 235–255.

Barron, J. E. (2017). Age-related diseases and clinical public health implications for the 85 years old and over population. *Frontiers in Public Health, 11*(5), 335. https://doi.org/10.3389/fpubh.2017.00335.

Berman, R. S., Patel, M. R., Belamarich, P. F., & Gross, R. S. (2018). Screening for poverty and poverty-related social determinants of health. *Pediatrics in Review, 39*(5), 235–255.

Caraballo, C., Ndumele, C., Roy, B., Lu, Y., Riley, C., Herin, J., & Krumholtz, H. (2022). Trends in racial and ethnic disparities in barriers to timely medical care among adults in the US, 1999 to 2018. *JAMA Health Forum, 3*(10), e223856. https://doi.org/10.1001/jamahealthforum.2022.3856.

CDC. (2021). *Racism and health.* https://www.cdc.gov/minorityhealth/racism-disparities/index.html.

CDC. (2022). *Intimate partner violence.* https://www.cdc.gov/ViolencePrevention/intimatepartnerviolence/index.html.

Center for Relationship Abuse Awareness. (2019). *Avoiding victim blaming.* http://stoprelationshipabuse.org/educated/avoiding-victim-blaming/

Child Trends. (2023). *Data on families with low incomes across America can inform two-generation approaches.* https://childtrends.org/publications/data-on-families-with-low-incomes-across-america-can-inform-two-generation-approaches.

Child Trends Data Bank. (2023). *Poverty and inequality.* https://www.childtrends.org/research-topic/poverty-and-inequality.

CNA. (2017). *Code of ethics for registered nurses.* https://cdn1.nscn.ca/sites/default/files/documents/resources/code-of-ethics-for-registered-nurses.pdf#:~:text=The%20Canadian%20Nurses%20Association%20%28CNA%29%20Code%20of%20Ethics,receiving%20care.%20The%20Code is%20both%20aspirational%20and%20regulatory.

Cohen, R. A., Cha, A. E., Terlizzi, E., & Martinez, M. E. (2022). *Health insurance coverage: Early release of the estimates from the national health interview survey, 2021.* National Center for Health Statistics. https://www.cdc.gov/nchs/data/nhis/earlyrelease/insur202205.pdf.

Colorado Coalition for the Homeless. (2022). *We will remember 2022: Homeless death review,* Denver, CO. https://www.coloradocoalition.org/sites/default/files/2022-12/2022%20Death%20Review_Digital_F.pdf.

Côté, P. -B., Flynn, C., Dubé, K., Fernet, M., Maheu, J., Gosslin-Pelerin, A., Couturier, P., Cribb, M., Petrucci, G., & Cousineau, M. (2022). "It made me so vulnerable": Victim-blaming and disbelief of child sexual abuse as triggers of social exclusion leading women to homelessness. *Journal of Child Sexual Abuse, 31*(2), 177–195.

Creamer, J., Shrider E. A., Burns, K., & Chen, F. (2022). *Poverty in the United States: 2021.* US Census Bureau. https://www.census.gov/library/publications/2022/demo/p60-277.html.

Cree, R. A., Bitsko, R. H., Robinson, L. R., Holbrook, J. R., Danielson, M. L., Smith, C., Kaminski, J. W., Kenney, M. K., & Peacock, G. (2018). Health care, family, and community factors associated with mental, behavioral, and developmental disorders and poverty among children aged 2-8 years: United States 2016. *Morbidity and Mortality Weekly Report, 67*(50), 1377–1383. Available from https://www.cdc.gov/mmwr/volumes/67/wr/mm6750a1.htm.

Davis-Young, K. (2022). Homelessness is aggravating harm caused by the Phoenix heat, medical personnel say. *NPR.* https://www.npr.org/2022/08/30/1119671257/homelessness-aggravating-harm-health-phoenix-heat-medical.

Du, Y., & Xu, Q. (2016). Health disparities and delayed health care among older adults in California: A perspective from race, ethnicity, and immigration. *Public Health Nursing, 33*(5), 383–394.

Eisler, R. (1987). *The Chalice and the Blade: Our history, our future.* Harper & Row.

Felson, R. B., & Palmore, C. (2018). Biases in blaming victims of rape and other crime. *Psychology of Violence, 8*(3) 16802–16207.

Fleary, S. A., Nigg, D. R., & Freund, K. M. (2016). An examination of changes in social disparities in health behaviors in the US 2003-2015. *American Journal of Health Behavior, 42*(1), 119–134.

Francis, L., DePriest, K., Wilson, M., & Gross, D. (2018). Poverty, toxic stress, and social determinants of health: Screening and care coordination. *Online Journal of Issues in Nursing, 23*, 2.

Futures Without Violence. (2023a). *Get the facts.* https://www.futureswithoutviolence.org/resources-events/get-the-facts.

Futures Without Violence. (2023b). *Human trafficking: A hidden problem.* https://www.futureswithoutviolence.org/human-trafficking-a-hidden-problem/.

Government Accountability Office. (2021). *Racial and ethnic health disparities.* https://www.gao.gov/assets/gao-21-105354.pdf.

Gundersin, C., & Ziliak, J. P. (2015). Food insecurity and health outcomes. *Health Affairs, 34*(11), 1830–1839. https://doi.org/10.1377/hlthaff.2015.0645.

Gutwinski, S., Schreiter, S., Deutscher, K., & Fazel, S. (2021). The prevalence of mental disorders among homeless people in high-income countries: An updated systematic review and meta-regression analysis. *PLOS Medicine, 18*(8). https://doi.org/10.1371/journal.pmed.1003750.

Harvard School of Public Health. (2016). *Health disparities between blacks and whites run deep.* https://www.hsph.harvard.edu/news/hsph-in-the-news/health-disparities-between-blacks-and-whites-run-deep/.

Hill, L., Ndugga, N., & Artiga, S. (2023). *Key data on health and healthcare by race and ethnicity.* https://www.kff.org/racial-equity-and-health-policy/report/key-data-on-health-and-health-care-by-race-and-ethnicity/#:~:text=One%20quarter%20of%20AIAN%20adults,fair%20or%20poor%20health%20status.

Hossain, M. M., Sultana, A., Tasnim, S., Fan, Q., Ping, M., Lisako, E., McKyer, J., & Purohit, N. (2020). Prevalence of mental disorders among people who are homeless: An umbrella review. *International Journal of Social Psychiatry, 66*(6), 528–541. https://doi.org/10.1177/0020764020924689.

ICN. (2021). *The ICN code of ethics for nurses.* https://www.icn.ch/system/files/2021-10/ICN_Code-of-Ethics_EN_Web_0.pdf

International Labour Organization. (2022). *Global estimates of modern slavery: Forced labour and forced marriage.* https://www.ilo.org/wcmsp5/groups/public/---ed_norm/---ipec/documents/publication/wcms_854733.pdf.

James, C. V., Moonesing, R., & Wilson-Frederick, S. M. (2017). Racial/ethnic health disparities among rural adults--United States, 2012-2015. *Morbidity and Mortality Weekly Report, 66*(23), 1–9. https://www.cdc.gov/mmwr/volumes/66/ss/ss6623a1.htm.

Kaiser Family Foundation. (2021). *Health insurance coverage of the nonelderly (0-14) with incomes below 100% federal poverty level.* https://www.kff.org/other/state-indicator/nonelderly-up-to-100-fpl/?currentTimeframe=0&sortModel=%7B%22colId%22:%22Location%22,%22sort%22:%22asc%22%7D

Kaiser Family Foundation. (2022). *Women's health insurance coverage.* https://www.kff.org/womens-health-policy/fact-sheet/womens-health-insurance-coverage/.

Kyunghee, L., & Liangliang, Z. (2022). Cumulative effects of poverty on children's social-emotional development: Absolute poverty and relative poverty. *Community Mental Health Journal*, *58*(5), 930–943.

LeCook, B., Trinh, H., Li, Z., Hou, S. S., & Progavac, A. M. (2017). Trends in racial-ethnic disparities in access to mental health care 2004-2012. *Psychiatric Services*, *68*, 9–16.

Leemis, R. W., Friar, N., Khatiwada, S., Chen, M. S., Kresnow, M., Smith, S. G., Caslin, S., & Basile, K. C. (2022). *The national intimate partner and sexual violence survey: 2016/2017 report on intimate partner violence.* https://www.cdc.gov/violenceprevention/pdf/nisvs/NISVSReportonIPV_2022.pdf.

Little, M. O. (2000). *Introduction to the ethic of care new century, new challenges.* Washington, DC: Intensive Bioethics Course XXVI, Georgetown University.

Lopez, L., Hart, L. H., & Katz, M. H. (2021). Racial and ethnic health disparities related to COVID-19. *JAMA*, *325*(8), 719–720.

Maguire-Jack, K., & Sattler, K. (2023). Neighborhood poverty, family economic well-being, and child maltreatment. *Journal of Interpersonal Violence*, *38*(5–6), 4814–4831. https://doi.org/10.1177/08862605221119522.

McCloskey, L. A., Lichter, E., Williams, C., Gerber, M., Wittenbert, E., & Ganz, M. (2006). Assessing intimate partner violence in health care settings leads to women's receipt of interventions and improved health. *Public Health Reports*, *121*(4), 435–444.

McCormick, E. (2022). 'Homelessness is lethal': US deaths among those without housing are surging. *The Guardian.* https://www.theguardian.com/us-news/2022/feb/07/homelessness-is-lethal-deaths-have-risen-dramatically

Murthy, V. H. (2016). Food insecurity: A public health issue. *Public Health Reports*, *131*(5), 655–657.

National Academies of Sciences, Engineering, and Medicine, Health and Medicine Division, Board on Population Health and Public Health Practice, Policy and Global Affairs, & Science and Technology for Sustainability Program, & Committee on an Evaluation of Permanent Supportive Housing Programs for Homeless Individuals. (2018). The history of homelessness in the United States: Permanent supportive housing: Evaluating the evidence for improving health outcomes among people experiencing chronic homelessness. National Academies Press. https://doi.org/10.17226/25133.

National Center for Health Statistics. (2021). *Demographic variation in health insurance coverage: United States, 2019.* National Health Statistics Reports. https://www.cdc.gov/nchs/data/nhsr/nhsr159-508.pdf

National Coalition Against Domestic Violence. (2023). *National statistics.* https://ncadv.org/statistics.

National Council on Aging. (2021). *Get the facts on elder abuse.* https://www.ncoa.org/article/get-the-facts-on-elder-abuse.

Ng, J. H., Bierman, A. S., Elliott, M. N., Wilson, R. L., Xia, C., & Scholle, S. H. (2014). Beyond black and white: Race/ethnicity and health status among older adults. *Journal of Managed Care*, *20*(3), 239–248.

Nickel, C., Arendts, F., Lucke, J., & Mooijaart, S. (2021). *Silver book II: Geriatric syndromes.* https://www.bgs.org.uk/resources/silver-book-ii-geriatric-syndromes.

Office of Disease Prevention and Health Promotion. (2020). *Healthy people 2030: Poverty.* https://health.gov/healthy-people/priority-areas/social-determinants-health/literature-summaries/poverty.

Pai, S., & Bahadur, K. (2020). The impact of food insecurity on child health. *Pediatric Clinics of North America*, *67*(2), 387–396. https://doi.org/10.1016/j.pcl.2019.12.004.

Phipps, E. J., Singletary, S. B., Cooblall, C. A., Hares, H. D., & Braitman, L. E. (2016). Food insecurity in patients with high hospital utilization. *Population Health Management*, *19*(6), 414–420.

Portela-Parra, E. T., & Leung, C. W. (2019). Food insecurity is associated with lower cognitive functioning in a national sample of older adults. *Journal of Nutrition*, *149*(10), 1812–1817. https://doi.org/10.1093/jn/nxz120.

Public Health Ontario. (2019). *Homelessness and health outcomes: What are the associations?* https://www.publichealthontario.ca/-/media/documents/E/2019/eb-homelessness-health.pdf.

Reich, W. R. (2003). Historical traditions of an ethic of care in healthcare In S. G. Post (Ed.), *Encyclopedia of bioethics* (pp. 349–367). Thomas Gale, Macmillan Reference.

Semborski, S., Henwood, B., Madden, D., & Rhoades, H. (2022). Health care needs of young adults who have experienced homelessness. *Medical Care*, *60*(8), 588–595. https://doi.org/10.1097/MLR.0000000000001741.

Singh, G. K., & Jemal, A. (2017). Socioeconomic and racial/ethnic disparities in cancer mortality, incidence, and survival in the United States, 1950-2014: Over six decades of changing patterns and widening inequalities. *Journal of Environmental and Public Health*, *2017*. https://doi.org/10.1155/2017/2819372.

Smith, M. C. (1999). Caring and the science of unitary human beings. *Advances in Nursing Science*, *21*(4), 14–28.

Soriano, J., Nakahata, M., & Baz, C. (2022). Deaths uncounted: Using local data to act on unnecessary tragedy. https://nhchc.org/wp-content/uploads/2022/10/Mortality-in-PEH-Marin-Co-10-22.pdf.

Steiner, J. F., Stenmark, S. H., Sterrett, A. T., Paolino, A. R., Stiefel, M., Gonzansky, W. S., & Zeng, C. (2018). Food insecurity in older adults in an integrated health care system. *Journal of the American Geriatric Society*, 66, 1017–1024.

Tolbert, J., Drake, P., & Damico, A. (2022). *Key facts about the uninsured population*. Kaiser Family Foundation. https://www.kff.org/uninsured/issue-brief/key-facts-about-the-uninsured-population/.

U.N. Women. (2020). *#MeToo: Headlines from a global movement*. https://www.unwomen.org/en/digital-library/publications/2020/08/brief-metoo-headlines-from-a-global-movement.

U.S. Census Bureau. (Revised 2019). *The graying of America: More older adults than kids by 2035*. https://www.census.gov/library/stories/2018/03/graying-america.html#:~:text=Starting%20in%202030%2C%20when%20all,add%20a%20half%20million%20centenarians.

U.S. Department of Homeland Security. (2022). *Indicators of human trafficking*. https://www.dhs.gov/blue-campaign/indicators-human-trafficking.

U.S. Department of Housing and Urban Development. (2022). *The 2022 annual homeless assessment report (AHAR) to Congress*. https://www.huduser.gov/portal/sites/default/files/pdf/2022-AHAR-Part-1.pdf.

U.S. Department of State. (n.d.). *About human trafficking*. https://www.state.gov/humantrafficking-about-human-trafficking/#human_trafficking_U_S.

United Nations Department of Economic and Social Affairs. (2023). *Poverty in all its forms everywhere*. https://unstats.un.org/sdgs/report/2021/goal-01/.

United Nations Office on Drugs and Crime. (n.d.). *What is human trafficking?* https://www.unodc.org/unodc/en/blueheart/

University of Nevada, R. (n.d.). *Homelessness in America: Statistics, resources, and organizations*. https://onlinedegrees.unr.edu/blog/homelessness-in-america/.

USDA. (2022). *Definitions of food security*. https://www.ers.usda.gov/topics/food-nutrition-assistance/food-security-in-the-u-s/definitions-of-food-security/.

Victims of Trafficking and Violence Protection Act of 2000, Pub. L. No. 106-386—Oct. 28, 2000. https://www.govinfo.gov/content/pkg/PLAW-106publ386/pdf/PLAW-106publ386.pdf.

Watson, J. (2002). Intentionality and caring-healing consciousness: A practice of transpersonal nursing. *Holistic Nursing Practice*, 16(4), 12–19.

Weeks, E. (2018). Medicalization of rural poverty: Challenges of access. *Journal of Health Politics, Policy, and Law*, 46, 651–657.

WHO. (2011). Intimate partner violence during pregnancy. WHO_RHR_11.35_eng.pdf.

WHO. (2021). Violence against women. https://www.who.int/news-room/fact-sheets/detail/violence-against-women.

WHO. (2022). *Ageing and health*. https://www.who.int/news-room/fact-sheets/detail/ageing-and-health#:~:text=By%202050%2C%20the%20world%27s%20population,2050%20to%20reach%20426%20million.

WHO. (2023a). *Abuse of older people*. https://www.who.int/health-topics/abuse-of-older-people#tab=tab_1.

WHO. (2023b). *Social determinants of health*. https://www.who.int/health-topics/social-determinants-of-health#tab=tab_1.

Xu, J., Murphy, S. L., Kochanek, K. D., & Arias, E. (2022). *Mortality in the United States 2021*. CDC. https://www.cdc.gov/nchs/products/databriefs/db456.htm#section_4.

Ziliak, J. P., & Gundersen, C. (2022). *The state of senior hunger in America in 2020: An annual report*. Feeding America. https://www.feedingamerica.org/sites/default/files/2022-05/The%20State%20of%20Senior%20Hunger%20in%202020_Full%20Report%20w%20Cover.pdf.

17

Gender Issues and Nursing Ethics

When we are committed to the ideal of concern for all others, it follows that this should inform our social and political policies.

(Dalai Lama, 1999)

OBJECTIVES

After completing this chapter, the reader should be able to:

1. Discuss how ethics relates to gender issues in nursing.
2. Explore how the title *nurse* contributes to gender stereotyping and gender bias in nursing.
3. Discuss how stereotyping and gender bias affect the nursing workforce.
4. Compare issues found in women's and men's health care.
5. Examine issues in the health care of LGBTQ+ individuals.

INTRODUCTION

Gender issues affect nursing as a profession as well as the face-to-face delivery of nursing care. You will recall from Chapter 1 that gender is one of the most critical factors influencing nursing practice. Throughout history, in nearly every culture, nursing has been a profession of women. As a small microcosm of the larger society, the healthcare workforce manifests many gender-related social issues such as pay equity, employment opportunities, sexual harassment, and gender stereotyping. Gender issues also affect the day-to-day patient care. According to the *Code of Ethics for Nurses with Interpretive Statements* (2015), "The nurse practices with compassion and respect for the inherent dignity, worth, and unique attributes of every person" (p. 1). Further, the interpretive statements affirm that "the need for and right to health care is universal, transcending all individual differences" (p. 1) and that "nurses consider the needs and respect the values of each person in every professional relationship and setting" (p. 1). Similarly, the ICN *Code of Ethics for Nurses* (2021) states that

nurses support and respect the dignity and universal rights of all people, including patients, colleagues, and families (p. 7). The CNA *Code of Ethics for Registered Nurses* (CNA, 2017) goes further, instructing nurses not to "discriminate on the basis of a person's race, ... gender, gender identity, gender expression, sexual orientation, ... lifestyle, ... or any other attribute" (p. 14). Recognizing that gender discrimination is pervasive and that nursing codes of ethics call for nurses to respect the rights of all people, this chapter explores gender issues in the workplace and issues of gender encountered in the patient care arena. We ask you to keep in mind the ethical principles of beneficence, autonomy, confidentiality, and justice as you read the chapter and thoughtfully answer the "Ask Yourself and Think About It" questions.

GENDER ISSUES IN THE WORKPLACE

Controversy remains concerning the derivation of the title *nurse* and how the title relates to the gender of the person providing care. Identifying written reference to the term *nurse* as early as the late Middle Ages, the *Oxford English Dictionary* cites an early use of the word in reference to a wet nurse, or a woman employed to take charge of children. Although this definition is obsolete, the current definition continues to suggest a gender bias: "A person (historically usually a woman) who cares for the sick or infirm. . . ." (Oxford English Dictionary). During the past few decades, the profession has made small strides to eliminate gender bias and recruit men into the profession.

Throughout the decades, nurses have struggled with a patriarchal ideology that continues to affect the profession. **Patriarchy** is defined as "[t]he predominance of men in positions of power and influence in society, with cultural values and norms favoring men" (Oxford English Dictionary). Coupled with an enduring cultural attitude that diminishes the status of the caring role in society, patriarchy has inhibited the profession. The negative outcomes of patriarchy affect both women and men in the profession. Historically, women chose nursing because it was among the very few professional options deemed appropriate for women. Men, on the other hand, were expected to select blue-collar trades or professions such as medicine, law, or politics, which perpetuated the male power base in society (Christensen & Knight, 2014). This patriarchal system extended into the healthcare professions and created certain gender stereotypes.

In what has been termed the *medicalization* of American society, nursing has struggled to overcome the prejudices that have historically embraced the biomedical curative model of health care. As diversified consumers of healthcare demand more sophisticated and culturally congruent care, nurses are in a prime position to provide ethical, cost-effective, high-quality care. If nursing is to be successful in this and other arenas, the profession must simultaneously address issues of gender stereotyping, gender bias, territoriality, power, and authority within its own ranks as well as with other healthcare professionals.

Gender and the Nursing Workforce

Throughout time, women comprised 95 to 98 percent of nurses. Data from the *National Nursing Workforce Survey* indicate that the overall percentage of females in the profession is decreasing slowly. Ninety-eight percent of nurses were female in 1970, compared with 90.5 percent in 2020 (Smiley et al., 2021; U.S. Census Bureau, 2013). Nursing leaders and professional nursing

organizations strive toward a nursing workforce that mirrors the population in general, yet progress toward increasing the number of men in nursing has been slow. Although the percentages have not changed dramatically, the overall increase in the number of men in nursing in the last 50 years has been significant. The number of men in full-time nursing positions jumped from 9500 in 1950 to 211,000 in 1990 and to 3,900,000 in 2020 (D'Antonio & Whelan, 2009; Smiley et al., 2021). Even with this dramatic increase in the number of men in nursing, their percentage of the total nursing workforce is still low. Schools of nursing must recruit and retain men, along with those from diverse cultural, ethnic, and socioeconomic backgrounds to create a nursing workforce that reflects the characteristics of the general population. This is congruent with the Institute of Medicine's recommendation that nursing "leaders should partner with education accrediting bodies, private and public funders, and employers to ensure funding, monitor progress, and increase the diversity of students to create a workforce prepared to meet the demands of diverse populations across the lifespan" (IOM, 2010, p. 281).

In addition to overall percentages, studies show some other differences in men and women in nursing. Women who work in nursing are slightly older than men in nursing, they are less likely to work in hospitals, and they earn slightly lower wages. Men in nursing are more likely to earn a master of science (MSN) in nursing or doctor of nursing practice degree, whereas slightly more women obtain a diploma in nursing or a doctor of philosophy (PhD) (Smiley et al., 2021).

Pay Equity

Women have historically worked for lower pay than their male counterparts. Identified as a distributive justice issue, women's salaries in the US general population are approximately 20 percent lower than the salaries of men in similar occupations. This wage gap has remained steady over the past several years. When earnings are measured by gender and race, the wage gap is even larger, with White men's earnings significantly higher than Hispanic and Black women. Hispanic women earn just 50 percent and Black women earn just 60 percent of White men's average pay (Hegewisch, 2018). Salaries in nursing remain relatively low compared with other professions that require comparably high levels of skill, education, and responsibility. However, average nursing salary varies dramatically from state to state, with nurses in the metropolitan areas of highest paid state earning dramatically more than those in states with the lowest salaries (Smiley et al., 2021; U.S. Bureau of Labor Statistics, 2021). The increasing number of men in nursing may be one factor related to raising salaries, but other economic considerations, such as nursing shortages, local economies, labor legislation, and collective bargaining, may also be responsible.

Although a 20 percent pay gap exists between men and women in the general population, the pay gap between male and female nurses is less. Female nurses are paid 16 percent less than males, with differences seen among various specialties (Nurse.com, 2022; Smiley et al., 2021). Pay equity is generally protected by state laws. Issues of comparable worth associated with traditionally female-dominated professions such as teaching and nursing have not had the same protection. However, the fact that a gap exists at all is striking, in that men make up only a small percentage of the nursing profession. Men typically enjoy higher wages, faster promotions, and more prestigious positions in occupations such as nursing that are dominated by females (U.S. Census Bureau, 2013). Men's dominance in the higher-paying jobs and the patriarchal structure of the healthcare industry in which fewer women hold senior management positions may account for this. For example, although just nine percent of employed nurses are men, they constitute over 41 percent of nurse anesthetists—a specialty with significantly higher pay (U.S. Census Bureau, 2013). This is noteworthy because the mean annual salary of registered nurses in 2021 was $83,000 whereas nurse anesthetists earned an average of $202,000 (U.S. Bureau of Labor Statistics, 2021).

Closing the gap in wages does not require losses for men in nursing—it simply requires women's wages to rise faster than men's wages. This trend may have already started because women's earnings have increased in the last several years, whereas men's wages during the same period have remained virtually unchanged. One strategy to close the wage gap may be for women to negotiate salary. In a recent survey of nurses, 40 percent of men reported that they negotiate salaries most of the time or always, compared with only 31 percent of women (Nurse.com, 2022).

Stereotyping

A **stereotype** is a persistent idea about a person's characteristics that is preconceived, oversimplified, and often wrong. Gender stereotypes are stubbornly ingrained in nursing. Because characteristics vary significantly across a population, stereotypes can be vastly incorrect and harmful. Thus, stereotyping is unethical. The United Nations Human Rights Office of the High Commissioner (2023) defines gender stereotype as "a generalized view or preconception about attributes or characteristics, or the roles that are or ought to be possessed by, or performed by women and men. A gender stereotype is harmful when it limits women's and men's capacity to develop their personal abilities, pursue their professional careers, and make choices about their lives." Stereotypes of all kinds can be harmful. They can flow from hostile or negative beliefs such as "women are scatterbrained" and "men are aggressive" or from seemingly benign beliefs such as "women are caring" and "men are tough."

ASK YOURSELF

Is There Gender Stereotyping in Nursing?

- How can you distinguish between an accurate description of a personality characteristic and an inaccurate stereotype?
- In what ways do you think nurses can help dispel stereotypes in nursing?
- How would you respond if your son or daughter chose nursing as a profession? Would you encourage him or her? Why or why not?

Stereotyping of Women in Nursing

Much has been presented in previous chapters about stereotyping and the position of women in society and in nursing. Social and cultural customs, along with the masculinization of medicine, have contributed to a female stereotype. Female nurses are likely to suffer from stereotypes such as women are emotional, passive, naïve, nurturing, accepting, or scatter brained. These hyperfeminine stereotypes increase female nurses' struggles for acceptance particularly in spheres of power where it may be difficult for female nurses to attain a place at the table. Stereotypes may also have a detrimental effect on patient care when female nurses have difficulties, for example, convincing male physicians of patients' deteriorating conditions (Andrews & Waterman, 2005). Female stereotypes may influence the perceived value of female-dominated, caring, professions. England (2010) argues that professions dominated by women, such as nursing, teaching, and social work, are not valued as much as those dominated by men. This gendered devaluation has given women a strong incentive to enter male-dominated jobs but has given men little incentive to take on female-dominated jobs. Like women, though, men in nursing also suffer from pervasive stereotypes.

Stereotyping of Men in Nursing

Florence Nightingale may have set the stage for the near exclusion of men in the profession. In the preface to *Notes on Nursing*, Nightingale (1859) wrote, "Every woman, . . . has, at one time or another of her life, charge of the personal health of somebody, whether child or invalid—in other words, every woman is a nurse" (p. 1). She went on to write "if, then, every woman must, at some time or other of her life become a nurse, *i.e.*, have charge of somebody's health, how immense and how valuable would be the produce of her united experience if every women would think how to nurse" (p. 1). The assumption that it was natural for nursing to be provided by women may have had a dampening effect on men who wanted to join the profession. In fact, stereotypes may be men's biggest challenge when they choose the profession of nursing (Teresa-Morales et al., 2022). Villenueve (1994) identified the feminine imagery associated with the term *nurse* as a potential barrier for men considering a career in nursing. MacWilliams et al. (2013) agree with Villeneuve—the source of the term *nurse* and the evoked images remain a barrier to some men who are considering a career in nursing. Although female imagery may discourage men from becoming nurses, men in nursing have reported other harmful stereotypes such as men are not compassionate, men in nursing are studying to become doctors, or men in nursing are failed medical students (Teresa-Morales et al., 2022; Wojciechowski, 2016).

Some men in nursing may experience a form of gender discrimination because of the stereotypical belief that men in nursing are gay. This stereotype is rooted in gender-based role assumptions related to the caring attributes that many perceive as feminine. Because nursing has historically been viewed as "woman's work," men in nursing have been categorized as feminine and have subsequently been labeled as gay, thereby exposing them to homophobia in the workplace. Harding (2007) found that heterosexual men in nursing sometimes employ strategies to avoid the being stereotyped as gay. Their strategies include avoiding contact with gay colleagues and making overt expressions of their heterosexuality. Nurses must be alert for stereotyping that marginalizes persons who do not identify as heterosexual and creates issues for those who do.

As the number of men in nursing increases, research directed toward gender-related issues in the profession has emerged. For example, many authors have focused nursing research on caring as it correlates with gender. Ironically, a gender bias in the literature on caring predates much of the actual research. For example, Reverby (1987) offered a historical perspective of caring as it relates to women but did not address implications related to the addition of men to the profession. Despite an interest in the caring aspect of nursing, Chinn (1991) devoted an entire anthology to caring but did not explore gender in relation to caring, except as it related to economic gains (or lack thereof) for male faculty members in male-dominated academic centers. Begany (1994) perpetuated a nursing stereotype by equating the positive attribute of caring to images of nurturer or handmaiden. The exclusion of men by Grigsby and Megel (1995) as they explored the caring experiences of nursing faculty is another example of nursing research that did not include men.

Research about possible differences in the expression of caring as it relates to the gender of the student, educator, or recipient of care demonstrates the attention these and other issues in nursing have commanded. In a literature review on gender and caring, Zhang and Liu (2016) found that differences in caring by gender have been identified. Male nursing students are more restrained than female students as they learn caring behaviors. Zhang and Liu also found that men in nursing used more humor in nursing care, whereas women used more touch. Touch is associated with caring behaviors but presents a problem for men in nursing because of gender and social rules. Men in nursing may be in a defensive position because masculine touch has been associated with sexual abuse. This stereotype forces a dichotomy in nursing behaviors because intimate touch is an expression of caring among female nurses, whereas men in nursing feel restrained from intimate touching (Baker et al., 2022). Harding (2007) suggested that these stigmatizing stereotypes create a barrier to caring, deter men from entering the profession, and may affect their retention in the workplace.

The image of nursing as an all-female profession may be gradually changing as strides are made to resolve gender issues through research, direct recruitment of male students, and advocacy. MacWilliams et al. (2013) conducted a literature review and assert that changes in nursing education may be the first step in the process of increasing the number of men in the profession. They propose attention to several issues that contribute to discrimination against men in nursing schools. Among those are the following:

- Ubiquitous reference to nurses as "she"
- Scarce course content on men's contribution to the profession
- Gender bias in clinical assignments
- Anti-male remarks from nursing faculty
- Scarcity of male mentorship
- Lack of course content related to communication differences between the genders (p. 41)

Various organizations advocate for men in nursing. The primary advocacy group for men is the American Association for Men in Nursing (AAMN). AAMN addresses issues of gender stereotyping with the mission "[t]o shape the practice, education, research, and leadership for men in nursing and advance men's health" (American Association for Men in Nursing, nd). AAMN's objectives include (1) encouraging men to become nurses; (2) supporting men who are nurses to grow professionally; (3) advocating for continued research, education, and dissemination of information about men's health issues and men in nursing, and (4) supporting members' full participation in the profession. The Oregon Center for Nursing is an example of an organization that stepped up to the challenge to recruit more men into the profession with the campaign entitled "Are You Man Enough to Be a Nurse?" (Fig. 17.1). Ongoing since 2002 the recruiting campaign attempts to reframe men in the profession through posters that depict a group of men in nursing accompanied with masculine symbols such as a golf bag, a snowboard, a business suit, climbing attire, and

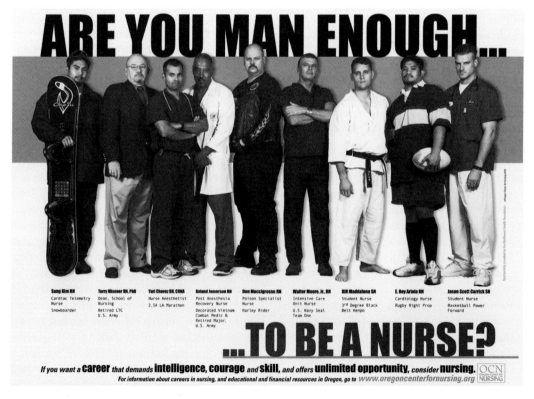

Fig. 17.1 Recruiting Poster From the Oregon Center for Nursing. (From the Oregon Center for Nursing archives. https://oregoncenterfornursing.org/store/)

a rugby uniform (Bridges & Mosseri, 2013). The incremental changes initiated by AAMN and the Oregon Center for Nursing are examples of a welcomed evolution of the profession.

Gender Bias

Whereas gender stereotyping refers to generalized preconceptions, **gender bias** suggests a preference or prejudice toward one gender over the other. Bias can be conscious or unconscious. It may manifest in many ways, both subtle and conspicuous, and can result in insignificant or significant consequences. In the workplace, gender bias may include the unequal treatment in such areas as promotion, pay, benefits, privileges, and expectations due to gender-based attitudes of an employer. In nursing practice, gender bias may also include patients' preference of one gender nurse over another.

Patients' Preference

A patient's preference of one gender nurse over another can emerge from culture, religion, or past experiences. For example, modesty is a fundamental precept of the Muslim faith. Muslim female patients may refuse to undress in front of or be touched by a male nurse. Likewise, Buddhist monks and nuns may prefer to be treated by a nurse of the same sex. In an intriguing study on patients' preferences of one gender physician over another, nearly 90 percent of patients had no gender preference regarding routine medical visits. However, patients who preferred male physicians were slightly more likely to be Black, and patients who preferred female physicians were slightly more likely to be White. Not surprisingly, patients who preferred a female were more likely to be female, and patients who preferred a male were more likely to be male (Nolen et al., 2016). The Nolen et al. study gives some insight into patients' preferences of physician gender, however, more nursing research is needed to determine patients' preferences regarding nurses. Although these preferences may be examples of gender bias, nurses should be sensitive to and respect patients' preferences when possible. The perception of appropriate relationships between genders is integral to human values and customs. The ICN *Code of Ethics for Nurses* (2021) states that nurses must acknowledge and respect the values, customs, and religious beliefs of the individual. Likewise, the American Nursing Association (ANA) *Code of Ethics for Nurses* (2015) is clear that patients have the "moral and legal right to determine what will be done with and to their own person" (p. 2). Congruent with the ICN, the CNA *Code of Ethics for Registered Nurses* (2017) enjoins nurses to respect the person receiving care, support them in maintaining their dignity, and take into account their values, customs, and spiritual beliefs.

Gender Bias in Nursing Education

Even though nursing education has been lauded for its efforts to bring men into the profession, gender bias still exists—particularly among students. Alex Miller wrote, "I know gender bias is alive and well in many ways, shapes and forms" (2014, p. 47). Miller reports that when he was in nursing school he was told that he was going to have an "easy ride up the ladder of progression in my career and would most likely end up in a critical care area because men were just more technically minded" (p. 47), a nursing stereotype that can be harmful to men's relationships with female nurses. Morgan et al. (2019) discovered instances of male graduate students being targeted in online classrooms because their opinions differed from female classmates. Some men in the study reported that they had difficulty connecting with the female students in online group assignments or sometimes were totally excluded from online work groups. Men in the study also described uncivil behaviors directed toward them in the clinical setting. In one instance a female student berated a male student who had been offered a nursing position, suggesting that he was offered the position only because he was male. Another student suggested that a male student was selected because "men are helpful for moving heavy patients" (Morgan et al., 2019). In one study, male nursing students perceive a higher level of gender bias in nursing education than their female faculty (Davidson, 2014), perhaps highlighting unintentional faculty bias. The same types of gender bias based on stereotypes have been reported in numerous other studies.

Although men may have hidden advantages in nursing, some areas, primarily in women's health, have remained closed to them. Many anecdotal stories involve men in nursing who were denied experiences in the care of women—particularly obstetrics and gynecology. This form of discrimination is reinforced in educational settings when faculty members seek permission for male student nurses to observe or participate in procedures with female patients, but do not seek permission of male patients when female students are involved.

Are Male Nurses Perceived as More Competent?

A number of studies over the past 30 years have shown that physicians view male nurses as more competent than their female counterparts and that female nurses are often ignored, whereas male nurses' opinions are valued.

- Have you observed this behavior in your clinical or classroom settings?
- How could you best deal with this form of modern sexism?

Sexual Orientation

Although we pointed out that heterosexual men in nursing are often incorrectly stereotyped as gay, nurses are likely to be practicing in every state and working in every hospital. Fearing sexual harassment and discrimination from coworkers, superiors, and bureaucratic systems, many remain reluctant to reveal their sexual orientation. Lesbian, gay, bisexual, transgender, queer (or questioning), and other (**LGBTQ+**) nurses face unique difficulties in the nursing workforce. Sexual harassment and bigotry are facts of life for many LGBTQ+ nurses. However, acceptance of the LGBTQ+ lifestyle is improving worldwide. There has been a general shift in many countries around the globe toward greater acceptance of homosexuality and gay rights. In fact, many of the countries surveyed since 2002 have seen a double-digit increase in acceptance of homosexuality (Pew Research Center, 2020). Although the United States has far from the highest acceptance rate, attitudes are improving. In 2022, 62 percent of a Gallup Poll survey respondents said they were satisfied with the acceptance of gays and lesbians in the nation. This was up from 55 percent in 2021 and 56 percent in 2020 (Gallup, 2022). Nevertheless, there are those in the United States who continue to hold a bias against individuals with nonheterosexual orientation.

A harmful, culturally insidious attitude against LGBTQ+ individuals can range from prejudice to homophobia. More extreme forms of bigotry include harassment and physical violence. In 1997 Zurlinden wrote, "Unmasked, homophobia is really hatred, willful ignorance, mean-spiritedness, and narrow-mindedness. People suffering from homophobia do not run screaming in terror when they encounter a lesbian or gay man.

Instead, they assume they are justified to be cruel; to discriminate in housing, employment, and education; and to pass laws to prevent gay men and lesbians from enjoying the civil liberties that other Americans take for granted" (p. 11). Further, prejudice at the institutional level leads to employment discrimination.

Within healthcare institutions, bigotry can be insidious, damaging, and difficult to change. Some employers systematically discriminate against LGBTQ+ nurses through hiring, promotion, and disciplinary practices. This may be the result of institutional policy, discriminatory administrative practice, punitive supervisors, or sexual bias of coworkers. For example, discrimination may be the basis of denying some employment benefits, such as spousal health insurance, to LGBTQ+ people while making the same benefits available to heterosexuals. In 2015 the Supreme Court guaranteed the right to same-sex marriage, and although most states have had contentious public battles defining marriage, most states now allow same-sex marriage. In a progressive move forward, many employers have agreed to extend spousal benefits such as health insurance, life insurance, and maternity leave to same-gender couples.

Though discriminatory practices remain in some places, most healthcare professions have publicly endorsed a nonjudgmental attitude toward sexual orientation. The ANA, the American Academy of Nursing, the International Society for Psychiatric-Mental Health Nurses, the National Association of School Nurses, the National Student Nurses Association, the American Psychiatric Association, the American Psychological Association, the National Association of Social Workers, and the American Medical Association all include statements related to nonjudgmental recognition of sexual orientation.

GENDER ISSUES AND NURSING PRACTICE

Issues in Women's Health Care

Health care provided to women has been different from that of men. In the past, women's healthcare issues were marginalized, medicalized, or ignored completely. For example, the word *hysteria* comes from the Greek word meaning *womb*. The term arose from an ancient medical misunderstanding of basic female anatomy that imagined a nomad uterus wandering aimlessly around the female body. During the 19th and most of the 20th centuries, medical research was conducted nearly exclusively on men—ignoring the unique aspects of and health needs of women. Childbirth and menopause, both of which are natural and healthy life transitions, were medicalized, and women were subjected to invasive and dangerous treatments.

Thanks to women's advocates, Western society has come a long way in recognizing the healthcare needs of women and closing many of the gaps. Medical research now includes women (with exceptions for pregnancy), and there has been a strong focus on the women's health care. In the United States, many federal assistance programs support women's health. These include Medicaid, which covers health insurance for certain categories of mothers; the Special Supplemental Nutrition Program for Women, Infants, and Children (WIC); the Family Planning Program; the Breast and Cervical Cancer Early Detection Program; and the Maternal-Child Health Block Grant. Numerous other federal programs benefit children. These and other programs are congruent with the World Health Organization's goal to ensure access to safe, respectful, high-quality sexual and reproductive health care, particularly contraceptive access and maternal health care, to reduce the global rates of maternal morbidity and mortality (WHO, 2015).

Many contemporary issues involve the ethics and distributive justice of women's health care. Nurses are witness to all of it. For example, because of recent policy changes, contraception is no longer available to many women. Some health insurance plans do not cover contraception, occasional physicians refuse to prescribe contraception, and a few scattered pharmacists refuse to dispense contraceptives. The same is true of abortion. Since the 2022 Supreme Court decided in *Dobbs v. Jackson Women's Health Organization* (2022) that women have no constitutional right to abortion, many states have passed legislation that ban abortion and some have laws that are so restrictive that abortion providers are no longer able to deliver the service (New York Times, 2023). In addition, women who have abortions could face potential criminal charges in some states (Ali, 2022).

Pregnancy and childbirth present many healthcare issues for women, most of which are imbued with moral overtones and ethical implications. Many are surrounded by partisan and policy discussions. As you recall, some of these issues have been discussed throughout this book. Issues include assisted reproductive technology, advanced maternal age, pregnancy and

substance abuse, elective cesarean birth, prenatal diagnostic procedures, abortion, and surrogacy. Ask yourself the following questions about these issues.

The questions that arise around issues of women's health, particularly pregnancy, are so value-laden that they spark contentious debate. Nurses are not immune to these moral and ethical controversies. Nurses' identities integrate the values of the profession with personal values, which sometimes collide with the values of the society, institution, or patient. When this happens, nurses must provide compassionate, respectful, and competent care. However, they also have a responsibility to preserve their own wholeness of character and integrity. According to the ANA *Code of Ethics for Nurses* (2015), when patients ask for help clarifying values, nurses are free to express their informed personal opinions if they do not coerce, manipulate, or unintentionally influence patients. When a decision or action is morally objectionable, the nurse may refuse to participate on moral grounds. Refusal to participate in the form of conscientious objection may not be arbitrary and must be based on moral values rather than personal preference, prejudice, bias, or convenience (ANA, 2015, p. 21). When nurses decide not to participate, they must communicate the decision in a timely manner so that alternative arrangements for patient care can be made. Both the ICN and CNA codes of ethics for nurses stipulate that while conscientious objection is ethically permitted, the nurse must provide continuity of care to the patient until an alternative professional is present. Even so, a nurse who exercises conscientious objection may not be protected from organizational consequences.

Issues in Men's Health Care

The ethics and issues surrounding men's health revolve more around general health disparities and healthcare access, rather than reproductive health. Even though men are thought to enjoy more privileges, opportunities, and power than women, they have a lower life expectancy. Men have a life expectancy six years shorter than women (CDC, 2022c) and the discrepancy widens with older age. By age 85 women outnumber men by a ratio of 2.6 to 1 (Harvard Medical School, 2019). The health disparity between men and women begins before birth and continues throughout the life span. Males are more likely to die before birth, be born prematurely, and die before their first birthday. Men are more likely to become ill and die at a younger age. Their rates of

ASK YOURSELF

What are your Thoughts About These Issues?

1. Assisted reproductive technology
   a. Is assisted reproductive technology, such as in vitro fertilization, a right or a privilege?
   b. Who should pay for assisted reproductive technology?
   c. Who should "own" unused embryos?
   d. Should there be a maximum age at which women can no longer receive assisted reproductive technology?
2. Advanced maternal age
   a. Pregnancy at advanced age presents questions about the risk to the fetus and the mother. At what age should planned pregnancy be discouraged?
   b. What about the effects of chronic illness or medication on a fetus?
   c. What may be the long-term social implications of geriatric pregnancy?
3. Pregnancy and substance use
   a. What is the nurse's role in caring for an addicted pregnant woman?
   b. Who should bear the cost for neonatal abstinence syndrome?
   c. Should a newborn be released to an addicted mother?
4. Cesarean birth
   a. Nearly one-third of all babies born in the United States are born via cesarean section (CDC, 2022a), and most of these are elective. Some blame the high infant mortality rate in the United States (which is higher than most other developed countries) on the high percentage of cesarean deliveries. Should physicians and nurses discourage elective cesarean delivery?
   b. Who should bear the cost of elective cesarean delivery?
5. Prenatal diagnostic procedures
   a. Prenatal diagnostic procedures can reveal fetal anomalies and allow parents the choice to terminate the pregnancy. What are the moral implications of the choices parents make based on prenatal testing results?
   b. If a pregnant couple has moral objections to abortion, should they have prenatal diagnostic testing?
   c. How can nurses support pregnant couples who have abnormal prenatal diagnostic test results?
6. Abortion
   a. Is abortion a right or a privilege?
   b. Who should have access to abortion, and who should pay?
   c. Should decisions about abortion rest solely with the pregnant woman? Both parents? The government?
   d. Should late-term abortions be allowed to save the life or health of the mother?
7. Surrogacy
   a. In the case of commercial contractual surrogacy, who should make decisions about the pregnancy and fetus?
   b. Should a contractual surrogate have the right to keep the child?
   c. Should the biological father share rights with the surrogate?
   d. What moral/ethical implications arise when a woman is paid to be a surrogate?

liver disease, heart disease, cancer, diabetes, hypertension, HIV/AIDS, inguinal hernias, aortic aneurism, gout, kidney stones, alcoholism, emphysema, and duodenal ulcer are all higher than in women. Men are also more likely to die from suicide, unintentional injuries, homicide, and toxic occupational exposure (Harvard Medical School, 2019; Heron, 2018; Moon, 2018). Men are four times more likely to have gout; three times more likely to develop kidney stones, become alcoholics, or have bladder cancer. Nevertheless, men are less likely to seek health care, particularly for mental health problems. Although women seek health care more often than men do, healthcare costs for men beyond the age of 65 exceeds that of women (Harvard Medical School, 2019).

Therefore, it is especially important that nurses are alert to gender-related healthcare disparities and focus on improving men's overall health through patient teaching and support of primary, secondary, and tertiary prevention efforts.

Even though men suffer more health problems in general, reproductive health is an important component of men's overall health. Infertility, pregnancy, and contraception have been perceived as female issues, so males have often been overlooked in discussions. The problem is compounded because most nurses are women, making it difficult for some male patients or some female nurses to raise issues of reproductive health. Ignoring reproductive health issues can be devastating. Prostate cancer is the second-leading cancer occurring in men and the second-leading cause of cancer death. One in eight men will be diagnosed with prostate cancer during his lifetime, and more than 34,000 men die from prostate cancer in the United States each year (American Cancer Society, 2023a). Also, many men will develop testicular cancer. The average age of diagnosis for testicular cancer is about 33 years, a time of life when many men avoid seeking health care (American Cancer Society, 2023b). Bioethics and the law agree that women have the right to make decisions about their own bodies, including pregnancy, but men are often part of the conversation. Issues of men's autonomy, accountability, and responsibility also surround reproductive issues such as infertility, contraception, pregnancy, sexually transmitted diseases, surrogacy, abortion, sperm donation, and erectile dysfunction. Discussion about reproductive issues should include rights and responsibilities of men as well as women (Fig. 17.2).

Even though men have overall poorer health and die younger than women, men's health gets little public attention. In fact, a review of national and state health assistance programs reveals that there is no program solely dedicated to men's health care. Benefits. gov (2023), an official US government website, lists nearly 300 healthcare and medical assistance programs that serve special populations such as veterans; Native Americans; women; children; children with disabilities; disabled adults; children of female Vietnam Veterans; and those who are homeless, indigent, or addicted. Even

though many very specific groups of people are targeted by these assistance programs, not one is solely dedicated to the care of men. The ethical principle of distributive justice demands that nurses advocate for men's health issues because inequality in healthcare delivery increases the incidence and burden of illness, trauma, suffering, and premature death of men (ANA, 2015). The ICN, ANA, and CNA codes of nursing ethics all call for nurses to work together with other health professionals to design ethical, respectful, and equitable approaches to reduce health disparities.

Issues in LGBTQ+ Health Care

Health care of LGBTQ+ patients is fraught with ethical issues, from stigmatization to health disparities and unfair and unethical distribution of healthcare resources. According to a Gallup poll, 7.1 percent of American adults identify as lesbian, gay, bisexual, or transgender (Jones, 2022). There are same-sex households in all 50 states and 99 percent of US counties (Ard & Makadon, 2012; Williams Institute, 2019). LGBTQ+ people are diverse. They include people of all races and ethnicities, all socioeconomic groups, all ages, and all walks of life. So, it is likely that every practicing nurse has encountered LGBTQ+ patients, whether aware of it or not. To deliver proper nursing care, nurses must set aside bias and prejudice when caring for LGBTQ+ patients and become sensitive to health issues surrounding sexual orientation.

Nurses must be aware that LGBTQ+ people have higher risk for and higher incidence of many disorders. LGBTQ+ people more commonly report being in fair or poor health than the general population, even though the LGBTQ+ population is younger. They also report higher rates of ongoing health conditions and disability or chronic disease. Proportionately more LGBTQ+ people have health problems that require regular monitoring, medical care, medication than their non-LGBTQ+ counterparts (Dawson et al., 2021). They are at a higher risk for sexually transmitted diseases, Tb, hepatitis, HIV, cancers, cardiovascular diseases, and obesity, (CDC, 2016a, 2022b; Hafeez et al., 2017). They are more likely to smoke, use alcohol and other illicit substances, and participate in risky sexual practices (Gonzales et al., 2016), which puts them at higher risk for a number of chronic diseases. LGBTQ+ people are also more likely to suffer social and mental health problems.

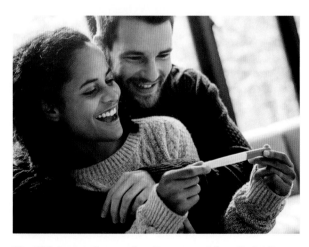

Fig. 17.2 Issues Surrounding Pregnancy Affect Both Women and Men. (©iStock.com/Rawpixel.)

LGBTQ+ people are more likely to face social and family problems and to experience mental health problems. Many face homophobia and stigma within their families and/or communities, which increases the probability of discriminatory acts such as rejection, bullying, teasing, harassment, and physical assault (CDC, 2016b). LGBTQ+ youths are more likely to be rejected by their families and to become homeless. In fact, more than a quarter of all LGBTQ+ youth report homelessness or housing instability at some point in their lives with the incidence rising to nearly half of all native/indigenous LGBTQ+ youth (The Trevor Project, 2022b). Depression, self-harm, and suicide attempts are more common among LGBTQ+ people (Medina-Martinez et al., 2021). One research study found that those who experienced stronger family and community rejection were six times more likely to report high levels of depression and eight times more likely to have tried to commit suicide (CDC, 2016b). Three-fourths of LGBTQ+ youth experience anxiety and more than half experience depression (The Trevor Project, 2022a). Even though LGBTQ+ people are known to have more physical and mental health problems, they encounter barriers to health care.

To deliver holistic, patient-centered care to LGBTQ+ patients, nurses must be aware of the unique psychosocial environment of bias, which has a dampening effect on health-seeking behaviors, and the specific health disparities that affect this population. Although the numbers of uninsured dropped after passage of the *Affordable Care Act*, LGBTQ+ patients face barriers when accessing health care such as stigma, discrimination, inequity in health insurance, and outright denial of health care because of sexual orientation. LGBTQ+ people are twice as likely to be uninsured (Baker & Durso, 2017), and they are more likely to receive substandard health care. Bias exists among some healthcare providers to the point of open hostility. Because LGBTQ+ patients are often aware of this bias, they may conceal their sexual orientation from providers. This leads to deficiencies in access to care, missed opportunities to identify domestic violence, and failure to diagnose diseases that are prevalent in the LGBTQ+ community (Ard & Makadon, 2012). In addition, LGBTQ+ patients in same-sex relationships are less likely to have preventive health care. Lack of access to employer-sponsored health insurance for same-sex partners and spouses accounts for some of these differences (Ard &

Makadon, 2012). Many have difficulty finding providers who will not pass judgment on their sexual orientation or gender identity. LGBTQ+ patients have said that providers have directed disrespectful, harsh, or abusive language toward them (Human Rights Watch, 2018). Some providers may not offer the services LGBTQ+ people need, particularly in rural areas or may refuse to refer them to other providers. LGBTQ+ people sometimes have trouble finding providers who will treat them at all. In one survey, as many as one-third of LGBTQ+ people seeking care experienced negative interactions with a healthcare provider because of their gender identity, and many avoided health care altogether because they were worried about being mistreated (Baker & Durso, 2017). Barriers to healthcare services cause or exacerbate disparities health, but ongoing efforts have improved healthcare access to this population. Healthy people 2030 addresses goals for LGBTQ+ health care (Box 17.1).

Nurses must honor the human rights of all people. Bias goes against the core values of nursing and is specifically addressed in nursing codes of ethics, which enjoin nurses to treat patients with sensitivity and respect regardless of their personal attributes. According to the ANA *Code of Ethics for Nurses* (2015), "When caring for patients, nurses must consider factors such as 'culture, value systems, religious or spiritual beliefs, lifestyle, social support system, sexual orientation, or gender expression, and primary language when planning individual [patient], family and population-centered care'" (ANA, 2015, p. 1). Language in the Canadian *Code of Ethics for Registered Nurses* (2017) is very similar, "Nurses do not discriminate on the basis of a person's race, ethnicity, culture, political and spiritual beliefs, social or marital status, gender, gender identity, gender expression, sexual orientation, age, health status, place of origin, lifestyle, mental or physical ability, socio-economic status, or any other attribute" (Element F.1). Likewise, the ICN (2021) *Code of Ethics for Nurses* states "Nursing care is respectful of and unrestricted by considerations of age, colour, culture, ethnicity, disability or illness, gender, sexual orientation, nationality, politics, language, race, religious or spiritual beliefs, legal, economic or social status" (p. 2). Recall that nursing codes of ethics are nonnegotiable standards which nurses must uphold. So, regardless of personal, cultural, or religious beliefs, nurses must deliver nursing care to LGBTQ+ patients that honors their human

BOX 17.1 **Healthy People 2030**

Healthy People 2030 sets national objectives to improve health and well-being over the next decade in the United States. Below is the goal of Health People 2030 as it relates to LGBTQ+ people.

LGBTQ+ Goal: Improve the health, safety, and well-being of lesbian, gay, bisexual, and transgender people.

Adolescents
- Reduce bullying of lesbian, gay, or bisexual high school students.
- Reduce bullying of transgender students.

Drug and Alcohol Use
- Reduce the proportion of lesbian, gay, or bisexual high school students who have used illicit drugs.
- Reduce the proportion of transgender high school students who have used illicit drugs.

Mental Health and Mental Disorders
- Reduce suicidal thoughts in lesbian, gay, or bisexual high school students.
- Reduce suicidal thoughts in transgender students.

Public Health Infrastructure
- Increase the number of national surveys that collect data on lesbian, gay, and bisexual populations.
- Increase the number of national surveys that collect data on transgender populations.
- Increase the number of states, territories, and DC that include sexual orientation and gender identity questions in the BRFSS.
- Increase the number of states, territories, and DC that use the standard module on sexual orientation and gender identity in the Behavioral Risk Factor Surveillance System (BRFSS) (CDC, 2023).

Sexually Transmitted Diseases
- Reduce the number of new HIV diagnoses.
- Increase linkage to HIV medical care.
- Reduce the syphilis rate in men who have sex with men.
- Reduce the number of new HIV infections.
- Increase knowledge of HIV status.
- Increase viral suppression (Office of Disease Prevention and Health Promotion, 2020).

rights and is sensitive to their unique problems and life circumstances.

When providing care, nurses must be aware of physical and mental health disparities of LGBTQ+ patients. Nurses who are alert to health risks of this population can deliver more compassionate and holistic care. They should learn about LGBTQ+ issues and current healthcare policies. They should create an inclusive environment with sensitivity and respect. For example, nurses might not understand that the terms *sexual orientation* and *gender identity* are different. **Sexual orientation** refers to sexual preference in a partner, including terms like gay, lesbian, or heterosexual, whereas **gender identity** refers to expressions of gender, including male, female, or nonbinary. This means that a nurse should address a patient and document nursing care according to the patient' stated gender identity, sexual orientation, chosen name, and preferred pronoun. Nurses' mistakes can present barriers to creating positive nurse/patient relationships, so communication basics are crucial. The nurse should avoid assuming a patient's gender identity or sexual orientation based on outward appearance because inferences may be incorrect. The nurse should never ask for a patient's "real" name, rather ask for the name listed on their insurance. Then, the nurse should refer to the patient by the preferred name. Respectful use of names and pronouns can open the door for productive communication.

Communication forms the basis of the nurse-patient relationship. So, nurses should encourage open dialogue that includes a nonjudgmental and compassionate attitude when caring for LGBTQ+ patients. They should assure privacy, especially when eliciting patients' health histories. The assessment of sexual and social history can be difficult for both the nurse and the patient. When talking about sexual relationships, nurses should ask specific questions about sexual practices, use gender-neutral language such as *partner*, assure patients that private information will be kept confidential, and be sensitive to patients' wishes about who may access their health records, who may visit, and who they have chosen to make healthcare decisions in case of their incapacity. Nurses should advocate for LGBTQ+ patients' rights, particularly if they witness patients being ignored, disrespected, bullied, or abused in other ways. Good communication and compassionate nursing care can establish the foundation of LGBTQ+ patients' experience of the healthcare system and set them on the path to better health.

CASE PRESENTATION

Lessons Learned From a Transgender Patient

Ryan K. Sallans (2016) published a commentary about his encounters in the healthcare system in the *AMA Journal of Ethics*. The commentary describes lessons from his experience as a transgender male. These lessons included the following:

Lesson 1: Understanding transgender health means understanding risks faced by transgender people.

Lesson 2: A healthcare professional's humility can be a source of relief to an anxious patient.

Lesson 3: Transgender patients are not all alike and need different things from health care.

Lesson 4: There is not a single right way to transition and not a single way to order events that need to happen for patients making transitions.

Lesson 5: Patients should not be required to conform to healthcare professionals' conceptions of what men and women are, have, or don't have.

Lesson 6: When personal pronoun usage mistakes happen (and they will), apologize sincerely and move on.

Lesson 7: Challenge uses of demeaning references ("he-she," "it," or other slang) to transgender patients.

Lesson 8: Being transgender might not be relevant to a particular clinical encounter, but references to a patient's gender identity in a health record can be relevant to all subsequent clinical encounters that patient has.

Lesson 9: Take care not to "out" patients who aren't "out" to everyone; ask patients about which information to document in their health records and preserve confidentiality.

Lesson 10: Transgender health literacy requires ongoing education and training.

Think About It

Issues related to transgender individuals evoke strong opinions, social discomfort, and political controversy. Lesson 2 is especially applicable to nursing: *A healthcare professional's humility can be a source of relief to an anxious patient.* This lesson alludes to an open and caring attitude nurses can assume when caring for transgender patients. When Ryan revealed to a healthcare provider that he was transgender, he feared the healthcare professional would reject him as a person. Instead, her response was, "I have never worked with someone who is transgender, but I am willing to learn." Ryan felt relief when he heard her nonjudgmental tone and sensed her humility and openness. He believed correctly that she would not reject him or his identity and that he could rely on her to listen, learn, and be a source of support (Sallans, 2016). Nurses must acknowledge that transgender individuals have inherent dignity, worth, unique attributes, and human rights. As a nursing student, please think about the following questions.

1. What ethical principles guide the care you deliver to transgender patients?
2. How will you, as a nurse, respond when a patient reveals to you that he or she is transgender?
3. What actions will you take when you hear other healthcare providers making negative remarks about a transgender patient?
4. Nursing codes of ethics call for nurses to engage in public policy focusing on the public's health. What legislative and regulatory policies that affect transgender individuals might benefit from nursing influence?

SUMMARY

Nursing has been faced with gender issues since the early days of the profession. The nursing role and status have been colored by societal expectations of women and paternalistic ideology permeating the healthcare arena. Considerations of gender can be related to lower salaries for nurses compared with primarily male professions, communication patterns with physicians and patients, perceptions of abilities to carry out nursing's caring imperative, and stereotypical expectations of how nurses should look and act. Although men in the profession face the challenge of dealing with societal stereotypes, they are also often tracked into higher-paying and more prestigious positions. Issues concerning discrimination based on sexual orientation occur on many fronts and may be underrecognized. Awareness of these issues enables nurses of both genders to be alert for inequities and to develop strategies for change. In addition to workforce gender issues, nurses must be sensitive to healthcare needs of men, women, and LGBTQ+ patients.

CHAPTER HIGHLIGHTS

- Social expectations of women and patriarchal ideology throughout history have led to gender discrimination for both women and men in nursing.

- Issues of comparable worth relative to gender are of concern in nursing, particularly in areas of salary and positions of prestige and responsibility.
- Gender stereotyping and bias can lead to rude and disruptive behavior, which diminishes cognitive and procedural skills—affecting the quality of nursing care.
- There are distinct issues in healthcare delivery, health-seeking behaviors, health needs, and available resources for men and women.
- Health care of LGBTQ+ patients is fraught with ethical issues, from health disparities to unfair and unethical distribution of healthcare resources.

DISCUSSION QUESTIONS AND ACTIVITIES

1. In what ways does your school curriculum address issues of improving gender equality in the nursing profession?
2. Read an article on how nursing students learn to care. Do men express caring differently than women? How does this relate to your experiences as a student nurse? How does this relate to Begany's (1994) images of nurses as nurturers or handmaidens?
3. What stereotypes of nurses are present in your community or the national media? What do you think it will take to change these and other stereotypes about nurses?
4. What is the gender makeup of your local nursing administration? How many women are in positions of authority or power within your healthcare setting? What are their salary ranges? How do their salaries compare with those of men in positions of similar responsibility?
5. Search the nursing curriculum in your nursing school for evidence of content related to men in nursing. Does the content seem relevant? Is the amount of content sufficient in your opinion?
6. Ask female and male students in your nursing class their perception of gender stereotyping and gender bias in nursing. Is their perception different?
7. Conduct an Internet search for "men and abortion decisions." Have a critical discussion with your classmates and course instructor about the issues raised.
8. Read the ANA position statement on nursing advocacy for LGBTQ+ populations. Discuss with your classmates how each will implement the position in your practice.

REFERENCES

Ali, S. S. (2022). Prosecutors in states where abortion is now illegal could begin building criminal cases against providers. *NBC News.* https://www.nbcnews.com/news/us-news/prosecutors-states-abortion-now-illegal-begin-prosecute-abortion-provi-rcna35268.

American Association for Men in Nursing. (n.d.). *Our values.* https://www.aamn.org/our-values.

American Cancer Society. (2023a). *Key statistics for prostate cancer.* https://www.cancer.org/cancer/prostate-cancer/about/key-statistics.html.

American Cancer Society. (2023b). *Key statistics for testicular cancer.* https://www.cancer.org/cancer/testicular-cancer/about/key-statistics.html.

ANA. (2015). *Code of ethics for nurses with interpretive statements.* Nursebooks.org. http://nursingworld.org/DocumentVault/Ethics-1/Code-of-Ethics-for-Nurses.html.

Andrews, T., & Waterman, H. (2005). Visualizing deteriorating conditions. *Grounded Theory Review, 4*(2), 63–94.

Ard, K. L., & Makadon, H. J. (2012). *Improving the health care of lesbian, gay, bisexual and transgender (LGBT) people: Understanding and eliminating health disparities.* https://www.lgbthealtheducation.org/publication/improving-the-health-care-of-lesbian-gay-bisexual-and-transgender-lgbt-people-understanding-and-eliminating-health-disparities/.

Baker, K., & Durso, L. E. (2017). *Why repealing the Affordable Care Act is bad medicine for LGBT communities.* https://www.americanprogress.org/issues/lgbt/news/2017/03/22/428970/repealing-affordable-care-act-bad-medicine-lgbt-communities.

Baker, M. J., Fisher, M. J., & Pryor, J. (2022). Potential for misinterpretation: An everyday problem male nurses encounter in inpatient rehabilitation. *International Journal of Nursing Practice, 28*(1), 1–10. https://doi.org/10.1111/ijn.12985.

Begany, T. (1994). Your image is brighter than ever. *RN, 57,* 28–35.

Benefits.gov. (2023). *Healthcare and medical assistance.* https://www.benefits.gov/categories/Healthcare%20and%20Medical%20Assistance.

Bridges, T., & Mosseri, S. (2013). "Are you man enough to be a nurse?" Campaign posters. In: *Inequality by (Interior) design.* https://inequalitybyinteriordesign.wordpress.com/2013/06/10/are-you-man-enough-to-be-a-nurse-campaign-posters/.

CDC. (2016a). *Gay and bisexual men's health.* https://www.cdc.gov/msmhealth/.

CDC. (2016b). *Stigma and discrimination.* https://www.cdc.gov/msmhealth/stigma-and-discrimination.htm.

CDC. (2022a). *Cesarean delivery rate by state.* https://www.cdc.gov/nchs/pressroom/sosmap/cesarean_births/cesareans.htm.

CDC. (2022b). *For your health: Recommendations for a healthier you*. https://www.cdc.gov/msmhealth/for-your-health.htm.

CDC. (2022c). *Life expectancy in the U.S. dropped for the second year in a row in 2021*. https://www.cdc.gov/nchs/pressroom/nchs_press_releases/2022/20220831.htm.

CDC. (2023). *Behavioral risk factor surveillance system*. https://www.cdc.gov/brfss/index.html.

Chinn, P. L. (1991). *Anthology on caring*. National League of Nursing Press.

Christensen, M., & Knight, J. (2014). Nursing is no place for men: A thematic analysis of male nursing student experiences of undergraduate nursing education. *Journal of Nursing Education and Practice, 4*(12), 95–104.

CNA. (2017). *Code of ethics for registered nurses*. https://cdn1.nscn.ca/sites/default/files/documents/resources/code-of-ethics-for-registered-nurses.pdf#:~:text=The%20Canadian%20Nurses%20Association%20%28CNA%29%20Code%20of%20Ethics,receiving%20care.%20The%20Codeis%20both%20aspirational%20and%20regulatory.

D'Antonio, P., & Whelan, J. C. (2009). Counting nurses: The power of historical census data. *Journal of Clinical Nursing, 18*(19), 2717–2724. https://doi.org/10.1111/j.1365-2702.2009.02892.x.

Dalai Lama. (1999). *Ethics for the new millennium*. Riverhead.

Davidson, R. M. (2014). *Female faculty and senior male student perceptions of gender bias in nursing education*. Capella University.

Dawson, L., Frederiksen, B., Long, M., Ranji, U., & Kates, J. (2021). *LGBTQ+ people's health and experiences accessing care*. https://www.kff.org/report-section/lgbt-peoples-health-and-experiences-accessing-care-report/

Dobbs v Jackson Women's Health Organization (U.S. Supreme Court 2022). https://supreme.justia.com/cases/federal/us/597/19-1392/.

England, P. (2010). The gender revolution: Uneven and stalled. *Gender and Society, 24*(2), 149–166.

Gallup. (2022). *Americans offer gloomy state of the nation report*. https://news.gallup.com/poll/389309/americans-offer-gloomy-state-nation-report.aspx.

Gonzales, G., Przedworski, J., & Henning-Smith, C. (2016). Comparison of health and health risk factors between lesbian, gay, and bisexual adults and heterosexual adults in the United States: Results from the National Health Interview Survey. *Journal of the American Medical Association, 176*(9), 1344–1351. https://doi.org/10.1001/jamainternmed.2016.3432.

Grigsby, K. A., & Megel, M. E. (1995). Caring experiences of nurse educators. *Journal of Nursing Education, 34*(9), 411–418.

Hafeez, H., Zeshan, M., Tahir, M. A., Jahan, N., & Naveed, S. (2017). Health care disparities among lesbian, gay, bisex-ual, and transgender youth: A literature review. *Cureus, 9*(4), e1184. https://doi.org/10.7759/cureus.1184.

Harding, T. (2007). The construction of men who are nurses as gay. *Journal of Advanced Nursing, 60*(6), 636–644. https://doi.org/10.1111/j.1365-2648.2007.04447.x.

Harvard Medical School. (2019). Mars vs. Venus: The gender gap in health. *Harvard Men's Health Watch*. https://www.health.harvard.edu/newsletter_article/mars-vs-venus-the-gender-gap-in-health.

Hegewisch, A. (2018). *The gender wage gap: 2017 earnings differences by gender, race, and ethnicity*. https://iwpr.org/publications/gender-wage-gap-2017/.

Heron, M. (2018). *Deaths: Leading causes for 2016*. https://www.cdc.gov/nchs/data/nvsr/nvsr67/nvsr67_06.pdf.

Human Rights Watch. (2018). *You don't want second best: Anti-LGBT discrimination in US health care*. https://www.hrw.org/report/2018/07/23/you-dont-want-second-best/anti-lgbt-discrimination-us-health-care.

ICN. (2021). *The ICN code of ethics for nurses*. https://www.icn.ch/system/files/2021-10/ICN_Code-of-Ethics_EN_Web_0.pdf.

IOM. (2010). *The future of nursing: Leading change, advancing health*. N. A. Press. https://www.nap.edu/read/12956/chapter/1.

Jones, J. M. (2022). *What percentage of Americans are LGBT*. https://news.gallup.com/poll/332522/percentage-americans-lgbt.aspx.

MacWilliams, B. R., Schmidt, B., & Bleich, M. R. (2013). Men in nursing. *AJN American Journal of Nursing, 113*(1), 38–44. https://doi.org/10.1097/01.NAJ.0000425746.83731.16.

Medina-Martinez, J., Saus-Ortega, C., Sanchez-Lorente, M. M., Sosa-Palanca, E. M., Garcia-Martinez, P., & Marmol-Lopez, M. I. (2021). Health inequities in LGBT people and nursing interventions to reduce them: A systematic review. *International Journal of Environmental Research and Public Health, 18*(3–16). https://mdpi-res.com/ijerph/ijerph-18-11801/article_deploy/ijerph-18-11801-v4.pdf?version=1637139418.

Miller, A. (2014). Gender equality in nursing? *Australian Nursing & Midwifery Journal, 22*(1), 47.

Moon, D. G. (2018). Changing men's health: Leading the future. *World Journal of Men's Health, 36*(1), 1–3. https://doi.org/10.5534/wjmh.18101.

Morgan, B. T., Smallheer, B. A., Gordon, H. A., & Malloy, M. A. (2019). *Starting the conversation: Gender and incivility in nursing education*. Reflections on Nursing Leadership. https://www.reflectionsonnursingleadership.org/features/more-features/starting-the-conversation-gender-and-incivility-in-nursing-education.

New York Times. (2023). *Tracking the states where abortion is now banned*. https://www.nytimes.com/interactive/2022/us/abortion-laws-roe-v-wade.html.

Nightingale, F. (1859). *Notes on nursing: What it is, and what it is not.* Harrison & Sons. http://digital.library.upenn.edu/women/nightingale/nursing/nursing.html.

Nolen, H. A., Moore, J. X., Rodgers, J. B., Wang, H. E., & Walter, L. A. (2016). Patient preference for physician gender in the emergency department. *Yale Journal of Biology and Medicine, 89*(2), 131–142. https://www.ncbi.nlm.nih.gov/pubmed/27354840.

Nurse.com. (2022). *Nurse salary research report.* https://www.nurse.com/blog/wp-content/uploads/2022/05/2022-Nurse-Salary-Research-Report-from-Nurse.com_.pdf.

Office of Disease Prevention and Health Promotion. (2020). *Healthy People 2030: Building a healthier future for all.* https://health.gov/healthypeople.

Oxford English Dictionary. *Nurse.* http://www.oed.com/view/Entry/54060?redirectedFrom=discrimination.

Oxford English Dictionary. *Patriarchy.* http://www.oed.com/view/Entry/54060?redirectedFrom=discrimination.

Pew Research Center. (2020). *The global divide on homosexuality persists: But increasing acceptance in many countries over the past two decades.* https://www.pewresearch.org/global/2020/06/25/global-divide-on-homosexuality-persists/.

Reverby, S. (1987). A caring dilemma: Womanhood and nursing in historical perspective. *Nursing Research, 36,* 5–10.

Sallans, R. K. (2016). Lessons from a transgender patient for health care professionals. *American Medical Association Journal of Ethics, 18*(11), 1139–1146. https://doi.org/10.1001/journalofethics.2016.18.11.mnar1-1611.

Smiley, R. A., Ruttinger, C., Oliveira, C. M., Hudson, L. R., Allgeyer, R., Reneau, K. A., Silvestre, J. H., & Alexander, M. (2021). The 2020 national nursing workforce survey. *Journal of Nursing Regulation, 12*(1), S1–S96. https://doi.org/10.1016/S2155-8256(21)00027-2.

Teresa-Morales, C., Rodríguez-Pérez, M., Araujo-Hernández, M., & Feria-Ramírez, C. (2022). Current stereotypes associated with nursing and nursing professionals: An integrative review. *International Journal of Environment, Research, and Public Health, 19*(13). https://doi.org/10.3390/ijerph19137640.

The Trevor Project. (2022a). *2022 National survey on LGBTQ youth mental health.* http://thetrevorproject.org.

The Trevor Project. (2022b). *Homelessness and housing instability among LGBTQ youth.* https://www.thetrevorproject.org/research-briefs/homelessness-and-housing-instability-among-lgbtq-youth-feb-2022/.

U.S. Bureau of Labor Statistics. (2021). *Occupational employment and wage statistics.* https://www.bls.gov/oes/current/oes291141.htm#nat.

U.S. Census Bureau. (2013). *Men in nursing occupations: American community survey highlight report.* https://www.census.gov/content/dam/Census/library/working-papers/2013/acs/2013_Landivar_02.pdf.

United Nations Human Rights Office of the High Commissioner. (2023). *Gender stereotyping.* https://www.ohchr.org/en/issues/women/wrgs/pages/genderstereotypes.aspx.

Villenueve, J. J. (1994). Recruiting and retaining men in nursing: A review of the literature. *Journal of Professional Nursing, 10*(4), 217–228.

WHO. (2015). *The prevention and elimination of disrespect and abuse during facility-based childbirth.* https://apps.who.int/iris/bitstream/handle/10665/134588/WHO_RHR_14.23_eng.pdf;jsessionid=C114B-94F026A0869543A4E18D6B5B241?sequence=1.

Williams Institute, UCLA School of Law. (2019). *LGBT data & demographics.* https://williamsinstitute.law.ucla.edu/visualization/lgbt-stats/?topic=LGBT#density.

Wojciechowski, M. (2016). *Male nurses confronting stereotypes and discrimination: Part 1, The issues.* Minority Nurse. https://minoritynurse.com/male-nurses-confronting-stereotypes-and-discrimination-part-1-the-issues/.

Zhang, W., & Liu, Y. -L. (2016). Demonstration of caring by males in clinical practice: A literature review. *International Journal of Nursing Sciences, 3*(3), 323–327. https://www.sciencedirect.com/science/article/pii/S2352013215300351.

Zurlinden, J. (1997). *Lesbian and gay nurses.* Delmar.

18

Ethical Issues Related to Transcultural and Spiritual Care

God is a spirit, a mystery beyond human understanding, and therefore we can only approach that mystery through metaphor. Our metaphors come, of course, from human and cultural understandings of the good, the loving, the just. . . . More surely than anything else, we are defined by our stories—the cultural myths we hear from our earliest days.

(Sewell, 1991, pp. 237, 261)

OBJECTIVES

After completing this chapter, the reader should be able to:

1. Describe factors associated with cultural competence within nursing.
2. Discuss the influence of culture on health and healthcare decisions.
3. Identify ethical approaches for addressing transcultural care issues in nursing.
4. Discuss ethical concerns related to the use of complementary and traditional therapies by patients.
5. Identify legal/ethical considerations related to transcultural issues.
6. Discuss the relationship between spirituality and health.
7. Describe potential ethical concerns associated with spirituality and religion.
8. Identify the nursing role in addressing patients' spiritual concerns.
9. Discuss considerations regarding nurturing one's spirit.
10. Identify components of codes of nursing ethics that provide an ethical imperative to incorporate transcultural and spiritual considerations in nursing care.

INTRODUCTION

The influence of culture, religion, and spirituality is a major factor in the development of values. Nurses come from many cultural and spiritual perspectives and deal with people, both patients and colleagues, from varied cultural and spiritual backgrounds. The complexity of living and working in a multicultural-spiritual society requires nurses to be alert for ethical issues related to these areas. Addressing transcultural and spiritual differences and needs in care is grounded in respect for the inherent dignity and uniqueness of each person and the nursing imperative to provide compassionate and

safe care for each person. This chapter presents general considerations regarding culture and spirituality and discusses related issues that may arise when caring for patients.

TRANSCULTURAL ISSUES

The multicultural society in which we live is alive with diversity. Such diversity of people and backgrounds provides richness to our lives, yet it challenges our abilities to appreciate differences rather than to judge or fear them. Diversity is encountered wherever there are differences among people, such as gender, age, socioeconomic position, sexual orientation, health status, ethnicity, religious or spiritual perspective, race, or culture. Because dealing with diversity is an essential component of nursing care, nurses are expected to demonstrate competence in providing culturally congruent care (ANA, 2021; ANA, 2015, Provisions 1.2, 1.4 CNA, 2017, Part I.A.2, I.C.3, I.D.2, I.F.1; ICN, 2021, Element 1.2, 1.3).

Cultural competence and providing culturally congruent care are grounded in nursing standards of practice and ethical imperatives that include: principles of respect for persons, autonomy, beneficence, nonmaleficence, and right to self-determination; respect for human dignity, values, customs, and beliefs; promoting human rights, equity, inclusion and social justice; and providing competent and compassionate care in a nonjudgmental manner. Cultural competence includes **cultural awareness**, **cultural sensitivity**, **cultural humility**, **cultural safety**, and **linguistic competency** (Ackerman-Berger, 2022; ANA, 2021; Doutrich et al., 2014; Engebretson & Ahn, 2022; Fowler, 2015; Spector, 2017; Srivastave, 2023). **Cultural awareness** begins with recognizing that another person's culture is different from one's own. It includes knowledge about the values, beliefs, behaviors, and the like of the other cultures. **Cultural sensitivity** starts with acknowledging that the values, beliefs, and behaviors of another culture are legitimate, even though different from one's own. It includes the ability to incorporate the patient's cultural perspective into nursing assessments and to modify nursing care to be as congruent as possible with the patient's cultural perspective.

Cultural humility involves approaching people from other cultures with dignity and respect, a willingness to learn from the wisdom and knowledge of their worldview, honoring their values, beliefs, customs, and healing practice, and respectfully acknowledging differences between personal beliefs and those of the other person. Integral to cultural humility is a life-long commitment to reflect on and challenge personal cultural viewpoints, biases, prejudices and ethnocentrism and being comfortable in the role of a learner rather than the expert in relation to understanding the other person's culture, experience, and needs.

Cultural safety implies that nursing care is provided in a manner that enables the patient or family to feel safe in discussing and incorporating their cultural values, behaviors, and beliefs into their care. It considers all that makes them unique; avoids actions that diminish, demean, or disempower the cultural identity and well-being of the patient; and ensures that what is safe and effective care is defined by the patient or family (Nursing Council of New Zealand, 2011). **Linguistic competency** is evident when healthcare services are provided in the language best understood by the patient. Assuring that patients and families have competent interpreters when their first language is different from the dominant culture is essential to culturally safe care.

Our culture teaches us to understand a particular perception of reality. Because of this, the same phenomenon may be viewed differently by people from different cultures. For example, the man in the moon that most people in Western cultures have been taught to "see" is identified in other cultures as a frog in the moon, a woman in the moon, or a rabbit in the moon (Tafoya, 1996). Another way of appreciating different perspectives is to consider what we see when we are in the valley, compared with what we see from halfway up the mountain or the view from the top of the mountain. Different perceptions of the same reality derive from the perspectives from which it is viewed. One view of reality is not more correct than the other; the different views merely come from different perspectives.

Understanding Culture

Self-awareness is a component of cultural competence and a key factor in dealing with transcultural issues. The best starting point for becoming sensitive to the culture of another is to understand our own culture and its influence on our perceptions and behaviors. As noted in Chapter 5, culture refers to the totality of lifeways of a

---

ASK YOURSELF

How Do You Deal With Diversity?

Consider a situation in which you were afraid of or judged someone you did not know because she or he was different from you.

- What was it about the person or situation that triggered your judgment or fear?
- Why do you think you reacted to the person or situation the way you did?
- How and from whom did you learn to react in this way?
- What has helped you understand diversity and overcome fear?
- How can nurses learn to appreciate rather than fear diversity among colleagues and patients?

group of interacting individuals, consisting of learned patterns of values, beliefs, behaviors, and customs shared by that group (Engebretson & AHN, 2022; McFarland & Wehbe-Alamah, 2015; Ray, 2016; Spector, 2017 Srivastave, 2023). These learned patterns are transmitted from one generation to the next in formal ways, such as through educational settings, and in informal ways, such as through role modeling. Unique cultural expressions can be observed within many groups of interacting individuals—for example, the culture of the deaf community, prison culture, the culture of a religious group, or the culture of health care. When we recognize that each of us is part of a culture and identify the values, beliefs, and behaviors that we hold dear, we become clearer about our own cultural perspective. In this process, it is important that we must be alert to our own ethnocentrism, reflected in our tendency to judge the beliefs and behaviors of someone from another culture by the standards of our own culture. People from the dominant culture are often blind to their own ethnocentrism and unaware that their values, practices, and beliefs derive from a cultural perspective. This may engender perceptions of other cultures as inferior and lead to various forms of prejudice, stereotyping, and even violence against members of the other culture. Cultural humility and safety, as noted earlier, require that we engage in ongoing reflection of our own cultural identity and ethnocentric assumptions and behaviors and how these affect our personal interactions and professional practice. Because cultural attitudes and behaviors are often unconscious, this reflective practice enables us to become more aware of culturally based power relationships, sense of privilege, prejudices, structural violence, and various forms of oppression that can lead to health inequities and disparities for patients and families. **Health disparities** refer to discrimination or perceived discrimination in the delivery of health care to individuals and groups of people that leads to a delay in seeking health care, lesser quality of care, and poor healthcare outcomes. These inequities in health outcomes are often based on race, ethnicity, cultural background, immigrant status, gender, socioeconomic status, and the like. "All nurses must recognize the potential impact of unconscious bias and practices contributing to discrimination, and actively seek opportunities to promote inclusion of all people in the provision of quality health care while eradicating disparities" (ANA, 2018, p. 1).

Through reflection, we become more alert to tendencies to impose our cultural values on others and

---

ASK YOURSELF

How Might Ethnocentrism Affect Nursing Care?

Consider the varied meanings the following behaviors may have depending on the cultural context in which they occur: direct eye contact may connote honesty or intrusion, a firm handshake may be viewed as confidence or as hostility, and frequent bathing may be considered necessary or unhealthy.

- How might behaviors such as these be judged by people within the dominant culture in your country? How are they perceived within your own culture?
- How do practices and expectations within healthcare settings reflect ethnocentrism regarding behaviors such as these?
- How might ethnocentrism or stereotyping affect interaction with others, especially within a nursing setting? Have you ever experienced a reaction toward your beliefs or behaviors from another person that you felt was ethnocentric? How did you feel?
- What do codes of nursing ethics say about ethnocentrism, stereotyping, and discrimination in nursing care? Give specific examples.

---

to ways we may stereotype those from other cultures. Stereotyping is expecting all persons from a particular group to behave, think, or respond in a certain way based on preconceived ideas. Every culture contains variation, and some people within the group may not ascribe to all beliefs and values attributed to that culture. With awareness, nurses can be more alert to the impact of cultural issues on health care, learn from patients about their beliefs and culturally accepted practices, and work with patients and families to ensure a culturally safe care experience.

Cultural Values and Beliefs

Culture is one of the key organizing concepts of nursing. Thus, we need to be knowledgeable about how patients and cultural groups with whom we interact understand life processes, define health and illness, and maintain wellness within the context of their own culture. This includes understanding what members of the groups believe to be the causes of illness and how healers within the group cure and care for members (AHNA, 2019). It is important to appreciate what members of the cultural group expect of healthcare practitioners and of the

CASE PRESENTATION

Sociocultural Barriers to Care

Juan is a 52-year-old man who comes to the local clinic accompanied by his wife. When the nurse asks him what brings him to the clinic, he points to the left lower side of his abdomen, looks away, and tells her he has pain. In a mixture of Spanish and English his wife indicates that Juan has been sick for a long time and keeps saying it was just something he ate. When Jolene, the nurse, asks about other symptoms, Juan doesn't say much and looks a bit embarrassed. Jolene is aware that some Hispanic men are reluctant to discuss sensitive issues with a woman, so she asks the nurse practitioner, Ricardo (who speaks fluent Spanish), to complete the health history as part of his examination. Ricardo discovers that Juan is an immigrant from Mexico who has been here for 20 years. He knows enough English to get by. He has a green card and works long days at several part-time manual labor jobs. He has no health insurance and has rarely sought health care for any reason, other than with a local traditional healer. Even though he has some physical pain, he feels that he is healthy as long as he can work and take care of his family. For the past six months or more, he has been having pain in the left lower quadrant of his abdomen. He also describes having tenesmus, having some blood in his stool every few days, particularly if he strains, and having lost around 15 pounds. He said he is only here today because his wife made him come. He is worried about missing work because he needs to support his family. He also indicates that he doesn't like coming to the clinic because of the way some staff treat Latinos as if they are dirty and don't deserve to be there.

Because of Juan's symptoms, Ricardo is concerned about the possibility of colorectal cancer. He is aware that colorectal cancer is the second-leading cause of death among Hispanic men and that diagnosis may be delayed due to a lack of regular health care. He understands that Juan's cultural background may make him resist having a rectal examination, so he acknowledges this and takes time to explain the importance of doing the examination. On examination, he palpates a firm nodule. Ricardo tells Juan what he found and that it is important to have more tests done to determine what is going on. Juan says he'll have to talk with his wife and family about it. He also indicates he is not sure he can afford to take time from work and is concerned about how much everything will cost. Ricardo gives Juan an appointment to come back in a week and hopes he will keep the appointment.

Think About It
Sociocultural Influences on Health and Health Care
- What sociocultural health issues do you see in this situation?
- What cultural healthcare–seeking behaviors and family dynamics are evident?
- How might bias or discrimination based on ethnicity influence the care Juan receives?
- What evidence of potential health disparities do you see in this situation?
- Where do you see efforts to provide culturally safe care in this situation?
- How does the care Jolene and Ricardo provide for Juan reflect directives in the codes of nursing ethics? Give specific examples.

conventional healthcare system. Awareness of how the cultural background and attitudes of nurses and other health team members influence the way in which care is delivered is also essential.

Cultural values and beliefs guide our thinking, being, and doing in patterned ways. Beliefs about health and practices related to health and healing are some of the patterns influenced by culture that are significant in providing health care. Such beliefs and practices manifest in both direct and subtle ways, and sensitivity to them can affect patient outcomes and satisfaction with care. It is helpful to recognize a distinction between disease, which is the biomedical explanation of sickness, and illness, which is a personal response to the disease that flows from how our culture teaches us to be sick.

Transcultural issues are often present in nursing situations but may not be identified as such. Instead, patients may be labeled as stoic, uncooperative, noncompliant, strange, or "crazy" because of choices they make, and their health and care may be compromised. For example, a patient who asks for a vegetarian diet may have cultural-religious reasons for such a request, such as an observant Jewish person who keeps kosher (dietary practices that include prohibition of mixing meat or poultry with milk products), a person who follows traditional Hindu or Buddhist dietary practices, or a person who is Seventh-day Adventist. This simple request provides an opportunity for the nurse to explore cultural beliefs and practices that may affect patient care. Madeline Leininger (1991), considered the "mother" of transcultural nursing, delineated principles of transcultural care, human rights, and ethical considerations that offer guidance for nurses in dealing with transcultural issues. These principles, listed in Box 18.1, are still pertinent and continue to offer a framework for providing culturally sensitive and safe care.

Incorporating cultural assessment into care with patients is an important part of a comprehensive nursing assessment. This assessment facilitates a better understanding of sometimes overlooked factors that influence health behaviors and decisions. Cultural assessment helps nurses appropriately identify and understand the meaning of behaviors that might otherwise be judged negatively or be confusing to the nurse. We recognize that each person is culturally unique and that not all persons in a particular cultural group believe or respond similarly. Various approaches to cultural assessment are found in the nursing literature (Giger & Haddad, 2020; McFarland & Wehbe-Alamah, 2015; Ray, 2016; Spector, 2017; Srivastave, 2023). One example is Geiger and Davidhizar's Transcultural Assessment Model (Giger & Haddad, 2020). This model includes exploration of cultural phenomena that are evident in all cultural groups: communication, personal space, social organization, time, environmental control, and biological variation. The application of this model to nursing care and practice is illustrated in Fig. 18.1 and Fig. 18.2 provides a schematic of the model. Students are encouraged to become familiar with a process of cultural assessment that they incorporate into every nursing assessment.

BOX 18.1   Transcultural Care Principles, Human Rights, and Ethical Considerations

1. Human beings of any culture in the world have a right to have their cultural care values known, respected, and appropriately used in nursing and other healthcare services.
2. Human cultures have diverse and universal modes of caring and healing practices that need to be recognized and used by professional nurses to function effectively and therapeutically with people of different cultures.
3. Care is the essence of nursing and a basic human need for growth, healing, well-being, recovery, and survival.
4. Cultural care is a critical component influencing human health, well-being, and recovery from illnesses or disabilities.
5. Every culture has at least two major types of healthcare systems, namely, the *folk (generic, lay, or indigenous) care system* and the *professional care system*, which influence their health outcomes, and the transcultural nurse is challenged to use this knowledge to guide nursing care decisions and actions.
6. All professional nurses are challenged to respect common human needs and humanistic aspects of people care worldwide and also the divergent care expressions, meanings, and practices.
7. Transcultural nurses are expected to respect Western and non-Western cultures, which often have different values, beliefs, and norms, to assess and understand human beings.
8. Transcultural nursing principles and practices are the arching framework for all nursing care practices, which differ from nursing practices that rely on traditional medical symptoms, diseases, and treatment regimens.
9. Because transcultural nursing focuses on comparative cultural care values, beliefs, and practices of cultures, the nurse is expected to work with individuals, families, groups, cultures, subcultures, and institutions that reflect cultural care variabilities.
10. Nurses with transcultural knowledge are expected to respond appropriately to culture care differences and similarities to ease or ameliorate a human condition or lifeway and to help clients face death.
11. Ethical and moral differences and similarities exist among human cultures, which necessitates that nurses recognize, respect, and respond appropriately to such variabilities.
12. It is essential that transcultural nurses be open-minded and willing to learn from cultural informants about their human values, beliefs, needs, and practices to make appropriate nursing care plans, judgments, and actions.
13. The ability of the nurse to listen, use silence, and envision the client's or family's human condition or cultural circumstance with its positive or less positive features is important in transcultural nursing.
14. Transcultural nursing often requires that nurses communicate with clients in their native language to know, learn, and understand individuals, families, and groups of different cultures.
15. Transcultural nurses are challenged to identify what constitutes ethical or moral principles and norms of cultures and not assume that all cultures are alike.
16. Transcultural nurses are expected to guide other nurses who have not been prepared in transcultural nursing to prevent marked ethnocentrism, cultural imposition practices, and inappropriate ethical and moral judgments about clients.

17. Transcultural nursing reflects that individuals or groups of a designated culture are active participants and decision makers in culture care practices to develop and maintain creative and effective professional care practices.
18. Clients of diverse or similar cultures have a right to have their caring lifestyles and expressions known and used in transcultural nursing to promote client health or well-being.
19. Transcultural nursing considers the worldview, environmental context, ethnohistory, social structure features (including the religious, kinship, philosophic, economic, political, technological, and cultural values), language, expressions, gender, and age differences of people.
20. Transcultural nursing is concerned with the assessment of caregiver and care-receiver expressions, beliefs, and lifeways that often go beyond nurse-client dyadic relationship to that of care relationships with families, groups, institutions, and communities to facilitate congruent care practices and to avoid unfavorable culture care conflicts, stress, and negligent care practices.
21. Because ethical, moral, and legal systems of human values and rights exist in all cultures, it is the task and responsibility of transcultural nurses to discover these dimensions with key and general informants and in diverse cultural contexts.
22. Human care rights tend to be covert and embedded in the social structure, cultural values, and worldview of clients, so the transcultural nurse is challenged to discover these dimensions mainly through qualitative research methods.
23. Transcultural nurses recognize that cultures are complex, dynamic, and change over time and in varying ways.
24. Transcultural nurses recognize that many cultures and subcultures in the world have not been studied and yet nurses are expected to care for all peoples, including minorities.
25. Transcultural nursing is a major breakthrough for new nursing knowledge and practices that do not follow the traditional nursing or medical disease, symptom, and illness models.

(From Leininger, M. (1991). Transcultural care principles, human rights, and ethical considerations. *Journal of Transcultural Nursing*, 3, 21–23. Reprinted with permission from the *Journal of Transcultural Nursing*.)

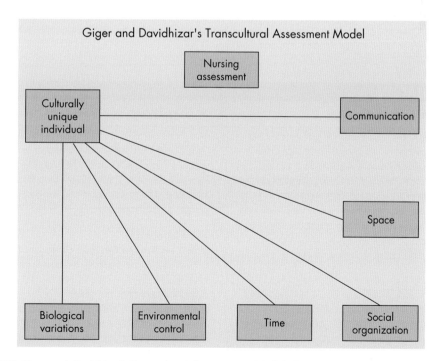

Fig. 18.1 Giger and Davidhizar's Transcultural Assessment Model: Application of Cultural Phenomena to Nursing Care and Nursing Practice. (From Giger, J. N., & Haddad, L. (2020). *Transcultural nursing: Assessment and intervention.* 8th ed. Elsevier.)

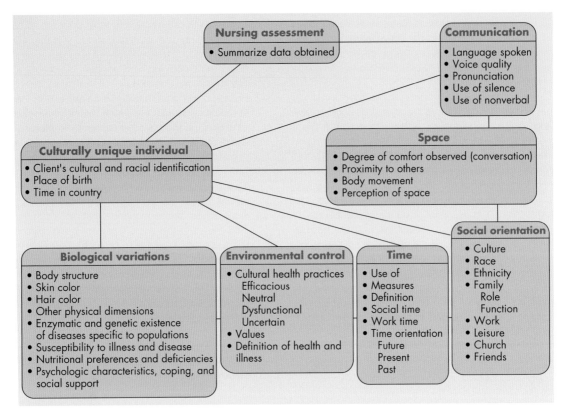

Fig. 18.2 Schematic of Giger and Davidhizar's Transcultural Assessment Model. (From Giger, J. N. & Haddad, L. (2020). *Transcultural nursing: Assessment and intervention.* 8th ed. Elsevier.)

CASE PRESENTATION

Cultural Misunderstanding

Brenda White is a home health nurse caring for 72-year-old Mrs. Cortez, who is living with her daughter and family while recovering from a stroke. Part of the care involves working with the patient on coordination and strengthening exercises. Brenda speaks some Spanish and thinks that Mrs. Cortez understands most of what she says, although she does not always understand what the patient says to her. She has found Mrs. Cortez to be very cooperative and uncomplaining in doing the exercises under her direction, indicating that she would do what was needed to get well. One day Brenda's supervisor, Maria Lopez, tells her that the agency has received a complaint from Mrs. Cortez's family that Brenda is being too rough on the patient. Brenda responds that she does not understand this because Mrs. Cortez has never complained. Brenda further explains that she was trying to have the patient work to her maximum capability and to

give her instructions in a clear and direct manner. Ms. Lopez says that in her culture elders are considered very precious and are treated with gentleness and respect. Perhaps the family perceived that Brenda's direct ways indicated disrespect for their mother, even though the patient did not indicate this.

Think About It
How Can Nurses Develop Cultural Competence?
- How is cultural diversity evident in this situation?
- Where is there evidence of a lack of cultural sensitivity and linguistic competence?
- What might Brenda do to make her care more culturally safe?
- How do you think you would respond in a similar situation?
- How can nurses develop cultural competence?

Such exploration enables nurses to identify areas where modifications in care can be incorporated so that care is more culturally congruent. Although the process may also reveal divergent beliefs that are difficult to accommodate within the current healthcare system, acknowledging differences may help the patient and family feel more comfortable within the system. For example, when assessing eating patterns and food preferences, the nurse might discover that the patient commonly eats only two meals a day, consisting of burritos in the morning and rice and beans in the evening. Typical hospital food and a three-meals-a-day pattern might not be appetizing for this patient. The patient's nutrition may suffer, and she or he may perceive that she or he is not being fed. By arranging for the patient to have culturally similar foods at similar times, the nurse provides more culturally congruent care.

Culture and the Healthcare System

Concepts of health and healing, of right and wrong, of what is proper and what is not, are rooted in culture. Cultures have different explanatory models regarding health and illness that reflect their beliefs about the causes, symptoms, and treatments of illness and their response to dying and death (AHNA, 2019). Our explanatory model helps us recognize, respond to, interpret, cope with, and make sense of illness and other life experiences.

Transcultural issues arise when nurses, patients, and families hold differing views of what is important or necessary regarding health, recovery, illness, or the dying process. Providing culturally competent nursing care may help address concerns before they become serious ethical issues (Fig. 18.3). Addressing cultural issues within some areas of the contemporary healthcare system can be a challenge. Increasing diversity among nurses, physicians, and other health practitioners can lead to cultural differences and misunderstandings in professional interactions and in approach to patient care. For example, a nurse may find her input regarding a patient's situation is brushed off by a male physician from a culture in which women are considered subservient to men. At the same time, the female patient in this situation may be upset by the physician's ethnocentric attitude that he knows what is best for her and the way he addresses the discussion of her care options to her husband and not to her.

The healthcare provider's perspective generally derives from a combination of two cultural orientations.

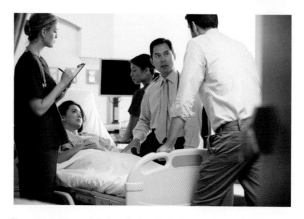

Fig. 18.3 How Might Cultural Differences Affect Patient Care and Professional Interactions? (©iStock.com/monkeybusinessimages.)

The primary cultural orientation is the biomedical model, and the secondary cultural orientation is the provider's personal cultural background. If the patient's perspective is different from this model and is not taken into account by healthcare providers, ethical dilemmas may emerge. Consider, for example, a situation in which the physician, who is schooled in the Western biomedical model, views death as "the enemy" to be overcome at all costs. The patient, who comes from an indigenous culture, views death as a part of life that one prepares for by being in harmony with one's surroundings. Medical or surgical interventions that may prolong the patient's life a few weeks, which would be very important in the physician's worldview, may be low on the list of considerations for this patient. Another patient who believes the suffering from his illness is a way of atoning for his sins may resist taking pain medication that health professionals deem important for his recovery.

The healthcare system is a different culture from that of most of the patients served by the system. The medical language and the values, norms, behaviors, rituals, and overall environment are generally unfamiliar to those who seek its services. Even people who belong to the same dominant culture in society as their healthcare providers are often strangers when they enter the institutions of the system. For those who do not belong to the dominant culture, negotiating the system can be a formidable task. Lack of understanding of the language, procedures, expectations, and other elements of the dominant culture can lead to miscommunication, unclear decisions, and a sense of powerlessness or lack of control. Ethical or legal dilemmas may arise due to misunderstandings. Consider again the case of Mrs. Cortez. Misunderstanding of the nurse's intent might lead the family to decide to terminate nursing care or to bring legal action against the nurse because of their perception that their mother is being mistreated. Another example is a mentally alert 90-year-old Appalachian woman who, after her doctor of 35 years retired, sought care from a new young physician. After a few visits she stopped going to see him, even though she was having serious health problems, because, in her perception, he did not do anything for her. Essentially, he did not talk with her, do the kind of examination she expected, or spend the kind of time with her that her former physician had. Instead, he gave her medicines that she felt made her sick and that she did not need.

When considering values such as autonomy, beneficence, justice, or the right to self-determination, we ask from whose perspective these values are understood—that of the nurse or that of the patient. This same question is appropriate regarding definitions of health. For example, some cultures place a higher emphasis on working together and loyalty to the group than on the self-reliance and individualism valued within the broader culture in the United States (Andrews et al., 2020; Giger & Haddad, 2020; Ray, 2016, Srivastave, 2023). Healthcare decisions in these cultures may be made by a group such as the family, community, or society, rather than by the individual. Cultural assessment provides insight into the congruence, or lack thereof, between patients' and nurses' values and understandings of health. Consider, for example, a situation in which the nurse believes that health includes being able to be a productive member of society and that health problems provide opportunities for one to grow and become more self-actualized. The patient, on the other hand, believes that his work-related injury is an act of *fate* and focuses on being free of pain and able to "get around." If the differing perceptions of health are not recognized and addressed, efforts to have the patient participate in rehabilitation and job retraining or to utilize nonpharmacological measures for pain control may meet with resistance and patient dissatisfaction.

Complementary and Traditional Therapies

Culture guides one's choice of when to go for health care, what kind of care to seek, to whom to go for care, and how long to participate in care. It is common knowledge that many people who utilize conventional healthcare settings also utilize therapies that are generally not part of the dominant healthcare system. Because they derive from models of health and healing that are different from the dominant system such therapies may be traditional or alternative (therapies that may be used instead of those in the dominant system), complementary (therapies that may be used along with conventional therapies), integrative (therapies that may be integrated into the dominant system). Often referred to as CAM (complementary and alternative medicine), they may derive from traditions in the patient's own culture or may be borrowed from traditions of another culture. CAM includes a wide variety of modalities, such as relaxation techniques, healing touch and other energy-based healing techniques, spiritual healing, biofeedback, nutritional practices, herbal treatments, massage and other body work, meditation, prayer, homeopathy, acupuncture, and biofeedback. Students are encouraged to explore health information regarding CAM therapies through the National Institutes of Health, National Center for Complementary and Integrative Health (https://nccih.nih.gov/health). Folk remedies and care provided by traditional healers are also included within the context of complementary therapies.

As noted above, these therapies are often used concurrently with conventional therapies, but may also be chosen in lieu of conventional therapies. Traditional healing systems prevalent in various cultures derive from explanatory models that, although different from the Western biomedical model, are based on knowledge, experience, skills, beliefs, and practices that have been helping people deal with health and illness for thousands of years. For people from nondominant cultures, their traditional healing system is often the norm and the conventional system of the dominant culture is the alternative. Nurses need to be alert to this, particularly with immigrant, indigenous, and other vulnerable populations.

To have a broad picture of the many factors affecting a patient's health and healing, we need to be aware of various therapies being utilized by the patient. We should incorporate discussion of CAM therapies into nursing assessment in an open way, because patients may be hesitant to bring up the subject. We do not need to use or support such therapies to become knowledgeable about them. CAM therapies often derive from paradigms that differ from and may not make sense in the conventional medical model yet may be very useful in the healing process. When patients are interested in or already using CAM therapies, we can assist them in determining whether there are risks associated with their use alongside conventional therapies. If significant risks are involved and the patient is committed to using the therapy, we can work with other health team members to minimize risks and maximize benefits. When conventional healthcare providers can work with traditional systems and their healers, the overall care becomes more culturally congruent, promoting the health and safety of the patient.

The principle of patient self-determination directs us to honor the right of persons to use both conventional and CAM therapies to address their healthcare needs. Respect for persons calls us to be open to views other than our own and to appreciate that there are many paths to healing. CAM modalities should never be discounted merely because they are not understood within the Western biomedical frame of reference. Codes of nursing ethics direct nurses to respect convictions that derive from belief systems that are different from their own and to be open to the contributions to health offered by other explanatory models. A nonjudgmental approach that respects differing values and beliefs and is sensitive to ethnocentric bias of nurses and other healthcare providers enhances the opportunity to explore jointly the efficacy of all options with the patient.

The area of informed consent presents some important questions relative to CAM therapies. Because listing alternative treatments is an important element of an informed consent, consider whether it is an ethical duty for biomedical practitioners to include discussion of CAM therapies in discussion of therapeutic alternatives. Similarly, do you think that practitioners of other healing modalities should make certain that their clients are aware of biomedical alternatives? Those who offer CAM therapies should explain the intervention and discuss risks, expected effects and benefits, and treatment options before initiating therapy. It is prudent to apprise other health team members of the use of CAM therapies because these therapies can affect conventional interventions in varying ways.

Practitioners of both conventional and CAM therapies need to be alert to potential threats to patient autonomy that flow from practitioner attitudes. When we assume that patient values and thought processes are the same as ours, we may believe that what we suggest is the only reasonable course of action. When patients choose another course of action, we may question their decision-making capacity or label them as unreasonable. In conventional practice, this is evident in references to nonconventional therapies as quackery or nonscientific in trying to dissuade patients from using them, and even in deriding the patient for making such choices. Remember that a patient's choice of an option that may seem unreasonable from our perspective does not necessarily mean that the patient has not thought it through. Such differences often merely reflect a difference in values.

Factors important for the healing process are often culturally prescribed. For example, the involvement of family in the care of a sick member may be very important in some cultures. It can be quite distressing for nursing staff on a hospital unit when multiple family members "camp out" in a patient's room or the nearby hallway or bring food from home that is not on a patient's diet. Providing culturally congruent care in such situations may include relaxing visiting regulations and collaborating with the family regarding appropriate foods from home. If the needs of one patient are different from those of the roommate, dilemmas may arise that require diplomatic interventions by the nurse.

ASK YOURSELF

How Should Nurses Deal With Complementary or Traditional Therapies?

Conventional medicine and medical practitioners tend to be skeptical of healing modalities that have not been subjected to empirical scientific study; thus, discussion of nonconventional modalities is rarely included in lists of alternatives for patients, nor are these modalities generally available in most conventional healthcare settings.

- What do you think about this attitude toward traditional healers or complementary therapies?
- What experiences have you had with complementary or traditional therapies?
- How might attitudes toward traditional healers or complementary therapies affect the ability of nurses to provide culturally congruent care for their patients?
- What are the ethical implications related to limiting a patient's access to traditional healers or complementary therapies and practitioners within conventional healthcare institutions?
- How have you experienced complementary or traditional therapies within nursing practice?

Legal-Ethical Considerations Related to Transcultural Issues

Cultural and linguistic misunderstandings can provide fertile ground for litigation. Communication—verbal, nonverbal, and written—is always of utmost importance in providing competent and ethical nursing care. Codes of nursing ethics direct nurses to respect approaches to decision making based on cultural understanding, assuring that patients receive accurate and understandable information that is appropriate to their linguistic, cultural, and cognitive needs (ANA, 2015, Provision 1.4; CNA, 2017, Part I.C.1; ICN, 2021, Element 1.3). When a patient's first language is different from our own, **linguistic competency** is a prime consideration. We must determine the extent to which the patient understands our language as well as the extent of our understanding of the patient's language. When the patient uses another language (including sign language), having an interpreter fluent in the patient's language is essential. If the interpreter is a member of the patient's family, the translation may be filtered through the perspective of the family member. Consider, for example, an elderly Cambodian man who is in the hospital and not doing well. His grandson serves as an interpreter. The grandson was born in this country and is embarrassed by his grandfather's "old" ways. When the man says that he needs a particular traditional herbal tea each afternoon to get well (which is available in a local international foods store), the grandson translates this generically as "tea." Even though the nurse responds by making sure that the patient has tea each afternoon, the patient's needs are not met. Utilizing a professional interpreter when possible ensures a more nonbiased and accurate interpretation.

Srivastave (2023) notes a distinction between **linguistic interpretation** that focuses on the spoken word, and **cultural interpretation** that includes knowledge of cultural context and meaning of both verbal and nonverbal communication. Linguistic interpretation includes **interpretation**—verbally communicating a message from one language to another while making every effort to faithfully preserve the message; **translation**—transposing a written text from one language to another while retaining elements of meaning and form; and **sight translation**—verbal translation of material written in one language to spoken word in another language (Ontario Council on Community Interpreters [OCCI], 2023). Ensuring that interpreters are engaged when needed and act ethically is part of a nurse's responsibility for protecting the health and safety of patients and advocating for their rights. Readers are encouraged to review ethical standards of practice for interpreters at https://www.occi.ca/_files/ugd/8d6ad0_d427c489a313431b83bf89d4b919edab.pdf; https://www.ncihc.org/assets/documents/publications/NCIHC%20National%20Standards%20of%20Practice.pdf; https://www.ncihc.org/assets/documents/publications/NCIHC National Code of Ethics.pdf.

The language used to explain procedures and the language of consent forms may also present issues. We need to ensure that the patient or family member is able to read the language in which the form is written and that all terms used are understood. This includes assessing the patient's literacy level, even if the patient speaks English and the form is in English. If the form needs to be interpreted for the patient, it is essential that the interpreter understands the procedure and that an appropriate person is available to clarify any areas of uncertainty. People may indicate that they understand the information in the form when they do not to avoid offending the nurse or being considered ignorant. One way of dealing with this is having patients describe in their own words what they have been told.

ETHICAL ISSUES RELATED TO SPIRITUALITY AND RELIGION

Spirituality is a universal human experience that transcends culture, although it may be conditioned and shaped by cultural experiences. A basic part of nursing practice is being attentive to spirituality and recognizing the individual as a body-mind-spirit being who experiences health concerns in all these dimensions (ANA, 2021; ANA, 2015, Provisions 1.2,1.3; CNA, 2017, Part I.D.3; ICN, 2021, Element 1.2). In the midst of advances in technology and scientific discoveries that have increased our understanding of the nature of illness and disease, awareness of the role of spirituality in health and healing has diminished. Perhaps the limited scientific knowledge of former times made the role of the spirit and the intangible forces deriving from that spirit more apparent. Many persons were cared for in their homes, even in the case of serious illness. Touching, praying, and presence were a natural part of such environments. Historically, institutions such as hospitals were often staffed by religious orders concerned for both spiritual and physical needs.

Healing and health care have long been connected with the spirituality of a people. With indigenous peoples, healing rituals frequently are spiritual in nature. People seeking medical care continue to incorporate spiritual and religious rituals and practices into their care for self and others. It is noteworthy that the words *health, holy*, and *whole* all derive from the same Old Saxon word Hal and the Greek word Holos, both meaning "whole." By their nature, then, health and healing are associated with that which is holy and whole. A question to ponder is whether contemporary healthcare culture, now vested in technology, managed care, medical home, corporate structure, mergers, and the like, can once again incorporate spirituality within its vision of healing.

Addressing Spirituality

By nature, humans are body-mind-spirit beings. The uniqueness of each person a nurse encounters encompasses the spiritual as well as physical, mental, and emotional manifestations of that person. **Spirituality** is the animating force, life principle, or essence of being that permeates life and is expressed and experienced in multifaceted connections with self, others, nature, and God or Life Force (AHNA, 2019; Blasdell, 2015; Burkhardt & Nagai-Jacobson, 2002, 2022; Rykkje et al., 2011). Meaning and purpose in life and life events flow from the spirit and are manifested in open or private ways. All persons are spiritual, whether they ascribe to a religious tradition or deny the existence of the Divine. Beliefs and values are molded and shaped by our spirituality as well as by societal and cultural conditioning.

Nursing espouses a holistic view of persons. Understanding that persons are indeed body-mind-spirit beings, we recognize that spirituality is part of every encounter whether we are conscious of it or not (Burkhardt & Nagai-Jacobson, 2002, 2022). Holistic nursing care impels us to address the spiritual as well as physical and mental concerns of patients. We strive to become more aware of our own and others' spirituality to bring this essential aspect of care consciously into every nursing interaction.

Because spirituality is at once universal and very personal and private, we may find this area difficult to approach. Developing competence in addressing spiritual needs is an important area of nursing practice. The

recommendations for integrating spirituality into care that were derived from the Consensus Conference on Improving the Quality of Spiritual Care in Palliative Care (Puchalski et al., 2009) apply to nursing care in all settings. These recommendations include:

- Making spiritual care integral to all patient-centered healthcare system models of care
- Basing spiritual care models on honoring the dignity of all people and providing compassionate care
- Treating spiritual distress or religious struggle with the same urgency or importance as treating other medical or social problems
- Considering spirituality as a patient vital sign that is routinely screened
- Implementing interdisciplinary spiritual care models that include board-certified chaplains in clinical settings (Puchalski et al., 2009, p. 891)

Recognizing that spirituality is both basic to health and an essential component of nursing care enables us to listen for language, observe behavior, and gather information related to spiritual concerns in every encounter with patients and families.

Spirituality assessment can provide us with information about how patients view life, death, health, and health concerns. Such assessment provides insight into important connections, beliefs, practices, or rituals that may influence a person's choices or affect healing. Processes that incorporate open-ended questions and allow patients to tell their stories facilitate spirituality assessment (Burkhardt & Nagai-Jacobson, 2002, 2022; Hughes, et.al., 2017; Liehr & Smith, 2018). Although expression of spiritual concerns may include talk of God or faith, patients communicate their spiritual needs and concerns in many other ways as well. They may express questions related to the meaning of present or past experiences, fears or worries about what is happening, or how they will find the strength they need. They may talk about important relationships, the need for reconciliation, experiences of peace or anxiety, or the desire to put their lives in order. Religious articles may be evident, or the nurse may observe the patient engaging in practices such as prayer or meditation.

Opportunities to explore spirituality with patients are present in many situations. Effective spirituality assessment requires us to attend with our whole beings to indicators of spirituality occurring within routine interactions with patients. The white paper titled *Spiritual Care and Nursing: A Nurse's Contribution and*

Practice (Hughes, et.al., 2017) notes that spiritual needs are revealed within trusting interpersonal relationships between patients and nurses. Focused spirituality assessment processes can help guide nursing observations and communication with patients related to spiritual issues and care.

One process for spiritual assessment is the FICA Spiritual History Tool (Puchalski, 1996/2020). This process incorporates open-ended questions regarding four key elements of spirituality:

- Faith, belief, meaning—whether the person considers self to be spiritual or religious and what is meaningful to the person
- Importance and influence of these in one's life and what might be supportive in times of stress
- Community—spiritual and other groups to which the person belongs and that provide meaning and support to the person
- Address/action in care—how would the person like the health practitioner to address the first three components in care?

This spirituality assessment guide is available at https://gwish.smhs.gwu.edu/sites/g/files/zaskib1011/files/2022-06/FICA-Tool-PDF-ADA.pdf.

Spirituality and Religion

Although spirituality may be expressed through religious beliefs and practices, it is not synonymous with these terms. **Religion** is the codification of beliefs and practices concerning the Divine and one's relationship with the Divine that are shared by a group of people. Religion may be quite intertwined within a dominant culture, as with Judaism in Israel or Hinduism in India, or it may be a counterculture, as with the Amish in the United States. Some religions, such as many Christian sects, include people from different cultures. Religious teachings generally include rules regarding right and wrong and guidelines for dealing with issues related to these areas.

Because religious beliefs and teachings flow from a particular worldview, rules and values can be quite variable among different religions. A minor consideration within one religion or sect may constitute a serious dilemma in another. Norms for proper dress for women is one example. Although most Christian denominations have few, if any, restrictions regarding how women dress, certain Christian sects teach that women should wear only skirts or dresses and not use makeup or cut their hair. Amish women dress in a particular fashion,

---

ASK YOURSELF

Recognizing Spiritual Concerns

Spiritual issues reflect core experiences that often defy explanation. Such experiences may relate to suffering, forgiveness, hope, love, or mystery. In the midst of care with patients, nurses often hear comments or questions or observe behaviors reflective of spiritual concerns. Consider the following examples:

A patient or family member says,
"I don't know why God is doing this to me (or her)."
"I should have locked the gate."
"Will you pray for me?"
"I don't know why, but having surgery worries me."
"I wish I had been willing to go to the beach when he wanted to."
"I think I need to trust God and not take chemotherapy. God wants me to trust Him completely."
"Without my income, I don't know how my family will make it."
"We told him not to buy that motorcycle."
"Do you believe in miracles?"

Patients or family members may be observed:
Reading a sacred text.
Wearing religious jewelry or articles of clothing.
Praying or meditating.
Staring out a window with a worried or pensive expression.

In each of *these* examples:
- Describe a potential spiritual concerns reflected in each the comment or behavior.
- What personal beliefs or experiences might affect your feelings and responses to comments or behaviors such as these?
- Describe aspects of each comment or behavior that might raise questions or concerns for you.
- How might you respond to each of these comments or behaviors? In which circumstances would you feel more comfortable or less comfortable?

---

and orthodox Muslims and Jews have strict rules regarding how women are to dress in public.

What is considered right or wrong within a particular religion is not always congruent with the ethical perspectives of the greater society. Consider, for example, an infant girl brought to a hospital in the United States with severely infected wounds from trauma to her labial area after a clitorectomy procedure performed by a family member. From the perspective of

CASE PRESENTATION

Respecting Spiritual-Cultural Practices

Nasira is a 26-year-old woman from Syria who has been admitted to the hospital with severe abdominal cramping and vaginal bleeding. She wears a head covering and has been reluctant to change from her own clothing into a hospital gown. She appears frightened. She speaks English fairly well, although it is not her first language. She told Elena, her nurse, that she thought she might be pregnant but had not yet been to the clinic to confirm this. Her friend who brought her to the hospital had to go home. She said that she called her husband, who was on his way back from being out of town and should be there in an hour or so. She has no other family in the area. Dr. Jones, the hospitalist physician, tells you that when he went in to take a history and examine Nasira, she looked away, would barely respond to him, and pulled back when he tried to examine her. He said he would like to order some diagnostic tests but wasn't sure she understood what he was telling her. He asked Elena to explain the tests again and get the consent forms signed and to see if she could get the patient into a hospital gown so he could examine her.

Think About It
Integrating Spiritual-Cultural Beliefs and Practices Into Nursing Care

- What spiritual-cultural issues are evident in this situation?
- How might cultural misunderstanding compromise Nasira's care?
- How might Nasira experience discrimination or health disparity because of her beliefs and practices?

- Review the American Nursing Association's (ANA's) ethics and human rights position statement, *The Nurse's Role in Addressing Discrimination*, and reflect on nursing's role in preventing discrimination in nursing practice (https://www.nursingworld.org/~4ab207/globalassets/practiceandpolicy/nursing-excellence/ana-position-statements/social-causes-and-health-care/the-nurses-role-in-addressing-discrimination.pdf).
- What do you think about Dr. Jones's directives to Elena?
- What would you include in a spiritual-cultural assessment of this patient?
- Mujallad and Taylor (2016) note that in Islamic life, modesty is a fundamental value that is evident in both behavior and mode of dress. Modesty for Muslim women is understood as religious devotion. For married women, this includes practices such as wearing clothing that covers all of the body except the hands when with men other than family; generally not exposing the body from the navel to the knees; refraining from touch or conversation with a man other than her husband unless for professional, health-related, or educational reasons; and avoiding eye contact with unrelated men and women. A conservative Muslim woman is likely to defer to her husband to give consent for elective procedures. Knowing this information, what factors need to be considered to provide spiritually, culturally, and linguistically sensitive and safe care for Nasira?
- What would you include in your nursing care plan to address the spiritual-cultural issues in this situation? How would nursing codes of ethics provide guidance in developing your plan of care?

the nurse and the institution, this would be viewed as severe mutilation, constituting abuse, whereas the family would consider this an important cultural-religious practice. Another example is the Jehovah's Witness belief that prohibits blood transfusion, and the ensuing dilemma when a transfusion is medically indicated as a lifesaving measure. In situations where there is a significant conflict between a nurse's moral beliefs and values and patient decisions or the care they require, codes of nursing ethics note that the nurse may conscientiously object to caring for the patient. In such a situation the nurse must communicate the objection in a timely and appropriate manner and continues to provide safe, compassionate, and respectful care until

other arrangements are made for care that meets the patient's needs (ANA, 2015, Provision 5.4; CNA, 2017, Part I, G.7; ICN, 2021, Element 2.8). Such conscience-based refusals must be clearly based on moral grounds and not on personal preference, convenience, bias, or prejudice.

Religiosity refers to beliefs and practices that are the expressive aspects of religion. These include, among others, prayer, ritual, dietary practices, modes of dress, and study of sacred texts. Awareness of religious practices and beliefs that are important to patients and families enables nurses to incorporate religious needs into care planning. Being familiar with beliefs and practices of different religions that may affect health care enables nurses

How Does Spirituality Affect Your Nursing Practice?

- What religious or spiritual beliefs or practices are important to you?
- How has your spirituality or religious perspective been influential in your choice of nursing as a profession?
- How do you think your spirituality or religious perspective might affect or be incorporated into your nursing practice? Give specific examples.

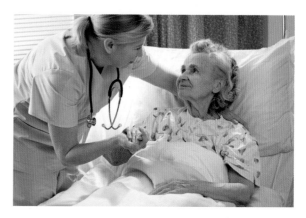

Fig. 18.4 Addressing Spiritual Needs Through Compassionate Presence. (©iStock.com/AlexRaths.)

to be better able to incorporate particular needs into patient care (Hanson & Andrews, 2020). This information provides a basis from which nurses can explore with patients what is necessary to support or meet their spiritual needs, taking care not to presume a need until it is verified with the patient. For example, a Catholic patient may not wish to have a priest called, a Jewish patient may have no problem with eating ham, or a patient who lists no religious affiliation may practice daily meditation.

Although many people express their spirituality through religion, spiritual expression is not limited to this context. Many people will note that they believe in God but do not go to church. Instead, they pray on their own, or experience the Divine through nature, or relate to a Higher Power or Universal Being that is found in all of life. We must plan nursing care according to how each patient expresses and experiences spirituality.

Creating Sacred Space

Addressing religious concerns within a healthcare setting does not require us to share the same religious perspective as our patients. What is necessary is that we create an environment that is open to a variety of religious and spiritual expressions. Creating sacred space in the midst of science and technology can challenge our creativity. Nursing care may include providing the quiet a patient needs for meditation or prayer, arranging a private space for a particular ritual, contacting an appropriate spiritual support person, or ensuring that specific dietary requirements are met. The most basic way of integrating spiritual care into nursing care is through love, hope, compassion, empathy, listening, and holding space (Hughes, et.al., 2017). This involves emotionally connecting with and communicating with the patient and family on a personal and human level.

Such compassionate care is the moral way to address the needs of the whole person (Fig. 18.4).

Praying with or reading sacred scripture to patients may be included in nursing care, provided it is based on an assessment of the patient's spiritual needs and done with the patient's permission and within the context of the patient's tradition. The literature provides evidence for the therapeutic value of prayer and that prayer can be an important intervention (Breslin & Lewis, 2008; Hughes, et.al. 2017; Helming, 2011; Narayanasamy & Narayanasamy, 2008). As with any therapeutic intervention, obtaining permission from patients before praying for them is an important part of nursing care. Unsolicited prayer by health practitioners may make patients or family members uncomfortable or reflect a goal different from that of the patient, and may be considered unethical (French & Narayanasamy, 2011). If a patient asks the nurse to pray for her or him, the nurse can ask what the patient would like to pray for and whether the patient would like to say a prayer together or have the nurse pray for the patient throughout the day. Clarifying the request in this way shows respect for the patient and supports self-determination by allowing the patient to choose how and when the prayer should occur (Hughes et.al., 2017). Asking the patient to begin the prayer helps fashion the prayer within the patient's spiritual tradition. For nurses who are so inclined, it is good to include prayer for patients in their personal prayer, with the intention of what is for the patient's highest good. Overall we need to be aware of acting out of our own spiritual or religious perspectives while taking care not to impose our views on another.

Dilemmas Related to Religious Beliefs

When patients refuse conventional medical treatments based on religious beliefs or spiritual perspectives, dilemmas can arise. Patients who decide to rely on prayer for healing, rather than chemotherapy for treatment of cancer, for example, may be considered irrational, and their competence to make decisions may be questioned. If an adult refuses a blood transfusion due to religious beliefs after all risks have been explained, it is considered an informed decision. If a parent refuses a transfusion for a child based on the same belief, it may be taken to court as neglect or abuse. A woman who refuses to leave a dangerously abusive marriage because of religious convictions may find that frustrated healthcare providers are less responsive to her cries for help.

CASE PRESENTATION

When Religious Beliefs and Medical Care Conflict—Part 1

Suella is a 33-year-old, unmarried woman who belongs to a Holiness church that includes the practice of snake handling. Three days ago she was bitten twice during a church service. After the service, she stayed with the preacher, who prayed with her for healing, as is the custom in this church. The religion does not believe in taking antivenom. Suella's parents and siblings, who do not belong to the same church, brought her to the hospital in renal failure. On admission, she was alert but lethargic and repeatedly informed nurses that she did not want any blood, dialysis, feeding tube, or life support. She kept saying, "My King will take care of me," insisting that her reliance was on God and that she did not want antivenom. On her move to the intensive care unit, the attending physician documented the conversation with the patient, indicating that she did not want blood, dialysis, feeding tubes, cardiopulmonary resuscitation (CPR), or life support. The attending physician also consulted a renal physician, who ordered dialysis. A nurse who was getting ready to do the second dialysis treatment read the attending physician's note and recognized the ethical dilemma.

Think About It
Dealing With Conflicts Between Religious Beliefs and Medical Care
- What do you think the nurse should do in this situation? Give rationale.
- How do you think you would react to this patient's decision?
- What principles would guide you in dealing with dilemmas arising from religious convictions? What guidance is given by codes of nursing ethics? Be specific.
- What personal religious or spiritual practices are important to your health?
- What personal convictions might affect your healthcare decisions?

CASE PRESENTATION

When Religious Beliefs and Medical Care Conflict—Part 2

The nurse in this situation requested an ethics consult, and members of the hospital's ethics committee talked with the patient. Although the patient was lethargic, she could nod and reply "yes" and "no" when questioned. The patient reaffirmed her same wishes as noted on admission. When asked if she knew what would happen without treatment, she stated, "I'll die." The primary physician spoke to the patient again in the presence of an ethics committee member, at which time she once again reiterated her previous wishes. The physician discontinued all dialysis and set up a meeting with the family, after which the family spoke to the patient. Later that day the patient said she changed her mind and now wanted everything done. Ethics committee members were again called. When they asked the patient why she changed her mind, she responded, "My family." Further exploration of what "everything" meant to the patient revealed that she was willing to have dialysis, blood, and tube feedings but no CPR or intubation.

Think About It
When Family Members Have Different Religious Beliefs
- How would you, as the nurse, feel about following this patient's new directives?
- Do you see any possible new dilemmas resulting from the current situation?
- Is there any evidence of possible coercion in this situation? If so, how would you respond to that?
- How would your own spiritual perspective influence your care for this patient and family?

Nurturing Spirit

Caregiving is influenced by a nurse's spiritual, as well as physical and emotional, well-being. The ability to attend to spirituality with another requires that nurses first attend to their own spirits (Burkhardt & Nagai-Jacobson, 2002, 2020; Hughes, et.al., 2017). Self-awareness, which includes appreciation of ourselves as unique body-mind-spirit beings, underlies our recognition of this same wholeness in others.

Just as sustenance and care are necessary for the health of body and mind, so too does the spirit require nurture. Caring for our spirit includes mindfulness and taking time to attend to our inner being. The spirit can be nurtured in many ways, and we must each discover what our own spirit needs to thrive. Prayer, meditation, music, religious worship, or shared ritual may be important. The spirit may be nurtured through special time with friends or family, or by giving ourselves alone time at home, in nature, or in some other sacred space. Attending to our need for rest, play, or creative activity are other ways to care for spirit. The spirit can be nurtured in a very profound way through sharing our stories. As we become more adept at nurturing our spirits, we are better able to recognize and support this process with patients and families.

■ SUMMARY

Attentiveness to spiritual and cultural aspects of care with patients is an important part of holistic nursing care. Providing safe, compassionate, and ethical care requires nurses to incorporate the diversity of cultures and spiritual expressions into patient care. An important component of this care is the ability to identify ethical issues and concerns and to address them competently and confidently. Familiarity with the values, beliefs, and practices of various cultures, religions, and spiritual traditions is a useful adjunct to careful cultural and spiritual assessments with patients. Self-awareness regarding our own cultural and spiritual values, beliefs, and expressions is necessary to address these areas with patients in open and nonjudgmental ways. Such awareness allows us to act from our own spiritual or cultural perspectives, while taking care not to impose these views on others. In this way, care planning more readily flows from assessments that identify issues and needs based on the patient's cultural and spiritual expressions and experiences.

■ CHAPTER HIGHLIGHTS

- Because culture influences beliefs and behaviors regarding health and healing, cultural assessment is integral to a comprehensive nursing assessment.
- Providing effective nursing care within the diversity of our multicultural society requires cultural competence on the part of nurses. Cultural competence can help prevent ethical dilemmas in care when there are differences in cultural perspectives between patient and nurse.
- The culture of healthcare institutions may vary greatly from that of the people served by these systems. Values such as autonomy, beneficence, and the right to self-determination must be considered from the cultural perspectives of patient, family, and healthcare providers.
- CAM therapies are used by many people seen in conventional healthcare settings. Nursing care is enhanced when nurses are aware of various therapies being utilized by patients. Knowledge of and working with traditional healing systems and healers can help nurses promote more culturally congruent care.
- Communication is a key factor in providing culturally congruent and spiritually sensitive care and in averting associated legal and ethical dilemmas.
- Health and healing are associated with that which is holy and whole. Spirituality has long been a component of healing and health care, because, by nature, humans are body-mind-spirit beings.
- Grounded in a holistic view of persons, nursing care includes spirituality assessment and interventions addressing spiritual needs, recognizing that a religious or spiritual perspective may influence healthcare choices.
- Expressions of spirituality are many and varied and may include but are not limited to the context of religion. Religious values are not always congruent with the ethical perspectives of the greater society.
- Providing spiritual care requires that nurses be attentive to both their own spirits and the spiritual concerns of patients and create an environment that is open to a variety of religious and spiritual expressions. Nurses need to be aware of acting from their own cultural, spiritual, or religious perspectives, while not imposing these views on others.
- Codes of nursing ethics provide an ethical imperative to incorporate transcultural and spiritual considerations in nursing care.

DISCUSSION QUESTIONS AND ACTIVITIES

1. Consider how your cultural, spiritual, or religious values affect personal choices regarding health and healing. Discuss this with other students, noting similarities and differences.

2. What aspects of the culture of the healthcare system are difficult for you as a nurse? Identify personal conflicts and the beliefs and values underlying them.

3. Recall a time when you or someone you know experienced a conflict with persons within the healthcare system. What values, beliefs, or understandings contributed to this conflict?

4. Discuss with other students CAM or traditional/folk remedies that you or someone you know have used. Why was the therapy used? How did you know about the therapy? Was it used in place of or along with conventional therapies? What was the outcome? Research a complementary therapy through the National Center for Complementary and Integrative Health (http://www.nccih.nih.gov).

5. List 10 things that nurture you spiritually. Consider how often you have done these in the past day, week, or month. Make a plan to include at least one each day for the next week.

6. Choose a religious tradition or CAM therapy with which you are unfamiliar. Explore this tradition or therapy through readings and discussions with members, practitioners, or persons who have practiced the religion or utilized the therapy. Share your findings with classmates. The Religious Movements Project is one resource for beginning this exploration: http://web.archive.org/web/20060907005952/http://etext.lib.virginia.edu/relmove/

7. Review the white paper *Spiritual Care and Nursing: A Nurse's Contribution and Practice* (Hughes, et.al., 2017) found at https://www.spiritualcareassociation.org/docs/resources/nurses_spiritual_care_white_paper_3_22_2017.pdf Discuss nursing's role in providing spiritual care. Discuss how nurses can create sacred space within healthcare settings.

8. Discuss patient healthcare choices or behaviors that are based on religious beliefs that might present a dilemma for you. Consider how you would approach the situation in a professional manner, and describe the ethical stance that would guide your decisions. Include specific directives from the ANA (2015), the CNA (2017), or the ICN (2021), whichever is most appropriate for your situation, that would support your choices.

9. Expand your knowledge of cultural competency, diversity, and spiritual care by exploring some of the following websites:

   https://www.nursingworld.org/practice-policy/nursing-excellence/official-position-statements/

   http://nccc.georgetown.edu/ (National Center for Cultural Competence)

   http://www.hrsa.gov/culturalcompetence/index.html (Health Resources and Services Administration)

   http://ethnomed.org/ (EthnoMed)

   https://minorityhealth.hhs.gov/omh/browse.aspx?lvl52&lvlid534 (Center for linguistic and Cultural Competency in Health Care)

   https://tcns.org/standards/ (Standards of Practice for Culturally Competent Nursing Care)

   https://tcns.org/resources/ (Transcultural Nurses Society)

   https://cccm.thinkculturalhealth.hhs.gov/ (USDHHS Office of Minority Health)

   http://www.gwumc.edu/gwish/clinical/fica-spiritual/index.cfm (Institute for Spirituality and Health, George Washington University)

   http://www.ish-tmc.org/ (Institute for Spirituality and Health, Texas Medical Center)

   https://www.csh.umn.edu/education/online-modules-and-resources (Center for Spirituality and Healing—University of Minnesota)

   http://www.spiritualityhealth.com

   http://www.ahna.org/ (The American Holistic Nurses Association)

   https://nccih.nih.gov/health (National Institutes of Health, National Center for Complementary and Integrative Health).

REFERENCES

Ackerman-Berger, P. (2022, June 6–11). *The intersection of cultural humility and health equity [plenary presentation].* Albuquerque, NM, United States: American Holistic Nurses Association Annual Conference.

ANA. (2015). *Code of ethics for nurses with interpretive statements.* http://nursingworld.org/DocumentVault/Ethics-1/Code-of-Ethics-for-Nurses.html.

American Holistic Nurses Association (AHNA). (2019). *Holistic nursing: Scope and standards of practice* (3rd ed.). American Nurses Association.

American Nurses Association (ANA). (2021). Nursing: Scope and standards of practice (4th ed.). American Nurses Association.

American Nurses Association (ANA). (2018). *Ethics and human rights position statements: The Nurse's role in addressing discrimination: Protecting and promoting inclusive strategies in practice settings, policy, and advocacy.* https://www.nursingworld.org/~4ab207/globalassets/practiceandpolicy/nursing-excellence/ana-position-statements/social-causes-and-health-care/the-nurses-role-in-addressing-discrimination.pdf.

Andrews, M. M., Boyle, J. S., & Collins, J. W. (2020). *Transcultural concepts in nursing care* (8th ed.). Wolters Kluwer.

Blasdell, N. D. (2015). The evolution of spirituality in the nursing literature. *International Journal of Caring Science, 8*(3), 756–764.

Breslin, M. J., & Lewis, C. A. (2008). Theoretical models of the nature of prayer and health: A review. *Mental Health, Religion & Culture, 11*(1), 9–21.

Burkhardt, M.A., & Nagai-Jacobson, M.G. (2002). *Spirituality: Living our connectedness.* Delmar.

Burkhardt, M. A., & Nagai-Jacobson, M. G. (2022). Spirituality and health In M. A. Blaszko Helming., D. A. Shields, K. M. Avino, & W. E. Rosa (Eds.), *Dossey & Keegan's holistic nursing: A handbook for practice* (8th ed., pp. 121–143). Jones & Bartlett Learning.

CNA. 2017). *Code of ethics for registered nurses.* https://cdn1.nscn.ca/sites/default/files/documents/resources/code-of-ethics-for-nurses.pdf#:~:text=The%20Canadian%20Nurses%20Association%20%28CNA%29%20Code%20of%20Ethics,receiving%20care.%20The%20Codeis%20both%20aspirational%20and%20regulatory.

Doutrich, D., Dekker, L., Spuck, J., & Hoeksel, R. (2014). Identity, ethics and cultural safety: Strategies for change. *Whitireia Nursing Health Journal, 21*, 15–21.

Engebretson, J. C., & AHn, H. (2022). Transcultural Engagement In M. A. Blaszko Helming., D. A. Shields, K. M. Avino, & W. E. Rosa (Eds.), *Dossey & Keegan's holistic nursing: A handbook for practice* (8th ed., pp. 417–426). Jones & Bartlett Learning.

Fowler, D. M. (2015). *Guide to the code of ethics for nurses with interpretive statements.* American Nurses Association.

French, C., & Narayanasamy, A. (2011). To pray or not to pray: A question of ethics. *British Journal of Nursing, 20*(18), 1198–1204.

Giger, J. N., & Haddad, L. (2020). *Transcultural nursing: Assessment and intervention* (8th ed.). Elsevier.

Hanson, P. A., & Andrews, M. M. (2020). Religion, culture, and nursing In M. M. Andrews & J. S. Broyle (Eds.), *Transcultural concepts in nursing care* (8th ed, pp. 373–415). Walters Kluwer.

Hughes, B., DeGregory, C., Elk, R., Graham, D., Hall, E. & Ressallat, J. (2017). *Spiritual Care and Nursing: A Nurse's Contribution and Practice.* https://www.spiritualcareassociation.org/docs/resources/nurses_spiritual_care_white_paper_3_22_2017.pdf.

Helming, M. B. (2011). Healing through prayer: A qualitative study. *Holistic Nursing Practice, 25*(1), 33–44.

ICN. (2021). *The ICN code of ethics for nurses.* https://www.icn.ch/system/files/2021-10/ICN_Code-of-Ethics_EN_Web_0.pdf.

Leininger, M. (1991). Transcultural care principles, human rights, and ethical considerations. *Journal of Transcultural Nursing, 3*, 21–22.

Liehr, M. P. R., & Smith, M. J. (2018). Story theory In M. J. Smith & P. R. Liehr (Eds.), *Middle range theory for nursing* (4th ed.). Springer.

McFarland, M. R., & Wehbe-Alamah, H. B. (Eds.). (2015). *Leininger's culture care diversity and universality: A worldwide nursing theory* (3rd ed.). Jones & Bartlett.

Mujallad, A., & Taylor, E. J. (2016). Modesty among Muslim women: Implications for nursing care. *Medsurg Nursing, 25*(3), 169–172.

Narayanasamy, A., & Narayanasamy, M. (2008). The healing power of prayer and its implications for nursing. *British Journal of Nursing, 17*(6), 394–398.

Nursing Council of New Zealand. (2011). *Guidelines for cultural safety, the Treaty of Waitangi, and Maori health in nursing education and practice.* https://online.flippingbook.com/view/960779225/4/.

Ontario Council on Community Interpreters (OCCI). (2023). *OCCI Frequently asked questions: Community interpreters.* https://www.occi.ca/faqs.

Puchalski, C. M., Ferrell, B., Virani, R., Otis-Green, S., Baird, P., Bull, J., … Sulmasy, D. (2009). Improving the quality of spiritual care as a dimension of palliative care: The report of the Consensus Conference. *Journal of Palliative Medicine, 12*(10), 885–904.

Puchalski, C. M. (1996/2020). The ©FICA spiritual assessment tool: A guide for spiritual assessment in clinical settings. https://gwish.smhs.gwu.edu/sites/g/files/zaskib1011/files/2022-06/FICA-Tool-PDF-ADA.pdf.

Ray, M. A. (2016). *Transcultural caring dynamics in nursing and health care.* F. A. Davis.

Rykkje, L., Eriksson, K., & Råholm, M. (2011). A qualitative metasynthesis of spirituality from a caring science perspective. *International Journal for Human Caring, 15*(4), 40–53.

Sewell, M. (Ed.), (1991). *Cries of the spirit: A celebration of women's spirituality.* Beacon Press.

Spector, R. (2017). *Cultural diversity in health and illness* (9th ed.). Pearson.

Srivastave, R. H. (2023). *Health care professional's guide to cultural competence* (2nd ed.). Elsevier.

Tafoya, T. (1996, May). *Embracing the shadow: Mending the sacred hoop.* San Antonio, TX: Paper presented at the South Texas AIDS Training (STAT) for Mental Health Providers: The Human, Transcultural, and Spiritual Dimensions of HIV/AIDS.

Power to Make a Difference

Part V discusses the importance of empowerment of nurses and patients. To deal with the complex issues facing nursing today, nurses are required to exercise integrity, accountability, and moral courage. Nurses' professional responsibility, authority, and power to make principled choices are embedded in professional codes of nursing ethics. These codes express nursing's own understanding of its commitment to society and the ethical basis from which nurses, individually and collectively, in all roles and practice settings, can advocate for safe and ethical practice settings and safe, equitable, competent, and compassionate care for patients and communities. The ethical values, responsibilities, duties, professional ideals of nurses, and expectations regarding ethical behavior stated in these codes reflect attributes of empowerment and attitudes and skills that facilitate empowerment of nurses and patients. Empowerment of patients is grounded in nursing's ethical imperative of advocacy for patient rights, health, and safety and derives from an appreciation that patients have the ability to discern their needs and make decisions about their lives and health. Being a facilitator of empowerment requires nurses to relinquish power and embrace the patient as an equal partner. Nurses are called to facilitate empowerment by working directly with patients and by addressing social, political, and environmental factors affecting the health, rights, and safety of individuals and communities. Directives in codes of nursing ethics also impel nurses to deal in principled ways with issues and dilemmas arising in health care settings, foster personal health and safety, advocate for healthy and collaborative work environments, promote moral communities, and maintain ethical competence.

19

The Power of Ethical Nursing

Copper Woman warned Hai Nai Yu that the world would change and times might come when Knowing would not be the same as Doing. And she told her that Trying would always be very important.

(Cameron, 1981, p. 53)

OBJECTIVES

After completing this chapter, the reader should be able to:

1. Discuss the effect of mindset and metaphors for nursing on expectations regarding nursing practice and ethical stances.
2. Explain the impact on nursing practice of perceptions about nursing, both from within and from outside the profession.
3. Describe the concepts of power and empowerment.
4. Discuss the relationship among personal and professional empowerment, principled behavior, and nursing practice.
5. Relate nursing's role of patient advocate to patient empowerment.
6. Describe nurse attitudes, knowledge, and skills that facilitate patient empowerment.
7. Describe factors that enhance or inhibit patient empowerment.
8. Describe nursing's vision of nursing reflected in professional codes of nursing ethics and position statements.
9. Discuss the practical application of professional codes of nursing ethics in empowering nurses to practice according to nursing's vision for nursing.

INTRODUCTION

Dealing in a principled way with issues facing nursing requires integrity, accountability, and moral courage. Discussion of issues in this book is grounded in the belief that (1) as moral agents, nurses have the power to make choices and to act in responsible and principled ways, and (2) nurses have the authority to make decisions and recommendations regarding activities that are within the scope of their practice and grounded in professional codes of nursing ethics. The parameters of nursing's power and authority, however, are not always clear. The moral identity that grounds a nurse's ability to be a moral agent is linked to personal and professional self-identity. This self-identity is influenced by

factors such as how nurses perceive themselves personally and professionally, how the public perceives them, traditional views and expectations of women and nursing, cultural values, work environment, and healthcare systems. Many nurses feel constrained by the systems within which they work, by stereotypes that diminish the value of nursing judgments and care, and by persisting paternalistic attitudes that promote disempowerment. The concept of empowerment relates to the principle of autonomy. This chapter discusses the concept of empowerment as a process and an outcome through which nurses are enabled to clarify and claim their role as moral agents in making decisions regarding issues related to nursing practice, and to facilitate empowerment with patients. Fostering empowerment in others requires nurses to be attentive to both personal and professional empowerment. Supporting patients to feel empowered to make decisions about their own health and care is grounded in nursing's ethical imperative of advocacy for patient rights, health, and safety. Nursing attitudes, knowledge, and skills that foster empowerment are discussed; processes that facilitate patient empowerment are addressed; and factors associated with professional empowerment are considered.

INFLUENCES ON NURSING'S PERCEPTIONS OF PRINCIPLED PRACTICE

Nurses, patients, and other healthcare providers may vary greatly in their perceptions of ideals for nursing and nursing practice. These perceptions influence expectations and decisions regarding care, authority, and accountability. Expectations regarding good nursing care and ethical nursing practice flow from such perceptions. We recognize that factors in our internal and external environments affect both personal and professional decision making. External environmental factors include the norms, ideals, and expectations of patients; families; the nursing profession; other healthcare providers; public perceptions; and the professional, social, and cultural systems within which we interact. The internal environment includes our mindset or inner world of personal beliefs and perceptions, as well as our personal values and moral identity.

Influence of Mindset

Our attitudes, views, and beliefs about the healthcare system influence how we identify and respond to ethical issues and dilemmas in practice. For example, when nurses view healthcare in terms of medical cases focused on the cure of disease, the physician is seen as the dominant authority. In this view of healthcare, following the physician's orders (whether or not the nurse agrees with them) and loyalty to the physician and institution are considered the legitimate and ethical focus of nursing activities. This mindset is contrary to the independent, ethical practice of nursing that requires nurses to be accountable for their own actions and decisions. If nurses view healthcare as a commodity in which nursing and medical care are sold to patients by institutions, the nurse's primary responsibility is to the employing institution. Within this view, needs of individual patients may be subordinated to the utilitarian goal focused on the good of the greatest number of people or the institutional goal of making a profit. Nurses who hold this view may not challenge the rightness or wrongness of nursing actions or the impact on patient care, provided they are congruent with the goals and policies of the institution. This mindset finds fertile ground in large corporate institutional settings and managed care arenas. When nurses view healthcare as a basic human need and a right for each person, the nurse's primary responsibility is to the patient. The legitimate and ethical focus of nursing activities within this mindset is grounded in professional codes of nursing ethics and must include advocacy for patient rights, safety, and overall well-being.

Ethical Accountability and Nursing Self-Image

Metaphors help us understand a concept by comparing two things that are different yet share common characteristics. People often use metaphors to focus attention on particular aspects of reality to enhance understanding of roles, events, and experiences. Metaphors may also influence our perceptions of these events and experiences. For example, likening nurses to angels in white calls attention to the nursing roles of caring, protecting, and serving; yet viewing nurses as angels may set up the expectation that they should be somewhat distant, above human frailties, self-sacrificing and willing to work out of the goodness of their hearts regardless of compensation. Metaphors that have been associated with nursing reflect different ideas about nursing roles and responsibilities in healthcare. These metaphors also suggest different approaches to determining an appropriate ethical stance for nursing care delivery.

The military metaphor for nursing that was grounded in Florence Nightingale's model for nursing and was common from the late 19th into the mid-20th century is associated with obedience to higher authority, a view of disease as the enemy, discipline, respect for those of higher rank, uniform dress, and, above all, loyalty. Loyalty to patients was considered part of being loyal to the institutions and to the physicians under whom nurses worked. Ethical imperatives that flow from this metaphor include following physician orders, even if the nurse questions the appropriateness of these orders; upholding the patient's faith in the physician, even if the nurse questions the doctor's competence;

and being loyal to healthcare colleagues, even at the expense of the patient.

In the early history of nursing, following the physician's order without question would have absolved the nurse from guilt, even in the event of a harmful outcome for the patient. Today, however, this is not the case. Nursing's transition from vocation to profession requires that nurses be personally accountable for their actions. Court rulings have held nurses legally responsible for their decisions and actions. Legal decisions, changes in the healthcare delivery system, and feminist awareness within the nursing profession have encouraged the transition from the metaphor of loyal soldier to that of patient advocate. Beginning in the 1960s and 1970s, a significant revision in nursing's self-image emerged that included the legal metaphor of patient advocacy and the academic metaphor of rational thought regarding ethical dilemmas (Milton, 2009; Sharoff, 2009; ten Hoeve et al., 2014). Greater emphasis on consumerism and patient rights, coupled with growing dissatisfaction with increased costs and depersonalization of healthcare, helped open the door for nurses to expand their roles as patient advocates and professional colleagues. Professional nursing codes of ethics and standards of practice stress responsibility to patients through collegial membership in the healthcare team and reflect ethical imperatives flowing from the stance of advocacy and professional accountability. As advocates for patient rights, nurses are responsible to those who require nursing care. This obliges nurses to establish caring and trusting relationships with patients and be alert to situations in which patients may be endangered by incompetent, unethical, or illegal practices by any member of the healthcare team or the healthcare system and to take appropriate actions to safeguard the patient (ANA, 2015a, Provisions 2, 3, 6; CNA, 2017, Part I.A, I.B; ICN, 2021, Elements 1,2).

Loyalty remains a valued virtue for nurses within the focus on advocacy. Although ideally the nurse's first loyalty is to the patient, circumstances of conflicting loyalty may occur. Loyalty to colleagues and to employers is also important, and nurses may at times be faced with making difficult decisions between advocacy for patients or loyalty to colleagues. Such situations require personal integrity, knowledge, and moral courage on the part of the nurse.

Nursing's self-image is evident in the images nurses use to describe their roles and their practice. These images illuminate the complexities and ambiguities of nursing practice, as well as the influence of social, organizational, and cultural constraints on nurses. How nurses picture nursing and the vision they hold of their role in healthcare influence their ability to practice in a holistic, patient-focused way. Personal self-image affects how one lives in the world, relates to self and others, thinks, acts, behaves, and makes decisions. Influences on nursing self-image evident in the literature include personal thoughts and experiences; education; work environment; work values; social, cultural, and environmental feedback; reference groups; roles and value of women in society; and media and other public images of nurses (DiGregorio, 2023; Fletcher, 2007; ten Hoeve et al., 2014). Constraints engendered by negative self-images may prompt nurses to feel unable to practice nursing in a way that is consistent with their values. Awareness of factors that influence self-image enables nurses to work to counter negative influences and to enhance and claim their professional self-image (Fletcher, 2007; Gordon, 2010; Grinberg & Sela, 2022; Liaschenko & Peter, 2016; ten Hoeve et al., 2014).

Perception of Others and Nursing Ethical Accountability

Factors such as mindset and metaphors influence our perceptions of and choices regarding principled behavior. The perceptions of others also affect our considerations regarding appropriate or ethical nursing actions. Although nursing as a profession has now claimed the role of advocate in lieu of that of loyal soldier, there are nurses within the profession who have not fully embraced the change. Operationalizing the advocacy role may put nurses at risk in some institutions and situations, as demonstrated in cases such as that of Jolene Tuma discussed in Chapter 11, and in cases of whistleblowing discussed later in this chapter. Although nursing has made a paradigm shift regarding its role and responsibilities, awareness of nursing's current professional and ethical imperatives is often lacking among patients, families, physicians, and healthcare administrators. The role of nursing as perceived by many outside of the profession remains embedded in the loyal soldier metaphor and in mindsets that view healthcare as a collection of medical cases or as a commodity. As a result, many physicians still expect nurses to follow their bidding and take offense when nurses challenge their decisions or actions. The hierarchical system remains the norm in many healthcare institutions. Because physicians are perceived to be of higher rank, their influence often holds more sway than that of nurses who may challenge them. Although patients and families often have more continual and direct contact with nurses, they may not fully understand the breadth and depth of the nurse's role and responsibility in their care, including the role of their advocate. Instead, they often function from the mindset that the physician is the captain of a ship on which the nurse is a member of the crew. Images in the media that depict nurses in ancillary, subordinate roles also affect the perceptions of patients and others regarding the expectations of nurses.

CASE PRESENTATION

Conflicting Views of Nursing's Role

Inga is the vice president of nursing at a large medical center. Recently one of the physicians, who holds a lot of power in the system and is generally very open and easy to work with, expressed considerable displeasure about the refusal of a particular nurse to carry out a medical order. He was irate when she decided to refer her concerns about certain of his medical practice decisions to the ethics committee. The physician says that Inga should fire the nurse for insubordination. Inga is aware that the nurse's decisions were reasonable, in the patient's interest, and aligned with ethical codes and standards of nursing practice. She is also aware that the physician in question is well known nationally and brings a lot of money to the hospital.

Think About It
A Need for Moral Courage
- Where do you see the potential for conflicting loyalties in this situation?
- Discuss how differing perceptions of nursing might affect this situation. What do you think is the physician's image of a moral nurse? How would you describe the nurse's self-identity as a moral agent? How does she exhibit moral courage?
- How do you think Inga should address the physician's complaint and request? What factors would be important for her to consider before responding? What specific sections of codes of nursing ethics should she incorporate into her response?
- Describe what you see as the most realistic outcome in this situation. What about the ideal outcome?

UNDERSTANDING POWER AND EMPOWERMENT

Nurses have the power to make a difference by acting in principled ways in all areas of their lives and practice. However, as has been evident throughout the discussions in this book, many factors mitigate against nurses claiming this power. Nurses need to develop skills in dealing with these factors to function fully in their legitimate roles within healthcare. Nurses must be aware of values, beliefs, and other influences affecting personal decision making and must expand their knowledge of ethical principles, contextual factors, legal considerations, and other issues facing nursing. Understanding power and empowerment can help in developing strategies for action in this regard.

Although the word *power* is often understood in terms of strength, force, or control, dictionary definitions of the term, derived from its Latin root "potere," refer as well to the ability to do or act, which includes the capability of doing or accomplishing something. To have power, then, implies having the ability to do or act; and to empower would be to facilitate the ability of another person to do or to act. A key aspect of empowerment, then, is developing or promoting the ability for autonomy or self-determination (Tengland, 2016). This applies both to nurses and to patients.

Seeking a better understanding of both the concept of empowerment and how empowerment (or its lack) affects nurses, patient care, and patient self-determination has been a topic in the nursing literature for many years. Intrapersonal, interpersonal, and environmental factors all play a role in empowerment. These factors include self-esteem; personal values and perceptions; moral identity; sense of self in relation to others; self-determination or sense of control over the situation; and an environment that fosters access to information, resources, and support.

A Participative Process

Empowerment is understood to be a participative process between individuals or within a group. This process may be evident in collaborative efforts by nurses to improve patient care and support a healthy work environment on a hospital unit or the partnership between a nurse and patient that supports patient well-being and facilitates choices that promote healthy behaviors (Ellis-Stoll & Popkess-Vawter, 1998; Friend & Sieloff, 2018; Hewitt-Taylor, 2004; Linnen & Rowley, 2014; Shearer & Reed, 2004; Williamson, 2007; Watson, 2018).

This collaboration is viewed by some as a social process of recognizing, promoting, and enhancing nurses' or patients' abilities to meet their own needs, solve their own problems, and mobilize the necessary resources to feel in control of their own lives and work (Akpotor & Johnson, 2018; Friend & Sieloff, 2018; Fulton, 1997; McCarthy & Freeman, 2008). Another understanding of empowerment is the capacity of disenfranchised people to understand and become active participants in the matters that affect their lives, suggesting that a personal attitude that affirms change as possible is important for empowerment to occur (Bolton & Brookings, 1998; Rao, 2012; Tengland, 2016). Empowerment may be viewed as a philosophy or worldview flowing from a belief in each person's inherent worth and a belief in the process of self-discovery that involves creating a vision, taking risks, making choices, and behaving in authentic ways (Gurka, 1995; Rao, 2012). Empowerment requires respect for an individual's personal beliefs and goals and trust in the person's ability to make decisions, take action, and be accountable for the actions. Although sharing knowledge through education is important for empowerment, the literature clearly indicates that emotional and social support is essential as well.

Collaborative and Transactional Process

In-depth analyses of the concept of empowerment suggest that it is both process and outcome, taking different forms within different people and contexts (Akpotor & Johnson, 2018; Ellis-Stoll & Popkess-Vawter, 1998; Gibson, 1991; McCarthy & Freeman, 2008; Rao, 2012; Rodwell, 1996; Ryles, 1999; Tengland, 2016). Because of this, empowerment needs to be defined by the people concerned. It is a transactional process involving relationship with others. This relationship includes mutually beneficial interactions aimed at strengthening rather than weakening; power sharing through mutual sharing of knowledge, resources, and opportunities; and respect for self and others. Empowerment is nurtured by collaborative efforts that focus on solutions rather than problems, and on strengths, rights, and abilities rather than deficits. Empowerment derives from a feminine perspective of power with or power to, which implies sharing responsibility, knowledge, and resources; collaboration for goal achievement; incorporating diversity; valuing the contributions of each person; and valuing the process. In contrast, the masculine view of power over incorporates a sense of paternalistic control, struggle for and protection of limited resources, separation of leaders and followers, expediency, and results, even at the expense of persons (Chinn, 2013).

Attributes of Empowerment

Empowerment can seem like a rather abstract term, and you may be wondering what being empowered looks and feels like. Certainly, two people in the same circumstances can have different experiences of empowerment. Nurse scholars use a variety of descriptive terms when discussing people who are empowered (Akpotor & Johnson, 2018; Bolton & Brookings, 1998; Ellis-Stoll & Popkess-Vawter, 1998; Friend & Sieloff, 2018; Fulton, 1997; Hartrick & Schreiber, 1998; Jones et al., 2000; Kuokkanen & Leino-Kilpi, 2000; Laschinger et al., 2006; Linnen & Rowley, 2014; McCarthy & Freeman, 2008; Rodwell, 1996; Ryles, 1999). These attributes of empowerment (noted in Table 19.1) are reflected throughout

TABLE 19.1 Attributes of Empowerment		
Autonomy/Freedom	**Self-Efficacy**	**Sense of Mastery Regarding Self and the Environment**
Courage	Self-development	Sense of control
Authority	Self-determination	Sense of connectedness
Caring, enabling	Self-confidence	Capability of social intercourse
Endurance, resilience	Self-control	Decision-making ability
Expertise	Positive self-concept	Freedom to make choices
Participation, solidarity	Personal satisfaction	Ability to make changes
Influence	Feeling of hope	Action orientation
Sturdiness	Assertiveness	Taking a position
Visionary	Strength	Power sharing

codes of nursing ethics in descriptions of ethical values, responsibilities, duties, professional ideals of nurses, and expectations regarding ethical behavior and patient care. Not all of these attributes are necessarily part of every experience of empowerment; however, they provide markers that help us identify characteristics of nurses and patients that support the process and presence of empowerment.

Empowerment implies choice on the part of those being empowered. We cannot empower another, because to presume to do so removes the element of choice. Empowerment requires both inner motivation and environmental factors that support the process. As noted earlier, this process requires self-awareness, positive self-esteem, a commitment to self and others, and the desire and ability to make decisions. Responsibility and accountability for our actions and having the authority to act are implicit in the ability to choose.

Through the empowerment process we can enable others to develop awareness of areas that need change; foster a desire to take action; and share resources, skills, and opportunities that support the change. Self-empowerment derives from self-awareness and resources that support self-determination more than services provided to persons (Akpotor & Johnson, 2018; Rao, 2012; Rodwell, 1996). Enhanced self-esteem, personal satisfaction, a sense of connectedness, the ability to set and reach goals, a sense of control over life and change processes, and a sense of hope and direction are all outcomes of empowerment.

ASK YOURSELF

What Makes You Feel Empowered?

- Consider a situation in which you felt empowered. Describe factors contributing to your sense of empowerment.
- Recall a time when you felt disempowered. What contributed to this sense? How might you have felt more empowered in the situation?

PERSONAL EMPOWERMENT AND MORAL IDENTITY

Nursing's power to make a difference in care with patients derives from many factors. To serve as credible models of empowerment for others, we must demonstrate congruence between values and behaviors in our own lives. Personal integrity implies an ability to be honest with and care for ourselves, as well as respond to the needs of others. Often nurses, and especially women, have learned to value care for others before or instead of care for self. A true value for human life must include value for our own lives as well. The biblical adage is "Love thy neighbor as thyself," not instead of thyself or before thyself (Leviticus 19:18). We must attend to ourselves and treat ourselves with the same respect and dignity with which we treat others. Recall that Provision 5 of the American Nursing Association (ANA) *Code of Ethics for Nurses with Interpretive Statements* (2015a) states "the nurse owes the same duties to self as to others, including the responsibility to promote health and safety." Similarly Element 2.4 of the *ICN Code of Ethics for Nurses* (2021) states that "nurses value their own dignity, well-being and health". Personal empowerment begins with actions that support the meeting of our own needs and self-actualization. It is from our personal stores of creativity, empowerment, and health that we are able to inspire, teach, and assist others in achieving their potential.

In principle, many nurses would agree with the concept of care for self, however, actions often conflict with this acknowledged belief. Nurses often agree to work additional hours even when they are exhausted; consume large amounts of caffeine and sugar to boost waning energy; go home to care for children, spouse, and friends; and collapse into bed only to get up and do it all again the next day because they feel limited power to do otherwise. What causes a person to behave in ways that conflict with his or her stated values? Often the person has learned conflicting messages. A belief in caring for ourselves may conflict with a learned belief that caring for others is more admirable or more important than caring for ourselves.

Some people feel very little control over any area of their lives. Others may feel empowered to make decisions in some situations but not in others—for example, a nurse may actively make decisions in the home environment while feeling like a pawn of the system at work. The sense of power that nurses have in their personal lives may affect their perception of empowerment in the professional arena. Moral distress, burnout, workplace incivility, job dissatisfaction, and limited professional commitment affect the quality of patient care and are often associated with feelings of powerlessness

(Laschinger et al., 2014; Leiter & Laschinger, 2006; Linnen & Rowley, 2014; Ning et al., 2009; O'Brien, 2011). Attributes of empowerment noted in Table 19.1 reflect important considerations for self-empowerment on both personal and professional levels.

Self-Awareness, Personal Accountability, and the Empowered Person

The ability to facilitate empowerment in others requires us to attend to personal empowerment. This means valuing ourselves as we listen inwardly to our own senses, as well as carefully listening to trusted others, consciously taking in and forming strength (Chinn, 2013). Self-awareness is necessary because self-perception is linked to quality of patient care (Fletcher, 2007; Grinberg & Sela, 2022; ten Hoeve et al., 2014). Such awareness requires attentiveness to the many things that influence our thoughts, feelings, actions, and reactions in the present circumstance and reflective consideration of such influences on past experiences. Empowerment involves taking ownership of our inner lives and recognizing that we have full control over our thoughts, feelings, and actions.

Owning our thoughts involves recognizing old or repetitive thought patterns and changing those that are no longer supporting a creative, actualizing life. Self-critical, judgmental, and negative thinking is particularly confining. Old thinking can be updated with new knowledge. Questioning the origin of particular thoughts can reveal ideas that were true at one time but now are no longer true. For example, a child who was always told that she did not know enough to make a decision and that her Mother knew best may become an adult who still consults her mother before making decisions; or a person who was frequently criticized as a young adult may react to any suggestion about a way to do things differently as a personal affront. Seeking alternative views of situations and learning logical or critical thinking skills are other ways to restructure thought patterns. Journaling about our thoughts, feelings, and reactions related to situations in our personal and professional lives may help provide insight into old patterns so we can begin conscious change.

Feelings are transient signals that alert us to what is supportive or offensive in a situation. Owning feelings means acknowledging and investigating the internal source of the message, rather than blaming other persons or situations for our feelings. People may experience different feelings in similar situations. For example, a death can elicit feelings of sadness, despair, hope, relief, joy, and others, depending on the unique inner response of each person. Feelings and the reactions they elicit are in the person, not in the event.

We need to name and take ownership of personal values and to claim our ability to make choices. When experiencing a lack of control in life, we should identify both internal and external barriers to having control, consider whether we want control, and explore what we need to do and are willing to risk to take control. Consciously acting based on a clear evaluation of the current situation, rather than acting automatically, is one way to own our behavior. Taking ownership of behavior requires being able to see options. Believing that there are no options can result in feeling powerless, trapped, or victimized. Even when we do not believe we can change a current unacceptable situation immediately, we can plan for change and set that plan into motion one step at a time. A victim waits and hopes something or someone else will change; makes excuses for not acting (time, cost, fatigue, and the like); blames people, places, or things for the situation; and is trapped and unaware of options. An empowered person decides to be accountable for personal responses, makes plans, considers options, develops strategies for change, and acts on plans by doing what is necessary to succeed.

Personal Moral Identity and Moral Courage

Personal empowerment requires growth of personal strength and power, and includes the ability to enact our own will and love for ourselves in the context of love and respect for others. This can only happen when individuals express respect and reverence for all forms of life and appreciate that the energy of the self is interconnected with the energy of the whole of life (Chinn, 2013; Watson, 2018). A commitment to personal growth and self-care, developing a positive sense of self and awareness of strengths and abilities as well as limitations, and drawing on our supports and sources of connectedness foster this process. Empathy with others, appreciation of diversity, tolerance, flexibility, and willingness to compromise empower a person.

Personal moral identity profoundly influences moral agency. Enacting personal moral agency requires that we trust ourselves and our knowledge and abilities and be courageous in taking risks. **Moral courage** reflects a high degree of personal empowerment. Moral courage means the willingness to stand up for personal and professional core values and ethical beliefs, even when we stand alone (ANA, 2015a; CNA, 2017; ICN, 2021; Kritek, 2017; Liaschenko & Peter, 2016; Murray, 2010). Implicit in moral courage is being willing to do what is right even when faced with the risk of ridicule, social rejection, shame, unemployment, and emotional anxiety. Moral courage requires the ability to determine the right thing to do, how to handle one's fears, and the course of action needed to maintain one's integrity (Kritek, 2017; Lachman, 2007). This implies thoughtful consideration of the issues inherent in the situation and the risks involved and requires being true to ourselves and our values when faced with morally distressing situations. The personal integrity essential to moral courage requires congruence among our being, knowing, and doing. This means that our actions flow from our essence, and our choices derive from what we know to be good and true.

PROFESSIONAL EMPOWERMENT AND ETHICAL NURSING PRACTICE

Professional empowerment is built on the foundational elements of personal accountability and support of nursing colleagues. To deal in a principled way with ethical issues and dilemmas arising within healthcare settings, nurses must feel personally and professionally empowered to act on sometimes difficult choices. Many factors affect nursing actions in the professional arena, including personal attitudes and self-concept; knowledge of and grounding in professional nursing codes of ethics, the structural and functional interrelatedness of healthcare systems; political, economic, social, and cultural forces; and interactions with patients and colleagues. Barriers to empowerment may exist within the community or imposed from external sources.

Empowerment requires nurses to become knowledgeable about and address system issues as well as interpersonal issues that affect patient care and nursing practice. Such issues include recognizing the need for changing the power base within the current healthcare system; moving from a paternalistic, hierarchical model of control toward one that values collaboration; addressing incivility in the workplace; and drawing on the power of the collective. Developing and supporting processes for nurses to become involved in shared decision making and in forming institutional policies is part of this process (ANA, 2015a, Provisions 8,9; CNA, 2017, Part II; ICN, 2021, Elements 1.6, 1.73.1, 3.4, 3.5; Edmonson, 2010; Laschinger et al., 2014; Liaschenko & Peters, 2016; Linnen & Rowley, 2014; Mathes, 2005).

Building Moral Communities

The effect of nurses' empowerment in the healthcare environment can have personal, institutional, and patient care implications. In terms of nursing management and health systems, some authors view empowerment as a method for delegating authority and sharing power and a strategy for improving the productivity of nurses. The literature suggests a link between nurses' perceptions of job satisfaction, their work effectiveness, quality of patient care, and workplace empowerment (Fig. 19.1). Empowered nurses are more likely to initiate and sustain independent behaviors that foster a healthy and collaborative work environment, increase work effectiveness, and promote moral community (Grinberg & Sela, 2022; Laschinger et al., 2009; Liaschenko & Peters, 2016; Linnen & Rowley, 2014; Marturano & Narva, 2023; Ning et al., 2009). Liaschenko and Peter (2016) discuss the important role of nurses in building *moral communities* within healthcare settings. These communities foster moral identities as they nurture and develop moral agency. They describe moral communities as places where moral language is a natural part of conversations that reflect our identities as moral agents. Moral communities create spaces for moral discourse that include and value the unique role of all who contribute to patient care outcomes. Within this context, codes of nursing ethics encourage nurses to be deliberative

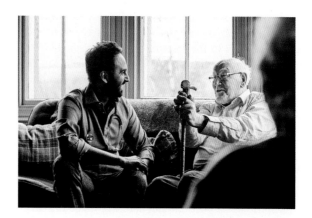

Fig. 19.1 Respect and Mutual Trust—Key Elements in Fostering Empowerment. (©iStock.com/Dean Mitchell.)

in exercising power in a way that assures nursing input into decisions about all aspects of nursing practice. This includes holding others accountable for taking nursing concerns seriously by demonstrating skilled and intelligent care that reflects the ethical grounding of the nursing profession.

Workplace Empowerment

Factors that have a positive impact on empowerment include access to the structures of information, support, and resources (Laschinger et al., 2014; Linnen & Rowley, 2014; Purdy et al., 2010). Studies indicate that workplace empowerment relates to job satisfaction, nurse retention, organizational commitment, reduced incivility and burnout, and better patient care (Grinberg & Sela, 2022; Laschinger et al., 2014; Ning et al., 2009; Purdy et al., 2010). In contrast, feelings of powerlessness are associated with job dissatisfaction, low levels of professional commitment, increased incivility, and burnout, which are barriers to quality patient care (Laschinger et al., 2014; Ning et al., 2009; O'Brien, 2011). Nurses who are burned out and dissatisfied are more inclined to give only the most routine care. Only an empowered workforce can be effective in today's healthcare system with its innovations of patient-focused care, case management, and shared governance (DiGregorio, 2023; Edmonson, 2010; Friend & Sieloff, 2018; Linnen & Rowley, 2014; Marturano & Narva, 2023). Inherent in this perspective is a sense that each person is free to make choices and that those who are empowered, both internally and by the system, feel more in control of their lives; are able to act in appropriate, meaningful ways; and are able to do what they truly want to do.

When nurses feel disempowered in their work settings, they can choose the victim stance, which relinquishes power to the system, or they can challenge the system. Dealing with the system requires skills in conflict management, negotiation, and effective communication, as well as moral courage. Challenging the system can take many forms. Being a change agent begins with the nurse's personal presence and attitude. For example, one nurse described how her commitment to caring for the whole person was challenged when she began working in a Level III trauma center. Feeling constantly criticized by coworkers as she incorporated emotional and spiritual support into her care, she made the choice to act out of her values as a holistic nurse and return a loving spirit to the injustice of their criticism. She noted

that this choice came as a great challenge and that it was often difficult to go to work under the scrutiny focused in her direction. However, she used each opportunity of conversation with coworkers to suggest that they work together to unite the staff with an attitude of mutual caring, support, and nurturance. Her presence was reflected in her choice to stand in her power and speak her truth. Although this was not easy, living her values contributed to a change in attitude within the whole staff, particularly regarding how they supported and cared for each other.

Nurses can address social and economic constraints on nursing and healthcare through their involvement in professional organizations and through becoming politically active. Participation on institutional boards or committees that focus on patient care and professional practice concerns is another way to challenge the system, as is speaking out about unsafe or questionable practices. Informing authorities within or outside of one's work setting about practices or situations that are unethical, unsafe, questionable, or unlawful, particularly when these practices are being overlooked by others, may be considered whistleblowing.

Moral Agency: Speaking Up

Empowerment incorporates divergent and conflicting solutions to problems based on value in support of others rather than in divisiveness (Chinn, 2013; Friend & Sieloff, 2018; Kritek, 2017). It implies embracing diversity and moving away from fear of that which is different to appreciation of the strength derived from and unity contained in diversity. Nurses need to recognize that systems exert control, in part, by fostering divisiveness among workers to deter unity of opposition to system policies. When nurses unite with and support colleagues who challenge harmful or potentially harmful practices, they are personally and professionally empowered.

Advocating for and making every effort to protect the rights, health, and safety of patients is a nursing responsibility that is clearly delineated in the ANA (2015a), CNA (2017) and ICN (2021) codes of ethics for nurses. Challenging unjust, unprofessional, or unethical practices is not an easy decision and may entail risk for nurses. The decision to do so may put the nurse in a difficult position of being labeled as a troublemaker, potentially victimized and ostracized, and subject to reprisals by colleagues or management. Although it may feel safer to remain silent, we need to consider whether we become complicit in the action or behavior of concern by doing so (Curtin, 2013; Fitzgerald et al., 2017). Moral courage is needed for nurses to choose to speak up about situations within their work settings that pose a serious threat to patient or staff health, safety, or rights. These situations include incivility, bullying, and workplace violence, as well as unsafe, unethical, or illegal practice by any member of the healthcare team. The complexity of factors related to speaking up or remaining silent requires thoughtfulness and careful consideration on the part of the nurse. Nurses need to be aware of institutional policies and procedures for reporting such situations and to follow appropriate channels within the organization to rectify them. If the organization has no policies, nurses are obligated to participate in the development of relevant policies (ANA, 2015a, 2015b; CNA, 2017, 2019; ICN, 2012, 2021). Guidelines and considerations related to seeking a solution to unethical practice are noted in Box 19.1.

Whistleblowing

When every effort has been made to have the situation corrected and the danger still persists, a nurse may decide to "blow the whistle" on the person or institution. **Whistleblowing** is the exposure of observed wrongdoing that affects the rights or safety of patients and others in clinical, academic, research, institutional, or other settings. Whistleblowers attempt to expose the wrongdoing through warning the public about negligence, professional misconduct, incompetence, or other factors that may endanger patients or staff, violate standards of academic honesty, or affect the integrity and truthful reporting of research (Fowler, 2015; Lachman, 2008; Mannion & Davies, 2015; Mansbach et al., 2014; Ray, 2006). Situations that prompt whistleblowing can involve ethical dilemmas related to a conflict between loyalty to coworkers or the institution and loyalty to patients, or the benefit of the action (to the patient) versus risk to the nurse. Although whistleblowing is considered a last resort in advocating for the rights and safety of patients and others, professional codes of nursing ethics and position statements provide guidance and support for nurses in taking such action if necessary (ANA, 2015a, Provision 3; CNA, 2017, Part I.B.5, I.F.8; ICN, 2012; ICN, 2021, Element 2.10, 2.11). A nurse who feels that being a whistleblower is the necessary course of action needs to be clear that it is being done for the correct moral reason and needs to be aware of potential consequences

> **BOX 19.1 Guidelines and Considerations for Addressing Unjust, Unethical, and Unsafe Practice**
>
> - Be familiar with your organization's policies and procedures for reporting occurrences of incivility; bullying; workplace violence; and unsafe, unethical, or illegal practice.
> - Do not let the complexity of the situation obscure your responsibility to assure safe and ethical patient care.
> - Unless a patient is in immediate danger in the situation, think it through for a day or several days. Reflect and perhaps journal about what you have observed or experienced with the intent of seeking a solution. Include your own feelings, reactions, fears, and sense of ethical responsibility. Write an account of the incident, how often it has occurred, and specific dates. The account should include details of what happened, pertinent names, and any witnesses to the incident. Keep your written account in a secure location.
> - Seek input and guidance from others such as trusted colleagues, those with different perspectives, chaplains, and those who are knowledgeable about your professional and legal responsibilities.
> - When you feel clear about the situation and your responsibility in addressing the issue, report it as soon as possible through appropriate channels in your organization, following established policies and procedures. If there were witnesses to the incident, you should ask them to document their observations and give you a signed copy of the written document to include with your written report of the situation. Keep a copy of the report you submit to the appropriate persons in your organization.
> - If the situation is not addressed fully at one level of management, work up the management chain to seek resolution.

(Data from ANA. (2015b). *Incivility, bullying, and workplace violence. (Position statement).* https://www.nursingworld.org/practice-policy/nursing-excellence/official-position-statements/id/incivility-bullying-and-workplace-violence/; Fitzgerald, E. M., Myers, J. G., & Clark, P. (2017). Nurses need not be guilty bystanders: Caring for vulnerable immigrant populations. *The Online Journal of Issues in Nursing*, 22, 1. http://ojin.nursingworld.org/MainMenuCategories/ANAMarketplace/ANAPeriodicals/OJIN/TableofContents/Vol-22-2017/No1-Jan-2017/Articles-Previous-Topics/Nurses-Need-Not-Be-Guilty-Bystanders.html).

of the action (Fitzgerald et al., 2017; Jackson et al., 2010; Lachman, 2008; Ray, 2006; Rice, 2015). Feeling empowered to take a stand requires personal integrity and support from others. Support that enables nurses

CASE PRESENTATION

Confronting Destructive Workplace Behaviors

Expansion of a case presented in Chapter 13.

Sabrina works at a hospital that serves a multiracial and multiethnic population, many of whom are immigrants. She is caring for Mrs. H., a middle-age Middle Eastern woman who was just admitted with severe pneumonia. Several family members are in the room with her. A nursing colleague, Louella, comments to Sabrina, "This is another ignorant foreigner who let things go too long" and tells her "to be careful because there may be terrorists in the room." Louella adds that they should all be arrested and sent back to where they came from. Sabrina feels offended by Louella's comment but hesitates to say anything because Louella is good friends with the charge nurse, and she is concerned about repercussions.

Consider that you are a nurse on this unit and observe this interaction. You talk to Sabrina in private about how upsetting Louella's comments were to you and wondered why no one said anything. Sabrina says most of the staff feel the same way, but when something has been said in the past the person got terrible schedules and did not get requested vacation. In the six months that you have been working there, you have heard Louella making disparaging comments about other patients related to race, physical characteristics, and socioeconomic status. She flatters the physicians to their faces while making comments like "he's a womanizer" or "she's not very bright" behind their backs. Your classmate, Meili, who was top of your class and started working the same time you did, has been the brunt of Louella's jokes and harsh words. One time when Meili asked a question about a procedure that was new to her, Louella replied that she thought all Asians were supposed to be smart and if she didn't know how to do this simple procedure, how was she ever going to become a real nurse. Then she tossed a procedure manual at her to read. You also notice that there is always tension among the staff when Louella is working a shift, and even patients have commented about her attitude; however, there is much more collaboration and collegiality when she is not there.

As you reflect on the situation, you wonder whether you can continue to work in this environment and even question whether you made the right choice in becoming a nurse. You feel you need to say something, yet know your position might be put in jeopardy. You decide to talk to a former faculty mentor about the situation and get some guidance. After sharing your observations and concerns and talking the situation through with him, he suggests that you write down what you have observed in as much detail as possible and continue to document incidences as you observe them. He suggests that you meet with him again in two weeks and bring both your documentation and a copy of the hospital's policies and procedures for reporting occurrences of incivility, bullying, workplace violence, and unsafe practice. He also suggests that you journal about your concerns, including thoughts, feelings, fears, hopes for resolution, and what kind of risks you might be willing to take to address this situation.

Think About It
The Challenge of Speaking Up

- What is your personal reaction to the described situation?
- What ethical issues are evident?
- Would you consider taking any different course of action at this point?
- What do you think about your faculty mentor's suggestions?
- What thoughts, feelings, and concerns would you include in your journal? Be specific.
- How would professional ethical codes and position statements inform your reflections? Be specific.
- What risks might you be willing to take?
- Presume that when you meet again with your faculty mentor you decide that your moral agency impels you to speak up. What would guide you in moving forward? Would you seek other input or support? What would be your next step in taking action to speak up?
- Following the advice of your faculty mentor, you talk to Sabrina, Meili, and another trusted colleague about your decision and ask if they would be willing to document what they have observed. They all agree to do so. Why would this be important?
- Your faculty mentor also suggests that you ask one of these colleagues to be with you when you report these concerns to someone in management. Why might this be a good thing to do?
- Your hospital's procedure for reporting situations of incivility and unsafe practice gives three options for an initial report. You may take it to the nursing supervisor, to the human resources director, or to the ethics and compliance officer. Who would you consider approaching first and why? How would you prepare for the meeting? How would you present the information about your concerns in a professional manner?

to be true advocates for patients may come from colleagues, from professional organizations, and from the legal protection of whistleblower laws. Most states have enacted or introduced whistleblower legislation or regulations in recent years, and federal regulations also provide legislative protection for whistleblowers. Empowered nurses work with state, provincial, and national nurses' associations to continue to strengthen whistleblower protection legislation. Information regarding state whistleblower protection laws for healthcare workers in the United States can be found at https://www.nationalnursesunited.org/whistleblower-protection-laws-for-healthcare-workers. US federal regulations can be found through the Occupational Safety and Health Administration whistleblower protection program at https://www.whistleblowers.gov/. Whistleblowing is a very serious matter that should

only be done after careful reflection individually and with others. Guidance for nurses who are considering acting or speaking up is delineated in Box 19.2. You will note that the process includes making every effort to address the issue within the organization before contacting an outside agency; thus, there is some overlap with the content of Box 19.1.

ADVOCACY AND PATIENT EMPOWERMENT

The ethical imperative to facilitate empowerment with patients is a nursing directive grounded in its ethical focus of advocacy for patients. Adherence to the principles discussed throughout this book, particularly respect for persons, autonomy, justice, and beneficence, makes it incumbent upon nurses to involve patients in

---

BOX 19.2 WhistleBlowing: Important Considerations for Nurses

- If you identify a situation of unsafe, illegal, or unethical practice, document instances that give you concern, including dates, times, and outcomes of unsafe or inappropriate care. Hold off on final judgment until you have sufficient documentation to establish wrongdoing. Keep copies of all documentation in a secure location.
- Seek input and guidance from others outside of the situation to give you an objective perspective, such as trusted colleagues, those with different perspectives, chaplains, and those who are knowledgeable about your professional and legal responsibilities.
- Engage in personal reflection and consultation with others to determine whether you are ready, both personally and professionally, to act.
- Before acting, consult a lawyer and your state nurses association for information about whistleblower legislation in your state, guidance regarding the whistleblower process, and guidance regarding how best to document your concerns.
- Follow your institution's established policies, procedures, and chain of command to the letter before contacting an outside agency. Document all interactions related to the situation of concern, including interactions with those to whom you are reporting the situation, keeping copies for your personal file.
- Be professional when dealing with those in management, remain calm, and refrain from making it personal. Keep documentation and interactions factual and

objective, and do not become upset or lose your temper, even if others try to provoke you. Administrators with integrity should act on your concerns quickly. Seek guidance from legal counsel or your state nurses association regarding how long it is reasonable to wait for results.
- If you are continuing to work in situations that are unsafe, submit "assignment despite objection" forms to the appropriate persons in your organization.
- Blowing the whistle is a very serious matter and should never be done frivolously. Make sure you have the facts straight and have legal, professional, and personal support before acting.
- Be aware that in a whistleblower situation, you are not protected from retaliation by your employer until you blow the whistle. Also groups such as The Joint Commission and the National Committee for Quality Assurance do not provide protection even if they are made aware of the situation.
- If you decide to blow the whistle and contact an outside agency, report your concern to the national and/or state agency that regulates the organization for which you work. If criminal activity is involved, you need to report to law enforcement agencies as well. Always send all documents via certified mail with a return receipt, being sure to keep a copy for your files. Seek advice from legal counsel and your professional organization before considering contacting other agencies such as media.

(Data from American Nurses Association. (n.d.). *Things to know about whistleblowing.* https://www.nursingworld.org/practice-policy/workforce/things-to-know-about-whistle-blowing/ and Tressman, 2000).

making decisions about their health and care. Some patients have both the desire and skills to take charge of their life, some have desire but need to improve their skills, and others have limitations in ability and desire. Negotiating within a system that has traditionally placed decision-making authority and power primarily within the hands of physicians requires skill, support, and a strong sense of personal empowerment. Factors discussed above regarding personal empowerment for nurses apply to patients as well. Patient empowerment is both a process and outcome in which nurses have an active role.

Speaking of empowering another suggests that power is a commodity given by one person to another. Such a view of empowerment strips patients of their ability to choose. Empowerment as reflected in codes of nursing ethics and described in nursing literature is a dynamic, interactive, and reciprocal process that is an inherent facet of the nurse–patient caring relationship (ANA, 2015a; CNA, 2017; ICN, 2021; Akpotor & Johnson, 2018; Jerofke et al., 2014; McCarthy & Freeman, 2008; Nieuwboer et al., 2017; Watson, 2018). Facilitating the empowerment process requires a paradigm shift away from the attitude that healthcare providers know what is best for the patient to recognizing and accepting that patients are essentially responsible for their own health. Most patients have the ability to discern what they need, make decisions, and direct their own destinies. To make appropriate decisions, however, patients may need information, resources, encouragement, and support. An important consideration in facilitating empowerment with patients is to understand that empowerment is contextual and the sense of control over one's health and healthcare decisions may vary in different cultures and situations. As you recall from previous discussions of cultural considerations regarding patient decision making, family and even the wider community may need to be involved.

Nurses Attitudes, Knowledge, and Skills That Facilitate Empowerment

Empowerment is a social process arising from reciprocal interactions among people through which the ability to meet needs, solve problems, and mobilize resources is recognized and enhanced (East & Roll, 2015; Gibson, 1991; Johnsen et al., 2017; McCarthy & Freeman, 2008; Moran et al., 2017). As a process of assisting people in asserting control over the factors that affect their health, empowerment links autonomy with accountability in a way that promotes greater access to needed resources (Gibson, 1991; McCarthy & Freeman, 2008; Nieuwboer et al., 2017; Rohatinsky et al., 2017). Attitudes, knowledge, and skills basic to facilitating the empowerment process with patients, families, and communities are embedded in codes of nursing ethics. Readers are encouraged to identify specific sections of these codes that speak to the attitudes, knowledge, and skills discussed in the following sections.

Collaboration, Respect, and Mutual Decision Making

A view of the nurse as a partner, facilitator, and resource rather than merely one who provides services for patients is basic to facilitating empowerment with patients (Akpotor & Johnson, 2018; Jerofke et al., 2014; Laschinger et al., 2010). Nurses must learn to surrender their need for control, developing instead attitudes of collaboration and mutual participation in decision making. This requires self-reflection on the part of the nurse, through which the nurse confronts personal values and the subtle—and not so subtle—benefits gained from being in a position of power. It is essential that nurses make a commitment to being with patients as they struggle with their questions and issues and seek meaning in the process. Relinquishing control also means that nurses need to accept decisions made by patients and families, even when they are different from what the nurse might do or suggest. Respect for persons, which includes valuing others and mutual trust, is key (Akpotor & Johnson, 2018; Ho et al., 2010; Jerofke et al., 2014; Laschinger et al., 2010; Rohatinsky et al., 2017).

Information presented throughout this book provides a foundation for facilitating the empowerment process. Attention to ethical principles and processes of decision-making fosters empowerment (Fig. 19.2). Awareness of the development of values and their impact on choices allows nurses to clarify their own perspectives so as to foster integrity and avoid imposing personal values on others. Knowledge of social, cultural, political, economic, and other forces affecting a person's options and health choices is essential.

Knowledge, Skills, and Resources

As already noted, empowerment is an interactive process. Attitudes and skills that foster patient empowerment flow from basic elements of holistic nursing practice. As in all areas of nursing, effective communication is necessary for facilitating empowerment. The ability to listen with our whole being and to trust intuitive as well as intellectual understandings is important. Reflective listening allows us to help people recognize their own strengths, abilities, and personal power. Active listening also helps people develop awareness of root causes of problems and determine their readiness to act for change. When it

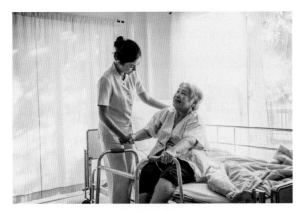

Fig. 19.2 The Nurse Supports the Patient in Reaching Her Goal to Become More Mobile. (©iStock.com/Jcomp.)

seems patients are hesitant about being involved in setting goals and actively participating in decision making, nurses can provide interventions in a style of empowerment rather than of control (Akpotor & Johnson, 2018; Johnsen et al., 2017; Ho et al., 2010; Watson, 2018). This means approaching patients with an attitude of trust in their ability—at some place within themselves—to know what they need, as well as incorporating behaviors, such as offering choices about aspects of care over which they can have control. As noted above, approaching patients as equal partners is a key factor in patient empowerment. Skillful collaboration and negotiation that incorporate power sharing and mutually beneficial interactions facilitate empowerment. Relinquishing professional power returns power to the patient (Box 19.3).

Having the opportunities and resources necessary for understanding and changing our world is part of the empowerment process. Nurses must have knowledge of factors affecting a patient's health and healthcare decisions to help provide or share the necessary resources. Such knowledge includes awareness of patient and family values and decision-making style; cultural context; social determinants of health, health disparities, social,

---

BOX 19.3 Nurse Attitudes and Skills That Enable Patient Empowerment

Attitudes of the Nurse
- Nonjudgmental
- Respect
- Empathy
- Caring
- Viewing patients as having strengths and abilities

Skills of the Nurse
Communication, including:
- Attentive, intentional listening, including therapeutic use of silence
- Ability to listen for and share stories
- Enabling responsive, reflective, respectful, and trusting interactions

Therapeutic nurse–patient relationship, including:
- Caring presence—the ability to be with patients as well as do for them
- Patient-centered focus
- Collaboration, including balance of control and shared power
- Cultural congruence

Assessment and intervention processes, including the include ability to:

- Assess patient readiness to make decisions or changes
- Promote patient self-awareness and self-determination
- Support/build patient self-esteem
- Focus on patient strengths and abilities
- Prioritize patient needs with patient
- Identify goals with patient
- Support patient's ability to achieve goals
- Encourage patient to actively participate in care (consensus decision making)
- Support choices—enabling and motivating patients to take needed steps
- Give autonomy and flexibility in decision making
- Provide emotional support and build on prior knowledge and skills
- Provide pertinent information, including knowledge of resources and support
- Provide access to resources and assist patient in developing collaborative relationships with other providers and support people
- Remove barriers where possible.

political, and economic influences on our options; and healthcare system constraints. Nurses recognize that individual responsibility for health is necessarily tempered by cultural, social, familial, and environmental factors. In addition to addressing individual patient concerns, nurses need to focus health promotion efforts on the macro-social level, attending to conditions that control, influence, and produce health or illness in people (DiGregorio, 2023; East & Roll, 2015; Moran et al., 2017; Murdaugh et al. 2018; Rohatinsky et al. 2017). Efforts as individuals, within professional organizations, and within communities, aimed at providing access to healthcare for all, provide a broad base of support for empowerment.

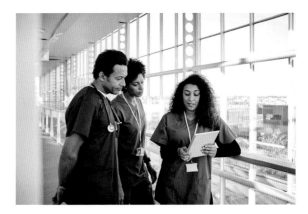

Fig. 19.3 Empowered Nurses Foster Healthy and Collaborative Work Environments. (©iStock.com/Dean Mitchell.)

Supporting Patient Capacity for Decision Making

As noted previously, a belief that patients have the right and ability to make choices regarding their health, and other areas of their lives, is basic to empowerment. Patients need to be given opportunities for choice regarding small as well as large decisions. This means that there needs to be participatory decision making, involving collaboration and negotiation, in all areas of healthcare. For example, involving patients in making decisions about when they will bathe, what foods to include in their diet, or when to take their medications is as important to empowerment as their participation in decision making regarding life-support measures. Because of social, environmental, and other factors, some people have had limited opportunities for making choices and may need education, practice, and nurturing in this area. Offering options and developing strategies to enhance the patient's ability to set and reach goals are important parts of the nursing role (Fig. 19.3). Support is an important part of the encouraging process.

The ability to make decisions regarding our lives and destinies requires a basic level of cognitive functioning and a sense of control over life and change processes. Empowerment originates in self-esteem; is developed through love, a sense of connectedness, responsibility, and opportunities for choice; and is supported through perceived meaning and hope in life (Akpotor & Johnson, 2018; Johnsen et al., 2017; McCarthy & Freeman, 2008; Moran et al., 2017; Watson, 2018).

Facilitating Self-Awareness

Helping patients know who they are facilitates empowerment. Because empowerment flows from a deep understanding of self, the process of self-discovery enables patients to decide what they want to do based on an appreciation of who they are. Supporting patient empowerment may require facilitating a patient's self-awareness on many levels, such as identifying personal values, the sources of these values, where and with whom they feel connected, and where and how they experience control in life. Utilizing the decision-making process discussed in Chapter 7 can facilitate empowerment with patients as they make health choices and deal with difficult decisions.

Support can take many forms. Nurses provide support by determining what patients identify as empowering to them and by encouraging these choices, behaviors, or attitudes. Caring relationships, in which experiences are shared and patients are accepted for who they are, offer support. Having at least one other person who supports a choice made or a stance that a person takes enhances the likelihood that the person will follow through on the decision.

Identifying Barriers to Empowerment

Empowerment involves a willingness to take risks and move beyond that which is known, and perhaps comfortable, to the unknown. It often requires a change in self-perception, developing a different vision of who we are. This can stimulate anxiety and fear. Nurses need to recognize such barriers and appreciate that not everyone wants to or knows how to take the risks and assume the responsibility that empowerment demands. Assisting others in identifying barriers to feeling empowered within themselves and within the system may be an important step in facilitating empowerment. For example, social, cultural, economic, or political factors can present barriers such as limited resources, control of knowledge about options, locking people into traditional roles and expectations, social labeling that stereotypes and devalues certain people or behaviors, and restriction of access to resources. Healthcare provider attitudes and sociocultural role expectations within the healthcare system have fostered reliance on healthcare providers to determine what patients need for health, contributing to patient lack of knowledge of resources or strategies that promote empowerment, dependency, apathy, and mistrust. (Akpotor & Johnson, 2018; Johnsen et al., 2017; Moran et al., 2017). Inability or unwillingness to share decision-making power with patients on the part of healthcare providers affects patient empowerment as well. Additionally, honoring patient decisions may be very threatening to nurses who do not appreciate that patients know what they need.

Developing Skills That Support Empowerment

Nurses can develop skills that support the empowerment of patients in many ways. The emerging nursing specialty of *nurse coaching* is a focused process that incorporates attitudes and skills essential to promoting empowerment with patients (Avino et al., 2022; Southard et al., 2021). Nurse coaches partner with patients in a creative process that assists patients in identifying health goals and focusing on their strengths and potentials in achieving these goals. Appreciating that patients are the experts on their own needs and choices, nurse coaches provide guidance and resources that support them in achieving their goals. The purposeful and structured interactions of the coaching process focus on increasing patient self-awareness, identifying where change is needed, developing action plans, and providing resources focused on particular outcomes. The overall focus is to support and facilitate patient growth, healing, and well-being. The nurse coaching process involves six simultaneously occurring steps that mirror the nursing process (Box 19.4). These steps outline a process similar to that which nurses would follow as they promote empowerment with patients.

Considering options and making choices implies having both knowledge and availability of needed resources. Facilitating empowerment may require nurses to provide, or help patients discover how to access, resources. In some instances, this may mean becoming politically and socially active regarding healthcare issues affecting vulnerable populations. Nurses need to develop strategies that enhance a patient's ability to acquire necessary knowledge. This may mean working with patients

---

> **BOX 19.4 Steps of the Nurse Coaching Process**
>
> 1. Establish the relationship and assess the client's readiness for change (Assessment)
> 2. Identify client concerns, strengths, opportunities, and issues (Diagnosis)
> 3. Assist client in establishing goals that focus on the desired change (Set outcome goals)
> 4. Structure the coaching interaction focused on attaining goals (Plan)
> 5. Support client's plan for reaching their goals (Implementation)
> 6. Assist clients in determining the extent to which their goals were achieved (Evaluation)

(Data from Southard, M. E., Bark, L., Dossey, B. M., & Schaub, B. G. (2021). *The art and science of nurse coachwing: The provider's guide to coaching scope and competencies* (2nd ed.) American Nurses Association; Avino, K. M., McElligot, D., Dossey, B. M., Luck, S. Nurse coaching. In: M. A. Blaszko Helming, D. A. Shields, K. M. Avino, W. E. Rosa (Eds.), *Dossey & Keegan's holistic nursing: A handbook for practice* (8th ed., pp. 389–400). Jones & Bartlett Learning)

> **ASK YOURSELF**
>
> ***Outcomes of Patient Empowerment***
>
> Upholding the view that patients know what they need opens nurses to the probability that some patients will make decisions that are not consistent with what the nurse or other health team members think is best. Such decisions may have a relatively minor impact on a patient's or family's health and well-being or may be judged to have potentially serious outcomes for the patient or family.
>
> - What factors need to be considered when dealing with decisions involving differing values between patients and nurses?
> - Give examples of situations in which patient empowerment might pose an ethical dilemma for you.
> - If you feel a patient is making an unwise decision, how would you respond?
> - Discuss your views regarding any limits or constraints on patient empowerment.

---

or communities to identify both health concerns and culturally relevant approaches to dealing with these concerns. Nurses foster empowerment by promoting processes that encourage mutually respectful exchange of ideas and analysis of concerns and potential solutions. Success in achieving goals must be defined from the perspective of the patient or community.

Determining whether a person functions primarily from a sense of **internal** or **external locus of control** can be useful. Locus of control refers to beliefs about the ability to control events in our lives. People who believe that they are able to influence or control things that happen to them are considered to have an internal locus of control. On the other hand, people who feel that forces outside of themselves direct or rule their lives—whether these be generalized forces such as fate or other persons who are perceived as more powerful—are considered to have an external locus of control. Persons who are internally motivated are more likely to perceive themselves as having the power to make choices and control their lives and to be motivated to make necessary changes. Those who are externally motivated tend to be more fatalistic, expecting their lives to be controlled by powerful others,

ASK YOURSELF

How Does Locus of Control Affect Empowerment?

- Reflect on how you have thought through significant decisions in your life. Do you consider that you are more internally or more externally motivated? Give specific examples to support your self-assessment.
- In working with patients or collaborating with classmates, what would you consider indications of internal and external locus of control?
- How would your approach to facilitating empowerment be different with persons who exhibit an internal locus of control compared with those with an external locus of control?

CASE PRESENTATION

Fostering Patient Empowerment

Kalinda, a 42-year-old patient, is being seen to initiate treatment for her newly diagnosed type 2 diabetes. When her nurse, Trey, takes her to the examination room, he notices that she looks worried and seems upset. When he weighs her, she says, "Oh no" and looks distressed. After taking her vital signs, he sits down and reflects to her, "You seem worried today. I wonder if there is something bothering you." Kalinda tells Trey she is upset because she has gained so much weight and now she has diabetes and has to take medicine. She says her grandmother had diabetes and had problems

with her eyes and her circulation and was in the hospital a lot. Kalinda says she needs to be healthy to take care of her two children and does not want to end up like her grandmother. She tells Trey she read on the Internet that if she lost some weight she might not have high blood sugar, adding that she had tried diets in the past but found it hard to stick to them. Trey acknowledges her concerns about having diabetes and her frustrations with past efforts to lose weight. He also notes that even though she has not lost the weight she would like in the past, she at least made the effort. He reflects that her desire to take better care of herself so that she is there for her children is a positive motivation. He then asks if she would like him to work with her in designing a diet and exercise program. Kalinda agrees, and they develop a plan that includes her desired outcome of a 40-pound weight loss and intermediate goals of losing 5 pounds each month. Trey discusses her eating habits with her, and they review information he gives her about healthy meal planning that supports her weight loss goal. They discuss the importance of regular physical exercise and incorporate activities into the plan that she feels she can do on a daily basis. Trey gives her information about some resources in the community, such as the diabetes cooking class at the community center and some walking groups, yoga, and exercise classes. Together they decide that she will make an appointment for three weeks to review how things are going with her plan and make adjustments if needed.

Think About It
Empowerment: A Collaborative Process

- In what way does Kalinda indicate that she feels a lack of power in this situation? What is the particular issue of concern?
- What attitudes and skills that foster patient empowerment does Trey demonstrate? Give specific examples of all those you identify.
- Do you think Kalinda indicates a readiness for change? How does Trey address this?
- In what ways are Kalinda's strengths identified and included in this process? Give specific examples.
- How does Trey incorporate collaboration into his interactions with Kalinda?
- If you were Trey, how would you approach the process of assisting Kalinda in identifying goals and designing an action plan? In what ways do you think you could support her in moving toward her goals?
- If you were Kalinda, what do you think you would need to support you in moving toward your goal? What do you think you would expect from Trey?

and less likely to enact personal power (Brincks et al., 2010; Moran et al., 2017).

EMBRACING NURSING'S VISION OF NURSING

Nurses need to be willing to struggle with difficult questions and arrive at decisions that flow from their internal values and perspective and are congruent with codes of nursing ethics, rather than looking for the right answer from an external source. Empowerment implies accountability for our own choices and actions. Jameton (1984) reflects that people pretend they are forced to do things when they are not. He gives the example of a nurse who instructs a patient to take medication because the physician ordered it, noting that both patient and nurse pretend that they must act because of the physician's order, although each could make another choice. Reflecting that nurses who choose to work in systems such as hospitals and other organizations are accountable for their actions despite the existence of systemic problems affecting healthcare, Jameton (1984) writes,

If one fails to resist exploitation, incompetence, and corrupt practices, one becomes responsible for them. If one resists them, one enters into conflict with conventional conceptions of behavior for employees and thereby risks reprisals. One has to choose between complicity and self-sacrifice, or enter the uncomfortable middle ground of irony. Ethics does not give a clear answer as to which one must choose. Instead, one is free to move in the direction of the kind of world one personally desires to create.

(p. 289)

We must decide whether we prefer a world in which we are empowered in the professional arena or one in which we are controlled by others. The choices we make influence the outcome.

Empowerment within the profession requires a clear vision of nursing. As nurses, we need to define nursing according to our own vision, rather than accepting definitions imposed by the dominant groups in healthcare such as physicians and institutions. When nurses draw pictures of their vision of nursing, what emerges are images of caring, light, comfort, and love. These images reflect the heart of the vision of nursing within nurses. Making choices based on the vision and values of the profession fosters congruence between nursing's knowing and doing, which strengthens personal and professional effectiveness. In contrast, nurses who work in situations in which they feel a lack of synchronicity with their values often experience burnout, become nasty, take on attributes and values of the dominant group, and look for someone to blame (behaviors reflective of oppressed groups). Remaining in a victim role involves a choice to give away our power and allow someone else to define our reality. Defining nursing according to nursing's own vision is an act of empowerment.

Empowerment involves risk and commitment and requires both courage and compassion. Curtin (1996) illustrates this through a parable about a baby eagle that fell from its nest and broke its wing. The eagle was found by a mountain climber who took it home, nursed the wing, and put the eagle in with the chickens. Not knowing what to eat, the baby eagle followed the chickens pecking the feed on the ground. As he grew larger and stronger, he continued to peck like the chickens, forgetting that he was an eagle. A friend of the climber noted that the eagle should be flying in the mountains with other eagles. The climber responded that the eagle had a good situation with free food and a warm coop and would not fly away even if he could. The friend offered to teach the eagle to fly and took him to the barn roof, told him he was an eagle, and explained that he could fly freely. The eagle heard this but remembered what happened the last time he tried to fly. Seeing the chickens below, he remembered the food and shelter and would not fly. The friend decided to take the eagle to the mountains, taught him how to flap his wings, encouraged his efforts, and told him repeatedly that he was an eagle and could fly. Finally, the eagle took the risk and flew, delighting in the experience; but as he flew over the chicken yard, he remembered that he was hungry and returned to peck for food with the chickens. The friend disparaged the eagle for continuing to act like a chicken when he could be free. A new plan was devised. The friend crept up to the eagle, put a hood over his head, and carried him to an area where there were other eagles. The eagle saw their nests and watched them hunt, eat, and fly. The friend showed the eagle the beauty of his homeland, encouraged him to hunt and fly, and reminded him that he was an EAGLE (Fig. 19.4). After several days the eagle got the idea, and when the friend took him to the top of the highest mountain, he took off and soared high, never looking back, and never eating

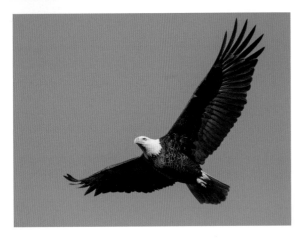

Fig. 19.4 Empowered to Fly. (©iStock.com/Jganz.)

chicken feed again, because he was an EAGLE, and he knew it (summarized from Curtin, 1996).

Curtin relates the insights of this parable to empowerment for nurses. The story demonstrates that empowerment is not easy for either the one trying to empower or the one being empowered but that it is important not to give up. We must also realize that empowerment costs money, time, and effort.

"It (empowerment) isn't easy." Telling the eagle to fly wasn't enough. It isn't easy. Changing the eagle's environment and even teaching him to fly wasn't enough. It isn't easy. You have to start at the beginning and re-create an attitude in a new environment. It's tough on the eagle too. The eagle was frightened: he had been hurt. The eagle knew the old, safe ways of pecking and free grain and warm nest. And he could have that with no effort! It was hard for the eagle to believe that the easy way sooner or later would destroy him. And it was really tough on the eagle when (the friend) blamed him for being what he'd been taught to be all his life.

(Curtin, 1996, p. 210)

Curtin notes that neither freedom nor risk is easy and that they are not for everyone. It is important, however, not to "blame the chickens for what they are. It's unfair—and it's a waste of time. But never give up on the eagles. They can fly—and they will" (p. 210). Empowerment for nurses means recognizing who we are, knowing

that—like the eagle—we have the ability, the freedom, and the responsibility to fly!

SUMMARY

Empowerment is a multifaceted concept. Awareness of attitudes about nursing's role in healthcare and factors that shape these attitudes enables nurses to identify more effectively that which supports or diminishes both personal and professional empowerment. Attentiveness to personal empowerment, which includes integrity, accountability, and moral courage, is foundational for addressing empowerment issues with patients and within the profession. Patient empowerment, an important element of nursing care, is grounded in nursing's advocacy role and derives from an appreciation that patients have the ability to discern their needs and make decisions about their lives and health. No one can empower another. Facilitating empowerment requires that nurses learn to relinquish power and embrace the patient as an equal partner. Nurses can facilitate the inner process of empowerment when knowledge and resources are offered within an environment of mutual respect and support, by working directly with patients, and through addressing social, political, and environmental factors affecting empowerment of individuals and communities. In the midst of an ever-changing and challenging healthcare environment in which issues of power and control continue to affect nursing practice and patient care, it is essential that all nursing practice be aligned with and grounded in directives provided in professional codes of nursing ethics and standards of care.

CHAPTER HIGHLIGHTS

- Mindset regarding healthcare influences how nurses identify and respond to ethical issues and dilemmas in practice settings.
- Nursing's contemporary self-perception reflects the legal metaphor of patient advocate rather than the military metaphor of loyal soldier. Each of these metaphors implies different ethical imperatives for nursing.
- Current nursing codes and standards of practice reflect ethical imperatives that flow from the advocacy metaphor and ground professional empowerment.

- Patient empowerment relates to ethical principles and flows from nursing's focus on patient advocacy.
- Empowerment, which is both process and outcome, derives from a feminine perspective of power to or power with, reflecting a supportive partnership based on mutual love and respect that enables people to change situations given the necessary resources, knowledge, skills, and opportunities. Empowerment comes from within a person and involves choice; we cannot empower another.
- Facilitating patient empowerment requires recognition and acceptance that patients have the ability to discern what they need, to make decisions, and to direct their own destinies.
- The ability to deal with healthcare issues and dilemmas in a principled way derives from personal and professional empowerment and requires attentiveness to intrapersonal, interpersonal, and systems issues.
- Personal empowerment requires self-awareness and is characterized by maintaining personal integrity in the midst of a loving response to the choices of others. Self-concept and sense of power in a nurse's personal life affect nursing care and a nurse's ability to enable empowerment in others.
- Empowerment is interactive and requires of nurses self-knowledge of personal values and needs for control, mutual trust and respect, effective communication and reflective listening skills, and a willingness to accept patient decisions, regardless of whether the nurse thinks they are best.
- Fostering patient empowerment requires knowledge of social, political, cultural, economic, and environmental factors affecting a person's options and health choices and may involve addressing health promotion efforts on the macro-social level.
- Empowerment is fostered through self-discovery; enhanced self-esteem; a sense of connectedness; support; opportunities for choice; and having needed resources, knowledge, and skills.
- Empowerment strategies that mesh with a person's or a community's sociocultural context are more effective.
- Moral courage is necessary for nurses to speak up about situations of incivility; bullying; workplace violence; and unsafe, unethical, or illegal practice. Nurses need to be aware of factors to consider in addressing these concerns and appropriate

policies and procedures to follow when reporting the situation.
- Defining nursing according to nursing's own vision is an act of empowerment that implies accountability for our own choices and actions, with awareness that each choice helps create the kind of world and environment within which nurses must practice.

DISCUSSION QUESTIONS AND ACTIVITIES

1. Reflect on the attributes of empowerment noted in Table 19.1. Working with a partner, list five attributes that you feel are evident in your life and five attributes you see in your partner. Share with each other, giving specific examples of why you chose these attributes. Incorporate into the discussion examples of where in your life you feel most personally empowered and the circumstances surrounding your feelings of empowerment.
2. Describe a situation in which you took ownership for your own thoughts, feelings, or actions. Describe a time when you found yourself blaming others or assuming a victim stance. Describe a situation in which you felt you acted with moral courage. Discuss with classmates factors prompting each stance and how you felt in each situation.
3. Describe a patient or family with whom you have worked who exhibited empowerment. Give specific examples of evidence of empowerment from your perspective. What would indicate to you that a patient might not be ready to be empowered?
4. With two other classmates, role-play the situation in the case presentation *Fostering Patient Empowerment*. Take turns being the patient, nurse, and observer (whose role is to give feedback). Integrate various attitudes and skills noted in Box 19.3 into your interactions. Use elements of the coaching process noted in Box 19.4 to guide the process of identifying readiness for change, strengths, concerns, goals, the plan for achieving goals, and the process of evaluation. Be specific and realistic. Discuss how you feel when in the role of nurse and of patient. Include discussion of the relationship between patient empowerment and principled behavior in nursing.
5. What aspects of empowerment do you think are most important in nursing practice settings? Which

are the most challenging? Support your perspective. Include a discussion of factors within the healthcare system that inhibit nurse or patient empowerment.

6. Explore issues related to whistleblowing in your state or province, including the status of whistleblower legislation. Discuss with classmates specific situations in which a nurse's ethical responsibility directs the nurse to speak up about unjust, unprofessional, or unethical practices.

7. Discuss with another classmate the case presentation *Confronting Destructive Workplace Behaviors* and share your responses to the *Think About It – The Challenge of Speaking Up*. Work together to decide on a course of action you think you would take in this situation. How would nursing codes of ethics and specific position statements guide and support your proposed actions?

8. Interview practicing nurses regarding personal and professional power, including situations in which they feel empowered to make decisions and those in which they have experienced dilemmas around the issue of power. Discuss how they derive authority to make decisions and how they exhibit ethical empowerment.

9. Illustrate your vision of nursing in words or as a drawing. Share with classmates and develop strategies for making nursing's self-vision better known to others. Implement one strategy.

10. Re-read the professional codes of nursing ethics pertinent to you and make a list of each section and sub-section that reflects attributes of empowerment, and attitudes and skills that enable empowerment of nurses and patients.

REFERENCES

Akpotor, M. E., & Johnson, E. A. (2018). Client empowerment: A concept analysis. *International Journal of Caring Science, 11*(2), 743–750.

American Nurses Association (ANA). (2015a). *Code of ethics for nurses with interpretative statements.* American Nurses Association.

ANA. (2015b). *Incivility, bullying, and workplace violence. (Position statement).* https://www.nursingworld.org/practice-policy/nursing-excellence/official-position-statements/id/incivility-bullying-and-workplace-violence/.

Avino, K. M., McElligot, D., Dossey, B. M., & Luck, S. (2022). Nurse Coaching In M. A. Blaszko Helming., D. A. Shields, K. M. Avino, & W. E. Rosa (Eds.), *Dossey & Keegan's holistic nursing: A handbook for practice* (8th ed., pp. 389–400). Jones & Bartlett Learning.

Brincks, A. M., Feaster, D. J., Burns, M. J., & Mitrani, V. B. (2010). The influence of health locus of control on the patient-provider relationship. *Psychology, Health & Medicine, 15*(6), 720–728.

Bolton, B., & Brookings, J. (1998). Development of a measure of intrapersonal empowerment. *Rehabilitation Psychology, 43*(2), 131–142.

Cameron, A. (1981). *Daughters of copper woman.* Press Gang.

CNA. (2017). *Code of ethics for registered nurses.* https://cdn1.nscn.ca/sites/default/files/documents/resources/code-of-ethics-for-registered-nurses.pdf#:~:text=The%20Canadian%20Nurses%20Association%20%28CNA%29%20Code%20of%20Ethics,receiving%20care.%20The%20Codeis%20both%20aspirational%20and%20regulatory.

CNA. (2019). *Joint position statement: Patient safety.* https://hl-prod-ca-oc-download.s3-ca-central-1.amazonaws.com/CNA/2f975e7e-4a40-45ca-863c-5ebf0a138d5e/UploadedImages/documents/2019_Joint_Position_Statement__Patient_Safety.pdf.

Chinn, P. (2013). *Peace and power: Building communities for the future* (8th ed.). Jones & Bartlett.

Curtin, L. (1996). *Nursing into the 21st century.* Springhouse.

Curtin, L. (2013). When nurses speak up. *American Nurse Today, 8*(10). https://www.americannursetoday.com/when-nurses-speak-up-they-pay-a-price/.

DiGregorio, S. (2023). *Taking care: The story of nursing and its power to change our world.* Harper-Collins.

East, J. F., & Roll, S. J. (2015). Women, poverty, and trauma: An empowerment practice approach. *Social Work, 60*(4), 279–286.

Edmonson, C. (2010). Moral courage and the nurse leader. *Online Journal of Issues in Nursing, 15*(3) Item Number: 2010889995.

Ellis-Stoll, C. C., & Popkess-Vawter, S. (1998). A concept analysis on the process of empowerment. *Advances in Nursing Science, 21*(2), 62–68.

Fitzgerald, E. M., Myers, J. G., & Clark, P. (2017). Nurses need not be guilty bystanders: Caring for vulnerable immigrant populations. *The Online Journal of Issues in Nursing, 22*(1). http://ojin.nursingworld.org/MainMenuCategories/ANAMarketplace/ANAPeriodicals/OJIN/TableofContents/Vol-22-2017/No1-Jan-2017/Articles-Previous-Topics/Nurses-Need-Not-Be-Guilty-Bystanders.html.

Fletcher, K. (2007). Image: Changing how women nurses think about themselves. Literature review. *Journal of Advanced Nursing, 58*(30), 207–215.

Fowler, D. M. (2015). *Guide to the code of ethics for nurses with interpretive statements.* American Nurses Association.

Friend, M. L., & Sieloff, C. L. (2018). Empowerment in nursing literature: An update and look to the future. *Nursing Science Quarterly, 31*(4), 355–361.

Fulton, Y. (1997). Nurses' views on empowerment: A critical social theory perspective. *Journal of Advanced Nursing, 26,* 529–536.

Gibson, C. H. (1991). A concept analysis of empowerment. *Journal of Advanced Nursing, 16,* 354–361.

Gordon, S. (2010). Nursing and health policy perspectives. *International Nursing Review, 57*(4), 403–404.

Grinberg, K., & Sela, Y. (2022). Perceptions of the image of the nursing profession and its relationship with quality of care. *BMC Nursing, 21*(57). https://doi.org/10.1186/s12912-022-00830-4.

Gurka, A. M. (1995). Transformational leadership: Qualities and strategies for the CNS. *Clinical Nurse Specialist, 9,* 169–174.

Hartrick, G., & Schreiber, R. (1998). Imaging ourselves: Nurses' metaphors of practice. *Journal of Holistic Nursing, 16*(4), 420–434.

Hewitt-Taylor, J. (2004). Challenging the balance of power: Patient empowerment. *Nursing Standard, 11*(18), 33–37.

Ho, A. Y. K., Berggren, I., & Dahlborg-Lyckhage, E. (2010). Diabetes empowerment related to Pender's health promotion model: A meta-synthesis. *Nursing & Health Sciences, 12,* 259–267.

ICN. (2012). *Position statement: Patient safety.* https://www.icn.ch/sites/default/files/inline-files/D05_Patient_Safety.pdf.

ICN. (2021). *The ICN code of ethics for nurses.* https://www.icn.ch/system/files/2021-10/ICN_Code-of-Ethics_EN_Web_0.pdf.

Jackson, D., Peters, K., Andrew, S., Edenborough, M., Halcomb, E., Luck, L., … Wilkes, L. (2010). Understanding whistleblowing: Qualitative insights from nurse whistleblowers. *Journal of Advanced Nursing, 66*(10), 2194–2201.

Jameton, A. (1984). *Nursing practice: The ethical issues.* Prentice-Hall.

Jerofke, T., Weiss, M., & Yakusheva, O. (2014). Patient perceptions of patient-empowering nurse behaviors, patient activation and functional health status in postsurgical patients with life-threatening long-term illness. *Journal of Advanced Nursing, 70*(6), 1310–1322.

Johnsen, A. T., Eskildsen, N. B., Thomsen, T. G., Grønvold, M., Ross, L., & Jørgensen, C. R. (2017). Conceptualizing patient empowerment in cancer follow-up by combining therapy and qualitative data. *Acta Oncologica, 56*(2), 232–238.

Jones, P. S., O'Toole, M. T., Hoa, N., Chau, T. T., & Muc, P. D. (2000). Empowerment of nursing as a socially significant profession in Vietnam. *Journal of Nursing Scholarship, 32*(3), 317–321.

Kritek, P. B. (2017). Reflections on moral courage. *Nursing Science Quarterly, 30*(3), 218–222.

Kuokkanen, L., & Leino-Kilpi, H. (2000). Power and empowerment in nursing: Three theoretical approaches. *Journal of Advanced Nursing, 31*(1), 235–241.

Lachman, V. D. (2007). Whistleblowers: Trouble makers or virtuous nurses? *MEDSURG Nursing, 17*(2), 126–134.

Lachman, V. D. (2008). Whistleblowing: Role of organizational culture in prevention and management. *Dermatology Nursing, 20*(5), 394–396.

Laschinger, H. K. S., Leiter, M., Day, A., & Gilin, D. (2009). Workplace environment, incivility, and burnout: Impact on staff nurse recruitment and retention outcomes. *Journal of Nurse Management, 17,* 302–311.

Laschinger, H. K. S., Wong, C., & Greco, P. (2006). The impact of staff nurse empowerment on person-job fit and work engagement burnout. *Nursing Administration Quarterly, 30*(4), 358–367.

Laschinger, H. K. S., Gilbert, S., Smith, L. M., & Leslie, K. (2010). Towards a comprehensive theory of nurse/patient empowerment: Applying Kanter's empowerment theory to patient care. *Journal of Nursing Management, 18,* 4–13.

Laschinger, H. K. S., Wong, C. A., Cummings, G. G., & Grau, A. L. (2014). Resonant leadership and workplace empowerment: The value of positive organizational culture in reducing workplace incivility. *Nursing Economics, 32*(1), 5–15.

Leiter, M. P., & Laschinger, H. K. S. (2006). Relationships of work and practice environment to professional burnout: Testing a causal model. *Nursing Research, 55*(2), 137–146.

Liaschenko, J., & Peter, E. (2016). Fostering nurses' moral agency and moral identity: The importance of moral community. *Hastings Center Report, 46*(Suppl. 1), S18–S21. Nurses at the table: nursing, ethics, and health policy, special report. https://doi.org/10.1002/hast.626.

Linnen, D., & Rowley, A. (2014). Encouraging clinical nurse empowerment. *Nursing Management, 45,* 44–47. https://doi.org/10.1097/01.NUMA.0000442640.70829.d1.

Mannion, R., & Davies, H. T. (2015). Cultures of silence and cultures of voice: The role of whistleblowing in healthcare organisations. *International Journal of Health Policy Management, 4*(8), 503–505.

Mansbach, A., Kushnir, T., Ziedenberg, H., & Bachner, Y. G. (2014). Reporting misconduct of a coworker to protect a patient: A comparison between experienced nurses and nursing students. *The Scientific World Journal.* https://doi.org/10.1155/2014/413926. Article ID 413926, 6 pages.

Marturano, E., & Narva, A. (2023). Nursing ethics and shared governance model. *American Nurse Journal, 18*(4). https://doi.org/10.51256/ANJ042306.

Mathes, M. (2005). On nursing, moral autonomy, and moral responsibility. *MEDSURG Nursing, 14*(6), 395–398.

McCarthy, V., & Freeman, L. H. (2008). A multidisciplinary concept analysis of empowerment: Implications for nursing. *Journal of Theory Construction and Testing, 12*(2), 68–74.

Milton, C. L. (2009). Common metaphors in nursing ethics. *Nursing Science Quarterly, 22*(4), 318–322.

Moran, T. E., Gibbs, D. C., & Mernin, L. (2017). The empowerment model: Turning barriers into possibilities. *Palaestra, 31*(2), 19–26.

Murdaugh, C. L., Parsons, M. A., & Pender, N. J. (2018). *Health promotion in nursing practice* (8th ed.). Pearson.

Murray, J. S. (2010). Moral courage in healthcare: Acting ethically even in the presence of risk. *Online Journal of Issues in Nursing, 15*(3) Item Number: 2010889996.

Nieuwboer, C. C., Fukkink, R. G., & Hermanns, M. A. (2017). Analysing empowerment-oriented email consultation for parents: Development of the guiding the empowerment process model. *Child & Family Social Work, 22*, 61–71.

Ning, S., Zhong, H., Libo, W., & Qiujie, L. (2009). The impact of nurse empowerment on job satisfaction. *Journal of Advanced Nursing, 65*(12), 2642–2648.

O'Brien, J. L. (2011). Relationship among structural empowerment, psychological empowerment, and burnout in registered staff nurses working in outpatient dialysis centers. *Nephrology Nursing Journal, 38*(6), 475–481.

Purdy, N., Laschinger, J. H. S., Finegan, J., Kerr, M., & Olivera, F. (2010). Effects of work environments on nurse and patient outcomes. *Journal of Nursing Management, 18*, 901–913.

Rao, A. (2012). A contemporary construction of nurse empowerment. *Journal of Nursing Scholarship, 44*(4), 396–402.

Ray, S. L. (2006). Whistleblowing and organizational ethics. *Nursing Ethics, 13*(4), 438–445.

Rice, A. J. (2015). Using scholarship on whistleblowing to inform peer ethics reporting. *Professional Psychology: Research and Practice, 46*(4), 298–305.

Rodwell, C. M. (1996). An analysis of the concept of empowerment. *Journal of Advanced Nursing, 23*, 305–313.

Rohatinsky, N., Goodridge, D., Rogers, M. R., Nickel, D., & Linassi, G. (2017). Shifting the balance: conceptualising empowerment in individuals with spinal cord injury. *Health & Social Care in the Community, 25*(2), 769–779.

Ryles, S. M. (1999). A concept analysis of empowerment: Its relationship to mental health nursing. *Journal of Advanced Nursing, 29*(3), 600–607.

Sharoff, L. (2009). Expressiveness and creativeness: Metaphorical images of nursing. *Nursing Science Quarterly, 22*(4), 312–317.

Shearer, N. B. C., & Reed, P. G. (2004). Empowerment: Reformulation of a non-Rogerian concept. *Nursing Science Quarterly, 17*(3), 253–259.

Southard, M. E., Bark, L., Dossey, B. M., & Schaub, B. G. (2021). *The art and science of nurse coaching: The provider's guide to coaching scope and competencies* (2nd ed.). American Nurses Association.

Tengland, P. (2016). Behavior change or empowerment: On the ethics of health-promotion goals. *Health Care Annals, 24*, 24–46. https://doi.org/10.1007/s10728-013-0265-0.

ten Hoeve, Y., Jansen, G., & Roodbol, P. (2014). The nursing profession: Public image, self-concept, and professional identity. A discussion paper. *Journal of Advanced Nursing, 70*(2), 295–309.

Tressman, S. (2000). Speaking out: Two nurses tell their stories. *The American Nurse, 32*(4), 1–2, 22.

Watson, J. (2018). *Unitary caring science: Philosophy and praxis of nursing.* University of Colorado Press.

Williamson, K. M. (2007). Home health care nurse's perceptions of empowerment. *Journal of Community Health Nursing, 24*(3), 133–153.

20

The Empowered Nurse

The most common way for people to give up power is by thinking that they don't have any.
(Walker, n.d)

OBJECTIVES

After completing this chapter, the reader should be able to:

1. Define and discuss ethical competence.
2. Describe ways that nurses maintain ethical competence.
3. Identify and discuss exemplars of empowered nurses.
4. Discuss how codes of nursing ethics inform the development and maintenance of both personal and professional empowerment.

INTRODUCTION

As noted in the preface, we believe that the ethically prepared and competent nurse is an empowered nurse. This belief has grounded the content of this text since the first edition was published in 1998 and continues to provide a framework for this current edition. This final chapter includes a brief discussion of the importance of developing and maintaining ethical competence, offers selected resources and suggestions for maintaining ethical competence, and provides exemplars of empowered nurses who have made and continue to make a difference in nursing and healthcare. It is our hope that these exemplars will inspire you to step into your own power to make a difference.

DEVELOPING AND MAINTAINING ETHICAL COMPETENCE

Ethical competence is necessary for providing ethical nursing care. Nursing codes of ethics clearly state that providing ethically competent care in every nursing act and encounter is a nursing responsibility. This includes interactions with patients, families, coworkers, communities, and others. These codes reflect that "the nurse has authority, accountability, and responsibility for nursing practice; makes decisions; and takes actions consistent with the obligation to promote health and to provide optimal care" (ANA, 2015, Provision 4); that "these responsibilities apply to nurses' interactions with all persons who have healthcare needs or are receiving care as well as with students, colleagues and other healthcare providers" (CNA, 2017, Part I); and that "these responsibilities and professional accountabilities... apply to nurses in all settings, roles and domains of practice" (ICN, 2021, p. 2). The directive that nurses have the responsibility to both develop and maintain ethical competence is also clear in the nursing codes of ethics (ANA, 2015, Provision 5; CNA, 2017, Part I.G; ICN, 2021, Element, 2.1).

Ethical Competence

Nursing literature provides insight into elements of the evolving concept of ethical competence. In their review of nursing literature, Lechasseur (2018) and colleagues identified six terms most frequently associated with

BOX 20.1   Weblinks to Nursing Ethics Resources

American Nurses Association (ANA) Center for Ethics and Human Rights: https://www.nursingworld.org/practice-policy/nursing-excellence/ethics/about-the-center/

ANA Position Paper (2021) *Nurses' professional responsibility to promote ethical practice environments*. https://www.nursingworld.org/~4ab6e6/globalassets/practice-andpolicy/nursing-excellence/ana-position-statements/nursing-practice/nurses-professional-responsibility-to-promote-ethical-practice-environments-2021-final.pdf

Georgetown University free course *Introduction to Bioethics*: https://www.edx.org/course/introduction-to-bioethics

Professional Journals that feature ethical content such as:

The American Nurse: https://www.myamericannurse.com/

The American Journal of Bioethics online: https://bioethicstoday.org/

Canadian Journal of Bioethics: https://cjb-rcb.ca/index.php/cjb-rcb

Nursing Ethics: https://journals.sagepub.com/home/nej

A list of other journals can be found at the Kennedy Institute of Ethics Bioethics Research Library: https://bioethics.georgetown.edu/bioethics-journals/

National or State/Provincial Centers for Ethics— examples

The Hastings Center: https://www.thehastingscenter.org/

Clinical Ethics Network of North Carolina: https://cennc.org/

West Virginia Center for Health, Ethics & Law: http://wvethics.org/

West Virginia Network of Ethics Committees: http://www.wvnec.org/

Canadian Bioethics Society: https://www.bioethics.ca/bioethics-centres

---

ethical competence in nursing: *ethical sensitivity, ethical knowledge, ethical reflection, ethical decision making, ethical action, and ethical behavior.* Three ethical values that are the pillars of Koskinen (2022) and colleagues proposed model for multiprofessional ethical competence are ethical attitude (personal desire to do good), ethical basis (what is best for the patient is a common goal), and ethical culture (sharing common goals and values in the organization).

As with any area of nursing practice, developing ethical competence begins as you incorporate basic knowledge, skills, and professional identity into your developing role as a nurse. As you have studied and worked with the various features of this text you have gained ethical knowledge, learned an ethical decision-making process, utilized processes for developing ethical sensitivity, engaged in ethical reflection, and deepened your understanding of expectations for ethical behavior and action grounded in nursing codes of ethics. These are all elements related to ethical competence identified by Lechasseur (2018) and colleagues. Additionally, you have incorporated the values that ground ethical competence identified by Koskinen (2022) and colleagues as you identified your own ethical attitude and values, learned to focus on what is best for the patient, and explored the importance of understanding and promoting ethical culture.

Maintaining Ethical Competence

Ethics & Issues in Contemporary Nursing has provided you with the basics necessary for becoming an ethically competent nurse. Maintaining competence requires building on these basics through ongoing education, self-development, and refinement of ethical skills, attitudes, and behaviors. This book can be a valuable resource for maintaining ethical competence as you find yourself confronting ethical questions, challenges, and dilemmas. Revisiting chapters or sections of chapters will help you deepen your knowledge of the content and perhaps see situations from a different perspective. Exploring resources and websites related to particular issues and topics referenced throughout the text can enable you to expand your knowledge and support you in developing more confidence and competence in bringing ethical awareness into your nursing practice. As you continue to review and apply your professional code of nursing ethics to your everyday practice as well as to challenging situations, living and practicing in alignment with the code will become second nature.

Nursing codes of ethics and position statements are key resources for ongoing development and maintenance of ethical competence. Web addresses for these are included in the appendix. There are many resources available online that provide education, resources, and support in maintaining ethical competence and we list selected examples in Box 20.1. You are encouraged to explore these resources and to seek out others that are pertinent to your needs.

THE EMPOWERED NURSE: EXEMPLARS

Ethical competence and nurse empowerment are closely linked. The empowered nurse is someone who sees a nursing need and takes actions consistent with the nursing obligation to promote health and to provide optimal care for people in any settings, role, and domains of practice. Koskinen (2022) and colleagues note that ethical competence is linked to the core of caring ethics and is strengthened by reflection, teamwork and leadership, and ethical role models and support. In this section we offer brief exemplars of nurses in a variety of roles, settings, and domains of practice who have made a difference by acting with power and moral authority to address health and healing needs of people directly or to support other nurses in doing so. It is our hope that these examples will serve as role models and inspire you to step more fully into your own empowerment as an ethically competent nurse.

Jean Watson PhD, RN, AHN-BC, FAAN

As faculty at the University of Colorado in the 1970s, Dr. Jean Watson had a vision of nursing as a human science concerned with how nurses express care to their patients. She articulated this vision in her book *Nursing: The Philosophy and Science of Caring*, first published in 1979, which "presented a human caring framework as the foundation, the soul, the core and essence of nursing as a discipline and a profession" (Watson, 2018, p. xv). Her *Human Caring Theory* stresses the primacy of relationship between nurse and patient, transpersonal and whole person caring, and the humanistic aspects of nursing as they intertwine with scientific knowledge and nursing practice. The evolution of her theory to include a better understanding of a global perspective of human-healing and health that is anchored in a unitary transformative worldview is presented in her book *Unitary Caring Science: The Philosophy and Praxis of Nursing* (2018). Watson writes that she has "shifted the language of caring from Carative to Caritas…to give caring a deeper, more ethical, human-to-human meaning" (p. 45). She notes that the word Caritas unites Love and caring and "makes more explicit unitary of oneness connections among caring, Love, and healing" (p. 45). She created the *Watson Caring Science Institute* to help nurses and healthcare institutions better understand and more effectively incorporate *caring*

science and *caritas practices* into nursing care (https://www.watsoncaringscience.org/). The Institute offers professional development for nurses globally that helps to translate caring theory into practice, thus enabling nurses to better live the theory in their personal and professional lives. Watson's theory has been instrumental in shaping and grounding nursing's vision of nursing and continues to be a source of empowerment for nurses worldwide in practicing from this vision.

Charlotte McGuire MA, RNC, HNC

As corporate Vice President of Patient Care for 19 hospitals in Texas in the 1970s, Charlotte McGuire, MA, RN witnessed burnout among nurses due to or resulting in a lack of caring, compassion, respect, and support within healthcare institutions. She particularly noted that nurses had little time to focus on their own health and well-being, and recognized the need for change. As she began to explore concepts of holism, she had a vision of a new paradigm for nursing that would support nurses in caring for themselves and help to heal a broken healthcare system. In 1981 she brought together nurses from eight states to share their own stories and frustration about working in the current healthcare system as well as their visions of a nursing profession and healing system that focused on wellness rather than illness and nurtured the caregiver. This gathering became the founding meeting of the American Holistic Nurses Association (AHNA). Holistic nursing is a philosophy and way of being in the world that is grounded in holistic principles and modalities and promotes healing of the whole body/mind/spirit person. AHNA continues to emphasize the need for nurses to care for self as well as others, to provide education and support for nurses in understanding and developing competence in caring for the whole body/mind/spirit person, and to support holistic research. The influence of AHNA and holistic nursing has expanded globally. Through the efforts of AHNA, the ANA now recognizes holistic nursing as an official nursing specialty with its own defined scope and standards of practice (ahna.org).

Taking Care: The Story of Nursing and Its Power to Change Our World

In her book *Taking Care: The Story of Nursing and Its Power to Change Our World* (2023), journalist Sarah DiGregorio (who is not a nurse) recognizes that "nursing is a profession, an independent scientific discipline, a practice, and a way of interacting with the world…[that] draws its power and effectiveness from the relationship between nurse and patient; it is the indispensable foundation of all healthcare" (pp. xii–xiv). The following are brief synopses from her book of a few of the many stories about empowered nurses who are making a difference.

Tobi Ash BSN, RN, and Colleagues: In 2018, in response to an outbreak of measles cases in ultra-Orthodox Jewish communities in New York and New Jersey where children had not been vaccinated, Tobi Ash and colleagues in the Orthodox Jewish Nurses Association responded to a need to address this serious health issue affecting these communities. These nurses formed the "EMES (Yiddish for "truth") Initiative to reach these mothers and to counteract anti-vaccine propaganda" (p. 89). Recognizing that nurses with roots in the community and culture would be more effective in reaching those in the community than those from the outside, they established caring trusting relationships with the women. They listened to the women's questions and fears, responded to them with empathy, and provided accurate information about vaccines. Their work within the community is ongoing.

Stephen Wickham RN and Karen Wickham RN: Stephen and Karen Wickham are married and are both nurses who recognized the impact of diabetes on the health of people in their community. To address this concern they conduct seminars on achieving better control of type 2 diabetes. They hold these group sessions in churches, libraries, city halls, and other easy-to-access community spaces across Tennessee. Their approach is based on their nursing awareness of the need to meet people where they are, provide culturally congruent care, and mobilize community support to help people succeed in achieving health goals.

Roxana Chicas, PhD, RN: The awareness that the incidence of kidney failure among migrant farmworkers has increased significantly over recent years spurred Roxana Chicas and her colleagues to study the connection among these kidney problems, heat-related illness, and needed protections that can slow or prevent kidney failure. Their research indicates a link to climate change, showing that the odds of a person sustaining an acute kidney injury on a given day increases for every five-degree increase in the heat index. The research also indicates that kidney failure can be slowed or prevented by regular access to water, shade, and rest, which employers do not always provide. She recognizes health disparities within this population and views the participants as people with health needs, not merely research subjects.

Understanding that she may be the only healthcare provider that they see regularly, when she meets with each worker she takes the opportunity to share with them information from their blood and urine analysis, address questions, provide culturally congruent health education, and point out areas that might need follow-up.

Nursing Ethics Core Council

In their article *Nursing ethics and shared governance model*, Maturano and Narva (2023) describe the creation of a Nursing Ethics Core Council (NECC) designed to support ethical competence among nurses at the Hospital of the University of Pennsylvania in Philadelphia (HUP). This council was established by a clinical nurse and a nurse leader and is embedded into the HUP shared governance structure. The NECC is aligned with the ANA's *Code of ethics for nurses with interpretive statements*, and promotes and provides "education that enhances ethical competence in nursing practice, which can lead to empowered, autonomous nurse and excellent patient outcomes." (p. 8).

Ethics Champion Programs

Responding to the need to mitigate moral distress, promote moral courage, and develop moral resilience among nurses, Fitzgerald et al. (2018) discuss *Ethics Champion Programs* established by and for nurses. Nurses who become *Ethics Champions* participate in educational forums that provide them with ethical resources, address moral distress, deepen moral sensitivity, and increase confidence in recognizing and responding to ethical issues. They take these skills back to their work settings and help clinical colleagues better understand and deal with ethically complex issues and to utilize other hospital ethics resources, such as the ethics committee.

Empowered Nurses During COVID-19

This is one example of many hundreds of situations in which nurses identified health needs of patients and communities and took action during the COVID-19 pandemic. During the initial outbreak of the COVID-19 pandemic two members of the African-American community in Fairmont, WV, Tiffany Walker-Samuels and Romelia Hodges (who are not nurses), noticed growing numbers of people infected with COVID within their community and traced it to one church event (Tiffany Walker-Samuels, personal communication). Because of initial lack of support from their local health department, and their knowledge of who had the symptoms, Tiffany and Romelia started contact tracing from the event. By the time they were able to obtain an initial round of COVID tests, there was the third-generation spread. Realizing they were not reaching enough people they set up a task force and approached state health officials to obtain what was needed to host large-scale testing events in Black communities and for the homeless. Nurse volunteers from surrounding counties came forward to do the testing, and nurses and other community volunteers went door to door to encourage people to get tested. When the COVID vaccine became available health disparities were evident again as they realized the African-American community was being missed. When they were able to get 300 doses of the vaccine, the nurse at the health department worked with them to coordinate the process of vaccine administration by volunteer nurses. This same nurse later helped them design the health clinic they were able to establish within the African-American community with the support of CARES funding. This clinic is coordinated and staffed primarily by African-American nurses who are culturally competent individuals who can advocate for and address the healthcare needs of the people within the community.

Francis Boyle BSN

Francis Boyle, BSN, a nurse at West Virginia University's Ruby Memorial Hospital, is an example of the many nurses who act to address health disparities at a global level by volunteering to participate in medical missions in remote and underserved areas of developing nations. Working through Project Helping Hands, he has frequently served as team leader on 2-week medical missions. He and other healthcare providers set up clinics in remote areas where they provide primary care for hundreds of patients and may offer educational seminars as well (WVU Nursing, 2015, pp. 4–6).

Aaron Santmyire DNP, RN

Addressing health and healing needs of people through caring for and loving them has been a primary focus of Aaron Santmyire's nursing and faith path. He has worked as a nurse practitioner in challenging and underserved areas of Madascar and Burkina Faso. His understanding of the primacy of care and love in doing healing work has focused his nursing practice as he learned from, adapted care for, and addressed healthcare needs of people with different cultural expectations, fears, and physical and emotional issues. He noted as he traveled, lived

---

BOX 20.2 Ethical Decision-Making Model

Step 1: Articulate the Problem and a Realistic Goal
- What is the current undesirable situation?
- What is the desired state (goal) that is possible or reasonable in this situation?

Step 2: Gather Data and Identify Conflicting Moral Claims
- What makes this situation a moral problem? Are there conflicting obligations, principles, duties, rights, loyalties, values, or beliefs?
- Who is legitimately empowered to make this decision, and who are other key participants?
- Who is affected and how? What is most important to each?
- What is the level of competence of the person most affected?
- What are the rights, duties, authority, context, and capabilities of participants?
- What are the moral perspectives and level of moral development of the participants?
- What are the issues of conflict and agreement among participants?
- What facts seem most important?
- What emotional and cultural factors are important?
- What information is missing?

Step 3: Explore Potential Strategies
- What potential realistic strategies emerge from discussions?
- What are the risks and benefits of each identified strategy?
- How does each strategy fit the lifestyles and values of the people affected?
- What are the professional, institutional, and legal considerations of each strategy?
- How are alternative strategies weighed and prioritized?
- What alternatives are unacceptable to one or all involved?

Step 4: Select and Implement a Strategy
- Choose the strategy that seems the best.
- Give oneself permission to set aside less acceptable alternatives, remaining attentive to the emotions involved in the process.
- Implement the chosen strategy.

Step 5: Evaluate Outcomes and Revise the Plan if Needed
- Has the ethical dilemma been resolved?
- Have other dilemmas emerged related to the action?
- How has the process and outcome affected those involved?
- Are further actions required?

in, and provided healthcare in different countries he that contemporary society seems to be less interested in caring for others and self than was prevalent in the past. His commitment to caring led him to further explore the concept of caring and to write the book *A Caring Life: How Each of Us Can Change the Trajectory of an Uncaring World* (Santmyire, 2022; WVU Nursing, 2015, pp. 16–19).

MOVING FORWARD

As you continue to develop and expand your personal and professional ethical competence, we encourage you to find other examples of empowered nurses in your own community, in articles in nursing publications, and in the media. Share these examples with classmates and colleagues and discuss how they demonstrate ethical competence, moral courage, and nurse empowerment. Engage in dialogue with these nurses and other colleagues when possible. Take advantage of the resources for ethical development listed in this chapter and others that are available in your area and online. Utilize the *Ethical Decision-Making Model* discussed in Chapter 7 and summarized again in Box 20.2. It is wise to keep this process where you can refer to it regularly. Most importantly, remember that you have the power to make a difference.

REFERENCES

ANA. (2015). *Code of ethics for nurses with interpretive statements.* http://nursingworld.org/DocumentVault/Ethics-1/Code-of-Ethics-for-Nurses.html.

CNA. (2017). *Code of ethics for registered nurses.* https://cdn1.nscn.ca/sites/default/files/documents/resources/code-of-ethics-for-registered-nurses.pdf#:~:text=The%20Canadian%20Nurses%20Association%20%28CNA%29%20Code%20of%20Ethics,receiving%20care.%20The%20Code is%20both%20aspirational%20and%20regulatory.

DiGregorio, S. (2023). *Taking Care: The story of nursing and its power to change our world.* Harper-Collins.

Fitzgerald, H., Knackstedt, A., Trotochaud, K. (2018). Novel ethics champion programs. *American Nurse.* https://www.myamericannurse.com/novel-ethics-champion-programs/

ICN. (2021). *The ICN code of ethics for nurses.* https://www.icn.ch/system/files/2021-10/ICN_Code-of-Ethics_EN_Web_0.pdf.

Koskinen, C., Kaldestad, K., Rossavik, B. D., Jensen, A. R., & Bjerga, G. (2022). Multi-professional ethical competence in healthcare – An ethical practice model. *Nursing Ethics,* 29(4):1003–13. https://doi.org/10.1177/09697330211062986.

Lechasseur, K., Caux, C., Dollé, S., & Legault, A. (2018). Ethical competence: An integrative review. *Nursing Ethics,* 25(6), 694–706. https://doi.org/10.1177/0969733016667773.

Maturano, E., & Narva, A. (2023). Nursing ethics and shared governance model: Building an infrastructure that supports competence and professional growth. *American Nurse Journal,* 18(4). https://doi.org/10.51256/ANJ042306.

Santmyire, A. (2022). *A caring life: How each of us can change the trajectory of an uncaring world.* Clarity Podcast.

Walker, A. (n.d.). *Alice Walker quotes.* BrainyQuote.com. https://www.brainyquote.com/quotes/alice_walker_385241.

Watson, J. (2018). *Unitary caring science: Philosophy and praxis of nursing.* University of Colorado Press.

West Virginia University School of Nursing. (2015). https://nursing.wvu.edu/media/74943/winter_2015final_web.pdf.

Appendix

ONLINE RESOURCES

Throughout this text and in the reference lists at the end of the chapters, we have included web links for numerous online resources pertinent to ethical nursing practice and that support and expand the content in the book. We encourage readers to explore all of these resources. The websites and resources listed here are those that provide information all nurses should be able to access easily at any time.

Codes of Nursing Ethics
American Nurses Association
Code of Ethics for Nurses With Interpretive Statements
https://www.nursingworld.org/practice-policy/
nursing-excellence/ethics/code-of-ethics-for-
nurses/

Canadian Nurses Association
Code of Ethics for Registered Nurses:
https://www.crns.ca/wp-content/uploads/2018/11/
Code-of-Ethics-2017-Edition.pdf

The International Council of Nursing
Code of Ethics for Nurses:
https://www.icn.ch/system/files/2021-10/ICN_Code-
of-Ethics_EN_Web_0.pdf

Position Statements
ANA Position Statements
https://www.nursingworld.org/practice-policy/nursing-
excellence/official-position-statements/

ICN Position Statements
https://www.icn.ch/nursing-policy/position-statements

Canadian Nurses Association Position Statements
https://www.cna-aiic.ca/en/policy-advocacy/policy-
support-tools/position-statements

US Government Laws, Regulations, and Documents
US Constitution
https://constitutionus.com/

Patients' Rights (Code of Federal Regulations)
https://www.ecfr.gov/current/title-38/chapter-I/
part-17/subject-group-ECFR8cadb005766bd82/
section-17.33

The Civil Rights Act of 1964
https://www.eeoc.gov/laws/statutes/titlevii.cfm

Americans With Disabilities Act of 1990
https://www.ada.gov/pubs/adastatute08.htm#12102

The Civil Rights Act of 1991
https://www.eeoc.gov/statutes/civil-rights-act-1991

HIPAA Privacy Rule
https://www.hhs.gov/hipaa/for-professionals/privacy/
index.html

Title IX and Sex Discrimination
https://www2.ed.gov/about/offices/list/ocr/docs/tix_
dis.html

National Practitioner Data Bank
https://www.npdb.hrsa.gov/

National Resources, Hotlines, and Guidelines

Never Events (Agency for Healthcare Research and Quality)

https://psnet.ahrq.gov/primer/never-events

Physician Orders for Life-Sustaining Treatment: Form Used in Several States

https://polst.org/

International Society of Nurses in Genetics

https://www.isong.org/

Self-Care for Nurses—American Holistic Nurses Association

https://www.ahna.org/Resources
ANA Health Nurse Healthy Nation
https://www.healthynursehealthynation.org/

American Academy of Pediatrics Policy Statement: Informed Consent in Decision Making in Pediatric Practice

https://publications.aap.org/pediatrics/article/138/2/e20161484/52512/Informed-Consent-in-Decision-Making-in-Pediatric?searchresult=1

Advance Directive Forms and Instructions

Hospice and Palliative Care Organization's Caringinfo
https://www.caringinfo.org/planning/advance-directives/by-state/

Health Law Institute, Dalhousie University End-of-life Law & Policy in Canada http://eol.law.dal.ca/?page_id=231

West Virginia Center for End-of-Life Care at https://wvendoflife.org/media/1292/2022-new-mpoa-faq.pdf

Legal Process for Choosing a Health Care Surrogate

United States: http://www.caringinfo.org/i4a/pages/index.cfm?pageid=3289.

Canada: http://eol.law.dal.ca/?page_id=231

HIV Laws by State US CDC

https://www.cdc.gov/hiv/policies/law/states/index.html

HIV Self-Test Information

https://www.cdc.gov/hiv/basics/hiv-testing/hiv-self-tests.html

Academic Honesty

https://ori.hhs.gov/avoiding-plagiarism-self-plagiarism-and-other-questionable-writing-practices-guide-ethical-writing

Disaster Preparedness—American Nurses Association

https://www.nursingworld.org/practice-policy/work-environment/health-safety/disaster-preparedness/

Institute of Medicine Crisis Standards of Care

https://www.nursingworld.org/~4ad845/globalassets/docs/ana/stds-of-care-letter-report-2.pdf

US Department of Homeland Security—Human Trafficking Awareness Training

https://www.state.gov/guide-for-introductory-human-trafficking-awareness-training-non-binding/

Department of Health and Human Services Human Trafficking Hotline

Website: https://www.dhs.gov/blue-campaign?gclid=Cj0KCQiAxbefBhDfARIsAL4XLRpcEd2iOjSvurryxZVBjAEHxOQ9-D0pcMZ_P73l_FFgrjxCi-MM0ngaAsdmEALw_wcB
Telephone Hotline: 1-888-373-7888

National Domestic Violence Hotline

Website: https://www.thehotline.org/
Telephone Hotline: 1-800-799-SAFE (help available in numerous languages)

Eldercare Locator—Reporting Elder Abuse

Website: https://eldercare.acl.gov/Public/Index.aspx
Telephone Hotline: 1-800-677-1116. Monday through Friday, 9:00 a.m. to 8:00 p.m. EST

Hospital-Acquired Condition Prevention Program (CMS.gov)

https://www.cms.gov/Medicare/Medicare-Fee-for-Service-Payment/AcuteInpatientPPS/HAC-Reduction-Program#:~:text=The%20Hospital%2DAcquired%20Condition%20HAC,in%20the%20inpatient%20hospital%20setting

Hospital-Acquired Conditions

https://www.cms.gov/Medicare/Medicare-Fee-for-Service-Payment/HospitalAcqCond/Hospital-Acquired_Conditions

Research Ethics

US Department of Health and Human Services, Office of Research Integrity—Avoiding Plagiarism

https://ori.hhs.gov/avoiding-plagiarism-self-plagiarism-and-other-questionable-writing-practices-guide-ethical-writing

NIH Guiding Principles for Ethical Research

https://www.nih.gov/health-information/nih-clinical-research-trials-you/guiding-principles-ethical-research

The Belmont Report

https://www.hhs.gov/ohrp/regulations-and-policy/belmont-report/index.html

The "Common Rule," 45 CFR Part 46, *Protection of Human Subjects*

https://www.hhs.gov/ohrp/regulations-and-policy/regulations/45-cfr-46/index.html

WMA Declaration of Helsinki

https://www.wma.net/policies-post/wma-declaration-of-helsinki-ethical-principles-for-medical-research-involving-human-subjects/#:~:text=The%20World%20Medical%20Association%20WMA,identifiable%20human%20material%20and%20data

Nuremberg Code

https://www.ushmm.org/information/exhibitions/online-exhibitions/special-focus/doctors-trial/nuremberg-code

Institute of Medicine Publications

To Err Is Human

https://nap.nationalacademies.org/catalog/9728/to-err-is-human-building-a-safer-health-system

Crossing the Quality Chasm: A New Health System for the 21st Century

https://nap.nationalacademies.org/catalog/10027/crossing-the-quality-chasm-a-new-health-system-for-the

The Future of Nursing: Leading Change, Advancing Health

https://nap.nationalacademies.org/catalog/12956/the-future-of-nursing-leading-change-advancing-health

Other Important Resources

United Nations *Universal Declaration of Human Rights*

https://www.un.org/en/about-us/universal-declaration-of-human-rights

Florence Nightingale's *Notes on Nursing: What It Is and What It Is Not*

http://digital.library.upenn.edu/women/nightingale/nursing/nursing.html

American Hospital Association, *The Patient Care Partnership*

https://www.aha.org/system/files/2018-01/aha-patient-care-partnership.pdf

American Medical Association *Code of Medical Ethics*

https://code-medical-ethics.ama-assn.org/

Choosing Wisely

https://abimfoundation.org/what-we-do/choosing-wisely

Earth Charter

https://earthcharter.org/

Alliance of Nurses for Healthy Environments

https://envirn.org

GLOSSARY

Accountability involves a reciprocal relationship in which one is responsible and therefore answerable to others for judgment and action taken in fulfilling a duty.

Active voluntary euthanasia An act in which the physician both provides the means of death for a patient, such as a lethal dose of medication, and administers it.

Activism A passionate approach to everyday activities that is committed to seeking a more just social order through critical analysis, provocation, transformation, and rebalancing of power.

Act-utilitarianism A basic type of utilitarianism that suggests people choose actions that will, in any given circumstance, increase the overall good.

Administrative law The branch of law that consists mainly of the legal powers granted to administrative agencies by the legislature, as well as the rules that the agencies make to carry out their powers.

Advance directives Instructions that indicate which health care interventions to initiate or withhold, or that designate someone who will act as a surrogate in making such decisions in the event that a person loses decision-making capacity.

Advocacy The act of supporting, speaking for, defending, or interceding on behalf of another.

Alarm fatigue Sensory overload for nurses related to ever-present alarms of medical technology and attention to operating and monitoring the various devices resulting in desensitization to alarm sounds and their significance.

Allocative policies Policies designed to provide net benefits to some distinct group or class of individuals or organizations, at the expense of others, in order to ensure that public objectives are met.

Altruism A motivation for action that is displayed as a selfless concern for the well-being of others.

Antivaccination Vaccine refusal for self or one's child based on personal reasons that may include disinformation, conspiracy theories, personal liberty, or political choice.

Appeals to conscience Personal and subjective beliefs, founded on a prior judgment of rightness or wrongness, that are motivated by personal sanction, rather than external authority.

Assault The unjustifiable attempt or threat to touch a person without consent that results in fear of immediately harmful or threatening contact.

Assent Agreeing to or concurring with a decision or proposal (such as a child agreeing with a parent's decision related to participating in a research protocol).

Assisted death A situation in which patients receive the means of death from someone, such as a physician, but activate the process themselves.

Authority The state of having legitimate power and sovereignty.

Autonomy The word "autonomy" literally means self-governing and is sometimes called *the right to self-determination*. Autonomy denotes having the freedom to make choices about issues that affect one's life, free from lies, restraint, or coercion.

Axiology The branch of philosophy that studies the nature and types of values.

Battery The unlawful touching of another or the carrying out of threatened physical harm, including willful, angry, and violent or negligent touching of another's person, clothes, or anything attached to his or her person or held by him or her.

Belmont Report Policies developed by the US National Commission for the Protection of Human Subjects of Biomedical and Behavioral Research (1978) regarding ethical principles for research with human subjects.

Beneficence The ethical principle that requires one to act in ways that benefit another. In research, this implies the protection from harm and discomfort, including a balance between the benefits and risks of a study.

Breach of duty A failure to perform a promised act or obligation.

Bullying A health-harming, repeated abuse of power that reveals itself in actions intended to humiliate, offend, and cause distress.

Cartesian philosophy A widespread belief during the Renaissance related to Descartes's proposals that the universe is a physical thing, that all therein is analogous to machines that can be analyzed and understood, and that the mind and body are separate entities.

Case law The basis of the judicial system, also known as *common law*.

Categorical health insurance programs Publicly funded health care programs such as Medicare, Medicaid, the Medicaid Children's Health Insurance Program (CHIP), Veteran's Health Administration, and the Indian Health Service that are restricted to certain categories of people (the elderly, children, veterans, and so forth).

Categorical imperative The Kantian maxim stating that no action can be judged as right that cannot reasonably become a law by which every person should always abide.

Cauistry The lowest and most specific level of moral discourse. Casuistry resolves moral questions by drawing parallels between the case at hand and a paradigm or pure case in the past.

Causation A legal term denoting a causal relationship between an action and the resulting harm or injury.

Character ethics Theories of ethics, sometimes called virtue ethics, that are related to the concept of innate moral virtue.

Cheating Dishonesty and deception regarding examinations, projects, or papers.

Civil law (Also called *private law*.) The law that determines a person's legal rights and obligations in many kinds of activities involving other people.

Claims made liability policy A liability insurance policy that provides coverage for events that occur and are reported within the specific time period identified in the policy.

Cloning The process of using biotechnology to create a genetically identical copy of a cell or organism.

Code of nursing ethics Explicit declaration of the primary goals and values of the profession that indicate the profession's acceptance of the responsibility and trust with which it has been invested by society.

Coercion Actual or implied threat of harm or penalty for not participating in a research project or offering excessive rewards for participation in the project.

Common law A system of law, also known as *case law*, based largely on previous court decisions. In this system, decisions are based on earlier court rulings in similar cases, or precedents. Over time, these precedents take on the force of law.

Communitarian theories Theories of justice that place the community, rather than the individual, the state, the nation, or any other entity, at the center of the value system; that emphasize the value of public goods; and that conceive of values as rooted in communal practices.

Compassion A focal virtue combining an attitude of active regard for another's welfare with an imaginative awareness and emotional response of deep sympathy, tenderness, and discomfort at the other person's misfortune or suffering.

Competence A person's ability to make meaningful life decisions. A declaration of incompetence involves legal action with a ruling by a judge that the person is unable to make such life decisions.

Complementary therapies Therapeutic interventions that derive from traditions other than conventional Western medicine that are used by patients with or without the knowledge of conventional medical practitioners.

Confidentiality The ethical principle that requires nondisclosure of private or secret information with which one is entrusted. In research, confidentiality refers to the researcher's assurance to participants that information provided will not be made public or available to anyone other than those involved in the research process without the participant's consent.

Conscientiousness An internal acknowledgment of one's motives and actions and a sense of right and wrong, particularly as related to things for which one is responsible. It includes an ability to judge the moral quality of one's motives and actions.

Consent Agreeing to or approving a request, proposal, or decision.

Consequentialism A theory of ethics, sometimes called utilitarianism.

Constitutional law A formal set of rules and principles that describes the powers of a government and the rights of the people.

Contract An agreement between two or more people that can be enforced by law.

Contract law A type of law that deals with the rights and obligations of people who make contracts.

Cosmology A branch of philosophy that describes the structure, origin, and processes of the universe.

Covert values Expectations that are not in writing that are often identified only through participation in, or controversies within, an organization or institution.

Criminal law A type of law that deals with crimes or actions considered harmful to society.

Cultural awareness Knowledge about values, beliefs, behaviors, and the like of cultures other than one's own.

Cultural competence Skill in dealing with transcultural issues, which is demonstrated through cultural awareness and cultural sensitivity.

Cultural humility Approaching people from other cultures with dignity and respect, a willingness to learn from the wisdom and knowledge of their worldview, honoring their values, beliefs, customs, worldview, and healing practice, and respectfully acknowledging differences between personal beliefs and those of the other person. Integral to cultural humility is a life-long commitment to reflect on and challenge our own cultural viewpoints, biases, prejudices, and ethnocentrism.

Cultural interpretation incorporating knowledge of cultural context and meaning of both verbal and nonverbal communication in communicating messages from one language to another.

Cultural safety Implies that nursing care is provided in a manner that enables the patient or family to feel safe in discussing and incorporating their cultural values, behaviors, and beliefs into their care. It considers all that makes them unique; avoids actions that diminish, demean, or disempower the cultural identity and well-being of the patient; and ensures that what is safe and effective care is defined by the patient or family.

Cultural sensitivity The ability to incorporate a patient's cultural perspective into nursing assessments and to modify nursing care in order to be as congruent as possible with the patient's cultural perspective.

Culture The total lifeways of a group of interacting individuals, consisting of learned patterns of values, beliefs, behaviors, and customs shared by that group.

Damages Monetary compensation awarded by a court to an individual who has been injured through the wrongful actions of another person.

Decision-making capacity The ability of a person to understand all information about a health condition, to communicate understanding and choices, and to reason and deliberate, as well as the possession of personal values and goals that guide the decision.

Decisional privacy The right of an individual to control the disclosure of how personal choices are made, including cultural and religious preferences.

Declaration of Helsinki Principles issued by the World Medical Assembly in 1964 to guide clinical research; revised in 1975.

Defamation Harm that occurs to a person's reputation and good name; diminishes others' value or esteem of that person; or arouses negative feelings toward the person by the communication of false, malicious, unprivileged, or harmful words.

Defendant The person sued or accused in a court of law.

Delegating To appoint or assign particular responsibilities to another person.

Deontology Related to the term *duty*, deontology is a group of ethical theories based on the rationalist view that the rightness or wrongness of an act depends on the nature of the act, rather than the consequences that occur as a result of it.

Dilemma A problem that requires a choice between two options that are equally unfavorable and mutually exclusive.

Discernment A focal virtue of sensitive insight, acute judgment, and understanding that results in decisive action.

Disciplining to punish or reprimand another person with the intention of correcting or altering their subsequent behavior.

Discrimination Unjust or prejudicial treatment of a person or group on the grounds of race, gender, sexual orientation, or other characteristics.

Disease The biomedical explanation of sickness.

Disparate treatment A type of workplace discrimination that occurs when an individual is treated differently by a superior or by organizational policy.

Disparate impact A type of workplace discrimination that occurs when employers consistently apply policies that appear to be fair to all employees but actually adversely affect one group.

Distributive justice Application of the ethical principle of justice that relates to fair, equitable, and appropriate distribution in society, determined by justified norms that structure the terms of social cooperation. Its scope includes policies that allot diverse benefits and burdens such as property, resources, taxation, privileges, and opportunities.

Diversity The experience within nursing of differences among colleagues and patients in areas such as gender, age, socioeconomic position, sexual orientation, health status, ethnicity, race, or culture.

Do not resuscitate (DNR) orders Written directives placed in a patient's medical chart indicating that cardiopulmonary resuscitation is to be avoided.

Durable power of attorney Allows a competent person to designate another as a surrogate or proxy to act on her or his behalf in making health care decisions in the event of the loss of decision-making capacity.

Duty of care An overarching legal principle that calls for the nurse to act as an ordinary, prudent, reasonable nurse would act in similar circumstances.

Egalitarian theories Theories of justice that promote ideals of equal distribution of social benefits and burdens and that recognize the social obligation to eliminate or reduce barriers that prevent fair equality of opportunity.

Empirical Knowledge gained through the processes of observation and experience.

Empowerment A supportive process and partnership, enacted in the context of love and respect for self and others, through which individuals and groups are enabled to change situations and are given the skills, resources, opportunities, and authority to do so. It involves creating a vision, taking risks, making choices, and behaving in authentic ways.

Ethic A personal consciousness of the moral importance that guides personal actions in particular situations.

Ethic of caring An approach to ethical decision making grounded in relationship and mutual responsibility in which choices are contextually bound and strategies are focused on maintaining connections and not hurting anyone.

Ethic of justice An approach to ethical decision making, based on objective rules and principles, in which choices are made from a stance of separateness.

Ethic of responsiveness An approach that demonstrates respect for persons and a desire to do good for this particular patient on this particular day. The nurse with this quality responds with sensitivity to the concerns, needs, and preferences of each patient.

Ethical dilemma Occurs when there are conflicting moral claims.

Ethical principles Basic and obvious moral truths that guide deliberation and action. Major ethical principles include autonomy, beneficence, nonmaleficence, veracity, confidentiality, justice, fidelity, and others.

Ethical treatment of data Implies integrity of research protocols and honesty in reporting findings.

Ethics A formal process for making logical and consistent decisions based on moral beliefs.

Ethnocentrism Judging the behaviors of someone from another culture by the standards of one's own culture.

Eugenics Meaning "good birth," eugenics is based on the belief that some human traits are more desirable for society than others and that society should weed out what proponents consider to be undesirable traits. Proponents of eugenics advocate policies that encourage so-called "genetically superior" people to have children, while discouraging so-called "genetically inferior" people from having children through practices such as forced sterilization.

Euthanasia Causing the painless death of a person in order to end or prevent suffering.

Expertise The characteristic of having a high level of specialized skill and knowledge.

External locus of control The belief that forces outside of oneself direct or rule one's life, whether these be generalized forces such as fate or other persons who are perceived as more powerful.

External standards of nursing practice Guides for nursing care that are developed by non-nurses, legislation, or institutions.

Faith A generic feature of the human struggle to find and maintain meaning flowing from an integration of ways of knowing and valuing.

False imprisonment The unlawful, unjustifiable detention of a person within fixed boundaries, or an act intended to result in such confinement.

Felonies Serious crimes that carry significant fines and jail sentences. Examples of felonies include first- and second-degree murder, arson, burglary, extortion, kidnapping, rape, and robbery.

Fidelity   An ethical principle related to the concept of faithfulness and the practice of promise keeping.

Food insecurity   An economic and social situation in which a household lacks consistent access to adequate food due to limited financial or other resources.

Forgery   Includes fraud or intentional misrepresentation.

Formalism   A term often used to refer to deontology.

Foreseeability   The legal concept that a person has the ability to reasonably anticipate that damage or injury may result from certain acts or omissions.

Fraud   A deliberate deception for the purpose of securing an unfair or unlawful gain.

Full disclosure   Indicates that a research participant must be fully informed of the nature of a study, anticipated risks and benefits, time commitment, expectations of the participant and the researcher, and the right to refuse to participate.

Gender bias   A preference or prejudice toward one gender over the other.

Gender identity   Concept of self as male, female, a blend of both, or neither which is expressed in how people perceive and call themselves.

Genetics   The scientific study of genes, their effects, and their roles in inheritance.

Genetic diagnosis   A process of performing a biopsy on embryos to determine the presence of genetic flaws and gender prior to implantation.

Genetic engineering   The ability to genetically alter organisms for a variety of purposes, particularly to promote their health and strength.

Genetic screening   A process for determining whether persons are predisposed to certain diseases and whether couples have the possibility of giving birth to a genetically impaired infant.

Genomics   The study of all of a person's genes (the genome), including interactions of those genes with each other and with the person's environment.

Grassroots lobbying   Lobbying efforts that involve mobilizing a committed constituency to influence the opinions of policymakers.

Guardian ad litem   A court-appointed guardian for a particular action or proceeding; such a guardian may not oversee all of the person's affairs.

Health disparities   Refers to discrimination or perceived discrimination in the delivery of health care to groups of people that leads to a delay in seeking health care and poor health care outcomes. These inequities in health outcomes are often based on race, ethnicity, cultural background, immigrant status, gender, socioeconomic status, and the like.

Health policies   Authoritative decisions focusing on health that are made in the legislative, executive, or judicial branches of government and are intended to direct or influence the actions, behaviors, or decisions of others; their lifestyles and personal behaviors; and improvements in the availability, accessibility, and quality of their health care services.

Herd or community immunity   A critical threshold of immunity within a community that helps prevent spread of a communicable disease to those who cannot be immunized.

Hospital-acquired conditions   A Center for Medicare and Medicaid term for health consequences within a hospital setting that could reasonably have been prevented through the application of evidence-based guidelines.

Horizontal violence   Incivility or bullying behaviors that occur top-down or bottom-up.

Human trafficking   Modern-day slavery that involves the acquisition, harboring, and trade of persons through force, threats, deception, or other forms of coercion, with the aim of exploiting them for forced labor, for their organs, and/or for sexual services.

Hunger   A physiological response in an individual that may result from food insecurity.

Illness   A personal response to disease flowing from how one's culture teaches one to be sick.

Incivility   A term for social behavior that lacks respect and is rude, impolite, discourteous, and offensive.

Informational privacy   The right of an individual to control the disclosure of information both in writing, such as medical records, and given orally, even in casual conversation.

Informed consent   A process by which patients are informed of the possible outcomes, alternatives, and risks of treatments and are required to give their consent freely. This implies legal protection of a patient's right to personal autonomy by providing the opportunity to choose a course of action regarding plans for health care, including the right to refuse medical recommendations and to choose from available therapeutic alternatives. In research, this refers to consent to participate in a research study after the research purpose, expected commitment, risks and benefits, any invasion of privacy, and ways that anonymity and confidentiality will be addressed have been explained.

Injury   A wrong or damage done to another person, which may be physical or emotional harm, as well as damage to reputation or dignity, loss of a legal right, or breach of contract.

Integrity   Refers to adherence to moral norms that is sustained over time. Implicit in integrity is trustworthiness and a consistency of convictions, actions, and emotions.

Intentional torts   Willful or intentional acts that violate another person's rights or property.

Internal locus of control   The belief that one is able to influence or control things that happen in one's life.

Internally displaced persons   Individuals or groups of people who have been forced or obliged to flee or to leave their homes or places of habitual residence, in particular as a result of, or to avoid the effects of, armed conflict, situations of generalized violence, violations of human rights, or natural or human-made disasters and who have not crossed an internationally recognized state border.

Interpretation   Verbally communicating a message from one language to another while making every effort to faithfully preserve the message.

Intervening factors   Elements that appear in the situation in such a way as to interfere with, alter, or obstruct action.

Invasion of privacy Includes intrusion on the patient's physical and mental solitude or seclusion, public disclosure of private facts, publicity that places the patient in a false light in the public eye, or appropriation of the patient's name or likeness for the defendant's benefit or advantage.

Journals Personal written records kept on a periodic or regular basis containing factual material and subjective interpretations of events, thoughts, feelings, and plans.

Judicial decisions Authoritative court decisions that direct or influence the actions, behaviors, or decisions of others.

Justice An ethical principle that relates to fair, equitable, and appropriate treatment in light of what is due or owed to persons, recognizing that giving to some will deny receipt to others who might otherwise have received these things. In research, justice implies the rights of fair treatment and privacy, including anonymity and confidentiality.

Kantianism A deontological theory of ethics based on the writings of the philosopher Immanuel Kant.

Lateral violence Negative or harmful behavior that occurs when a person is uncivil or bullies another person who is otherwise an equal.

Law A system of binding rules of conduct formally recognized and enforced to ensure that individuals adhere to the collective will of society.

LGBTQ+ A symbol referring to lesbian, gay, bisexual, transgender, queer, and related communities.

Libel Printed defamation by written words and images that injures a person's reputation or causes others to avoid, ridicule, or view the person with contempt.

Libertarian theories Theories of distributive justice that propose that the just society protects the rights of property and liberty of each person, allowing citizens to improve their circumstances by their own effort.

Linguistic competency This is evident when health care services are provided in the language best understood by the patient.

Linguistic interpretation Verbally communicating a message from one language to another focusing on the spoken word including interpretation, translation, and sight translation.

Living will Legal document developed voluntarily by persons, giving directions to health care providers related to withholding or withdrawing life support if certain conditions exist.

Lobbying The art of persuasion. Attempting to convince a legislator, a government official, the head of an agency, or a state official to comply with a request, whether it is convincing them to support a position on an issue or to follow a particular course of action.

Locus of control Beliefs about the ability to control events in one's life.

Loyalty Showing sympathy, care, and reciprocity to those with whom we appropriately identify; working closely with others toward shared goals; keeping promises; making mutual concerns a priority; sacrificing personal interests to the relationship; and giving attention to these over a substantial period.

Malpractice The form of negligence in which any professional misconduct, unreasonable lack of professional skill, or nonadherence to the accepted standard of care causes injury to a patient or client.

Managed care An integrated form of health care delivery and financing that represents attempts to control costs by modifying the behavior of providers and patients.

Material rules Rules by which distributive justice decisions regarding entitlement are made.

Medical futility Situations in which medical interventions are judged to have no medical benefit or in which the chance for success is low.

Metaethics A highly abstract branch of philosophy that explores the foundations of moral values. Metaethics focuses on ways of philosophical thinking about morality, such as the source of morality and how people know what principles or virtues are correct.

Migrants Individuals who are moving or have moved across an international border or within a state away from their habitual place of residence, regardless of the person's legal status, whether the movement is voluntary or involuntary, what the causes for the movement are, or what the length of the stay is.

Misdemeanor A criminal offense of a less serious nature than a felony, usually punishable by a fine or short jail sentence, or both.

Modern era A somewhat arbitrary term often used in common language to refer to present or recent time. The term is used in this text and many others to refer to the historical period immediately following the Renaissance, generally thought to include the late 16th through the late 18th centuries.

Moral agency Refers to a nurse's ability to act morally and promote positive outcomes for patients, basing actions and decisions on internalized principles and knowledge of right and wrong, good and bad.

Moral communities Places within health care settings where moral language is a natural part of conversations that foster moral identities as they reflect, nurture, and develop moral agency. Moral communities create spaces for moral discourse that include and value the unique role of all who contribute to patient care outcomes.

Moral courage The willingness to stand up for personal core values and ethical beliefs, even when we stand alone.

Moral development A product of the sociocultural environment in which one lives and develops that reflects the intellectual and emotional process through which one learns and incorporates values regarding right and wrong.

Moral discourse Written or spoken reasoned discussion or argument pertaining to moral issues.

Moral distress The reaction to a situation in which there are moral problems that seem to have clear solutions, yet one is unable to follow one's moral beliefs because of external restraints. This may be evidenced in anger, frustration, dissatisfaction, and poor performance in the work setting.

Moral integrity A focal virtue that relates to soundness, reliability, wholeness, integration of character, and fidelity in adherence to moral norms sustained over time.

Moral outrage   A state that occurs when someone else in the health care setting performs an act the nurse believes to be immoral. In cases of moral outrage, the nurse does not participate in the act and therefore does not feel responsible for the wrong, but feels powerlessness to prevent it.

Moral particularism   Moral particularism utilizes the principles and rules of other moral theories, embracing the uniqueness of cases, the culturally significant ethical features, and the ethical judgment in each particular case.

Moral philosophy   The philosophical discussion of what is considered to be good or bad, right or wrong.

Moral reckoning   Moral reckoning is a three-stage process that includes a stage of ease, a situational bind (not considered a stage), resolution, and reflection. It may include other processes such as moral distress, moral agony, and moral outrage.

Moral thought   An individual's cognitive examination of right and wrong, good and bad.

Moral uncertainty   A state that occurs when one senses that there is a moral problem but is not sure of the morally correct action, when one is unsure what moral principles or values apply, or when one is unable to define the moral problem.

Moral values   Preferences or dispositions reflective of right or wrong, should or should not, in human behavior.

Naturalism   A view of moral judgment that regards ethics as dependent on human nature and psychology.

Necessity   In general, necessity refers to something being required or indispensable. As a defense to battery, necessity refers to touching a person with the purpose of helping them in an emergency, even though consent was not obtained.

Negligence   The omission to do something that a reasonable person, guided by those ordinary considerations that typically regulate human affairs, would do, or doing something that a reasonable and prudent person would not do.

Never events   A phrase sometimes used interchangeably with "serious reportable events" which include incidents involving preventable, serious, and unambiguous adverse events resulting from error or lapse in care, which should never occur within a health care facility.

Noncompliance   Denoting an unwillingness on the part of the patient to participate in health care activities that have been recommended by health care providers.

Noncontact unwanted sexual experiences   Unwanted sexual attention that does not involve physical contact (such as verbal or written sexual harassment or exposure to pornography). This type of sexual violence occurs without a person's consent and can occur in different settings such as school, the workplace, in public, or through technology.

Nonmaleficence   An ethical principle related to beneficence that requires one to act in such a manner as to avoid causing harm to another, including deliberate harm, risk of harm, and harm that occurs during the performance of beneficial acts.

Normative ethics   A form of moral discourse that seeks to set norms or standards for conduct. Normative ethics focuses on intrinsic values such as truth, moral goodness, and happiness; guides for right action such as principles of bioethics and duty-based ethics; and virtues, including professional, secular, and religious virtues. Deontology, utilitarian, and virtue ethics are competing theories of normative ethics.

Nuremberg Code   A set of principles for the ethical conduct of research against which the experiments in the Nazi concentration camps could be judged.

Nurse practice acts   Legislative statutes within each state that define nursing, describe boundaries of practice, establish standards for nurses, and protect the domain of nursing.

Nursing process   A model commonly used for decision making in nursing.

Obligation   Being required to do something by virtue of a moral rule, a duty, or some other binding

demand, such as a particular role or relationship.

Occurrence-based liability policy   A liability insurance policy that protects from a covered event that happens during the policy period, regardless of when a claim is reported.

Overt values   Values of individuals, groups, institutions, and organized systems that are explicitly communicated through philosophy and policy statements.

Palliative care   A comprehensive, interdisciplinary, and total care approach focusing primarily on comfort and support of patients and families facing illness that is chronic or not responsive to curative treatment.

Parentalism   A nongender term that parallels the meaning of paternalism, while avoiding gender bias.

Partisan   Adherence to the ideology of a particular political party.

Paternalism   Acting in a way that one believes will benefit, protect, or advance the interest of a person, even when this action goes against the person's expressed desires or limits his or her freedom of choice.

Patient Self-Determination Act   A federal law requiring institutions such as hospitals, nursing homes, health maintenance organizations, and home care agencies receiving Medicare or Medicaid funds to provide written information to adult patients regarding their rights to make health care decisions.

Patriarchy   The predominance of men in positions of power and influence in society, with cultural values and norms favoring men.

Philosophy   The intense and critical examination of beliefs and assumptions.

Physical privacy   The right of an individual to control the disclosure of the individuals' bodies and their personal space.

Plagiarism   Taking another's ideas or work and presenting them as one's own.

Plaintiff   The term used for the complaining or injured party in a lawsuit.

Policy formulation   A phase of the policymaking process that includes such actions as agenda setting and the subsequent development of legislation.

Policy implementation   A phase of the policymaking process that follows enactment of legislation and includes taking actions and making additional decisions necessary to implement legislation, such as rule making and policy operation.

Policy modification   A phase of the policymaking process that exists to improve or perfect legislation previously enacted.

Political   Relates to the complex process of policymaking within the government.

Political issues   Those issues that are regulated or influenced by decisions within the executive, judicial, or legislative branch of government.

Political parties   Organized groups with distinct ideologies that seek to control government.

Power   The ability to do or act; the capability of doing or accomplishing something.

Practical dilemma   A situation in which moral claims compete with nonmoral claims.

Practical imperative   The Kantian maxim requiring that one treat others always as ends and never as a means.

Precautionary principle   When an activity raises threats of harm to human health or the environment, precautionary measures should be taken, even if some cause-and-effect relationships are not fully established scientifically.

Precedents   Court rulings on which subsequent rulings in similar cases are based. Over time, these precedents take on the force of law.

Principles   Basic and obvious truths that guide deliberation and action.

Privacy   Privacy refers to the right of an individual to control the disclosure of personal information or secrets, images, motivations, and relationships.

Private law   (Also called *civil law*.) The law that determines a person's legal rights and obligations in many kinds of activities involving other people.

Problem   A situation in which there is a discrepancy between the status quo (what is actually happening) and

what one desires or what should be happening, that is, the situation is unwelcome, harmful, or wrong and needs to be overcome.

Profession   A complex, organized occupation preceded by a long training program geared toward the acquisition of exclusive knowledge necessary to provide a service that is essential or desired by society, leading to a monopoly that provides autonomy, public recognition, prestige, power, and authority for the practitioner.

Professional codes of ethics   Explicit, discipline-specific rules of behavior for members of a profession that are developed to protect the people the profession serves, ensure the competence of members, and safeguard the integrity and trustworthiness of the discipline.

Proprietary privacy   The right of an individual to control the disclosure of property interests including a person's image or biological materials.

Public law   Law that defines a person's rights and obligations in relation to government and describes the various divisions of government and their powers.

Quality of life   A subjective appraisal of factors that make life worth living and contribute to a positive experience of living.

Racism   The assumption that members of one race are superior to those of another.

Rationalism   A view of moral judgment that regards truth as necessary, universal, and superior to the information received from the senses, having an origin in the nature of the universe or in the nature of a higher being.

Refugees   Individuals who, due to a well-founded fear of being persecuted for reasons of race, religion, nationality, or membership of a particular social group or political opinion are outside the country of their nationality and are unable or, due to such fear, unwilling to avail themselves of the protection of that country; or who, not having a nationality and being outside the country of their former habitual residence as a result of such events,

is unable or, due to such fear, is unwilling to return to it. Refugees may be considered a subset of the migrant population.

Regulatory policies   Policies that are designed to influence the actions, behaviors, and decisions of others through directive techniques.

Relational privacy   The right of an individual to control the disclosure of personal relationships, which includes the family and similarly intimate relations.

Religion   The codification of beliefs and practices concerning the Divine and one's relationship with the Divine that are shared by a group of people.

Religiosity   Beliefs and practices that are the expressive aspects of religion.

Respect for autonomy   An ethical principle that denotes an obligation to honor the autonomy of other persons.

Respect for human dignity   Implies the rights of patients to full disclosure and self-determination regarding participation in research and in making health care choices.

Respect for persons   An attitude by which one considers others to be worthy of high regard.

Responsibility   Means being reliable and trustworthy in fulfilling an obligation or a duty.

Right to fair treatment   Ensures equitable treatment of participants in the research selection process, during the study, and after the completion of the study.

Right to privacy   The right to be left alone or to be free from unwanted publicity. In research, this is the right of research participants to determine when, where, and what kind of information is shared, with an assurance that information and observations are treated with respect and kept in strict confidence.

Rules or regulations   Policies that are established to guide the implementation of laws and programs.

Rule-utilitarianism   A type of utilitarianism that suggests people choose rules that, when followed consistently, will maximize the overall good.

Self-awareness   Conscious awareness of one's thoughts, feelings, physical and emotional responses, and insights into various situations.

Serious Reportable Events   Incidents involving preventable, serious, and unambiguous adverse events resulting from error or lapse in care, which should never occur within a health care facility. Serious reportable events are commonly referred to as "never events."

Sexism   The assumption that members of one sex are superior to those of the other.

Sexual harassment   All unwelcome sexual advances, requests for sexual favors, and other conduct of a sexual nature.

Sexual orientation   An inherent romantic or sexual attraction to other people of one gender, both, or neither. Sexual orientations include gay, lesbian, heterosexual, bisexual, or asexual.

Sexual violence   Intimate partner (or domestic) violence, rape, stalking, unwanted sexual contact, and noncontact unwanted sexual experiences.

Sight translation   Verbal translation of material written in one language to spoken word in another language

Situational bind   A moral problem in a particular situation in which core beliefs come into irreconcilable conflict with social or institutional norms or other claims.

Slander   Defamation that occurs when one speaks unprivileged or false words about another.

Spirituality   The animating force, life principle, or essence of being that permeates life and is expressed and experienced in multifaceted connections with self, others, nature, and God or Life Force.

Stage of ease   A time after the novice period in which the professional has confidence in technical skill and a sense of comfort with rules and expectations in the workplace. Internal and external values and expectations are congruent.

Stakeholders   Persons with interest in a given situation.

Standards of nursing practice   Written documents outlining minimum expectations for nursing care.

Statutes or laws   Legislation that has been enacted by legislative bodies and approved by the executive branch of government.

Statutory (legislative) law   Formal laws written and enacted by federal, state, or local legislatures.

Stem cell   Considered a "master cell" that can grow into a variety of other cells—a cell that is unspecialized (does not yet have a specific function) and has the capacity to divide and replace itself and to differentiate into various types of specialized cells.

Stereotype   A persistent idea about characteristics of a person that is preconceived, oversimplified, often wrong, and coupled with an attitude about the person based on the preconception.

Sympathy   Sharing others' feelings in one's imagination.

Theory   A proposed explanation for a class of phenomena.

Tail coverage   A provision or special liability insurance policy that permits an insured to report claims that are made after a policy has expired or been canceled.

Tort   A wrong or injury that a person suffers because of someone else's action, either intentional or unintentional. The action may cause bodily harm; damage a person's property, business, or reputation; or make unauthorized use of a person's property.

Translation   transposing a written text from one language to another while retaining elements of meaning and form.

Trustworthiness   A focal virtue that results in recognition by others of one's consistency and predictability in following moral norms.

Unintentional torts   Torts that occur when an act or omission causes unintended injury or harm to another person.

Unwanted sexual contact   Unwanted sexual experiences involving touch but not sexual penetration, such as being kissed in a sexual way or having sexual body parts fondled, groped, or grabbed.

Utilitarian theories   Theories of distributive justice that distribute

resources based on the premise of the greatest good for the greatest number of people. These theories place social good before individual rights.

Utilitarianism   A moral theory holding that an action is judged good or bad in relation to the consequence, outcome, or end result derived from it.

Utility   The property of usefulness in any object, whereby it tends to produce benefit, advantage, pleasure, good, or happiness or to prevent mischief, pain, evil, or unhappiness.

Vaccine hesitancy   Hesitant or refusing to be vaccinated often due to insufficient and sometimes misinformation, lack of availability of vaccines and health care providers, language barriers, and a consequence of social determinants of health care such as structural racism.

Values   Ideals, beliefs, customs, modes of conduct, qualities, or goals that are highly prized or preferred by individuals, groups, or society.

Values clarification   Refers to the process of becoming more conscious of and naming what one values or considers worthy.

Values conflict   Internal or interpersonal conflict that occurs in circumstances in which personal values are at odds with those of patients, colleagues, or the institution.

Veracity   Truth telling.

Victim blaming   Holding the people burdened by social conditions accountable for their own situations and responsible for needed solutions.

Virtue ethics   Theories of ethics, usually attributed to Aristotle, that represent the idea that an individual's actions are based on innate moral virtue.

Whistle-blowers   Persons who alert the public about serious wrongdoing created or concealed within an organization, such as unsafe conditions, incompetence, or professional misconduct.

Whistle-blowing   Speaking out about unsafe or questionable practices affecting patient care or working conditions. This should be resorted to only after a person has unsuccessfully used all appropriate organizational channels to right a wrong and has a sound moral justification for taking this action.

INDEX

Note: Page numbers followed by *f* indicate figures, *t* indicate tables, and *b* indicate boxes.